A SYNOPTIC KEY
Of The
MATERIA MEDICA

(A Treatise for Homeopathic Students)

includes
A Brief Repertory

C.M. BOGER, M.D.

Rearranged & Augmented Edition

B. JAIN PUBLISHERS (P) LTD.
An ISO 9001 : 2000 Certified Company
USA — EUROPE — INDIA

A SYNOPTIC KEY OF THE MATERIA MEDICA

Rearranged & Augmented Edition: 2007

Published by Kuldeep Jain
for

B. Jain Publishers (P) Ltd.
An ISO 9001 : 2000 Certified Company
USA — EUROPE — INDIA
1921, Street No. 10, Chuna Mandi,
Paharganj, New Delhi 110 055 (INDIA)
Phones: 91-11-2358 0800, 2358 1100, 2358 1300, 2358 3100
Fax: 91-11-2358 0471; *Email:* bjain@vsnl.com
Website: www.bjainbooks.com

Printed in India by
J.J. Offset Printers
522, FIE, Patpar Ganj, Delhi - 110 092
Phones: 91-11-2216 9633, 2215 6128

ISBN 978-81-319-0007-9
BOOK CODE : BB-2078

PUBLISHER'S NOTE TO REARRANGED & AUGMENTED EDITION

- Correct prescribing is the art of carefully fitting pathogenetic to clinical symptoms, and as such at present requires a special aptness in grasping the essential points of symptom images, great drudgery in mastering a working knowledge of our large Materia Medica or a most skilful use of many *Books* of reference.

- It is the aim of this Rearranged & Augmented Edition to simplify and introduce method into this work, so that the truly homeopathic curative remedy may be worked out with greater ease and certainty. For this purpose a combination of the analytic and synoptic methods has been thought best.

- The Synopsis, is intended to make clear the *general expression or genius* of each remedy, and thereby help the prescriber correct his bearings. The scope of its contents is much enlarged by bracketing the most nearly affiliated remedies after some of the more important symptoms; this also helps in making differentiations.

- The Repertory is only intended to orient the searcher.

- The supplementary repertory at the back of the book has been incorporated with the repertory at the front and has been placed at the end of the book.

- Included is an index of remedies with the latest accepted abbreviations.

Kuldeep Jain
CEO, B. Jain Publishers

FOREWORD

Correct prescribing is the art of carefully fitting pathogenetic to clinical symptoms, and as such at present requires a special aptness in grasping the essential points of symptom images, great drudgery in mastering a working knowledge of our large materia medica or a most skilful use of many books of reference.

It is the aim of this book to simplify and introduce method into this work, so that the truly homeopathic curative remedy may be worked out with greater ease and certainty. For this purpose a combination of the analytic and synoptic methods has been thought best.

The spirit of the clinical symptom picture is best obtained by *asking the patient to tell his own story*, whenever this is possible. This account is then amplified and more accurately defined by the questioner, who should first try to elicit the evident *cause and course* of the sickness, to which he will add all the things which *now seem to interfere* with the sufferer's comfort. Especially should the natural modifiers of sickness—*the modalities*—be very definitely ascertained. The following are the most vitally important of such influences : Time, *Temperature, Open Air, Posture, Being Alone, Motion, Sleep, Eating and Drinking, Touch, Pressure, Discharges, etc.*

A consideration of the *mental state* comes next in order of importance. Here the presence of *Irritability, Sadness* or *Fear* is the ruling factor.

The third step concerns the estimate to be put upon the patient's own description of his sensations. This is a very vital point and in order not to be misled it is always well to ascertain whether any of the following primary sensations are present: *Burning, Cramping, Cutting, Bursting, Soreness,*

v

Throbbing and *Thirst.* There may be many others, but the presence of any one of these often overshadows them, especially such as may be due to the play of the imagination ; which feature is in itself of more importance than the particular thing imagined.

Next in order comes the *entire objective aspect or expression of the sickness* : This should especially include the *Facial Expression, Demeanor, Nervous Excitability, Sensibility, Restlessness* or *Torpor, State of the Secretions* and any abnormal coloring that may be present.

Lastly the *part affected* must be determined; this also brings the investigation in touch with diagnosis.

By going over the above rubrics in the order named the contour of the disease picture will be pretty clearly outlined and will point fairly well towards the simillimum, and the prescriber has only to keep in mind the fact that the actual *differentiating factor may belong to any rubric whatsoever* and also that the scope of these rubrics reaches far beyond the appended synoptic text.

For ready reference the following diagram has been arranged :

MODALITIES {
CAUSATION. TIME. TEMPERATURE.
WEATHER. OPEN AIR. POSTURE.
MOTION. EATING AND DRINKING.
SLEEP. IF ALONE. PRESSURE.
TOUCH. DISCHARGES.

MIND {
IRRITABILITY.
SADNESS.
FEAR.
PLACIDITY.

SENSATIONS {
BURNING. CRAMPING.
CUTTING. BURSTING.
SORENESS. THROBBING.
THIRST.

vi

OBJECTIVE ASPECT {
DEMEANOR.
RESTLESSNESS.
NERVOUS EXCITABILITY
FACIAL EXPRESSION.
TORPOR. SECRETIONS.
COLOR. ODOR.

PART AFFECTED {
ORGANS.
RIGHT.
LEFT.

THE SYNOPSIS, is intended to make clear the *general expression or genius* of each remedy, and thereby help the prescriber correct his bearings. The scope of its contents is much enlarged by bracketing the most nearly affiliated remedies after some of the more important symptoms; this also helps in making differentiations.

What often makes a cure hard is the laying of too much stress upon some particular factor at the expense of the disease picture as a whole, thus destroying its symmetry and forming a distorted conception of the natural image of the sickness. This does not, however, mean that all symptoms stand on the same level, for certain effects must be more prominent than others, yet be part and parcel of them. This is the sense in which we must learn to know our remedies, just as we do our friends, *by their air or personality*; an ever changing, composite effect, but always reflecting the same motive.

Whenever the chosen remedy excites little or no reaction, the selection has either been faulty, or what is just as likely, one of the fundamental miasms which calls for either Psorinum, Sulfur, Medorrhinum or Syphilinum, is present.

Whenever the general benefit derived from a single dose lags, the remedy should be repeated in the next higher potency, instead of looking upon the new symptoms as

indicators for some other drug; for only the most inveterately rooted dyscrasia can, by varying its expression, resist the whole scale of an indicated remedy. Sometimes we can advantageously change to another potency scale of the same remedy, before attempting to scrutinize the remaining picture for those new developments which must point towards our next choice, nor should this successor be chosen until the new symptom picture — disease phase — takes on a fairly definite or settled form.

This new fifth edition of the Synoptic Key is herewith submitted to all brothers in the work. Only changes of proven value in co-ordinating and assembling the significant features of seemingly disassociated symptom groups, have been made. Upon these depends almost wholly the final choice of the similimum. They should reflect a speaking image, as it were, of the correctly indicated remedy. To this end rubrics from my private files have been freely drawn upon. The symptom features of many remedies have been clarified in order to increase their usefulness, especially in precisionizing differentiations. The Repertory is only intended to orient the searcher.

The possibilities that inhere in the contact of the similimum with the disordered vital force can not be foreknown. It therefore behooves every prescriber to use the utmost care in selecting the curative remedy. It will always remain true, as Paracelsus says in "Erste buch von blatern," chap. 8, 1528. "Just so, Mercury, (etc.), — cures — things Mercuric" only.

The strain which runs through every pathogenetic symptom complex has been called the "genius" of the drug. To give this its proper place in the prescription should be the ideal of every prescriber. To this end is this book written.

C. M. BOGER

Parkersburg, W. Va.

CONTENTS

PART - I

MATERIA MEDICA

PART - II
REPERTORY

xiii

PART - III

MISCELLANEOUS

xiv

PART ONE

MATERIA MEDICA

An exposition of the important and characteristic features of the most important remedies of the Homeopathic Materia Medica, with their physiological spheres of activities, modalities and relationships.

ABROTANUM

SPHERE OF ACTION
Nerves.
Nutrition.
Veins.

AGGRAVATION
Cold air.
Wet.
Checked secretions.
Night.
Fogs.
AMELIORATION
Loose stool (Nat-s., Zinc.).
Motion.

Numb, weak, tremulous and paretic. Can't hold up head.
Exudations, into pleura, joints, from navel, etc. **True metastases;**
receding gout, etc. **Alternations;** piles with rheumatism (Coll.,
Sabin.). Rheumatism, after diarrhea. **Emaciation;** ascending; of legs.
.... Cross, irritable children. Pale hollow eyed, old
face. Distended veins; on forehead. Nosebleed; of youths. Vomits
much offensive fluid. Stomach floats in water (Bufo). **Bloated
abdomen.** Pains in left ovary. Nightly backache. Weak joints; can't
hold up head. Face cold, dry and wrinkled. Cold, prickling, numb
fingers and toes. Flabby skin. Protruding piles; burn on touch.

Related to: Chin., Led.

F- 2

ACONITUM NAPELLUS

SPHERE OF ACTION

MIND
- **Brain.**

NERVES
- Medulla.
- Sympathetic.
- Vagus.
- Respiratory centre.

HEART
- **Arterial.**
- **Circulation.**
- **Viscera.**
- Larynx.
- **Chest.**
- Abdomen.

Joints.

AGGRAVATION

Violent emotions
- FRIGHT.
- SHOCK.
- Vexation.

Sleeping in the sun.
Chilled by
- COLD.
- **Dry winds.**
- While sweating.
Pressure and touch.
Noise.
Light.
Dentition.
During menses.
Night; in bed, P.M., lying on side.

AMELIORATION

Open air.
Repose.
Warm sweat.

Robust habit. **Sudden; violently acute, painful effects,** of a big storm that soon blows over. **Tension. Congestion;** often apoplectic. **Excited nervous and vascular systems. Inflammation.** Congestion to head and chest: acute. **Inflammation:** internal; rheumatic. **Bright red hemorrhage** (Bell.). **Acute senses. Sticking, tearing pains. Parts feel numb, big, burn, tingle,** prickle or crawl; remain sore or **numb after the pains.** Neuralgia. Crepitation. Painfully sore externally, with internal heaviness. **Collapse.** .... TERROR. ANXIETY. AGONIZING FEAR; of death, crowds, etc. RESTLESS, **excited, nervous, feverish, impatient and anxious.** Beside himself; **frantic from intensity of the pain; WITH FEAR; screams,** moans, **gnaws the fists,** bites the nails (Ars.), wants to die. Delirium. Convulsions. **Forebodings;** predicts time of death. Sensitive. Music saddens.

Anxiety, congestion and pain. Head heavy. As of a hot band about the head, or boiling heat in brain. Hair seems on end. Violent squeezing or bursting, in forehead or eyes; crackling in; throbs in left forehead (right Ant-t., Bell., Ign.); aches, with more urine; **burning in**. Shooting in eyeballs. Numb nose; with epistaxis (Bell., Med.). Nose runs hot water. Coryza. ANXIOUS LOOK (Spong.). **Eyes** glitter; stare; bleared; foreign bodies in. **Hot, red cheeks**. Face: ghastly look; alternately red and pale; one cheek red and hot, other pale and cold. Face pales on rising. Faintness. Toothache. Throbbing in teeth and in head. Everything tastes bitter. Water has a bad taste. Chokes on swallowing. BURNING THIRST; craves acids, beer; < after ices. Appetite: milk agrees. Projectile vomiting (Verat-v.). Violent bilious or bloody vomitus. **Stools of pure blood**; slimy, **grass green**, or white; < hot days and cold nights (Dulc., Merc-c.). Dysentery. Itching, sticking at anus. Retained, scanty, red or bloody urine. Agonizing dysuria. Cystitis. Urethral chill. Orchitis. Suddenly suppressed menses. Respiration short; during sleep; anxious; hard; sits erect. **Dry, hoarse, painful cough**, or short, barking, ringing, or whistling cough, < from every inspiration. Grasps larynx; < night or drinking. Laryngitis. **Croup with fever**. Violent rushes of blood to chest. Pneumonia. Stitches in chest. Oppression of left chest. Pleurisy. Heart feels swelled. Carditis. Complaints of heart worse from sitting erect. Palpitation, anxious; with pain down left arm. Red fingertips. Powerless legs. Red, shining swelling. DRY, HOT SKIN, or as if ice water on it. Miliary eruptions. **Sleepless and nervous**. Pulse fast, bounding, shaking, forcible and tumultuous or wiry. Pulse very irritable. Arterial tension (Verat-v.). CHILL; in waves; alternates with heat. HIGH FEVER. **Dry, burning heat**; in eyelids; nose, mouth, throat, **lungs; on palms**; must uncover. **Sweat**: on uncovered parts; wants covers; drenching. **Back** and sacrum feel bruised. Remote effects of fright (Op.). Cries out and grasps genitals.

Complementary: Sulph.

Related to: Bell., Cham., Coff.

ACTAEA SPICATA

SPHERE OF ACTION

Joints
- Wrist.
- Small.

AGGRAVATION

Change of weather.
Slight exertion.
Cold.
Night.
Touch.

Old age. Tingling. Weakness................. Joints swell; can not move. Paralytic weakness of affected parts. Hypersensitive to cold.

Complementary: Caul., Coloc., Sabin., Stict., Viol-t.

ADONIS

SPHERE OF ACTION

HEART.
Spine.
Epigastrium.
Kidneys.
Skin.

AGGRAVATION

Cold.
Lying.

AMELIORATION

Exertion.

Wandering pains .... Apprehension. Vertigo, < when in motion; with palpitation. Aching occiput. Tight scalp. Tongue as if scalded. Thirstless. Faint in epigastrium, with vertigo. Bowels as if to break; < bending. Urging to urinate. Albuminuria. Dropsy. Dyspnea; < touching back. Dry, tickling cough; from heart. Heart weak, fatty, arrhythmic. Spine and nape stiff; with a tired ache. Vesicles on skin. Sleepless; from rambling thoughts.

Related to: Bufo.

AESCULUS HIPPOCASTANUM

SPHERE OF ACTION

Veins
- Liver.
- Naso-pharynx.
- ABDOMEN (Right).
- RECTUM.

Mucous membranes
- Naso-pharynx

Occiput.
Sacro-iliac region.

AGGRAVATION

Morning, on waking.
After stool.
Lying.
Stooping.
Urinating.
Walking.

AMELIORATION

COOL
- Open air.
- Bathing.
Bleeding (piles).
Kneeling.
Continued exertion.

Reflex rectal symptoms. Rectum: painful constriction; as of a knife sawing up and down. HOT, DRY, STIFF, ROUGH or **full feeling internally;** throat, abdomen, **anus,** etc. Purple, puffy parts. Venosity. Pains, sticking; like hot lightning.............................Irritable. Crushing in occiput. Nose sensitive to cool inspired air; it burns. Congestive catarrh. Follicular pharyngitis. Throbs, deep in abdomen. **Stool, hard, dry;** of several colors. RECTUM: sore , as of a **burr** or **sticking pains** long after stool; as of a bug **crawling from anus** (Sulph.). **Piles, purple, painful, external;** with BACKACHE (Nux-v.), chest pains, etc. **Laming, dull, lumbar pain; small of back gives out;** repeated efforts at rising; < walking. **Lumbar region or back:** as if to break. Bruised pain in sacrum and hips. Paralytic heaviness: of arms, spine, feet.

Complementary: Carb-v., Lach., Mur-ac.

Related to: Aloe, Coll., Puls.

AETHUSA CYNAPIUM

SPHERE OF ACTION
BRAIN.
Nerves.
Digestion.
Occiput.
Neck.
Glands.
Liver.

AGGRAVATION
MILK.
Hot weather.
Dentition.
Frequent eating.
Over-exertion.

Violent onset, profound **exhaustion and lack of reaction,** even speechless; as in cholera infantum, convulsions, etc. Can't stand or hold head up. Weak, nervous and prostrated; from over-work. Can't fix attention. Parts feel screwed together. Lancinating pains. Distress in occiput and nape. Violent convulsions.......... **Weepy;** < as disease progresses. Dizzy and drowsy (Gels.). Squeezing headache, > passing flatus. Eyes turn down. Face sunken. Deathly aspect; blue white pallor about lips. **White linea nasalis.** Tongue feels too long. Nibbling appetite. Regurgitates food long after eating (Kreos.). Violent sudden vomiting of milk. DEATHLY NAUSEA. VOMITS LARGE, HARD CURDS, THEN LIMPNESS AND DEEP SLEEP. Retching. Digestion ceases from brain exhaustion. Stomach seems turned upside down. Bubbling at navel. Yellow-green, slimy diarrhea. Watery menses. Lymphatics swelled, like a string of beads. Eruptions that itch from heat. Ecchymoses. **Cool, clammy skin.** Heat without thirst. Sweat (cold) with aversion to uncovering.

Complementary: Calc.

Related to: Ant-c., Cic.

AGARICUS MUSCARIUS

SPHERE OF ACTION	AGGRAVATION
SPINAL AXIS	**Air**
- OCCIPUT.	- COLD.
- NERVES.	- FREEZING.
- **Lumbar region.**	- OPEN. Stormy.
Peristalsis.	- **Exhaustion**
Heart.	- **Mental.**
Circulation.	- **Coition.**
Respiration.	- Debauchery.
Chest.	**Alcohol.**
	Pressure.
	Touch.
	Morning.
	During menses.

AMELIORATION

Gentle motion.

Gradual onset. **Many symptoms** (Tub.). IRREGULAR, ANGULAR, UNCERTAIN AND EXAGGERATED MOTIONS (**Ign.**); he reaches too far, staggers or steps too high, **drops things,** etc. TREMBLING, TWITCHING, JERKING **or fibrillar spasm;** here and there; < EYELIDS or tongue. Shuddering. Nervous and restless. Chorea. As of cold needles, a cold drop or a weight on parts. Painful twitching, then parts stiff and cold..................................... Hilarious or dull and dizzy; as if drunk. **Turns head to and fro.** Headache, > after stool or urine. Oscillating eyeballs. Gum in canthi. Musca volitantes. Angle of mouth droops. **As of a lump in epigastrium.** Rumbling and fermenting in bowels. Hot flatus or semen; cold urine. Isolated coughing attacks, then sneezing; as if from spine; easy expectoration of flocculi or balls of mucus. Indistinct, jerky speech. Palpitation during coition; depressed afterward. Premature ejaculation. Pressure or burning sticking from heart to left scapula. Angina pectoris, has excessive pain only. Metastases from suppressed milk. Single vertebra sensitive to heat. **Spine sensitive,** > pressure or touch; shooting, burning along; seems short (Sulph.), < stooping; stiff. Restless arms. BURNING-ITCHING (Apis), < IN SKIN; AS IF FROZEN; changing place on scratching. Skin pains when cold. Chilblains. **Yawning;** before pains or spasms; as a concomitant. Chills or sweats easily. Sweats on alternate sides. Night sweats. Itching, over affected part. Cold buttocks.

Antidotes: Coff., Puls.

Complementary: Calc.

Related to: Phys., Tub.

AGNUS CASTUS

SPHERE OF ACTION	**AGGRAVATION**
SEXUAL ORGANS.	VENERY
MIND.	Sprains
Nerves.	
Eyes.	

IMPOTENCY AND PREMATURE OLD AGE. **Jaded rakes.** ....Distraction. BAD MEMORY. Sad and despairing; repeats that he will soon die. Cold, relaxed genitals. Spermatorrhea. Gnawing-itching; < eyes. Agalactia.

Related to: Olnd., Ph-ac.

AILANTHUS

SPHERE OF ACTION	AGGRAVATION
BLOOD.	Suppressions.
THROAT.	Raising up.
Skin.	Sight of food.
Mind.	**AMELIORATION**
	Hot drinks.

Aching. Rapid prostration. Advancing MALIGNANCY AND STUPOR. Fetor and LIVIDITY. Sepsis. Acridity. Thinness. .... Dulness. Sighing. Faint on raising up, or vertigo < lying. Bloody, nasal discharge. Face and **throat dark** and **swelled**. Sordes on teeth. Dry, foul fauces. Deep **ulcers stud tonsils**, < left, with loose pultaceous material. Lacunar tonsillitis. Irritative itching of posterior pharynx. Diphtheria. **Eruptions in dark, sparse patches**; tardy; return slowly after pressure. Mottled skin. **Scarlatina maligna; suppressed.** Petechiae. Crawling over body. Adynamic fever, with weak heart. Cold sweat.

Related to: Arum-t., Bapt., Lac-c.

ALETRIS FARINOSA

SPHERE OF ACTION	AGGRAVATION
	Loose of fluids.
Female organs (Right).	**AMELIORATION**
	Passing flatus.
Blood.	Bending backward.

Debility. Always tired. **Heaviness of parts.** Uterine reflexes. Hemorrhage. Anemia.....................Frothy saliva. Abdominal colic. Terrible pain during stool. Constipation. Early, profuse menses. Tendency to abortion.

Related to: Chin., Helon., Tril-p.

ALLIUM CEPA

SPHERE OF ACTION	AGGRAVATION
MUCOUS MEMBRANES	WARM ROOM.
- NOSE.	**Wet feet.**
	Singing.
- EYES.	**Damp.**
- **Larynx.**	N.E. winds.
	Spring.
- Bowels.	**AMELIORATION**
Nerves.	Cool, open air.
Left to right.	Bathing.
	Motion.

Acute colds, catarrhs or neuralgias. Shooting pains; as **fine as a thread.** ....Forehead aches; into eyes and face; > free coryza or menses. **Watery eyes,** < coughing; wants to rub them (Squil.). FREQUENT, VIOLENT SNEEZING, CORYZA; ACRID, FLUENT; **with burning, smarting.** Dripping nose or from uvula. Sensitive to odors. Raw throat or larynx. Flatulence; noisy; foul; painful. **Copious urine. Incessant, hacking, tickling cough;** holds it back; **as if to tear or split larynx;** must grasp it. Painful talking. **Hoarseness.** Senile bronchitis. Neuralgia of stump. Galled feet.

Complementary: Phos.

Related to: Euphr., Gels., Kali-i.

ALOE SOCOTRINA

SPHERE OF ACTION

ABDOMINAL VEINS
- RECTUM.
- **Liver.**
- Colon.
- Pelvis.

Lumbar region.

Head.

Female organs.

AGGRAVATION

HEAT.
Damp.
Summer.
Early A. M. (in Bed)
After dysentery.
Stepping hard.
Evening.

AMELIORATION

Cool, open air.
Cold applications.

Relaxation and VENOUS CONGESTION, < abdomen. **Parts seem full.** HEAVY DRAGGING, **as of a load.** Downward sensation. **Drawing.** Gelatinous secretions: post-nasal, stool, etc. ....Mental effects, < cloudy weather (Phos.) or constipation. Heavy pressure on vertex. Head, alternating with abdominal, or lumbar symptoms; > closing eyes. Pain from navel to rectum. Heavy hypogastrium; rectum. Prolapse recti. A plug seems wedged in pelvis. **Rumbling, gurgling in bowels, sudden urging,** SENSE OF INSECURITY, **then hurriedly passes a gushing, watery stool** (Kalibi.). Diarrhea; with rectal pain. ANUS WEAK; oozes mucus. Stool escapes with flatus (Olnd.) or when urinating; mushy; solid stool passes unnoticed; urging to, passes flatus only; **lumpy;** gelatinous. Piles, prolapsing; like a bunch of grapes; > cold bathing. **Internal heat,** not stool, flatus, urine, etc. Burning in anus, rectum, piles, etc. Sexual erethism (in children). Heavy, congested uterus.

Complementary: Sulph.

Related to: Lil-t., **Podo.,** Sep., **Sulph.**

ALUMINA

SPHERE OF ACTION

SPINAL CORD (Lumbar).

Abdomen (Left).

RECTUM.

Lower limbs.

Mucous membranes.

Skin.

AGGRAVATION

WARMTH; ROOM, bed.

Foods
- Artificial.
- Potatoes.

Speaking.

Dry weather.

Early on awaking.

Sitting.

After menses.

AMELIORATION

Evening.

Open air.

Moderate.
- Exertion.
- Temperature.

Thin, Inactive; inclines to lie down. Paretic effects. Talking is exhausting. Exhaustion after menses. DRYNESS; of mucous membranes, eyes, throat, rectum, etc., or irritability and relaxation. Scanty, thick, acrid discharges (Hydr.). Mucus discharges, profuse: before menses, leucorrhea runs to feet; expectoration. Induration. Chronicity .... Illusions of being larger, numb, smooth, heavy, time passing too slowly, etc. Hasty, but slow of execution, hence mistakes in speaking, writing, etc. Peevish. Depressive mental states. Depressed, on awaking. Timorous; fears his own impulses; the sight of knives; loss of reason, etc. Bad memory. Vertigo, < talking. Violent stitches in brain. Dry, falling hair. Weak eyelids. Double squint; < teething. Inflamed, burning eyes. Hot, red ear. Dusky wrinkled, old look. As of white of egg or a cobweb on face. Teeth feel long; pain extends to other parts (Kali-bi.). Twitching lower jaw (Gels.). Uvula hangs down. Throat feels full of sticks or constricted. Craves coarse foods (Calc.). Big bellied children. Pains from rectum to ankle. Inactive rectum and bladder; strains to pass a soft stool;

hard ones cause severe cutting. Stools of small balls, hard knots or bright clots of blood. **Must strain at stool to urinate;** slow flow. Tickling in sexual organs; increased desire. Profuse leucorrhea. Constant, dry, hacking cough; interrupts breathing; with sneezing. Sudden loss of voice. As of a hot iron thrust through lower spine. Heavy lower limbs; staggering. **Festination.** Locomotor ataxia. Totters, if eyes are closed. Painful soles. Gnawing under nails. Bones feel squeezed. Dry, rough, cracked skin. Itching burning over seat of pain. Intolerable itching from heat of bed. Eczema. Chilliness; > open air. Heat, with/itching.

Antidotes: Cadm-m., Jab.

Related to: Bry., Plb.

AMBRA GRISEA

SPHERE OF ACTION	AGGRAVATION
NERVES	**Slight causes**
- Pneumogastric.	- **Presence of others.**
- Solar plexus.	- Music.
- Spinal.	- Embarrassment.
Mind	- Agitation.
Female organs.	- Worry.
One side.	- Thinking of it.
Chest (Left).	**Old age.**
	Evening.
	Warmth.
	Milk.

Dry, nervous, meager habit. Early senility. Weakness of upper part of body with trembling of lower parts. **Worn out, yet over-impressionable;** slight things < the breathing, the heart, start the

menses, etc. **Symptoms suddenly change place;** asleep, numb feeling
(in spots), **twitching,** itching, trembling, ebullitions, etc. General
pulsation................... **Dreamy,** flitting ideas or fixed disagreeable
fancies. Slow grasp. Does not understand what she reads. Sad. **Bashful.**
Vertigo; senile. Nosebleed, during menses. Coldness in abdomen.
Confusion, in occiput; also sprained feeling in. Imaginations.
Coldness of body with twitching. Asthma: dry; senile; < coition.
Flatulence. Can't have others present when urinating (Nat-m.) or
during stool; < during pregnancy. Itching labiae. Spasmodic cough,
then eructations. Bluish, white expectoration. As a lump in chest
(left). Palpitation. Sweat on abdomen and thighs.

Related to: Bar-c., Ign.

AMMONIUM CARBONICUM

SPHERE OF ACTION

HEART
- **Circulation.**
- **Blood.**

RESPIRATION.

Lungs
- Bronchi.

Right side.

AGGRAVATION

COLD
- CLOUDY DAYS.
- DAMP.
- Locally.
- **Raw, open air.**
Falling asleep. 3-4 A.M.
DURING MENSES.
Motion.

AMELIORATION
PRESSURE.
Eating.
Lying on abdomen.

Low vitality. **Lacks reaction.** LIVID, WEAK AND DROWSY.
Lies down. Collapse of nerves and heart. **Averse to cold.** Old age.
Bruised, sore pain. Internal, raw burning. **Acrid, hot, adherent**

secretions. **Dark, thin hemorrhage.** Scorbutic states. Malignancy.
.... Active, but soon exhausted. Sad. Peevish. Mind
vacant. Depressed, with weakened intellect. Heedless, fretting and
unruly. Loss of memory; < vexation. Brain seems loose. Shocks
through head, on biting. Violent headache; full, bursting in forehead.
Floods of tears. **Nose stopped at night,** or bleeds, if hands or face are
washed or on waking. Continuous urging to sneeze. Profuse, watery
coryza. Catarrhs, starting in nose. Cracked, burning lips. Tender,
bleeding gums. Loose or blunt teeth. Dark, acrid diarrhea. Persistent
erections. Menses with choleraic symptoms (Sil.); dark, lumpy flow,
< night; then dyspnea or weakness. Copious leucorrhea. **Increasing
shortness of breath;** it wakes him; > cool air (Carb-v.). **Rattling in
chest, but gets up little.** Aphonia. WEAK HEART; **causing stasis,**
dyspnea, etc. **Palpitation;** with cold sweat and lachrymation. Numb
right foot (Sep.). Asleep feeling of part lain on. Ganglion. Bones
ache as weather changes. Red or mottled skin. Coldness. Burning
heat with thirst. Scarlatina.

Related to: Ant-t., Carb-v., Glon., Lach., Mur-ac.

AMMONIUM MURIATICUM

SPHERE OF ACTION

MUCOUS MEMBRANES
- CHEST.
- **Gall-ducts.**

Liver.

Blood.

Female organs.

Tips of fingers and toes.

Between scapulae.

AGGRAVATION

Morning (Head, Chest).

Afternoon. (Abdomen).

Evening (Skin, Fever, Limbs).

Sprains (Chronic).

Periodically.

AMELIORATION

Open air.

Rapid motion.

Fat and puffy, with thin limbs (Ant-c.). **Irregular circulation;
ebullitions, burning or localized throbbings.** Symptoms

accompanied by cough or PROFUSE SECRETIONS. GLAIRY
CATARRHS. Hemorrhage. **Tightness, as if too short; tendons,**
hamstrings, lumbar region, etc. Tired and sore. Festering pain.
.... Brain paralysis. A rough body obstructs upper
nares. Acrid, watery coryza; closing one nostril. Anosmia. **Slimy**
mouth and pharynx. Pulsation in tonsils. Tense, sprained feeling in
groins; must walk bent. Scanty, hard, crumbling stools; changing
color. Polyuria. Menses flow more at night. Albuminous leucorrhea.
Blood from anus or diarrhea during menses. Prolapsus uteri. Cough,
with salivation (Am-c.) or liver symptoms. Can't breathe for coughing.
Noisy, rattling, tenacious mucus in chest. Bronchitis. Hoarseness,
with burning in larynx. Pulsating, burning spots in chest. **Swelled**
cervical glands. Sore sprain or cold between scapulae. Lumbago.
Bleeding eruptions. Desquamation between fingers. Contracting
sciatica (left); < **sitting** > **lying.** Pain in or ulcer on heel. Chilly as
often, as he wakes. Sense of heat; > open air; alternating with chill.

Related to: Caust.

AMYLENUM NITROSUM

SPHERE OF ACTION
VASOMOTOR NERVES
- **Circulation.**
- HEAD.
- **Heart.**
Respiration.

AGGRAVATION
CLIMACTERIC.
SLIGHT CAUSES.
Emotions.
Heat.
Close room.

    Flushing heats; then drenching (unilateral) sweat. Dilated
cerebral vessels. **Throbbing;** < head. .... **Blood surges to-**
head; with fiery red face. Easy blushing. Migraine, with pallor (Ars.).
Aching, backward, along left floating ribs. Tumultuous palpitation.
Constriction at heart. Full, soft pulse. Stretching and yawning, with
hiccough.

Related to: Glon., Lach.

ANACARDIUM ORIENTALE

SPHERE OF ACTION

MIND

Nerves

- Stomach.
- **Skin.**
- Palms.

Muscles.

Joints.

AGGRAVATION

MENTAL EXERTION

Emotions

- **Anger.**
- Fright.
- Care, etc.

Stepping hard.

Motion.

Drafts.

Open air.

Cold.

Long after eating.

AMELIORATION

Eating.

Hot bath.

Mental and physical LACK OF POWER. **Tremulous;** on slight exertion, < knees (Staph.) or arms. **Repeated, DULL PRESSURE, as of a plug, or band. Dulled emotions,** sense of hearing, sight, touch, etc. Paralysis. .... BAD MEMORY; **suddenly forgets** names, etc. Brain-fag. As in a dream. **Illusions,** or fixed ideas; **of duality,** imagines others present, **behind her,** etc. Cowardly and neurotic. Vacillating; at odds with himself (Bar-c., Cann-i.); **contradictory impulses. Ill-natured. Profane.** Pressure in temples. Illusory smells. Bad breath and taste. Stiff, swelled tongue. Gastric pain > eating, but < again in 3 hours. Rectum feels **plugged;** can't evacuate even a soft stool. Breath stops on coughing or drinking. Cough with occipital pain; then yawns and sleeps. Double stitch at heart; passing into lumbar region. As of a heavy load on shoulders (Rhus-t.). Dry hands. **Skin, insensible;** itching, < scratching; yellow vesicles. Dermatitis. Eczema. Easily chilled, > sunshine (Stront-c.). Clammy sweat on palms.

Related to: Ign., Rhus-t.

F- 3

ANTHRACINUM

SPHERE OF ACTION
Cellular tissue.

Terrible burning pains, with great prostration. Malignancy. Sepsis. Suppuration. Carbuncle. **Abscess of septum.** Quinsy. Succession of boils. (Arn., Sulph.). **Black or blue blisters. Gangrene.** Hard cellulitis.

Related to: Ars., Tarent.

ANTIMONIUM CRUDUM

SPHERE OF ACTION	AGGRAVATION
STOMACH.	COLD
DIGESTIVE TRACT.	- **BATHING.**
	- Dampness.
MIND.	- WATER (on Head).
SKIN.	OVER-EATING.
Changing sides.	**Acids.**
	Sweets.
	HEAT
	- SUMMER, **of sun.**
	- **Overheating.**
	- Radiated.

Gross feeders (Abies-c.); **showing gastric, mental and skin symptoms. Lumpy** stools, leucorrhea, skin, nails, etc. Strange absence of pain. **Cracks,** in canthi, nostrils, angles of mouth, etc. Gouty metastases (Abrot.). ....**Fat, fretful, cross and peevish; cries if looked at, touched** (Stram.) **or washed. Loathing;** of life, food, bathing, etc. **Ecstatic, dreamy, sentimental.** Pustules in tarsi. Canthi red, raw, moist (externally). Sore, **scabby nostrils.** Pimples about mouth (Ast-r.). TONGUE THICKLY COATED, LIKE WHITEWASH (Ars., Bism., Bry., Kali-m., Phos.). Aphthae. No thirst. DISORDERED DIGESTION; food leaves an after-taste or causes belching. VOMITING < eating or drinking; without nausea (Chel.) or relief. Stomach is painful to pressure; gout of. **Fullness in abdomen.** Pappy or **watery stool**, mixed with lumps. Gastrointestinal catarrh. Voice lacks control, > using it. Aphonia from overheating. Violent cough, each bout a little weaker. Horny or split nails; ingrowing. Shiny elbows. Gouty pains in fingers. Footsweat; wilts the skin. Callosities on soles. Eruptive tendency. Warts; horny. **Sleepy and weary.**

Related to: Sulph.

ANTIMONIUM TARTARICUM

SPHERE OF ACTION

MUCOUS MEMBRANES.

Pneumogastric nerve
- **Bronchi.**
- **Lungs.**
- **Heart.**
- CIRCULATION.
- **Respiration.**
Stomach.
Bowels.
Sleep.
Lumbar region.
Skin.

AGGRAVATION

WARM
- **Room.**
- **Wraps.**
- **Weather.**
Anger.
Lying.
Morning.
Overeating.
Cold.
Dampness.

AMELIORATION

Expectoration.
Sitting erect.
Motion.
Vomiting.

Depression. LACKS REACTION. INCREASINGLY WEAK. DROWSY, SWEATY AND RELAXED. MUCH SECRETION OF MUCUS. Old people and children. Complaints arising in digestive sphere........................Icy finger-tips. Whines before attack, cough, etc. Crushing weight on chest. Won't be touched or looked at. Prostrated in mind and body. Stupid on awaking. Unwilling to be looked at or touched. Wants to be carried upright. Mucus in tarsi. One eye closed. Upper lip drawn up. Tongue: thick white pasty coat; very red or red streaks; dry down middle. Flow of saliva. Craves apples. Vomits or expectorates with great effort. Abdomen feels full of stones. Expectoration: gluey; suppressed. Feet go to sleep on sitting down. Shocks on dropping to sleep. Asphyxia neonatorum. **Apathy** or easily annoyed; wants to be let alone. Peevish, **whining** and moaning. Clings to attendants. Consciousness wanes on closing eyes (Cann-i.). As of a lump in forehead. **Sooty** or flapping nostrils. **Sickly,** sunken, **pale, bluish or twitching face;** covered with cool sweat. Papillae show through white coat on tongue. Tongue flabby, red in streaks. **Craves acids,** which disagree. Belchings, like bad eggs. NAUSEA; in waves; **with weakness and cold sweat** (Lob.,   Verat.), **loathing or anxiety. Forcible vomiting;** then exhaustion and **sleep** (Aeth.). Violent retching. Sinking at stomach. Mucus or grass, green stools. **Diarrhea;** of eruptive diseases. **Unequal breathing.** SUFFOCATIVE SHORTNESS OF BREATH; before cough or alternating with cough; a leaflet seems over trachea. LOOSE, COARSE, RATTLING COUGH; CHEST SEEMS FULL, YET LESS AND LESS IS RAISED; then vomiting or sleep (Aeth.); < **anger.** Must sit up to breathe or cough. Coughs and yawns alternately. Thick expectoration. Capillary bronchitis or bronchitis. Pleuro-pneumonia. Paralytic depression of heart and lungs (Bar-c.). **Violent** (lumbar) **backache;** < lifting; motion excites retching and cold sweat. Restless arms. **Dropsy** of legs. **Yawning;** with many complaints. SOMNOLENCY; with all complaints, or from warmth. **Torpid, cool,** SWEATY SKIN. Delayed or receding, blue or **pustular eruptions.** Sycosis barbae. Smallpox. Impetigo. Weak, quick pulse. Heat coming from heart. Burning sensation. Sticky sweat.

Complementary: Bar-c.

Related to: Am-c., Asc-t., Ip., Lob., Op.

APIS MELLIFICA

SPHERE OF ACTION

CELLULAR TISSUE
- EYES.
- FACE.
- FAUCES.
- OVARIES.

SEROUS CAVITIES.

SKIN.

KIDNEYS.

BLADDER.

Nerves.

Respiration.

Heart.

Blood.

Right side; Right to left.

AGGRAVATION

HEAT
- ROOM.
- Weather.
- **Drinks.**
- Fire.
- Bed.
- Hot bath (Op.).

Touch, even of hair.

After sleep.

4 P.M.

Pressure.

Suppressed eruptions.

AMELIORATION

COOL
- AIR.
- Bathing.
- Uncovering.

Slight expectoration.

Motion.

Stinging, burning, prickling, smarting, like hot needles. Must lie down. **Rapid onset.** SUDDEN; SHRILL CRIES **or pains, that extort cries;** nervousness, swelling, effusion, etc. SENSITIVE; **to pain.** Sharp STINGING **burning or bruised** SORENESS; of brain, ABDOMEN, ovaries, bladder, etc. PUFFINESS, **Shiny redness.** edema; of eyelids or lips; red; saccular. BURNING-itching. Infections. Inflammation. Stiffness. Numbness ....
Childish. Irritable, excitable, **jealous, fussy and fidgety** or apathetic. Foolishly suspicious. Nervous and awkward or absent-minded; drops things. SUDDEN, PIERCING SHRIEKS. Head pains; stabbing or as of a **blow;** < occiput. ROLLS THE HEAD. Numb, tired headache, > pressure. **Painful hair.** Musty head sweat. Cheeks hang down. **Eyes puffy;** conjunctiva or lids like water-bags; red; chemosed. Perforating

corneal ulcer. Profuse hot tears. Photophobia; yet can't bear coverings. Squint. Blindness, > stool. Myosis. **Face puffy or red, < about eyes; waxy pallor.** Scarlatinal otitis. Red nose. Cold nose. Red mouth or tongue. **Grinds teeth. Tongue: vesicles on edge;** swelled; raw; as if burnt; sore. Sandy, **glazed** or translucent pharynx, > cold things. Edema of uvula. Purpleness of throat. Meaty, red tonsils. Right tonsils, > cold drinks. Angina. Diphtheria; early prostration (Merc-cy.); dirty membrane. ADIPSIA; but thirst during chill. Ascites. Orange yellow or tomato-sauce stools; odorless; < motion. Anus sore, swelled; oozes blood or stands open (Phos.). Burning urination. Dysuria. Scant, foul urine; coffee-grounds sediment. Nephritis. Ovaries numb; tumor of right; cystic. Amenorrhea of puberty. **Panting breathing; feels as if every breath would be his last.** Air hunger. Larynx, drawn in. Thirstless and dropsical. Abdomen **tight,** as if to break, on straining at stool. Profuse urine, but drinks little. Ovaries congested, with suppressed menses. Heart, stitches backward from apex; beat shakes whole body. Hands and feet numb. Palms hot. Nails feel loose. **Skin** rosy red; sensitive; rough eruption on; sting-like spots on; pale. Large urticaria. Asthma from hives. Erysipelas. Scarlatina. Dry, hot skin, alternates with gushes of sweat. SLEEPY, but too nervous; when hot; and CRIES OUT. Kicks covers off. Weak, quick pulse. Chill: anticipates; with dyspnea, urticaria, desire to uncover; alternates with heat; right side. BURNING HEAT; but chilly if moved; **without thirst; at 4 P. M. Heat of one part, with coldness of another.** Sweat in gushes; partial.

Antidotes: Carb-ac.

Complementary: Arn., Bar-c., Merc-cy., Nat-m.

Related to: Ars., Canth., Puls., Urt-u.

APOCYNUM

SPHERE OF ACTION

URINARY ORGANS.

Heart.

Digestive tract.

Uterus.

AGGRAVATION

COLD
- Weather.
- **Drinks.**
- Uncovering.
- Lying.

AMELIORATION

Warmth.

Weak and dropsical. Scanty discharges. Irritation. ....
Bewildered. Can't think. Faint. Thirst, but water distresses; vomits
every drink. Uremic vomiting. **Sinking at epigastrium.** Noisy, yellow,
painless, gushing stools. Diarrhea; with dropsy. Bed-wetting of old
men. Enlarged prostate. Uterine hemorrhage, then dropsy (Chin.).
Oppression of chest. Rough, **dry skin.** Can't sweat. Sleepy. Pulse slow,
fluttering, irregular or intermittent.

Related to: Chinin-ar., Nux-v.

ARALIA RACEMOSA

SPHERE OF ACTION

Respiration.

Mucous membranes.

AGGRAVATION

After a short nap.

Drafts.

AMELIORATION

Lying with head high.

Sitting up.

Weak, relaxed and nauseated. Biliousness ....
Sneezing, < drafts. Aphthae. Pains from liver to right scapula. Dyspnea
or violent cough after first sleep, > slight expectoration. Whistling
breathing. Salty expectoration.

Complementary: Lob.

ARANEA DIADEMA

SPHERE OF ACTION
Nerves.

Blood.

Bones.

Right side.

AGGRAVATION
EXACT PERIODICITY

DAMPNESS

- **Cold.**
- During rains.
- **Bathing.**

AMELIORATION
Smoking.

Cold to very bones (Calc.); can't get warm. Every damp day chills. AS OF, ENORMOUS ENLARGEMENT or **numbness of parts**; on waking. Hemorrhage. Periostitis. .... Nervous temperament. Violent pain in all upper teeth at once, on retiring. Enlarged spleen. Malaria.

Complementary: Cedr.

ARGENTUM METALLICUM

SPHERE OF ACTION
NERVES.

Cartilages; mucous mem-
        branes.

- LARYNX.
- Bones.
- Condyles.
- Joints.
- Genito-urinary.

Left side; ovary.

Testes (Right).

AGGRAVATION
USING VOICE.

Mental strain.

Noon.

Cold damp.

3 to 5 A.M.

AMELIORATION
Motion.

Coffee.

Wrapping up.

Slow, deep, low grade processes, THICKENED SECRETIONS, cartilages, tarsi, etc. **Gray tenacious mucus. Sore rawness.** Increasing violent pains, suddenly cease; < touch; with polyuria. Arthralgia. **Loss of power;** mental, over limbs, etc. Epilepsy, then rage. ....Hasty; deceitful. Talkative and **forgetful.** Whirling vertigo. Emptiness or crawling in head. Itching canthi, eyelids or earlobes. Exhaustingly profuse coryza. **Pale, sallow and weak.** Sticky teeth (Lach.). Croaking in abdomen (left). Emissions. Chronic urethritis. Foul leucorrhea. **Easily raises gray, gelatinous or starchy mucus;** < laughing. Hoarseness or aphonia, < using voice. Weakness in chest (left). Heart stops, then trembles and throbs; > inspiration. Swelled ankles. Diabetes. Nervous itching. Shocks on dropping to sleep.

Related to: Sel., Stann., Zinc.

ARGENTUM NITRICUM

SPHERE OF ACTION

MIND.

NERVES.
- **Cerebro-spinal.**
- ABDOMINAL.

MUCOUS MEMBRANE
- STOMACH.
- **Bowels.**
- **Eyes.**
- Throat.
- Urethra.

Periosteum.
Skin.
Left side.

AGGRAVATION

EMOTIONS.
- ANXIETY.
- Suspense.

In room.
Sugar.
Shut in places.
Lying on right side.
Looking down.
Drinking.
Crowds.

AMELIORATION

COOL
- AIR; Open.
- Bath.

Hard pressure.
Motion.

Old, dried up, tremulous and weak. Progressive emaciation. Paralysis, ascending. Parts seem ENLARGED or bound up (Glon.). VIOLENT PAINS; LIKE DEEPLY STICKING SPLINTERS; sharp shooting, like lightning; < down the back or legs; cause starting; grinding or radiating. Sinking downward from head. Ulceration, with much yellow, bloody pus (Hep.). .... Conjoined mental and digestive symptoms. Tormented by strange ideas or emotions. Nervous, impulsive and hurried, yet timid and anxious (Ars.). Fearsome. Dreads ordeals, impending evil, passing a certain point, dark (Stram.), etc. Incoherence. Faltering speech, gait, erections, etc. Nervous headache and nervous diarrhea. Brain-fag. Head as if in a vise; > tight bandage. Vertigo; epileptic, < night. Compressive or deep head pains; loses his senses (Laur.). Boring in left frontal eminence, 11-12 A.M. Migraine. Scaly tarsi. Eyeballs feel big (Guaj.). Swelled carunculae; chemosis. Photophobia. Violent purulent ophthalmia. Dilated pupils. Sickly, grayish, muddy color. Painful, red tip of tongue, or (dry) aphthae on edge. Food lodges in pharynx. Throat sensitive; as of a rough stick (Phyt.) or splinter in, > cool drinks. Dark red fauces and uvula. Craves sugar, which <. Astringent sour or bitter-sour taste and vomitus. Alcoholic gastritis. Gastralgia; in a spot. Eructates ingests. FLATULENCE; bursting (Lyc.); loud, explosive belching (Coca), discharged upward and downward: noisy diarrhea. Emotional diarrhea. Shreddy, mucus stools, turning green; < drinking. Violent pains from kidneys to bladder. Cutting in urethra, with painful priapism. Yellow, bloody gonorrhea. Painful coition. Cough from laughing. Dyspnea; nervous or flatulent; < gastric pains. Palpitation, < lying on right side. Craves fresh air. Laryngitis. Throbbing or weak spine. Trembling limbs. Peripheral neuralgias. Ischias antica. Weakness, rigidity or twisting in calves. Ulcers, angry, deep; hard edges; warty granulations. Adherent crusts. Chill if uncovered, yet smothers when wrapped up. Shivers through bowels; up back.

Antidotes: Cina, Nat-m.

Complementary: Nat-m.

Related to: Lyc., Puls.

ARNICA MONTANA

SPHERE OF ACTION	AGGRAVATION
BLOOD.	INJURIES
BLOOD-VESSELS.	- BRUISES.
Nerves.	- **Shock.**
Muscles.	- **Jarring.**
Digestive organs.	- **Labor.**
	- Over-exertion.
	- Sprains.
	TOUCH.
	After sleep.
	Motion.
	Old age.
	Alcohol.

AMELIORATION
Lying
- Head low (Verat-v.).
- Out-stretched.

A very painful and offensive remedy. Progressive weakness. Has absorbent action. Shock: mental or physical. VERY PAINFUL BRUISED, SORENESS; **all over;** after the pains; of the bleeding part (Ferr.), etc. Crushing pain. BED FEELS HARD, or full of lumps. As of a **lump** back of stomach, etc. Suddenly shifting joint (Colch.) or paralytic pains. FOUL; **breath,** taste, flatus, stool, etc.. Typhoid. Sepsis. HEMORRHAGIC TENDENCY; **epistaxis,** etc. **Involuntary evacuations.** ....Nervous, sanguine temperament. FEARS; **being struck** or approached; sickness; instant death; on awaking, etc. Morose, repellant mood. Physically **restless,** but mentally prostrate or **apathetic; says nothing ails him** (Op.); reverse (Ars.) answers slowly, with an effort. Feels well, in dangerous cases. Brain feels tired. Vertigo; of old age. **Bloodshot eyes. Ruddy,** congested face. Apoplexy. Fevers. Bright red, puffy fauces. Red stripe down center of tongue. Post-nasal dropping. Catarrh of antrum. **Eructations tasting of bad eggs.** Anorexia by day, but canine hunger before midnight. Cramps from epigastrium down over bowels, then foul stools. Acrid, foamy, stools. Cutting in kidneys. Urine retained or dribbles; after labor. Must wait for urine to pass. After-pains; < suckling. **Hoarseness**; < exertion, colds, or getting wet. Coughs without waking, or cough causing cries. Heavy lower chest. Sore nipples. Arm pains, > hanging down. Heart-beat shakes whole body. Weakened heart muscle. Angina. Heart pains; left to right. Dusky, mottled skin. Every little hurt makes a black and blue spot. Petechiae. Erysipelas. **Symmetrical eruptions. Very sore acne or crops of small boils. Sopor**; drops to sleep as he answers. Troubles or frightful dreams; awakes in terror. Coldness of part lain on. Thirst during chill. Hot head with cool body. Must uncover, but it chills him (reverse of Nux-v.).

Complementary: Calc., Nat-s., Sul-ac.

Related to: Bell-p., Echi., Hyper., Rhus-t.

ARSENICUM ALBUM

SPHERE OF ACTION

MUCOUS MEMBRANES.

MIND.

RESPIRATION.

Lungs; Right apex.

Blood.

Heart.

Nerves.

SPLEEN.

Lymphatics.

Muscles.

SKIN.

Serous cavities.

Organs.

AGGRAVATION

COLD
- ICES, DRINKS
- FOODS.
- Air

PERIODICALLY
- MIDNIGHT; After.
- AFTER 2 A.M.
- 14 days.
- Yearly.

VEGETABLES

DRINKING.

TIPPLING.

Infections.

Bad meat.

Eruptions
- Undeveloped.

- Suppressed.
Quinine.
Lying on part.
Tobacco.
EXERTION.

AMELIORATION
HOT
- APPLICATIONS (dry).
- FOOD.
- Drinks.
- Wraps.
- Motion, walking about.
ELEVATING HEAD.
Sitting erect.
Company.
Sweating.

Sudden, intense effects. Restless, anxious and very weak.
Maddening pains; BURNING LIKE FIRE, hot needles or wires, >
heat, felt, even during sleep; **exciting shortness of breath** (Nat-s.) or
chilliness. Inveterate neuralgias. Multiple neuritis. VERY RESTLESS,
< affected part. **Increasingly irritable** (Cimic.) or SUDDEN GREAT
WEAKNESS, from trivial causes. **Rapid emaciation.** ACRID,
SCANTY, THIN SECRETIONS; coryza, saliva, sweat, etc.
PUTRID, CADAVERIC ODORS. Destructive processes.
Malignancy. Sepsis. Low vitality. **Pale, puffy, baggy** SWELLING.
Dropsy. Anemia. .... Anxious. **Oversensitive.**
Fastidious. EXACTING. Fault-finding. ANGUISH; **despairs of**
recovery (Acon.). AGONIZING FEAR OF DEATH; nightly; yet
tired of living. VIOLENCE; self-torture; pulls her hair; bites her
nails. **Suicidal impulses. Restless and suspicious.** Congestion to head,
> cold, but neuralgia, > heat. Pain alternates between head and
stomach or body. Pain over left eye. **Restless head.** Early graying.
Falling hair. Spasm of eyelids. Burning tears. Scrofulous ophthalmia.
Takes colds. Nose colds descend to chest. **Cold sores;** in nose.
Sneezing, with biting, watery coryza; but stopped nose. Hay fever,

sensitive smell; **loathes odor, sight or thought of food.** PALE, **anxious sunken, haggard or distorted countenance**; with cold sweat. Black lips. Bluish white tongue. Nightly toothache. INSATIABLE BURNING THIRST; CRAVES ICE COLD WATER BUT IT DISTRESSES STOMACH (Nux-v.) AND IS VOMITED AT ONCE; with anorexia; during heat. DRINKS LITTLE AND OFTEN. Gastritis. Swelled spleen. **Vomiting, with purging, from ptomaine poisoning.** Foul, rice water or small, acrid, burning, black, mucous or lienteric stools; < cold drinks. Scanty urine. Uremia (Pip-m.). Profuse, acrid leucorrhea. As of a vapor in larynx. SHORT BREATH; felt in nose; must sit up; < odors, **receding eruptions** or ascending. Whistling inspiration. Wheezing breathing. Cough alternately dry and loose; must sit up. Frothy expectoration. Acute pain through upper third of right lung. Asthma. Pulmonary edema. Cough; dry, nightly; < drinking. **Heart**; weak; trembles; **palpitates;** < slight causes. Stiffness, ascends from coccyx to nape. Alternate internal and skin symptoms. SKIN; LOOKS SEARED; dry, rough, dirty or shrivelled (Op.). Free desquamation. Eczema. Acuminate eruptions. Hives after eating fish. Ulcerative tendency; chronic; with burning. Phagedena. Gangrene. Shocks on dropping to sleep. **Restless sleep.** Dreams of death. COLD, externally, with internal, burning heat; in spots; sensitive to, yet > in open air (Aur.). **Chills;** irregular, shaking; craves hot drinks; and can't get his breath. Heat, as of hot water in veins or they burn like lines of fire; burning or coldness in chest (Bry., Lach., Nat-m., Sulph.). Hectic sweat; with insatiable thirst, dyspnea or exhaustion; cold. Atypical or larval malaria. Old cases of malarias. Waves of icy coldness in blood-vessels or intense boiling heat. Yellow fever (prophylactic).

Complementary : Nat-s., Puls., Thuj.

Related to: Sul-ac., Verat.

ARSENICUM IODATUM

SPHERE OF ACTION
MUCOUS MEMBRANES
- NOSE.
- **Digestive tract.**
- Lungs.

Heart.

Glands.

Skin.

Left side.

Nerves.

AGGRAVATION
Weather
- **Dry.**
- Cold.
- Windy.
- Foggy.

Exertion.

In room.

Apples.

Tobacco smoke.

AMELIORATION
Open air.

Erethistic weakness. BURNING. **Profuse, acrid discharges;** thin in acute, or thick, gluey, yellow (Hydr.) in chronic affections. Rawness. Scrofula. Consumptiveness (Tub.). **Heaviness.** Debility .... Dull, heavy headache, < occiput. Eyeballs feel heavy. Foul otorrhea. Persistent, but unsatisfactory sneezing. Nose drips water; **hot** (Iod.); green; **acrid; reddens upper lip** (Merc.). **Coryza;** with dyspnea (Nit-ac.), post-nasal catarrh. Hay fever. Colds, with hunger. **Aching malar bones. Raw throat. Hoarseness. Goitre. Air hunger. Short of breath.** Hacking cough. **Yellow-green, foul expectoration.** Asthma of phthisical or psoric persons. Beginning resolution (Sul-i.). Burning heat in chest. Tubercular pleurisy. Weak heart; with erethism. Dry, harsh or dusky skin. Psoriasis. Ichthyosis. Rapid, irritable pulse. Chilly. Night-sweats.

Complementary: Kali-i.

Related to: Kali-bi.

ARUM TRIPHYLLUM

SPHERE OF ACTION
Mucous membranes
- Mouth.
- THROAT.
- **Larynx.**

Kidneys.

Brain.

Blood.

Skin.

AGGRAVATION
Over-use of voice.
- TALKING.
- Singing.

Cold, wet winds.

Heat.

Irritation. PAINFULLY SORE, RAW AND BURNING PARTS. ACRID DISCHARGES. .... Excessively cross and stubborn (Tub.). NERVOUS; CHILD PERSISTENTLY BORES INTO NOSE or **picks at lips,** the fingers or at one spot; **until it is sore or bleeds. Acrid, fluent coryza.** Raw, cracked lips (angles) (Psor.). Painfully raw, *sore,* inflamed **mouth.** Aphthae. Raw sore throat; **painful on clearing** or coughing yet **grasps** or wants to scratch it. Hay asthma. Stools like corn-meal. Uremia. **Voice hoarse,** squeaky or breaks. Itching fingers and toes. Eruptions leave a brilliant red stain. Pemphigus. Impetigo contagiosa.

Complementary: Nit-ac.

Related to: Ars., Merc-c.

ASAFOETIDA

SPHERE OF ACTION
NERVES.

Mind.

Gullet.

Digestive tract.

AGGRAVATION
Night.

In room.

Rest.

Eating.

Suppression.

Periosteum
- Ears
- Nose.

Tibia.

Left side.

Mercury.

Noise.

Sitting.

Warm wraps.

AMELIORATION

Motion in **open air.**

Pressure.

Full, stout aspect, but intolerably nervous and OVERSENSITIVE. Fits of violent, hard throbbing, pressure, sharp sticking, etc. Clavus. Easy relapses. Bone aches. **Pains extend outward,** are associated with **numbness** and change place or are > by touch. Boring. Blueness. Foul, thin acrid secretions. .... Magnifies her symptoms. Craves sympathy. Fickleness. Fainting. Hysteria. Clutches throat. Occipital ache > stool. Eyelids stick to ball. Numb about eyes. Ozena. Puffy, purple face, as if heated. **Greasy taste. Everything presses towards throat.** Globus. Spasm of gullet and stomach. **Rancid or explosive belching.** Regurgitations. **Flatulence;** sudden; pushing upward, hysterical. Wind colic. Reverse peristalsis. Bowels seem knotted. Foul, dark watery diarrhea. Spasmodic tightness of chest. Heart seems full, distended. Reflex heart symptoms, of nervous origin. Dark red swelling. Eruption of air vesicles. Bluish ulcers; with high sensitive edges. Foul, burrowing pus. Caries.

Related to: Aur., Lach., Samb., Valer.

ASARUM

SPHERE OF ACTION

NERVES.

Mucous membranes.

Female organs.

AGGRAVATION

PENETRATING SOUNDS.

Dry.

Cold.

Emotions.

AMELIORATION

Cold bathing; of face.

(Fl-ac.).

EXCESSIVE NERVOUS SENSIBILITY; scratching on silk, rattle of paper, etc., is unbearable. Contractive sensations. .... Lightness, as if floating. Painfully sensitive hearing. Cold saliva. Violent vomiting. Gelatinous or shreddy mucus stools. Lientery. Asthmatic breathing, < odors or cold. Violent backache, takes her breath, < motion.

Related to: Arg-n., Castm., Ther.

ASCLEPIAS TUBEROSA

SPHERE IF ACTION	AGGRAVATION
SECRETIONS	Motion.
- SKIN.	Deep breathing.
- **Serous.**	Lying.
- Mucus.	Tobacco.
Chest (Right).	
Muscles.	

Colliquative states (Agar.). SWEATINGS; in pleuro-pneumonia, **diarrhea** or rheumatism. Body numb........................ Sticky, yellow nasal discharge. Tough, yellow coat on tongue. **Stools smell like rotten eggs, or burn like fire.** Dysentery. Flabby genitals. Short of breath and weak on walking. Chest pains, < lying or breathing. Pleurodynia. Pericardial effusion. Pleurisy.

Related to: Ant-t.

ASTERIAS RUBENS

SPHERE OF ACTION
Circulation.
Nerves.
Female organs.
Rectum.
Left side.

AGGRAVATION
Heat.
Menses.
Contradiction.
Cold wet.

Pulsations; in head, womb, chest, etc. Drawn back feeling in eyes, nipples, etc. Cancer. .... Mentally and physically flabby. Weeps from least emotion. Rushes of blood to head; it feels surrounded by hot air. Red face. Pimples about mouth. Stools of brown, gushing water. Sexual erethism.

Related to: Murx., Sep.

AURUM

SPHERE OF ACTION
MIND.
Nerves.
VASCULAR SYSTEM.
Heart (Right).
Bones
- NASAL.
- Skull.
- Patellae.
- Joints.
Glands.
Liver.
Kidneys.

AGGRAVATION
Emotions
- Depressing.
- Disordered.
- Affections.
Mental exertion.
Cold.
Night.
- Sunset to sunrise.
Abuse of Merc. or Kali-i.
Cloudy weather.

AMELIORATION
Cool; Open air.
Cold bathing.
Becoming warm.
Music.
Walking.

Vasomotor mobility; erratic ebullitions and venous congestion, more to head and chest. Vascularity. Weak, yet sensitive to pain. Pains wander, impel motion, finally, attack heart (Benz-ac., Colch.); boring, cutting osteotopic. Indurations; glandular. Sclerosis; coronary. Necrosis. Chronicity. Mercurio-syphilitic dyscrasia. Extremely violent symptoms. Heart feels loose on walking. As of air blowing on part .... Intense, hopeless depression and suicidal anguish. Brooding melancholy; alternating with irritability or moroseness. Praying and self-reproaches; starting from heart. Weak memory. Vexed mood; enraged by least contradiction. Loquacity. Rapid questioning. Fears the least noise. Violent confusing headache; syphilitic. Hemiopia upper horizontal. Sore orbits. Congested, bluish-red face. Pains in zygomae. Red knobby nose. Ozena. Foul breath. Bulimy. Soreness over liver. Hepatitis. Ascites. Jaundice, of pregnancy. Liver, with heart symptoms. Chronic orchitis. Crushing weight under sternum < ascending. Dyspnea; < laughing. Oppression at heart; as if to stop, then gives one hard thump. Violent palpitation; at puberty. Cardiac hypertrophy. Angina pectoris. Aortic disease. As if lower spine bulged backward. Pott's disease. Nightly leg pains. Painfully sensitive to cold. Sweat about genitals. Cold and damp all over.

Related to: Merc.

BADIAGA

Cough; excited by sweets, candy, etc. (Med., Spong., Zinc.). **Expectoration; flies from mouth** (Kali-c.)

BAPTISIA

SPHERE OF ACTION	AGGRAVATION
BLOOD.	**Humid heat.**
Mind.	Fogs.
Nerves.	In room.
Mucous membranes	Pressure.
- Digestive tract.	On awaking.
Left side.	

SORE, HEAVY, ACHING MUSCLES; gall-bladder, heart, etc. WITH RAPID PROSTRATION; the bed is too hard, yet he feels too sick to move. Dark; mucous membranes, exudates, hemorrhage, stools, spots in body, etc. Brown; sordes, stripe down center of tongue, stool, menses, etc. FOUL; odor of body; excretions, stool, sweat, etc. Grippe. Zymoses. Sepsis. Typhoid states. Bed sores, etc. Insensible to pain. Restless mind but lifeless body. Bewildered. Thick speech. Sensation as if a blow on occiput. Dull, drowsy, besotted look. SENSE OF DUALITY; PARTS FEEL SCATTERED ABOUT, SEPARATED, numb or too large. Dull and confused. Falls asleep while answering or does not complete his sentence. Eyes feel swelled. DUSKY, SODDEN, BESOTTED, STUPID COUNTENANCE. Dark red, tumid mouth and throat. Throat, numb inside but sensitive outside. Fetor oris. Tongue cracked, bleeds, feels thick or is heavily coated. Viscid saliva. Aphthae. Ragged ulcers in throat. Can't swallow solids. Spasm of gullet. Easy vomiting. Diarrhea; sudden, horribly foul, mushy, painless, dark or slaty. Symptoms radiate from small of back. Dyspnea from weakness in chest. Air hunger; on waking, > standing. Bronchial asthma. Drowsy, stupid and languid; slides down in bed and lower jaw drops (Mur-ac.). Hyperpyrexia. Livid spots on body. Uremia.

Related to: Arn., Gels., Hyos., Lach., Mur-ac., **Op.,** Rhus-t.

BARYTA CARBONICA

SPHERE OF ACTION

NUTRITION.
MIND.
GLANDS
- THROAT.
- Prostate.
HEART.

Nerves.
Blood-vessels.
Lungs.

AGGRAVATION

Company.
Thinking of it.
Cold.
- **Damp;** to feet.
- To head.
- Changes.
Lying on
- **Painful part.**
- Left side.
Odors.

AMELIORATION

Warm wraps.

Torpid, dwarfish (Med., Syph.) or marasmic. Weakly. **Senility;** early (Calc.). Adenopathies. Scrophula. Chronicity. Single effects (Agar., Con.). Burnings, localised. Numb parts; mouth, genitals, fingers, etc. **Forced through a narrow place, as if.** Vascular softening and dilatation. **Paralytic effects.** Apoplexy. Too tired to even eat. Wants to lie down. **Takes colds.** Inflamed mucous membranes...................... SLOW, INEPT AND BACKWARD. Childish, thoughtless behavior. Timid. **Cowardly.** Groans from every little thing. Increasing mental weakness. **Weak, beclouded mind. Bad memory.** Forgets her errand or the word in her mouth. Irresolute. **Mistrustful. Shy of strangers.** Brain feels loose; > cool air. Heavy pressure over eyes (Bell.). Baldness; < vertex. Hazy cornea. Eyes, > looking down. **Old, sickly, weazened look.** Crusty ears. Nose dry, < blowing it. Pendulous lips. Weak tongue. Burning soreness or vesicles on tip of tongue. **Throat (glands) affected by every cold;** < menses. **Chronic quinsy. Enlarged tonsils** (Calc-p.). Spasm of esophagus. Sore spot in stomach. Diarrhea, with lumbar ache. Flabby genitals. Erections when riding. Paralytic aphonia. Asthma, < wet, warm air; senile (Bar-m.). Chronic bronchitis. **Heart;** bruised sore; < suppressed footsweat. Trembling feet. Hot, bruised soles at night. **Cold, foul footsweat. Indurated glands;** tonsils; cervical, swelled like knotted cords. Cysts. Lipoma. Warts. Acne. Pulse slow and small. High blood-pressure. Arterio-sclerosis.

Related to: Kali-p., Med., Sil.

BELLADONNA

SPHERE OF ACTION

Nerve centres.

Brain.

Blood-vessels; Capillaries.

Mucous membranes
- **Eyes.**
- **Mouth.**
- **THROAT.**

Skin.

Organs.

Right side.

AGGRAVATION

Heat; of Sun; if heated.

Afternoon (3 P.M.).

DRAFTS; on head; Hair cut (Glon.).

Washing head.

After taking cold.

CHECKED SWEAT.

LIGHT.

NOISE.

JARRING.

Touch.

Company.

Pressure.

Motion.

Hanging down.

AMELIORATION

Light covering.

Bending backward.

Rest in bed.

Plethoric, brainy. SUDDEN, VIOLENT EFFECTS. DRYNESS, BRIGHT REDNESS-streaked (Phos.)—AND BURNING HEAT; WITH GREAT PAIN; FULNESS OR SWELLING. CONGESTION: TO HEAD. Dilated arteries. Inflammation. Heat in body, parts, discharges, etc.

CONSTRICTIONS. Parts are hot, swelled, red and dry. THROBBING, SHARP CUTTING, SHOOTING or clawing PAINS; of maddening severity; coming and going, in repeated attacks (Nit-ac.). Scant or hot discharges. JERKS. Shocks. TWITCHINGS. SPASM; of throat, vagina, etc. .... Over-active. Excited. WILDLY DELIRIOUS; ferocious, noisy, cries out. RESTLESS and talks fast. Tries to escape. Furibund. Biting mania. Violent delirium. THROBBING HEAD; < temples; < motion; > letting hair down. Brain rises and falls in waves. Rolls head. Pains go downward from head. HEAD SENSITIVE TO DRAFTS AND COLD, or washing hair. HAMMERING THROB. Pulls her hair. Meningitis. Sunstroke. DILATED PUPILS. Prominent, sparkling eyes. Red sclerotic. Lurid, red, terrifying hallucinations; on closing eyes. Blind attacks; then yellow vision. Sees red. Flashes before vision. PHOTOPHOBIA. Red nose. Fiery RED, turgid, hot FACE, or alternately pale and red. DRY, HOT MOUTH AND THROAT (Phos., Rhus-t.). Toothache, > biting. Swelled tongue. Strawberry tongue. Urging to swallow, with choking. Drinks in sips. Must drink to swallow. Craves lemonade. Pain from stomach or liver to shoulder and throat, < lying on it. Cutting epigastric colic, > bending backward. Distended transverse colon. Clawing or downward forcing in abdomen. Acute prolapsus ani (Ars.). Stools contain chalky lumps. Enuresis on lying-down; nocturnal. Fiery red urine. Early, profuse, hot (Sabin.), red, gushing menses. Rigid os. Metritis. Bearing down > standing, < lying. Red streaked mammae. Dry cough. Barking voice. Stiff right neck and shoulder in afternoon. Back feels broken. BRIGHT, RED, GLOSSY SKIN. Intense dermatitis. Scarlatina. Erysipelas. Sleepy, but can't sleep. Heavy, hot sleep. JERKS DURING SLEEP. Frightful dreams; of quarrels, fire, etc. Internal coldness with external, pungent, burning heat. HOT HEAD, with cold limbs (Sulph.). Hot sweat. Skin hot, but moist and dry alternately. Spasm, then prolonged unconsciousness.

Complementary: Calc., Hep., Merc.

Related to: Glon., Hyos., Stram.

BELLIS PERENNIS

SPHERE OF ACTION	AGGRAVATION
BLOOD-VESSELS.	INJURY; sprains.
Nerves.	TOUCH.
Spleen.	Cold baths or drinks.
Joints.	Wet.
Left side.	Becoming chilled when hot.
	AMELIORATION
	Continued motion.
	Cold (Local).

BRUISED SORENESS. Hard, aching, squeezing or throbbing pain. Tired, fagged. Deep trauma or septic wounds; especially abdominal, pelvic, etc. Acrid pus; destroys the hair. Bleeding. .... Impulse to move. Headache, ending in shooting. Fulness about spleen. Falls on coccyx (Hyper.). Boils. Wakeful; too early. Sensitive to cold. Senile blood stasis. Unbearable pains that drive to distraction, < heat and > cold. Senile vertigo.

Related to: Arn.

BENZOICUM ACIDUM

SPHERE OF ACTION	AGGRAVATION
URINE	Open air.
- Kidneys.	Cold.
- Bladder.	Changing weather.
JOINTS.	AMELIORATION
Heart.	Heat.
Bowels.	Profuse urine.
Left side.	

Strong urinous odor of patient. **Changing or gouty-rheumatic pains, < at heart or alternating with urinary symptoms.** Pains alternate with heart symptoms. Painful, gouty nodes. Hygromae (Am-c.). Bunion. Meniere's disease (Sal-ac.). .... Salty vomitus. **Copious, grayish stools;** like soap-suds; of a pungent urinous odor; very foul; white. STRONG, HOT, DARK-BROWN URINE; foul, ammoniacal or odor of horse urine. Gravel. Hard, dry cough. **Cracking joints;** in knees. Profuse sweat, without relief; night sweats.

Related to: Calc.

BERBERIS VULGARIS

SPHERE OF ACTION
Urinary and
Digestive tract
- KIDNEYS.
- Liver.
- Bladder.
Lumbar region (Hips).
Joints.
Uterus.
Spermatic cord.

AGGRAVATION
Motion
- **Jarring.**
- **Stepping hard.**
- Rising from sitting.
Fatigue.
Urinating.

Mentally and physically tired. Sees things in twilight. **Many, rapidly changing or alternating symptoms; shooting outward,** as in urethra, toes, etc., about or RADIATING **from one point;** lower spine, etc. **Sticking.** Soreness. **Burning-smarting.** Numbness; insensitive to extreme heat or cold. GURGLING or bubbling. **Dry mucous membranes;** mouth, vagina, etc. **Dirty-gray face,** gums, feces, etc. Lithemia. Calculi..................As of a tight cap on head. Cold temples. Suppurating acne. Sticky mouth. Foamy, cottony saliva (Nux-m.). Painful pimple at tip of tongue. Pains from stomach to back or the reverse. Torn loose feeling in epigastrium. Biliary and urinary calculi. **Colic**, pains from gall-bladder to epigastrium; bilious; along ureter, arresting breathing; **renal** (right). Stools, pale, smarting, tough; watery, with jaundice. Fistula ani. Burning kidneys. Clear discharge from meatus, before urinating. **Urine thick, turbid, yellow;** red, mealy, **sandy or slimy sediment.** Dysuria. Genitals : cold, sweaty, pains change sides. Gray or brown mucus replaces menses. **Backache with severe prostration.** Sore spot under (right) scapula (Chel.). Crushing, stitching, paralysing lumbar pain. Numb lumbar region. Pain from **iliac crests down front of thighs**; when urinating. Lumbago. Itchy skin. Eruptions leave a brown stain. Chilly. **Cold single parts.** Everything excites sweating.

Complementary: Mag-m.

Related to: Benz-ac., Coc-c., Kali-bi., Lyc., Puls.

BISMUTHUM

SPHERE OF ACTION

DIGESTIVE TRACT

- **Stomach.**

- **Intestine.**

AGGRAVATION

Eating; Overeating.

AMELIORATION

Cold; Drinks; Applications.

Bending back.

Motion.

Apathetic and prostrated. **Tearing, pinching pains.** Internal heaviness....................Swelled gums. **Craves cold drink, which is vomited at once, or in great quantities when stomach becomes full.** Foul belching. Vomits liquids only, or bilious after eating. Atrophia ablactatorum (Kreos., Ox-ac.). Gastric, alternating with head or face pains. Violent gastralgia (Atro., Chin.); with cramping or burning. Food presses like a load on one spot. Prostration; after stool. Cholera infantum, when the body remains warm. Black ulcers. **Dry palms and soles.**

Related to: Ars., Cadm-s.

BORAX

SPHERE OF ACTION
Occiput
NUTRITION.
- NERVOUS.
- MUCOUS MEMBRANES
MOUTH.
Skin.
Kidneys, bladder.

AGGRAVATION
DOWNWARD MOTION.
Sudden noises.
Cold; Wet.
Least uncovering.
Nursing.
Children.
Fruit.

AMELIORATION
11 P.M.

Tough, bloody mucus. Tousy persons (Med., Sulph.): frowsy hair, tangles at ends. Frightened at every noise; starts from sleep, as if to fall. Restless in afternoon. Gummy, crusty eyelids and nostrils. Raw tarsi. Acrid coryza. Red nose of young women. Dirty complexion. Puffy face. Dry cracked tongue. Palate hard and wrinkled. Eructations when painful parts are pressed. Poorly nourished, soft and flabby. **Aphthous, catarrhal tendency. Clear, thick, hot, biting discharges.** Heat in single parts; mouth, vagina, palms, etc. Sticking or drawing pains; **intercostal**, in soles, etc. **Shrivelled skin** or mucous membranes. Marasmus........................ **Nervous, anxious, fidgety**, fickle. **Fretful,** before stool. **Fears downward motion. Starts at trifles, sudden sounds,** etc. Anxious cries during sleep. Hot head of babies; they **cry and scream when nursing or before passing stool or urine.** Entropion. Red about eyes. Dry, tender, **aphthous mouth.** Puffy, indented tongue. Griping toothache, < wet weather. Nausea when thinking hard. Catch in groin on coughing. Stools: turning green; like boiled starch. Mucous diarrhea, then weakness. Loose, pappy, repulsive stools. Hot, acrid, smarting urine. Nephritis. Cystitis. Easy conception. Membranous dysmenorrhea. Albuminous leucorrhea. Clear, hot, pasty leucorrhea. Empty feeling in mammae, after child nurses. Averse to coition. Pain in opposite breast, as child nurses.

Mother's milk is thick and tastes badly. Blood-streaked or mouldy expectoration. Limbs tremble, at 10 A.M. Itching on back of hands. Eczema. Weak calves. DRY SKIN; **festers easily,** won't heal. Sweat on stomach. Stitch in right chest, < deep breath and > hard pressure. **Heart feels as if on right side.** Violent palpitation.

Related to: Bell.

BOVISTA

SPHERE OF ACTION	AGGRAVATION
CIRCULATION	**Menses.**
- HEART.	Full moon.
- **Uterus.**	**Getting warm**
- Kidneys.	AMELIORATION
SKIN.	Doubling up.
	Eating.

Hemorrhagic-herpetic diathesis. Oozing hemorrhage, < night **Laxness;** joints seem loose; **easy indentation. General puffiness. Enlarged feeling,** head, heart, etc.................. **Awkward in speech and action; drops things,** stutters, etc. Inattentive. Weak memory. Confusion on awaking. Weak jointed and nervous. A wedge presses into occiput. Nose stops on lying down. Numb mouth. As of a lump of ice in stomach. **Colic, > eating.** Bloating. **Diarrhea, < menses. Menses early; more at night, less if in motion;** flow between periods. Thick, pussy, acrid leucorrhea. Short breath on using hands. Visible palpitation. **Itching coccyx.** Weak hands. Heavy painful legs. **Itching eruptions;** oozing; forming **thick crusts or scabs,** with pus beneath (Mez.). Hives, with diarrhea or menorrhagia. Eczema. Chill during pains.

Related to: Apis, The Carbons, Ust.

BROMIUM

SPHERE OF ACTION

LARYNX.
RESPIRATION.
Heart.
Circulation.
Glands
- **Parotid.**
- **Thyroid.**
- **Ovaries.**
- Mammae.

AGGRAVATION
WARM
- DAMPNESS
- **Overeating.**
- Room.
Chilled while hot.
Sea bathing.
Until midnight.

AMELIORATION
Nosebleed (Vertigo, Head,
    Chest).
At sea.
Motion.

Scrophulous blondes. Constrictions, glandular induration or membranous formations. **Weak and easily overheated, then sweaty and sensitive to drafts** .... Head congested, fears a stroke. **Acrid, burning coryza.** Nosebleed. Face seems drawn to a point at nose. Flatus from vagina. Inhaled air seems smoky, cold or raw. Lungs feel coated with down. **Wants to take a deep breath,** but it excites cough. **Suffocative fits;** he starts up choked with **croupy or wheezing** cough, or with palpitation. Asthma. Spasm of glottis. Asthma of sailors going ashore. Deep hoarseness, < if heated. Diphtheritic croup. **Colds** start in larynx; **go upward** (Merc., Sep.) and downward. Thick, white expectoration. Even a small goitre oppresses. Nervous palpitation. Cardiac hypertrophy. Slow, glandular enlargement. Boring in bones.

Related to: Lach., Samb.

BRYONIA ALBA

SPHERE OF ACTION

Blood.

CIRCULATION.

Liver.

SEROUS MEMBRANES
- HEAD.
- CHEST.
- JOINTS.
- ABDOMEN.

Motor apparatus
- Nerves.
- **Muscles.**

Right side.

Lymphatics.

Cellular tissue.

AGGRAVATION

MOTION
- LEAST.
- RAISING UP.
- STOOPING.
- EXERTION.
- COUGHING.
- DEEP BREATHING.

Dry
- Heat.
- Cold.

HOT
- BECOMING.
- ROOM.
- **Weather.**
- **Drinking, while hot.**

EATING

Vegetables.

Acids.

Calomel.

VEXATION.

Touch.

Suppressions.

Taking cold.

Early A.M.

AMELIORATION

PRESSURE
- LYING ON PAINFUL PART
- Bandage, etc.

COOL OPEN AIR.

QUIET.

Cloudy, damp days.

Drawing knees up.

Heat to inflamed part.

Slowly advancing, forcible processes, localizing in unyielding tissues. **Very painful effects;** on coughing holds sides, chest or head; in joints, etc. BURSTING, STITCHING or **heavy, sore pain,** going backward. AVERSE TO LEAST MOTION, even of distant parts. Dryness everywhere. Dryness of the mucous membranes. **Scanty, adherent secretions. Congestion,** INFLAMMATION, **exudation.** Streaks of red. Gastro-**bilious**-rheumatic type.......................... Determined, taciturn, irritable and **ugly.** Wants to be let alone or **go home.** Dull. DIZZY OR FAINT ON RAISING UP. Vertigo; felt in occiput. BURSTING, SPLITTING OR HEAVY **crushing headache;** fronto-**occipital;** < moving eyes, **coughing,** straining at stool, etc. Pain over left eye. Sensitive scalp; every hair pains. Oily hair. Eyeballs sore; **pains behind.** Dark red face. Nosebleed; vicarious. Suppressions or non-appearing discharges, eruptions, etc. Wagging lower jaw. Descending colds. Chewing motions. Dry, parched, cracked lips. **Dry mouth.** Tongue very dry, rough, coated along center; red at base. Soapy saliva. BITTER TASTE, or vomitus. Hawks brown lumps from posterior nares. THIRST; FOR LARGE DRINKS. Craves what he can't relish. Loathing. Nausea, < lying on right side. Throbbing, tender epigastrium. **Heavy load in stomach.** Heavy, sore liver, > lying on it. Appendicitis. Peritonitis. LARGE, DRY, VERY HARD STOOLS, as if burnt. Constipation. Gushing diarrhea on rising, < cabbage; burning; < hot weather. Lumps of tough mucus after stool. Yellow, mushy stool. Vicarious menstruation. Right chest; rusty expectoration. Wants to take a deep breath, but can't, or it excites cough. DRY, HARD, VERY PAINFUL COUGH, as if from stomach; < eating or drinking. Blood-streaked or tough expectoration. Bronchitis. Pneumonia (right). SHARP STITCHES IN CHEST, or at right scapula. Dry, friction sound. Pleurisy. Stony, hard mammae; before menses. Milk fever. Heavy, hard breasts before menses. Interscapular numbness or pain going to epigastrium or from left to heart. Lumbago, < stooping. Delirium; dreams of hard work. FULL, QUICK, HARD PULSE. **Undeveloped measles.** Jaundice. Chill, with hot head and red face; < warm room. Dry, burning heat; with < of all symptoms, blood seems hot. Painful, continued fevers; typhoid, catarrhal, etc.; after suppressions. Sour or oily sweat. Groins sore before menses.

Complementary: Alum., Lyc., Nat-m.

Related to: Phyt., Rhus-t.

BUFO RANA

SPHERE OF ACTION
Heart
- **Blood.**
- **Circulation.**
Kidneys.
Sexual organs; Ovaries.
Groin.
Skin.

AGGRAVATION
In warm room.
Sexual excitement (onanism).
During sleep.
Least motion.
Injuries.
AMELIORATION
Bleedings (Lach., Meli., Sars.).
Cool air.
Bathing; Feet in hot water.

Obesity. **Depravities and bad inheritance. Low minded and low disease forms.** Early break-down. Bloody oozings; nipples, saliva, etc. (Bov.). Festering sensation. As of a peg in joints. **Burnings;** ebullitions of heat. Flushings. Feels swelled in A. M. Trembling and as of electric shocks through body. Sexual epilepsy. Dropsy. .... **Moral depravity.** Childish, silly tittering. Talks nonsense, then angry if not understood. Feeble minded. Fears animals and strangers. Duplicity. Pillow hurts occiput. As of cold balls running through bowels. Asthma. Suffocative cough. **Heart seems to float or beat in water or air.** Rapid heart action; in exophthalmos. Violent pain in mammae, < night. Lumbago, < raising up or least movement. Anesthetic spots. **Red streaks under skin.** Lymphangitis. Panaris. Bullae. Horripilation.

Antidote: Op.
Related to: Bar-c., Graph., Tarent.
Complementary: Calc-c.
F- 5

CACTUS GRANDIFLORA

SPHERE OF ACTION

HEART (muscle).

CIRCULATION.

Head; Right.

Chest.

Circular muscles.

AGGRAVATION

Lying
- On left side.
- On occiput.

Periodically.

Exertion.

10-11 A.M. or 11 P.M.

Night.

AMELIORATION

Open air.

Pressure on vertex.

CONSTRICTIONS; **heart**; chest; neck; **body feels tight** or wrapped, (Bar-c., Graph., Med., Nux-v., Sulph.). **Irregular circulation. Violent congestion.** Hot gushings into chest. **Localised pulsations**; behind stomach. HEMORRHAGE. Pains that extort cries. **Periodical neuralgias**.................. As of a weight on vertex or chest. **Red face.** Cough; from heart affections; rattling. Menses lumpy; **black**; cease on lying. HEART FEELS CLUTCHED AND RELEASED ALTERNATELY, BY AN IRON HAND; or feels it expand and contract; seems to turn over (Lach.); stitches; irritable; intermittent beat. As if an iron band about chest. Numb left arm. Fingers tingle. Chill, not > covering. Strong pulsations in odd places.

Related to: Acon., Coc-c.

CADMIUM SUPHURATUM

SPHERE OF ACTION

Stomach.

Respiration.

AGGRAVATION

Raising up.

Least motion.

Cold.

Faintness on rising. Ozoena. Craves little drinks of cold water, which are vomited at once. Nausea, that compels quiet to avoid vomiting. Suffocates on dropping to sleep. Chest contracted; with asthma.

Related to: Zinc.

CALADIUM

SPHERE OF ACTION

GENITALS.

NERVES.

Skin.

Mucous membranes.

AGGRAVATION
Sexual excesses.
Motion.
Sudden noises.
On falling to sleep.
Tobacco.

AMELIORATION
Cool air.
Short sleep.
Sweating.

DRYNESS; food eaten seems too dry; must drink to swallow. **Red, dry stripe down center of tongue, widening towards tip.** Inclines to lie down. **Dreads to move** .... **Nervous excitation.** Fear of going to sleep. Vertigo, as if rocked. Crawling or as of a cobweb on face. Flaccid, sweaty genitals; glans like a rag. Atonic pollutions. Impotency; after gonorrhea. PRURITUS VULVAE; with burning; from pinworms. Violent, sexual erethism, or neurasthenia. Respiratory, alternating with skin symptoms. Hard cough, with asthma; > expectoration. Numb hands. Cold single parts; feet. Heat during sleep, ceases on waking. Sweet sweat, attracting flies. Low fevers.

Related to: Caps.

CALCAREA FLUORICA

SPHERE OF ACTION	AGGRAVATION
Elastic fibre - Veins. - Glands. Periosteum. Left side.	Beginning motion. Cold; wet. Drafts. Changing weather. Sprains.

Numbness. Weak in morning. Discharges **turn grass green.**
Slow, processes. General stiffness. INDURATIONS; **of stony
hardness; glands,** tonsils, neck; piles, tumors, edge of ulcers, etc.
Nodes in breasts. **Rough and ragged,** tonsils, **exostoses,** periostitis,
enamel, hypertrophied nails, etc. **Vascular dilatation; varicoses,**
inflamed; aneurism. Arteriosclerosis. After apoplexy. **Struma. Fistula.**
Cataract .... Sluggish temperament. Gushing, watery stools
of carrion odor. Expectorates tiny, tough, yellow lumps. Lumbago.
Hip-joint disease. Bursitis. Chronic synovitis. Periostitis of lower
jaw, ribs, etc. Skin cracked; dry, hard and of alabaster whiteness (Ars.).
Stinking pus. X-ray burns. Birth-marks. Cold wrists and ankles.

Complementary: Rhus-t.

Related to: Graph., Hecla.

CALCAREA HYPOPHOSPHORICA

SPHERE OF ACTION	AGGRAVATION
Nutrition.	Vital losses.

Pale and weak, with violent drenching sweats. Rapid and extreme
debility or emaciation. Scrofula. Pedatrophy .... Excitable,
nervous and sleepless. Frying or sizzling in ears. Ravenous hunger, <

2 hours after meals; only > when stomach is full. Anorexia. Sore throbbing in spleen. Diarrhea. Bronchitis. Starts in sleep. Exhausting nightsweats.

Related to: Chin.

CALCAREA CARBONICA OSTREARUM

SPHERE OF ACTION

NUTRITION

- GLANDS.

- BONES.

- SKIN.

- Cervical.

- Mesenteric

BLOOD.

CHEST. Rright lung

HEART.

CHILDREN.

AGGRAVATION

COLD
- RAW AIR.
- Wet.
- BATHING.
- Cooling off.
- Change of weather.

EXERTION
- Mental.
- **Physical.**
- **Ascending.**
- Eyestrain.

DENTITION.

Puberty.

PRESSURE OF CLOTHES.

MILK.

Awaking.

Anxiety.

FAT, **flabby** BLONDES, WHO SWEAT EASILY, < ON HEAD OR CHEST; DURING SLEEP. PROFUSE, OFTEN SOUR DISCHARGES, stools, **sweats,** odor of body, saliva, etc. **Soft,** torpid, **scrophulous** habit. Numb parts lain on. Easily sprained. Grows fat, but not strong. **Cold, moist air chills through and through. Takes cold easily;** in chest. Malnutrition. **Faulty bony development.** OPEN FONTANELLES. Tardy teething and walking. Scrofula. Rickets.

Curvatures. Calculous tendency. .... Forgetful; learns poorly.
Depressed melancholic or doubting mood; fears disease, misery,
disaster, being observed, insanity, etc. (Lil-t., Nux-v., Sep., Verat.).
Cautious. Confused; misplaces words. Sad. Apathetic. Indolent;
suddenly. Vertigo. BIG HEAD, WITH LARGE, HARD
ABDOMEN. Deep head pains—beating, shattering, etc., < wind, >
dark; with eructations. Migraine. **Scalp itches;** on awaking. **Thick,
foul milk-crust** (Sulph.). DILATED PUPILS. Sees things on closing
eyes; beside visual field. Coryza, with polyuria. Senile catarrh. **Swelled
nose and upper lip** (Bar-c. Sulph.). Face pallid, pasty and puffy.
Swelled tonsils. Anorexia; from overwork. Craves eggs or coarse foods.
Averse to meat. Sour, curdled vomit (Nat-p.). STOMACH LIKE
AN INVERTED SAUCER. Thirst for cold water at night. Cramp
at navel. Biliary colic. Chalky, gray (Ph-ac.) or green, watery stools.
Lientery. Foul or **strong urine.** White urinary sediment. Hydrocele.
Thick, milky, gushing leucorrhea. Painless hoarseness. Everything
makes him **short of breath.** Emphysema. Cough, as from dust.
Purulent, loose, sweet expectoration. **Weak heart.** Palpitation. Sore
chest; breasts before menses. Neck pains, < lifting. Chapped hands.
Arthritic nodes. ENLARGED GLANDS; cervical, mesenteric, etc.
Cysts. Psoriasis. Polypi; nasal, uterine, etc. Skin cold, like a snake.
Nightmare. Sleepless; from rush of ideas. **Coldness; icy, on vertex;**
spots on head, hands, knees and feet; of affected part (Led.); objective.
Chill with thirst. Internal heat, with external coldness and sweat.
Hot head from mental exertion. Clammy hands (Sulph.). **Sweat;** cold;
partial; **head,** < occiput; **chest; on hands.** COLD, DAMP FEET.

Complementary: Bar-c., Lyc., Sil.

Follows: Nit-ac., Sulph.

Related to: Bar-c., Sil.

CALCAREA PHOSPHORICA

SPHERE OF ACTION

NUTRITION
- BONES.
- GLANDS.
- Nerves
  - SUTURES.
  - PERIOSTEUM.
  - Cartilage.
ABDOMEN.
Vertex.
Chest.

AGGRAVATION

Exposure to
- **Weather changes.**
- **Drafts.**
- **Cold, wet.**
- **Melting snows.**
- East wind.

DENTITION.
Mental exertion.
Loss of fluids.
Puberty.
Fruits.
Cider.

AMELIORATION
Lying down.

Delicate, erethistic, **tall or scrawny children;** with dirty, brownish skins. **Soft, thin bones.** Malassimilation. Scrofula. Rickets. **Spots; cold or sore, vertex,** eye-balls, tip of nose, or fingers, etc. **Crawling, numb, cold limbs.** Pains shift. Arthritis. Rheumatism. Albuminous discharges, leucorrhea, etc. Anemia; as a sequel. .... **Peevish, restless and fretful.** Idiotismus versatilis. Headache; in occipital protuberances; down spine; > cool bathing or **sneezing; of school children.** As of ice in occiput. Thin skull bones. Open fontanelles. Hydrocephalus. **Teeth; late;** soft; decay easily. Tonsils, large; mycosis (Kali-m.). Adenoids. Throat aches; feels hollow. Craves raw, salt, piquant foods or bacon. Weak digestion : every bite hurts the stomach. Persistently vomits milk. FLABBY, SUNKEN ABDOMEN; pains, then burning leucorrheal flow. **Festering navel.** Diarrheic tendency. Stools foul, **hot; lienteric;** spluttering and watery; < fruits. Fistula; alternating with chest symptoms. Addison's disease. School girl's headache. Abnormal cravings. Tumor in left mamma. Menses early, scanty; every two weeks. Crawling in genitals. Exalted sexual instinct. Eruptions, < during menses. Uterus heavy; weak or

aching. Child loses its breath on being lifted up (Borx.). Cough, >
lying. Cavernous phthisis; with night sweats. **Neck or chest pains
from drafts. Weak, thin neck;** the head bobs about. Sore fingertips.
As of a splinter under nails. Weak through hips. **Thin, brittle bones.**
Pain, burning, **along sutures** or edges of nails. Slow ossification; non-
union. Swollen glands. Pott's or hip-joint disease. Easily chilled; during
pains. Sickly sweat; < head and throat; at night. Cold limbs with
digestive trouble. Chills up back, but heats down back.

Related to: Carb-an., Chin., Nat-m., Ruta.

Follows: Ferr-p.

CALCAREA SULPHURICA

SPHERE OF ACTION

CONNECTIVE TISSUE.

Glands.

Mucous membranes.

Bones.

Skin.

AGGRAVATION
Drafts.
Touch.
Cold.
Wet.
Heat of room.

AMELIORATION
Bathing.
Open air.
Eating.
Heat (local).
Uncovering.

Cutting pains; (right) ovary. **Tendency to suppuration. Pus
thick,** yellow, lumpy, bloody. Catarrh. ABSCESS, **running;** ears;
teeth; recurrent (Pyrog.). Ulcers, malignant; corneal; deep. Fistulae.
Poor reaction.....................Hurried. Ears flow dark wax. Red,
itching tarsi. Infants with bloody coryza, diarrhea or eczema. Stool
coated white. Pyelitis (Berb.). Thick, white leucorrhea. Choking.
Croup. Cold, foul footsweat. **Skin won't heal.** Averse to covers, when

cold. Dry heat at night. Easy sweat, < coughing. Starts from sleep, as if wanting air.

Related to: Hep.

CALENDULA OFFICINALIS

SPHERE OF ACTION

SOFT PARTS.

Spine.

Liver.

AGGRAVATION

Weather; Damp; Cloudy.

During chill.

Excessively painful, open, torn, **cut, lacerated, ragged or suppurating** WOUNDS. Hemorrhages, in scalp wounds or after drawing teeth, etc. **Prevents pus.** Sensitive to damp or open air. Takes colds. .... Yellowish vision. Nausea, in chest. Curdy stools. Bruised pain at angle to right scapula. Jaundice.

Related to: Arn., Bell-p.

CAMPHORA OFFICINALIS

SPHERE OF ACTION

DIGESTIVE TRACT.

Cerebro-spinal nerves.

Urinary organs.

Nose.

AGGRAVATION
Cold.
Drafts.
When half asleep.
   (M-aust., Nit-ac.)
Mental exertion.
Shock.
SUPPRESSION.
Inattention.

AMELIORATION
Free discharges.
Sweat.
Thinking of it.

Algidity; can't get warm; at start of colds, **cholera**, etc. Bluish, old, pinched look. ICY COLD, YET AVERSE TO COVERS (Sec.), or wants them off, then on; **with internal burning heat; and anxious. Sudden weakness;** dry collapse. Cholera. **Scanty or retained discharges.** Violent tonic **spasm;** of bladder; then stupor, **with** coldness. .... **Insensibility or anxiety.** Head feels knotted up. Hammering in occiput. Inhaled air seems cold. **Coryza;** in old age. Retracted lips; upper. Cold tongue. Burning thirst. Burning in stomach. Strangury. Hematuria. Sexual excitement. Satyriasis. Hoarse, squeaking voice. Asphyxia neonatorum. Cold breath. Thumbs cramp backward. Cramp in calves. **Dry skin. Erysipelas. Very sensitive to cold air or taking cold.** Shaking chill, with **cold skin.** Wants covers during hot stage only. Sudden, inflammatory fevers with rapid alternation of heat and cold; followed by rapid prostration. Heat or sweat, > covers. Corrects spoiled cases and antidotes most remedies. Chilly, below scapula; before colds.

Antidotes: Coff., Op., Phos.

Related to: Carb-v., Cupr., Op., Sec.

CANCER FLUVIATILIS
(ASTACUS FLUVIATILIS)

SPHERE OF ACTION   **AGGRAVATION**
  Liver.   Air.
  Glands.   Uncovering.
  Vasomotors.

Stinging pains. Shiverings. .... Cough, > walking. URTICARIA; with hepatic symptoms, jaundice, etc.; with cramps in liver region; on right side only.

Related to: Calc., Rhus-t.

CANNABIS INDICA

SPHERE OF ACTION	AGGRAVATION
EMOTIONS.	URINATING.
MIND.	DARKNESS.
Nerves.	**Exertion.**
GENITO-URINARY	Talking.
ORGANS.	Walking.
	Gonorrhea.

Extreme psychic mobility. EXALTED IDEATION AND PERCEPTION, WITH MENTAL EXCITEMENT. Imaginations. Wonderful hallucinations; ecstatic; heavenly; of agonizing terror or pain; with loss of sense of proportion; or time and space (Onos., Stram.) Mania of grandeur. Levitation. Gaiety. Violence. Delirium tremens. Feels weak and all gone to nothing. **Trickling sensations; at heart.** .... **Loquacity.** Craves light. Violent headache, with hallucinations. **Vertex opens and shuts.** Head seems separated from body. Sees objects outside of visual field (Ign.). Weak vision. Corneal opacity. Skin of face seems tight. Alive feeling in abdomen : it throbs here and there. SCANTY, BURNING URINE, PASSED DROP BY DROP (Canth.); with pain going backward. Nephritic colic. Swelled prepuce. Priapism. Gonorrhea. Irritable caruncle. Profuse menses, with great pain. Can't control voice. Suffocative attacks. Pains in limbs, < deep breathing. Dreams, erotic; of the dead.

Antidotes: Apis.

Related to: Anh., Cocain., Nux-m., Op.

CANTHARIS VESICATORIA

SPHERE OF ACTION
MEMBRANES
(Mucous and Serous)
- URINARY ORGANS.
- **Bladder.**
- **Pharynx.**
- Brain.
- Pleura.
- **Lower bowel.**
Pomum adami.
Skin.
Right side.

AGGRAVATION
URINATING.
Drinking.
Cold; **Bright objects.**
Sound of water.
Touch; Larynx.

AMELIORATION
Warmth.
Rest.

Rapid and intense action. Excitement during the pains. CUTTING SMARTING or BURNING-BITING PAINS; **as if raw. VIOLENTLY ACUTE INFLAMMATION, or rapidly destructive.** Discharge of bloody, acrid water. Serous effusion. Gangrene. Weak attacks, that take the voice away. .... Amorous frenzy. Rage. Yellow vision. Swelled, tremulous tongue; **raw edges.** Throat: full of blisters; painful swallowing. **Throat** and larynx painfully constricted, and as if **afire. Burning thirst,** but averse to liquids. Violent retching and vomiting. **Sensitive over stomach and kidneys** (Solid.). **Shreddy, burning stools, with tenesmus of rectum and bladder.** BURNING, SCALDING URINE, WITH CUTTING, INTOLERABLE URGING AND FEARFUL TENESMUS OR DRIBBLING. **Strangury.** Dysuria. Bloody urine. Acute nephritis. Nephritic colic. Cystitis. Griping in bladder. Gonorrhea. Dropsy. Painfully swelled genitals. Painful priapism. Pulls at penis. **Sexual irritation.** Pollutions. Many, short, dry coughing spells. Chest pains, > eructations. Pleurisy. Pericarditis. Vesicular erysipelas; turning dark (Ran-b.). Bullae. Chill, during stool. Urinous sweat; on genitals.

Antidotes: Acon., Camph.

Complementary: Apis.

Related to: Apis, Ars., Merc-c.

CAPSICUM ANNUUM

SPHERE OF ACTION

MUCOUS MEMBRANES.

THROAT.

Kidneys.

Bones.

Mastoids.

AGGRAVATION

SLIGHT DRAFTS.
COLD
- AIR.
- Water.
Uncovering.
Dampness.
Bathing.
Empty swallowing.
Drinking: < Throat, or
excites urination.
Eating.
Drunkards.

AMELIORATION

Continued motion.

Lax, lazy, fat, red (Asaf.), **clumsy, unclean persons** (Sulph.), **who react badly and dread the cold. Old age.** Indolent and can't think clearly. BURNING-SMARTING; **tip of tongue; throat,** stomach, stool, **piles,** prostate. SORENESS. **Constriction;** of throat, with urging to swallow. Dark, red, spongy mucous surfaces or oozing bloody mucus. **Springing, thread-like pains** (All-c.). Neuralgias. Deep abscess. Foul secretions. .... Changeable. Capricious. **Homesick.** Splitting headache, > heat. Ears affected alternately. Mastoiditis. NOSE AND FACE RED, BUT COLD. Vesicles or flat, painful aphthae. **Tongue greenish at base. Swelled uvula.** Increased saliva. Smoker's sorethroat. Craves stimulating, pungent things; wants a bracer. Dipsomania. Waterbrash. **Acid dyspepsia.** Small, hot, mucus stools, with tenesmus, also of bladder; then thirst and lumbar pain; < **drinking.** Dysentery. Urging to urinate. Strangury. Thick, white, creamy gonorrhea. **Cough causes distant pains,** or raises foul air; too weak to cough out expectorate. Ribs seem dislocated. Sleepy after meals. **Chilly; with the pains;** begins in back; with violent thirst, but **shivers from every drink;** with excruciating backache; alternating with heats, mounting to head; then sweat. Coldness of affected parts. Sweats easily; cold on thighs.

Complementary: Nat-m.

Related to: Canth.

CARBO ANIMALIS

SPHERE OF ACTION

NUTRITION.

Glands.

VEINLETS.

AGGRAVATION
Slight causes
- Small depletions
- Sprains.
- Lifting.
- Cold taking.
WHILE EATING
Dry, cold air.
Shaving (Ox-ac., Rad-br.)
Old age.
After menses.

AMELIORATION
Laying hand on part.

Old and feeble. Susceptible to colds, sprains or overaffected by small losses, etc. Venosity. Gummae. Slow, hard painful processes; burning like fire (Ars.), or threatening malignancy. Sense of looseness. Foul acrid discharges. Hemorrhage .... Whining. Brain seems loose or as if crown would split, > eating. Pains down through (right) eyeball (Gels.). Can't locate sounds. Nose, hard, red, swelled; hot, brown stripe across, with itching pimples and desquamation. Goneness in stomach; while suckling. All food distresses stomach. Abdomen, distended after operations. Right ovary seems a heavy ball. Neglected bubo. Pelvic bones pain on sitting. Dark menses; in A.M. only; then great weakness. Sore, moist anus (Carb-v.). Indurated os (Sep.). Suffocation on closing eyes; nervous dyspnea. Hard, painful nodes in breasts. **Bluish skin;** cheeks, lips, affected parts, etc. Coppery eruptions on forehead. Crawling, as of bugs. **Hard, swelled glands.** Surgings or hot flushes. Foul, exhausting sweats; at night; **staining yellow.**

Complementary: Calc-p.

Related to: Calc-f., Graph.

CARBO VEGETABILIS

SPHERE OF ACTION

MUCOUS MEMBRANES
- DIGESTIVE TRACT.
- STOMACH.

HEART
- VENOUS CIRCULATION.
- **Blood.**
Occiput.

AGGRAVATION
WARMTH.
DEPLETIONS.
Cooling off.
EXHAUSTING DISEASES.
Old age.
HIGH LIVING.
Rich foods.
DISSIPATION.
Overlifting.
Walking in open air.
Pressure of clothes.
Weather.
- Extreme temperature.
- Cold.
- Night air.
- Frosty; Humid.
Air.
Wind on head.
Suppression.

AMELIORATION
ERUCTATIONS.
Cool air.
Elevating feet.

Low, grave, depraved, or cachectic states. Atony, failing reaction or obstinate sequelae. Complaints of old age. WEAKNESS, FLATULENCE, FETOR OR AIR HUNGER, with most complaints. Tremulous, WEAK, SICK AND EXHAUSTED; suddenly; with pulselessness. Fainting. Collapse. Easily chilled. Cold, yet wants air or to be fanned, or thirsts for cold water. BLUENESS and decomposition. Sepsis. Ulceration (aphthous). HEMORRHAGE; dark oozing. Overfulness. Venosity. Thick, acrid discharges (Hydr.). Old catarrhs. General bruised soreness or **heavy**

aching burning; in bones, ulcers, etc. Numbness, of parts lain on.
.... Slow, anxious and **irritable**. Dejected. Unhappy.
Dull, compressive, heavy (leaden) headache; < occiput; < overheating,
lying or pressure of hat. Sneezing from irritation in larynx; - < blowing
nose or sneezing. Colds go downward (Phos.). PINCHED,
HIPPOCRATIC **or** DUSKY FACE. **Twitching upper lip.** Mumps
with metastasis. Loose teeth. Scorbutic gums. Small, painful aphthae.
Black tongue. Loathes even the thought of food. BELCHINGS;
RANCID; **loud,** without >; with cough. EXCESSIVE
FLATULENCE; obstructed; distending; < **upper abdomen** (Puls.);
< lying. All food turns to gas. Dyspepsia. Colic. Burning in rectum.
Itching anus. Septic albuminuria. Sore, hot, itching, swelled vulva.
Hoarse in evening. Spasms of tormenting, hollow or choking cough,
with headache and vomiting; < cold drinks and in bed; expectorates
with retching. Pertussis and its effects. Heavy, sore or weak chest; on
awaking. Senile asthma. Destructive lung diseases. Continuous,
anxious palpitation. Sore ribs. As of a plug in back. Weak fingers.
Raw or mottled skin. Ulcers, foul, burning and bleeding. Varicosis.
Horrors during sleep. Thready pulse. Alternate chill and heat. ICY
COLD; tongue; **knees;** legs, at night; **breath;** foot (left); unilateral,
etc. Warm head, cold limbs. **Internal, burning heat;** at heart; in chest;
with icy skin, sweat, etc. Sweats easily; takes cold; sour; cold on face;
< coughing. Icy, but wants air.

Antidote: Nat-m.
Complementary: Chin., Kali-c.
Follows: Caust.
Related to: Am-c., Ars., Colch., Graph., Lyss.

CARBOLICUM ACIDUM

SPHERE OF ACTION	AGGRAVATION
MUCOUS MEMBRANES	Jar.
- Throat.	Reading.
- STOMACH.	Pregnancy.
- Bowels.	Combing hair (Bry., **Chin.,**
- Lungs.	Ign., Sel.).
HEART.	
Blood.	
Respiration.	

Painless, languid and PROSTRATE. FOULNESS. Burning secretions; expectoration, etc. Malignancy. **Sepsis.** Low fever. Pricking-burning or sudden pain. .... Tender scalp. As of a burning ball in forehead. Acute smell. PALE ABOUT NOSE AND MOUTH. **Dusky face. Fetor oris.** Glazed throat. Vomiting. Heartburn. Stomach sore. Flatulence. **Shreddy stools.** Passes mucus from anus when urinating. Urine, scanty, green or dark. Leucorrhea; thick, causing itching. Aching between scapulae. **Sopor. Thready pulse.** Collapse. Bloody exudations, vesicles or pustules. Erysipelas. Profuse, cold sweats.

Related to: Kreos.

CARDUUS MARIANUS

SPHERE OF ACTION	AGGRAVATION
	Lying on left side.
Liver (Right).	**Beer.**
	Eating.
Spleen.	Touch.
	Motion.
Veins.	Cellars.
	AMELIORATION
	Bleeding.

Hepato-hemorrhagic diathesis (Lept., Thlas.). Blood-stasis. Acidity. Fatigue. .... Hypochondriacal. Dull frontal headache. Dirty, yellow complexion. Weak upper lip and (right) tongue. Tongue has white center with red, indented edges. **Vomits acrid bile** or blood. High diaphragm. **Liver engorged;** swelled laterally. Gall-stones (Lept.). Meteorism. Knotty, **clayey stools. Golden yellow urine.** Asthma. Dropsy. **Broken or hard thrombosed veins.**

Related to: Calc., Sang.

CASTOREUM

SPHERE OF ACTION	AGGRAVATION
	Emotions.
	Cold.
NERVES	During menses.
	Debilitating diseases.
Female generative organs.	**AMELIORATION**
	Pressure.

Weak and lacks reaction. Nervous and spasmodic effects of uterine origin. Fibrillar twitchings. Hysteria. **Irritability.** .... Twitching in tongue. Abdominal symptoms, with yawning. **Colics, with sudden weakness,** > pressure. Summer diarrhea of green mucus stools (Asar.). Violent cutting dysmenorrheal **colic,** then **cold sweat.** Exhausting sweats after fevers.

Related to: Mosch., Valer.

CAULOPHYLLUM

SPHERE OF ACTION

FEMALE ORGANS.

NERVES

Muscles.

Neck.

Lower limbs.

Small joints.

AGGRAVATION

Pregnancy.

Suppressed menses.

Open air.

P.M.

Exhaustion. PAINS, ERRATIC, **drawing,** cramping, shooting, **rheumatic;** ending in neck, which gets stiff. Uterine reflexes. **Internal tremor**..............Fretful and fearsome. **Nervous;** excitable. Chorea. Vomiting of uterine origin. Albuminuria. Violent, intermittent, crampy pains, with little flow. Late menses. Dysmenorrhea. LABOR PAINS FLY ABOUT (to breasts), ARE WEAK, OR IRREGULAR; **false. Eases labor.** Often acts as prophylactic of false labor pains. After-pains. Uterine atony. **Habitual miscarriage.** Vaginal spasm. Profuse, acrid leucorrhea; of little girls. **Sore nodes on finger-joints. Rheumatism; of small joints.** Aching, sore lower limbs; before menses. Paraplegia, after child-birth. **Chloasma;** on neck. As if overfull of blood. High fever.

Related to: Cimic., **Puls., Sep.**

CAUSTICUM

SPHERE OF ACTION

NERVES

- **Motor.**

- **Sensory.**

MUSCLES

- BLADDER.

AGGRAVATION

Air

- DRY COLD.

- Raw.

- WINDS.

- **Drafts.**

Extremes of temperature.

Stooping.

- LARYNX.
- Limbs.

Respiration.

Skin.

Right side; Face.

Suppressions.
Coffee.
3-4 A.M. or EVENING.
Exertion.
Change of weather.

AMELIORATION
A COLD DRINK (EVEN
   CHILLS).
Washing.
Warmth; of bed.
Gentle motion.

Sensitive to both heat and cold. **Weakness,** increasing uncertainty of control, stumbling, etc., finally PARALYSIS; **of single parts,** Atony. Anesthesia. Stiff joints. Contracted tendons; palms (Nat-m.), hamstrings, etc. Deformities. Atrophy. Jerks of single muscles. Epilepsy, at puberty. **Trembling. Burning. Soreness. Rawness;** larynx, anus, etc.....................Broken down; worn out; wants to die. Hopeless, despondent. **Mental tire. Anxious forebodings** (felt in head), < in twilight. Reticent. Oversympathetic. Empty behind forehead. Tight scalp. To and fro or nodding motions. Paralysis : of one eyelid (right), throat, bladder, etc. Heavy, drooping eyelids. Continuous eye pain. Diplopia, > looking to right. Objects look large. Cataract. Profuse acrid tears. Much, foul earwax. Echo in ears. Tinnitus. Eruption on lower nose. Prosopalgia, > cold water. **Facial paralysis,** < opening mouth. Swelling at root of tongue. Throat, < stooping. Urging to swallow, or swallows the wrong way. Greasy eructations. Cramp in rectum on stooping. Anus, prolapses on coughing; small, hard pustules. Stool glistens; difficult, > standing. Stooling easier by standing, but piles < standing. Must sit down to urinate. Insensible urethra or rectum; to solid stools (Aloe). Piles, < walking. **Urine retained after labor.** URINE SPURTS ON COUGHING; dribbles or passes slowly > sitting. Menses by day, leucorrhea by night. Dry, hard cough. Cough from tickling in throat pit (Sep.), or left larynx; incessant; dry night and morning. Can't cough deep enough (Rumx.); **expectorate slips back again;** < heat of bed, stooping, cold air; > sips of cold water. Greasy, ropy, difficult expectoration. Aphonia or **hoarseness**, in A.M.; of speakers; < stooping; > talking. Sore streak in larynx. Sore chest; vest seems tight. Purring in chest. Wandering chest pains, > pressure. Stiff neck or back on rising; pain goes forward or to thighs. Pain in spine on swallowing. Bursting in fingertips. Cramps in calves, feet or toes. **Deep burns and their effects.** Skin : cracks; ulcers. Warts, on brows, lids, nose, fingertips; seedy; bleeding; ulcerating. Coldness, not > warmth; causes paralysis, cough, diarrhea, etc. Sweat about 4 A. M.; profuse, on slight exertion; < open air.

Complementary: Carb-v., Graph., **Lach.,** Staph.

Related to: Gels., Kali-bi., Phos., Rhus-t., Sep.

CEANOTHUS

SPHERE OF ACTION	AGGRAVATION
Spleen.	Cold weather.
	Lying on left side.

Periodical neuralgias. Pain in left side, with dyspnea, diarrhea or leucorrhea. Swelled spleen or liver. Green urine.

Complementary: Nat-m.

Related to: Chin., Polym.

CEDRON

SPHERE OF ACTION	AGGRAVATION
Nerves.	**Periodically,** at same hour.
Blood.	After sleep.

EXACT PERIODICITY. Orbital neuralgia (right). Brow ague. **Eyes burn like fire.** Numbness. Excitement before chill. Malaria.
Related to: Aran.

CHAMOMILLA

SPHERE OF ACTION	AGGRAVATION

SPHERE OF ACTION

MIND.

NERVES.

EMOTIONS.

Mucous membranes

- DIGESTIVE TRACT.

Liver.

Women and CHILDREN.

Left side.

AGGRAVATION

ANGER.

NIGHT.

DENTITION.

Cold.
- Air.
- Damp.

Wind.

Taking cold.

COFFEE.

Narcotics.

Alcohol.

AMELIORATION

BEING CARRIED.

Mild weather.

Heat.

Sweating.

Cold applications.

Bad temper. **Frantic irritability,** snappish **and intolerant of pain. Mad during pain.** Magnifies her pains. Unappeasable crossness. OVERSENSITIVE. Tosses about, cries out or walks the floor (Ars.); demands instant relief. **Beside himself or prostrated by pain.** Neuralgic or gouty-rheumatic subjects. **Spells of being irritable and restless;** OF COLIC; of dry, tickling cough, etc. **Cramps,** with bilious vomit; of muscles. **Numb,** on awaking; **after pain;** hands, when grasping objects. Repeated spasms; of face, arms, legs, etc. .... UGLY, CROSS, AND UNCIVIL. QUARRELSOME; **vexed at every trifle. Abrupt. Averse to being spoken to or touched.** WANTS TO BE CARRIED **or what is refused when offered.** Omits words. Sensitive to cold wind about ears. Sticking, **earache;** > warmth. **Swelling,** or REDNESS OF ONE CHEEK. Faceache (right), to ear.

Jaws feel tired. Bad, sour breath. Bitter taste. Thick, yellow-white fur on tongue. Eructations like bad eggs. Distended bowels. Colic going upward; < anger (Coloc.). **Cutting or wind colic;** < night. STOOLS, **hot,** ACID, GRASS-GREEN, SLIMY, HACKED, yellow-green, OR LIENTERIC; **smelling like bad eggs.** Irregular, labor-like pains; going up; down inner thighs. Cramps when child nurses. Dark, lumpy menses or lochia. Asthma, < dry weather. Jaundice. Dry palms. Sleepy, disturbed, by pain, starting up, etc. Chilly, yet easily over-heated, hence takes cold. Coldness of one part, with heat of another; < uncovering. Alternate chill and heat. **Hot and thirsty or hot sweat, with the pains.** Hot coryza; hot stools. Feverish, from suppressed discharges. Sweat on head. Sleepless from abuse of narcotics.

Antidotes: Com., Ign., Nux-v., Puls.

Complementary: Mag-c., Sanic.

Related to: Nux-v., Staph.

CHELIDONIUM MAJUS

SPHERE OF ACTION

Right side
- **Portal system.**
- **Abdomen.**
- Lungs (Lower).

Mucous membranes.

Bowels (Right).

Occiput.

Kidneys.

Knees.

AGGRAVATION

Motion.

Cough.

Touch.

Change of weather.

North easters.

4 A.M. and 4 P.M. (Ign.).

AMELIORATION

Hot food.

Eating; dinner.

Milk.

Pressure.

Hot bath.

Bending backward.

YELLOWNESS. **Bilious disturbances;** vomiting, jaundice, catarrhs, etc. Pains **shoot backward** or in all directions. **Stitches. Heavy,** stiff, sore, paralyzed, **dislocative** or broken **feeling.** Numbness. Horror of motion..... ....Lazy. Averse to mental exertion or conversation. Despondency. **Vertigo;** felt in vertex. Headaches extend backward. Heavy occiput. Supra-orbital pain. Mucus in eyes. Outward, blowing, crawling, etc., in ears. Dark red or **sallow, sunken face.** Red nose. **Flapping alae.** Bitter taste. **Yellow tongue;** with indented edges (Hydr.). Choking, as from too large a morsel. Left sided goitre. Craves milk, piquant or hot foods (Lyc.). Nausea. Sensitive epigastrium. Sensation as of a plug in stomach. Gnawing, scraping gastric pains, > **eating.** LIVER PAINS GOING BACKWARD, OR FIXED AT ANGLE OF RIGHT SCAPULA; (to right shoulder and occiput— Kali-c., Nux-v., Sep.). Rawness in liver. Gall-stones. As of a string about abdomen or neck. Stools pasty, **pale, bright yellow, clayey** or hard balls. Dyspnea, < urinating (Dulc.). **Cough, as from dust;** with much rattling, but **little expectoration,** or it **flies from mouth.** Hepato-pectoral symptoms. Like a **nail deep in right chest.** Bilious pneumonia (Merc.). Fluctuating temperature. Pain from neck to right temple. Itching, > eating. **Lethargic,** DROWSY **and chilly. Icy cold nape and occiput. Cold fingertips.** One foot cold. Burning heat, spreads from hands over body. Sweaty, with aversion to uncover and without relief; after midnight.

Complementary: Lyc., Merc-d.

Related to: Bry., Kali-bi., Merc., Op.

CHENOPODIUM

Deafness: variable; > high pitched voice.

CHIMAPHILLA

SPHERE OF ACTION
Bladder.
Kidneys.
Glands
- Liver.
- **Prostate.**
- Mammae (Right).

AGGRAVATION
Cold damp.
Standing.
Sitting.
Beginning urination.
AMELIORATION
WALKING.

ROPY or muco-purulent, foul, scanty, thick, turbid, urine. Feels as if sitting on a ball, in the perineum; after gonorrhea. Old nodes in or atrophy of glands. Fluttering in kidney region. Acute inflammation in urinary tract. Gravelly urine.

Complementary: Kali-m.

Related to: Berb., Coc-c., Sabal.

CHINA OFFICINALIS

SPHERE OF ACTION
BLOOD.

CIRCULATION.

SECRETIONS

- **Digestive organs.**

- **Liver.**

Spleen.

Nerves.

AGGRAVATION
VITAL LOSSES.
TOUCH.
Jar.
Noise.
PERIODICALLY
- **Alternate days.**
  (Ars, Nat-m.).
Cold; Drafts; Wind.
Open air.
Eating; **Fruit;** Milk
Mental exertion.
AMELIORATION
Hard pressure (Lach.).
Loose clothes.

INTERMITTENCY. PROFUSE, EXHAUSTING DISCHARGES, HEMORRHAGES, etc. (Abrot., Calc-hyp., Ph-ac.). **Weak, oversensitive and nervous;** everything upsets him, **light, noise, odors,** pain, etc. Hard swelling. **Bursting.** Rheumatism. Neuralgia. Emaciation, Anemia. Dropsy. .... Stubborn. Disobedient. Vertigo; falls backward. Throbbing, bursting, swashing, or bruised feeling in brain, < temples. **Sore scalp,** < touching hair. Hot, red ears. **Tinnitus;** then vertigo. Deafness. Pale, earthy, sickly look; bluish about eyes. Teeth throb; < sucking. Acute, sour or **bitter taste,** or eructations. Craves delicacies. Quick satiety. Anorexia. **Loud belching, without relief** (Arg-n.). Slow digestion. Sore stomach. Thirst for cold water that aggravates diarrhea. Periodical liver symptoms (Quas.). Gall-stones. Swelled liver and spleen. **Flatulent bloating.** Tympanitis. Pain from rectum into genitals. STOOLS; LIENTERIC; **dark; foul; watery;** BLOODY; **painless;** < eating; < night. Dark, profuse, clotted menses. **Blood spitting.** Puffing, rattling, breathing. Every motion excites palpitation and takes his breath. Suppurative phthisis (Hep.). **Painfully sore chest and interscapular spine.** Heavy pressure (load) on shoulders, between scapulas or on sacrum. Twitching in knees. As of a band about legs. Pain in marrow. Drowsy. Heavy, snoring sleep. Anxious dreams. Swelled veins (hands, face). **Marked prodrome.** Clearly staged chill, heat and sweat. Chill, then thirst, then heat, then thirst. Red, hot face, with cold hands. **Hectic.** Sleeplessness, as a prodrome. Thirst during apyrexia. DRENCHING SWEATS; AT NIGHT, < **least motion;** from weakness, etc. Tropical fevers. Sepsis.

Complementary: Carb-v., Ferr., Kali-c.

Related to: Carb-v.

CHININUM ARSENICOSUM

Nightsweats; profuse, exhaustive. Oscillating temperature.

CHININUM SULPHURATUM

SPHERE OF ACTION

NERVES.

CIRCULATION.

Dorsal spine.

AGGRAVATION

EXACT PERIODICITY.

Cold, 10-11 A.M.

Head to left.

AMELIORATION

Yawning.

Neuralgias..................... **Sensitive.** Nervous. A net, fog or mote before eyes. Tinnitus. Deafness. Brow ague. Granular, brick-red, urinary sediment. **Vertigo, with tinnitus.** (Sal-ac.). **Spine (cervico-dorsal) aches, or is tender.** Anticipating chills. Delirium during heat. Increasing fever and prostration, with profuse nightsweats. Profuse sweat which >, but exhausts. Thirst in all stages. Clear apyrexia. Typical malaria. Itching. Petechiae.

Related to: Chin.

CHIONANTHUS

SPHERE OF ACTION

LIVER.

Head.

AGGRAVATION

Jarring.

Motion.

Cold.

AMELIORATION

Lying on abdomen (Chel.).

Bruised soreness; liver, eyeballs, etc. Pains ascend from forehead, stomach, etc.......................**Bilious sick headaches;** periodical. Nose, pressure at root or squeezing on bridge (Ham.). Tongue, greenish-yellow or feels drawn up. Vomiting bitter-sour; hot; bilious; ropy; gushing; setting teeth on edge (Sul-ac.); with colic and **cold sweat**

on forehead and **back of hands.** Uneasy ache in liver. Choleo-cystitis. Gall-stones. Griping at navel. As of a band about abdomen. Weakness in hypogastrium. Stools tarry, clay-colored or undigested. Arrested menses. Astringent expectoration. Jaundice. Heat, with aversion to uncover. Cold sweat on back of hands.

Related to: Bry., Iris, Lept., **Merc.**

CHLORALUM HYDRATUM

SPHERE OF ACTION	AGGRAVATION
BRAIN.	**Alcohol.**
Heart.	Night.
Muscles.	Exertion.
Liver.	**AMELIORATION**
Skin.	Open air.

Muscle prostration .... Indifferent and sleepy or **cerebral excitement;** hears voices. Mania. Bileless stools. Bed-wetting. Wants to be fanned. Dyspnea. As of a weight on chest. Weak heart. **Urticaria.** Sleepless from fatigue. Night terrors.

Related to: Apis, Astac.

CHLORUM

SPHERE OF ACTION	AGGRAVATION
Respiratory organs.	**Expiration.**
	After midnight.
Mucous membranes.	Lying.
Nerves.	**AMELIORATION**
Skin.	Motion.
Glands.	Open air.

Rapid emaciation. **Constrictions**...... ....Fears insanity or losing senses. **Protruding eyes. Acrid coryza.** Putrid aphthae, **Dry tongue. DYSPNEA; CAN'T EXHALE.** Spasm of glottis. Laryngitis. Laryngismus stridulus. Asthma of hay fever. Throat-pit; aching, tickling or whistling in. As if air were forced into upper chest (Sabin.). Sensitive skin. Easy sweat.

Related to: Ars-i., Iod., Meph., Merc.

Antidotes: Lyc.

CICUTA VIROSA

SPHERE OF ACTION	AGGRAVATION
BRAIN.	INJURIES; TO BRAIN (Nat-s.).
NERVES.	Jar.
Skin.	Noise.
	Touch.
	Cold.
	Dentition.
	Suppressed eruptions.

Violent convulsive phenomena, then prolonged unconsciousness. **Jerks;** of head. Twitchings; of arms and fingers. Sudden shocks through body (Ign.) or head, then **rigidity** or shrieks; **a terrific spasm moves downward** (reverse—Cupr.); **the eyes jerk and stare;** OPISTHOTONOS **and frightful facial contortions,** with bloody foam from mouth; **then utter prostration.** Epilepsy. **Spasm of diaphragm; of gullet.** Rigid muscles....................Childish. Suspicious. Violent. Rash. Delirium. Congestion to head, with vomiting and purging (Verat-v.). Headaches, > passing flatus. Head twists to one side. **Vertigo.** Meningitis. Squint. Bleeding ears. Red, sweaty face. Grinds teeth. Trismus. Craves chalk, coal, etc. **Loud hiccough;** alternating with thoracic spasm (Stry.). Oppressed breathing. Tremulous palpitation. Heart seems to stop (Dig.). Turns

feet inward; or big toes up during spasm. Pustules coalesce into **thick,
yellow** (loose), massive crusts; < head and face. Impetigo.

Related to: Cupr., Stry.

CIMICIFUGA

SPHERE OF ACTION
  Mind.
  Occiput.
  Vertex.
  Nape.
  NERVES AND MUSCLES
  - **Cerebro-spinal.**
  - Eyeballs.
  - Ovario-**uterine**
  - **Heart.**
  FEMALES.
  Joints.
  Left side; ovary, chest, etc.
  Front of thighs.

AGGRAVATION
  Menstruation; Suppressed.
  During labor.
  Emotions.
  Alcohol.
  Night.
  Air
  - **Damp.**
  - **Cold.**
  - Wind.
  - Drafts.
  Change of weather.
  Heat and cold.
  Sitting.
  Puberty and climaxis.

AMELIORATION
  Warm wraps.
  Open air.
  Pressure.
  Continued motion.
  Grasping things.
  Eating.

A **depressing irritant,** causing exhaustion and **low spirits,**
combined with **oversensitiveness,** < during pain (Nux-v.). Plumpness.
Irregular, changeful or alternating symptom groups; **utero-rheumatic**
(Caul.), etc. Violent pains; **achings;** shooting, **here and there;** shock-
like, **with cries, faints,** etc.; **up nape,** about thorax, **ovary to ovary**

(Arn.); lumbar spine, etc.; or alternating with other states. Myalgia. Ovaralgia. Lumbago. **Bruised, sore or heavy, aching muscles; behind eyeballs, uterus, neck; with a general sick feeling.** Grippe. Variola. **Trembling,** twitching; of part lain on, tongue, fingers, etc. Chorea; cardiac. Compressive pain; temples, feet, etc. ....Insanity before menses. Melancholy. Agitation. Alternate mental and physical effects. **Nervous, fidgety, excitable** and jerky. Annoyances drive her crazy. Depressed and **talkative,** with constant change of subject. Suspicious. **Gloomy** forebodings; of death, insanity, etc. Sees rats. Sees various colors and forms. Mania; alcoholic, puerperal, etc. **Deathly fear,** of rats, etc.; agitated. Weak will. Waving in brain (Glon.). **Head retracted. Vertex; as if to fly off;** as of a cold draft or heat on. **Occiput; like a blow** or pressive pain, ascends to eyes (1eft). **Eyeballs ache;** feel big. Sees red flashes, with black borders. Tinnitus; violent with deafness. Pate, hot face. **Thick saliva.** Mucus on teeth, or coppery mucus hawked up. Burning in throat. **Nausea in A.M.;** of pregnancy or alcoholism; in bowels; < pressure on spine. Vomits green; holds head and groans. Profuse, clear urine; weakening; with yellow sand. Menses irregular in time and amount; **more flow more pain.** Slow labor with nervous shivers. Uterine atony (Alet.). After-pains. Sore and tender along track of pains. **Nervous;** urination, shuddering, cough, etc. Delicate, sensitive women. Spasms of cerebro-spinal fever. Thyroid aches before menses. Incessant, dry night cough; < speaking. Sharp stitches in left chest. Pleurodynia. Left inframammary pain. Heart sore; swelled; needle-like pains; backward from or to left arm. Muscles fatigue. **Neckache.** Throws head back. Arms numb, cramp down; left seems bound to side. **Irritable,** sensitive spine; < lying on it. Stiff, contracted neck, back (Agar.) or Tendo-Achilles. Pain at angle of left scapula (Chen.). Heavy, pulsative lumbar pain, through hips and down thighs. **Cramps in limbs;** in calves. Alternate mental and rheumatic symptoms. Itching soles. Sleepless or dizzy, drunken sleep; with arms over head or yawning. Pulse weak, irregular; drops every 3rd or 4th beat. Chilly females. Cold sweat on hands and feet.

Related to: Bapt., Caul., Gels., Ign., Puls.

CINA

SPHERE OF ACTION

NERVES

- Cerebro-spinal.

- ABDOMEN.

Digestive tract.

Eyes.

Mucous membranes.

Children (left side).

AGGRAVATION
TOUCH.
Worms.
Vexation.
Looked at.
DURING SLEEP.
Full moon.
Staring.
Yawning.

AMELIORATION
Lying on abdomen.
Wiping Eyes.
Motion.

The greater the emaciation the greater the hunger. Bruised soreness. Painfully sore to motion and touch. Stiffens out; < if crossed, looked at, during cough, etc. Twitchings. Spasms; < worms; unilateral.................... TOUCHY. Nervous. Ugly, cross, petulant and dissatisfied. Wants to be rocked. Dilated pupils. Squint. Colored vision. Eyes fatigue, > rubbing. Nostrils drawn in. PICKS AND BORES AT NOSE. Dark rings about eyes. BLUISH WHITE ABOUT MOUTH. Sickly, pale face; during cough. GRINDS TEETH; during sleep. Chews and swallows in sleep. Worms. Noisy swallowing. Canine or gnawing hunger; after eating; after vomiting; alternating with anorexia; precedes chill or follows sweat. Hard, distended abdomen. Twisting at navel, > pressure. White, watery stool. Bed-wetting; < every full moon. MILKY URINE. Regularly recurrent, choking cough, then gurgling down throat. Tosses arms and legs from side to side. Restless sleep; lies on abdomen; cries out; wakes in terror. Fever, with pale face (Bry.). Cold sweat about nose and forehead.

Complementary: Calc., Dros., Rat.

Related to: Cham., Nat-p.

CINNABARIS

SPHERE OF ACTION	AGGRAVATION
Blood.	Touch.
Naso-pharynx.	Light.
Neck.	Dampness.
Bones.	**AMELIORATION**
	Open air.
	Sunshine (Stroph).

Pain outward along brow, encircling eyes, or like a saddle at root of nose. **Nose; heavy pressure** at root; < pressure of glasses; discharges foul, acrid, burning serum or dark lumps. Dry mouth, wakes from sleep. Hawks down stringy mucus or lumps of mucus drop from posterior nares. Naso-pharyngeal catarrh. Thin, white diarrhea. Foul, acrid sweat between scrotum and thigh. Warts on prepuce. Old, hard chancres. Heart flutters, then rushes of blood to head. Nodes on shin bones. Cramp in calf, after walking. **Fiery red ulcers,** eruptions, etc. Sweat, < nose.

Complementary: Thuj.

Related to: Merc.

CISTUS CANADENSIS

SPHERE OF ACTION	AGGRAVATION
GLANDS	COLD
- **Naso-pharynx.**	- **Inspired air.**
- **Neck.**	- **Talking.**
- Mammae (left).	- **Drafts.**
Throat.	- Water.
Lungs.	Mental
Skin.	- **Exertion.**
	- Excitement.
	Touch.

Painfully sensitive to cold; to inspired air, Coldness of tongue, saliva, in throat, eructations, stomach, etc.; < sweating. Suppurations. Much thick, yellow or foul mucus, leaving painful rawness (Aesc., Ant-c.). Internal and external itching. Burning. Indurations. Callosities. Scrofula. .... Fear. Headache from missing the noon meal, > eating. As of a lump in naso-pharynx. Colds affect the throat; it feels spongy, sandy, itches or has a dry spot, > sips of water. Expectorates quantities of tenacious, glairy mucus. Hard, swollen glands; < on neck; left mamma. Crawling over body. Cracked tetters; canthi; lips; fingertips. Chilliness.

Related to: Calc., Helo., Hep.

CLEMATIS ERECTA

SPHERE OF ACTION	AGGRAVATION
MUCOUS MEMBRANES	GONORRHEA.
- EYES.	Heat of bed.
- URETHRA.	NIGHT.
GLANDS	Cold washing.
- TESTES.	Light.
- Epidydymis.	Moon, < and > with (Phel.,
- Mammae.	Tarent.).
- Ovaries.	Mercury.
Skin; Scalp.	**AMELIORATION**
Occiput.	Sweat.

Flaccid muscles. VERY HARD, PAINFULLY SWOLLEN GLANDS; TESTES (right). Burning, itching, stinging, crawling pains......................Indifference. Chronic conjunctivitis. Iritis. Lachrymation. Urine flows by starts, or dribbles; strains out a few drops, then full stream follows. Stricture (Con.). Mucus in urine. Swelled inguinal glands and spermatic cord; with cutting, sore pains.

Orchids. Loathes coition. Full, heavy, sensitive breasts; outward darts in. Skin itches violently, with profuse desquamation. Vesicles. Pustules. Corroding eruptions; ending in flat, eating ulcers; with thick crusts and eczema; < occiput and lower legs. Sleepiness.

Complementary: Merc.

Related to: Phos., Rhod., Staph.

COBALTUM

SPHERE OF ACTION
Spine (lumbar).

Genitals.
Kidneys.

Bones.

AGGRAVATION
Sexual losses.
Sitting.
Heat of bed or sun.

AMELIORATION
Hawking mucus.
Continued motion.

Frothy discharges. Soreness. Aching bones. Sour taste, stomach, etc............................ Sense of guilt. Vertigo or head feels big; < stool. Vernal photophobia. Cracks across tongue. Emptiness at navel (Flac.). Yellow spots on abdomen. Sweet, foamy, lumpy expectoration. Pain along spine and down both legs. Lumbar ache; < coition; < sitting, > walking; with weak knees; can't straighten up. Sudden weakness in left hip; < walking.

Related to: Eup-per.

COCA

SPHERE OF ACTION

NERVES
- BRAIN.
- **Respiration.**
- Heart.
Muscles.

AGGRAVATION

Ascending.

High attitudes.

Cold.

Mental exertion.

AMELIORATION

Rapid motion, in open air.

After sunset.

Dizzy, dyspneic and exhausted (Ars.). Muscle exhaustion. ....Mental prostration; alternating with brightness. **Timid,** craves solitude. Sense of impending death. Loquacious excitement, with blissful visions. Exhilaration; before menses. Flashes before eyes. Migraine. Carious teeth. Aphonia. Senile asthma. Palpitation; excessively rapid pulse, with violent sweating. Crawling numbness in arms. Like a worm under skin (Calc.), moving away when touched. Sleepless; awakes with a shock in brain.

Related to: Cann-s.

COCCULUS INDICUS

SPHERE OF ACTION

SENSORIUM.

Cerebro-spinal axis
- **OCCIPUT.**
- **Lumbar.**
- Muscles.

Female sexual organs

One side.

AGGRAVATION

Motion
- BOAT.
- CARS.
- **Carriage.**

Slight causes
- **Loss of sleep.**
- Exertion.
- Pain.
- Noise.
- Touch.

-   Emotions.
Anxiety.
Cold.
Open air.
Eating.
During menses.

Acute senses with heavy or paralytic, muscular relaxation. **Too
weak to hold up head, stand or even speak.** Paralysis. **Tremor;**
intention; of head; lower jaw. **Cramps;** in masseters; abdomen;
dysmenorrheal; in heart. **Benumbed.** Spasms. Alternations. **EMPTY,
HOLLOW FEELING.** Weak, nervous women, < menses. Vomiting
with syncope. Hysterical asthma. Hysteria. **Sensitive to cold.**
.... Dazed; things seem unreal. Slow grasp.
Easily offended. Extremely sad, taciturn and peevish. VERTIGO; in
forehead; in A. M.; with nausea; with palpitation; < raising head.
Heavy head. **Occiput;** aches; < lying on it; > bending backward;
OPENS AND SHUTS, Throat tickles; with lachrymation. Speaks
or swallows with difficulty. Loathing. Nausea; rising into head.
Retching. VOMITING. **Train and sea sickness. Abdomen seems
full of sharp stones;** bloated. **Colic;** twisting (wind); nervous;
hysterical; with faintness; with salivation. Clutching in uterus.
Depleting menses; < standing on tip toe; replaced by gushes of
leucorrhea. Weak neck. SPINAL WEAKNESS; < **lumbar;** < walking.
Paraplegia. Limbs go to sleep, < grasping objects. Alternations between
arms. Humerus feels broken. Hands numb; alternately hot and cold.
Knees weak; cracking. Clumsy gait. Sleepless, from mental or physical
exhaustion. Drowsy. Low fever. Sweaty.

Complementary: Petr.

Related to: Gels., Ign.

COCCUS CACTI

SPHERE OF ACTION

MUCOUS MEMBRANES

- FAUCES.
- Throat.
- **Larynx.**
- Chest.
- Genito-urinary.

Left side.

AGGRAVATION

IRRITATING FAUCES.

Periodically.

Heat.

Lying.

Awaking.

Cold exposure.

AMELIORATION

Washing in cold water.

Catarrh. Spasms. Hemorrhage. Uric acid. Gouty-rheumatic. STRINGY DISCHARGES, EXPECTORATION, hanging from mouth, urine, feeling in throat, black menses, etc. **Sensitive, fauces, vulva, skin, etc. Intolerable internal tickle. Pulsations;** in glans; as of a fluid forcing its way. Dark blood. .... Sad; on waking at 2-3 A. M. **Hawking,** brushing teeth, etc., **excites cough, retching** or vomiting. Profuse post-nasal discharge. Constricted throat. Violent kidney pain, with dysuria. Nephritic colic. Irritated bladder. Sticking along ureters. **Urging to urinate;** > bloody clots from vagina. Urine scanty, thick, heavy, sour; **sediment; sandy,** dark red, brown or white; bloody mucus. Nephritis. REGULAR PAROXYSMS OF VIOLENT TICKLING, RACKING COUGH, ENDING IN VOMITING OR RAISING MUCH CLEAR, ROPY MUCUS (Kali-bi.); **with a purple, red face and internal heat;** periodically; with kidney symptoms; slowly increasing, then gradually declining; > **cold air** or drinks. Whooping cough. Soreness or stitches in apices of lungs. Coldness in back. **Burning;** as of pepper in nostrils, at tip of tongue, etc. (Lach.).

Related to: Apis, Berb., Lach., Phos.

COFFEA CRUDA

SPHERE OF ACTION
NERVES; Cardiac.

CIRCULATION.

Sex organs.

Women.

AGGRAVATION
NOISE.

Touch.

Odors.

Air (open, cold, windy).

Mental
- **Emotions.**
- **Exertion.**

Overeating.

Alcohol.

Night.

AMELIORATION
Lying.

Sleep.

Warmth.

Emotions cause severe symptoms. EXCITABLE AND OVER-ACTIVE. OVERSENSITIVE; **to noise,** it may even be painful (Ther.); **to pain, pleasure, etc.** .... **Irritable and wakeful.** Resents sympathy. Rushing ideas. **Weeps, laments and tosses about.** Now joyous, now gloomy. Faints easily. Brain seems torn, shattered or crushed. Clavus. Bright eyes. **Acute hearing;** overhears distant sounds. Faceache (right). **Toothache; > ice water,** < as it warms; pains into fingertips; during menses. Stomach feels overloaded. Hot, itching genitals. After-pains. Cough incessant; of measles. **Nervous palpitation;** < sun heat. Trembling hands. **Painfully sensitive skin.** Itching—scratches until it bleeds. NERVOUS SLEEPLESSNESS; from rush of ideas; awakes at or hears every sound; after pleasurable excitement.

Antidotes: Cham., Ign., Nux-v.

Complementary: Acon.

Related to: Coca, Ign.

COLCHICUM AUTUMNALE

SPHERE OF ACTION

DIGESTIVE TRACT.

HEART; **Pericardium.**

Circulation.

Kidneys.

Tissues.

- **MUSCLES**
- **Ligaments.**
- Fibrous.
- **Serous.**

JOINTS; Small.

AGGRAVATION

MOTION.
Touch.
Night.
Stubbing toes.
Vibration.
WEATHER
- **Cold; Damp; Rooms.**
- **Changing.**
- Autumn.
Slight exertion.
Checked sweat.
Stretching.
Sundown to sunrise.

AMELIORATION
Warmth.
Rest.
Doubling up.
Sitting.

COLD AND WEAK, BUT SENSITIVE AND RESTLESS.
Irritable and sensitive to impressions, strong odors, etc. Tearing, digging, drawing pains. Many joints are attacked. **Rapid sinking.** Moist collapse. Creepings. Small, rapidly shifting areas of severe pain, but little swelling. Subacute states, that finally attack the heart. Cardio-arthritic affections. Dropsy. ....**Depressed. Irritable and sensitive;** every little hurt pains terribly. Sensitive to odors and impressions. Unequal pupils. Acrid tears. Dark nostrils. ACUTE SMELL; **odors nauseate**—even to fainting, etc. Pinched, sunken face. Mouth hangs open. Flow of saliva, with a sense of dryness. Glossitis. Thirsty, but LOATHES THE SMELL, **or sight of food;** > lying quietly. NAUSEA. Retching. Burning or **icy coldness in stomach.** Meteorism. Diarrhea, then gouty effects. Chloreic or shreddy, gelatinous, mucus stools, then tenesmus or spasm of anus. Mucous colitis; after dysentery.

Tenesmus. Urine sedimentitious; black. Nephritis. Chest seems squeezed by a band. Cutting or stinging at heart. Weak heart. Cold limbs. Heat on rump. Sweat, cold on face; sour at night.

Complementary: Ars., Spig.

Related to: Ars., Carb-v., Verat.

COLLINSONIA

SPHERE OF ACTION	AGGRAVATION
Pelvis	PILES
- **Anus, rectum.**	- **When suppressed.**
- Uterus.	**Night.**
- Bowels.	**Pregnancy.**
Heart.	Cold.
Pharynx.	Excitement.
Liver.	

Congestions; pelvic; **reflex from or combined with hemorrhoids,** especially cardiac (Lycps.). Constrictions. **Swelled feeling,** in limbs, vulva, clitoris, etc. .... Speaker's sorethroat or cough. Colic. Acrid diarrhea; destroying the hair. Light, knotty stools. **Rectum;** aches; burns, seems dry and full of sticks or sand; with **cardiac pains.** Constipation or piles of pregnancy. **Piles (bleeding); alternating with heart,** chest or rheumatic symptoms. **Prolapsus,** ani, uteri, etc. **Itching of vulva or anus.** Varicocele. Palpitation. **Flushes of heat;** with piles; with oppressed breathing.

Related to: Lycps-v., Nux-v., Sulph.

COLOCYNTHIS

SPHERE OF ACTION
NERVES (Large)
- TRIFACIAL.
- ABDOMINAL.
- **Spinal.**
- SCIATIC
DIGESTIVE TRACT
   (NAVEL).
INTESTINES.
Ovaries.
Kidneys.
Left side.

AGGRAVATION
EMOTIONS.
VEXATION.
Chagrin.
Anger.
Lying on painless side.
Night, in bed.
Drafts.
Taking cold.

AMELIORATION
HARD PRESSURE.
Coffee.
Heat.
Rest.
Gentle motion.
After stool or flatus.

Acts on digestive tract, then longer on spinal nerves. SUDDEN, ATROCIOUS CRAMPINGS, **gripings,** tearings, etc., making him TWIST, **turn or cry out in pain; with nausea** or diuresis. Convulsive jerks or constrictions during pain (Ign., Lyc.). Lightning-like pains. CUTTING, **pinching, clamping, gnawing or boring pain;** then numbness. Parts seem too short. **Constriction.** Neuralgia. ....
Anger; easily vexed; < pains. Tearing head pains, < moving eyelids. Faceache (left); with eye symptoms or alternating with coelialgia. **Distorted face.** Persistent bitter taste.   Gas colic (flatulent colic). WAVES OF VIOLENT CUTTING, GRIPING, GRASPING, CLUTCHING OR RADIATING ABDOMINAL COLIC DOUBLE HIM UP; > HARD PRESSURE; < least food. Cutting in bowels; at navel. Pressure > at first then <. **Intestines feel squeezed between stones.** Pains alternating between ovaries. Ovaralgia. Vomits from pain. **Yellow, frothy, watery, shreddy,** sourish or gelatinous **stools; with colic and gas.** Dysentery. Slippery bubbles escape from anus. Gelatinous, sticky or stringy urine. Heart feels pushed up by a distended stomach. Pain under right scapula, > pressure (Bry.).

Lumbar ache, > pressure. **Cramps in hips.** Screwing, band-like or shooting sciatic pains; < least motion, rotation or night, > lying on painful part. Limbs drawn up like a hedgehog. Urinous sweat.

Antidotes: Op.

Complementary: Caust.

Related to: Staph.

COMOCLADIA

SPHERE OF ACTION
Skin.
Eyes.
Nose.
Right side.

AGGRAVATION
Heat.

AMELIORATION
Open air.

EDEMA; of reduced skin. ....Burning, itching of eyes and nose, with violent sneezing. Sore eyeballs. Pain from under left breast through to scapula. Cough. Wandering rheumatic pains. Eczema; recurrent.

CONIUM MACULATUM

SPHERE OF ACTION
NERVES.
MUSCLES.
GLANDS
- MAMMAE.
- Ovaries.
Sexual organs.
Respiration.

AGGRAVATION
SEEING MOVING OBJECTS.
ALCOHOL.
Raising arms.
After exertion.
Injury.
Night.
Sexual excesses.
Cold; Taking.
Continence.
Old age.
Lying; Head low.

AMELIORATION
Letting part hang down.

Irregular action ending in progressive DEBILITY, as in old age; clothes distress, faints at stool, difficult articulation, uncertain gait, etc. Trembling; looks old. Chronicity. Early senility. Cachexy. Paralysis. Suddenly sick or weak; with numbness. STONY HARDNESS. As of a lump in brain, in epigastrium. New growths. Hard blood-vessels. Ascending symptoms. Tearings. Stabbings. .... Slow. Apathetic. Shy people, yet fear being alone. Weak memory. Can't think after using eyes. VERTIGO, whirling; on lying, turning over, least motion of eyes or head, etc.; senile. Eyes feel crossed; lids heavy, droop, < outer side. Photophobia. Vision, colored. Pulpy earwax. Sour saliva. Cold flatus. Constipation on alternate days. Urine stops and starts; > standing. Testes enlarged. Cutting, as semen passes; in ovaries, uterus, etc. Prostatic dribble; < stool, emotions, etc. Emissions, from mere contact. Menses irregular. Acrid leucorrhea. Tormenting cough from dry spot in larynx; from tickling in throat-pit; as if from abdomen. Palpitation; < exertion, drinking, at stool, etc. GLANDS HARDEN AND GET SORE. Mammae; nodes in; congested before menses; sticking in; shrunken; too much milk, < before menses or at every step. Hot spots on head. Spinal injuries. Heels; as if bone would push through; shooting in. Skin greenish, like an old bruise; spots on; foul or eczematous eruption. Hebetude. Coldness in nape, calf, etc. Hot flushes or sweat on dropping to sleep. Sweat under eyes, on chin, in poplitae; cold on nape or palms.

Complementary: Phos.

Related to: Arn., Bar-c., Calc-f., Caust., Gels., Iod.

COPAIVA OFFICINALIS

SPHERE OF ACTION
MUCOUS GLANDS
- **Genito-urinary.**
- Bronchial.
Rectum.
Skin.

AGGRAVATION
Morning.
Taking cold.

FOUL BLENORRHEA: **bronchorrhea,** suppuration, etc. .... Stools of masses of or covered with mucus. Pulsation in penis. Urethra feels wide open. Acrid, scanty, bloody urine; odor of violets. Dysuria. Catarrh of bladder. Purulent or acrid, milky gonorrhea. Suppuration ascends urinary tract. Painful cough, with **heat,** oppression of chest and foul, bloody expectoration. Burning in lungs. Rushes of blood to head and face. Urticaria.

Complementary: Sep.

Related to: Ter.

CORALLIUM RUBRUM

SPHERE OF ACTION
RESPIRATORY ORGANS.
NERVES.
MUCOUS MEMBRANES.

AGGRAVATION
AIR
- Change of.
- **Inhaling.**
Eating.
Towards morning.

Almost continuous paroxysms of extremely violent, spasmodic **cough,** which begin with **gasping for breath,** are accompanied by a purple face, and **followed by exhaustion,** and vomiting of stringy mucus. A reverberating, minute gun cough. Cough as soon as he eats. Whooping cough. Sleeps with head under covers. Very red (flat) venereal ulcer. Too hot if covered, but chilled by uncovering.

Complementary: Sulph.
Related to: Coc-c.

CORNUS CIRCINATA

SPHERE OF ACTION   **AGGRAVATION**
Blood.   Night.
Liver.   Taking cold.
Spleen.
Digestive tract.

Weak and depressed. **Liver symptoms, with aching eyeballs.** Dark, foul stools, with burning at anus. Diarrhea. Sallow skin. Sleepy before the chills, with the heat and after meals. Old malarias.

Related to: Eup-per.

CRATAEGUS OXYACANTA

SPHERE OF ACTION
HEART
Nerves

Weak and exhausted; suddenly. Cardio-hemorrhagic or lithemic cases (Lycps-v.). .... Irritable. Despairing. Cough, with albuminous expectoration. WEAK HEART MUSCLES (right); with oppression, stitches or **insomnia.** Cardiac dyspnea. Myocarditis. Incompetent valves. Cardiac dilatation. Angina pectoris. Pain under left scapula. Dropsies. Pulse rapid, irregular and small. Burning, smarting eruption in back of neck; axillae and chin; < heat and sweating; > washing. Sweaty palms.

Related to: Apoc., Stroph-h.

CROCUS SATIVUS

SPHERE OF ACTION

MIND.

NERVES.

Eyes.

Circulation.

Female organs.

AGGRAVATION

Motion.

Puberty.

Pregnancy.

Reading.

Heat.

AMELIORATION

Open air.

Rapidly changing or alternating symptoms; of opposite moods; of sides; of mind and body, etc. Single muscles twitch; upper eyelids, etc. Faint, drowsy and hysterical. Chorea. **Jumping about, as of something alive internally.** HEMORRHAGE, dark, stringy, tough. .... Impressionable, affectionate and moody. Involuntary laughter and weeping; < music. Hysteria. Climacteric hemicrania; instead of menses; > pressure. Dry, burning eyes, as after weeping, or as if in a cool wind. Winks or must close eyes tightly. Lachrymation when reading. Nosebleed, with faintness and cold sweat on forehead; of young girls. Sexual excitement. **Dark, foul, stringy menses.** Threatened abortion. Narcotic sleep. Singing during sleep.

Related to: Ign., Tarent.

CROTALUS HORRIDUS

SPHERE OF ACTION

BLOOD.

Heart.

Cerebro-spinal nerves.

Liver.

Throat.

Occiput.

Right side.

AGGRAVATION

Lying on right side.

Falling to sleep.

Warm weather.

Spring.

Alcohol.

AMELIORATION

Light.

Motion.

Deathly sick, tremulous and weak. HEMORRHAGE; slow; oozing of dark, thin blood; **pharyngeal.** Bloody pus or sweat. **Putridity,** rapid decomposition and MALIGNANCY. **Septic;** tonsils, goitre, ulcers, abscess, etc. Dark or **bluish parts.** Petechie. Gangrene. General burning. ....Plaintive speech. Timid; fears evil. Torpid. Forgetful. Mistakes in writing. Delirium. Faintings. **Occipital ache;** in waves from spine. Distorted face on waking. Epilepsy. Dark, besotted face. Grinds teeth. Mouldy breath. Swelled tongue. Stiff palate. Craves pork. Craves stimulants. Bilious vomit. Perineal abscess. Mouldy excretions. Anxious, labored breathing. HEART, weak, trembles, feels loose or turns over; sensitive to lying on left side. First one limb then the other is numb. Jaundice. **Blood-boils. Horrible dreams;** of the dead. Black-water fever. High fever; with scarlet skin. Edema about affected parts.

Complementary: Lycps-v.

Related to: Lach., Sul-ac.

CROTON TIGLIUM

SPHERE OF ACTION	AGGRAVATION
MUCOUS MEMBRANES	DRINKING.
- Bowels.	Eating.
- Eyes.	Washing.
Bladder.	Motion.
Mammae.	Receding eruptions.
Uterus.	
Skin	
- **SCROTUM.**	
- **FACE.**	

Drawn backward feeling; in eyes; nipples, etc. ....
Neuralgia of tongue. Pressure excites rectal pain or a stool. **Gargling or swashing as of water in bowels;** THEN SUDDEN, PROFUSE,

GUSHING STOOL OF YELLOW WATER, < DRINKING; then prostration. Diarrhea. Cholera infantum. **Can't inhale deeply enough.** Pain from nipple to back, as child nurses. Nodes in mammae. Neck and shoulders pain. Violently itching, tense burning, red skin; sore if scratched, > gentle rubbing. **Eruptions**; clustered; of blisters which burst and form crusts; **vesiculo-pustular** (Sep.), < genitals, temples and crown of head. Eczema. Zoster.

Related to: Rhus-t.

CUBEBA OFFICINALIS

SPHERE OF ACTION
Mucous membranes
- URETHRA.
- Bladder.
- **Vagina.**

AGGRAVATION
Night in bed.

AMELIORATION
Walking about.

Burning rawness. Violent inflammation, then acrid, yellow or green, offensive discharges. Catarrhs......................Veins of forehead distended. Gelatinous, cold stools; with grains like rice. Cramp or cutting-burning after urinating. Stringy gonorrhea.

Related to: Cist., Cop.

CULEX MUSCA

Edema. Vertigo; on blowing nose. Menses stain indelibly (Thlas.). Griping down over hips, then into womb. As of cold air blowing through a hole in clothes on chest or back.

CUPRUM METALLICUM

SPHERE OF ACTION

NERVES

- Cerebro-spinal.

- Axis.

Digestive tract.

Epigastrium.

Abdomen.

Muscles.

Blood

AGGRAVATION

Emotions: Anger

Suppressions.

Overtax.

Motion.

Hot weather.

Vomiting.

Loss of sleep.

Touch.

Raising arm.

AMELIORATION

Cold drinks.

Pressure over heart.

Sub-oxidation, affecting the centers of the medulla. **Violer** ₁t effects; in recurring symptom groups. CRAMPS AND SPASMS; of all kinds; radiating from or of single parts; **extort cries**; tonic, **knotting** the muscles; twisting the head awry; with **trismus** or hiccough; then deathly exhaustion, chills, spasmodic laughter, etc.; in chest; behind sternum; of fingers, **calves** > stretching leg out, or soles, etc.; nocturnal; < at menses; epileptic. **Jerkings**; during sleep. Pains; pressive, < **touch**; as from blows, being broken, etc.; in racking darts, through whole body. Continued weakness. Poor reaction. Easy relapses. Latency. **Blueness.** .... Hypersensitive: every drug overacts, without curing. **Uneasy.** Nervous. Sense of losing consciousness. Impulsive. **Piercing shrieks.** Delirium; loquacious; then cold sweat. Confusion. Melancholy; with spells of fear of death. Sullen; tricky; alternately yielding and headstrong. **Vertigo; with** internal tremor, > stool. Can't hold head erect or bores it into pillow. Crawling on vertex. Pulls her hair. Meningitis. Eyeballs oscillate behind **closed lids. Face livid,** pale or distorted. Closed mouth. Grinds teeth. **Metallic taste.** Puts tongue out like a snake. Loss of speech. Noisy swallowing. Nausea. Vomiting; violent; tormenting; > drinking; with **agonizing colic,** diarrhea and shrieks or convulsions. Painful transfixion cramp. Hard pressure in epigastrium. Lies on stomach and jerks buttocks up. Tense abdomen. **Frightful colic,** > pressure, < raising arms. Spurting stools; of green water. Cholera. Suppressed urine. Cramps prevent coition. After-pains. Spasm of glottis. Dyspnea; can't bear anything near mouth; < coughing or laughing. Asthma. Cough; in violent paroxysms; coughs herself out of breath; > **cold drinks** (Caust.), < deep breathing or bending back; with cramps, spasms (Zinc.) or lachrymation. Whooping cough. **Chest; loud rattle in;** painful, constriction of (lower). Jerking hands and feet. Clenches thumbs into palms. Heavy ankles. Repressed or undeveloped eruptions, discharges, etc. (Zinc.) Yellow, scaly eruptions. Slow pulse. Icy cold; afebrile. Chilly. Cold, clammy sweat; at night. Collapse.

Complementary: Calc.

Related to: Verat.

CUPRUM ARSENICOSUM

SPHERE OF ACTION	AGGRAVATION
DIGESTIVE TRACT.	Touch.
Muscles.	**Pressure.**
Nerves.	Dampness.

Violent cramps and colics; inflammatory; in chest, fingers, calves, toes, etc.; with obstinate hiccough or icy cold body. Convulsions. Chorea. Sharp, shooting abdominal pains. Visceral neuralgia. Intestinal catarrh. Cholera infantum. Vomiting and diarrhea; with **uremia.** Rice water stools. Weak heart. Cold, clammy, intermittent sweat. Leg cramps, > pressing foot on floor (Stry-p.). Numb, paralysed feeling in legs.

Related to: Cupr.

CYCLAMEN EUROPAEUM

SPHERE OF ACTION
Cerebro-spinal axis.
Vision.
Blood.
Digestive tract.
FEMALE SEX ORGANS.

AGGRAVATION
Cold.
Evening.
Fresh air.
Sitting.
Fats.

AMELIORATION
Motion.
During menses.
Weeping.

VISUAL EFFECTS **or vertigo,** from menstrual or gastric disorders. Dreads open air. Chlorosis. .... Dull, sad, sleepy and morose. Self-reproaches. Silent weeping. The room seems too small (Berb., Nat-c.). Brain feels wrapped up. **Pain in left temple.** Prolonged migraine. Convergent squint. Blurred vision (Nat-m.). **Fluttering, glittering or black vision.** Sees stars. Sneezing, with itching in ear. Anosmia. Lost or salty taste. **Hiccough;** < pregnancy; with yawning. Hiccoughy eructation. Nausea in throat. Craves lemonade. Quick satiety. Loathing and nausea from the least food. Hyperemesis. Diarrhea, < coffee. **Menses;** excessive, early, dark or changeable; clotted; membranous; less if in motion. Dysmenorrhea. Coughs, without waking. Air seems to stream from nipples. Swelled breasts; < after menses. Milk in virgin breasts. Weakness; < in knees. Burning, sore heels. Pains in thinly covered bones. Chilly all over. Chilly, not > covers. Offensive sweat.

Related to: Puls.

DAPHNE INDICA

SPHERE OF ACTION
Muscles.

Bones.

Left side.

AGGRAVATION
Cold air.

Waning moon.

Evening in bed.

Parts—head, arms, etc.—seem separated from body (Bapt., Psor.). Bruised pain. **Fetor.** Exhaustion.................... Sad. Head feels big. **Tongue, coated on one side only** (Irid-m., Rhus-t.). Sleepless; from **bone aches.** Clammy sweat.

Related to: Rhus-t.

DICTAMNUS

SPHERE OF ACTION
Female organs.

Nerves.

Sleep.

AGGRAVATION
Standing.

Increased secretions. .... A lump rises in throat. Bearing down, with bilious vomiting, < standing on feet. **Menses early;** of black clots; preceded by blindness. Sensation of milk flowing into mammae. Cramps from anterior thighs into uterus, before menses. **Somnambulism** (Phos.). Dreams of piercing bodies of her children together (Phos.).

Related to: Puls.

DIGITALIS PURPUREA

SPHERE OF ACTION
Vagus.
HEART; Muscle.
CIRCULATION
- Liver.
- Lungs.
- Stomach.
Occiput.
Genito-urinary organs.

AGGRAVATION
Raising up.
Exertion.
Heat.
Lying on left side.
Motion.
Smell of food.
Cold drinks.
Excesses: Sexual.

AMELIORATION
Rest.
Cool air.
Lying flat on back.

WEAKNESS, faint-like; can hardly talk. Heart slow, with indefinite or causeless symptoms. HEART SLOW, weak or irregular; quick, on motion,; with liver or sexual symptoms; at puberty. Must walk about, with precordial anxiety; with teasing to urinate...................... Anxious solicitude. Dizzy. Crashes in head; on dropping to sleep. Spastic hemicrania. Yellow-red conjunctiva. Seething in ears. Face pale; bluish, also lips and tongue. Thick, flabby tongue. Much thirst, little appetite (Sulph.), but no fever. Deathly nausea or with faint sinking at pit of stomach. Liver sore, swelled. White, putty-like stools. Dribbling urination. Dropsy. Throbbing in neck of bladder. Early morning erection. Swelled prostate; senile. Atonic night losses. Glans inflamed; gonorrhea of (Jac-c.). Profuse, thick, yellow-white gonorrhea. Slow breathing. Cough, with pains in shoulders and arms. HEART; weak; feels like stopping; sprains; palpitation. Slow, intermittent pulse. Numb or weak left arm. Drowsy. Dreams of falling; wakes with a shock. Cold skin. Flushes of heat, then great weakness. Cold, clammy sweat.

Related to: Glon., Spig.

DIOSCOREA VILLOSA

SPHERE OF ACTION
NERVES
- Spinal cord.
- **Abdominal.**
- Sciatic.
Nevel.
Gall-bladder.
Right side.

AGGRAVATION
Doubling up.
Lying.
Tea; Eating.
AMELIORATION
Stretching out or bending back.
Motion; in open air (Mag-c.,
 Puls.).
Hard pressure.

A remedy of **pains**, of all kinds. UNBEARABLY SHARP, CUTTING, TWISTING, GRIPING OR GRINDING PAINS; **that dart about or radiate;** to distant parts, arms, etc.; **in paroxysms;** cease suddenly, then start in different place; periodical. **Shudderings,** from pain, etc. .... Nervous and easily troubled. Confused, full head. Sensation as if head were crushed down (Dios.). Eructations; with hiccough. Cardialgia. Pains shoot from liver to right nipple. Violent **abdominal colic,** > motion; pains go into back, chest or arms. Flatulence. Darting, from anus to liver. Piles like a bunch of cherries. Weakening morning diarrhea, without relief. Erections lasting all night. Cold, relaxed sexual organs. Atonic emissions, then weakness; < knees. Violent dysmenorrhea. Chest or cardiac pains radiate into both arms. Felon. Burning, numb, sciatic (right) pain, < motion. Hamstrings seem too short. Cold, clammy sweat; of strong odor on genitals.

Related to: Coloc., Mag-c.

DIPHTHERINUM

SPHERE OF ACTION
Blood.
THROAT.

AGGRAVATION
Lying.
Cold.
Milk.

Weak and restless, but without pain, or aching, breaking joint pains, > lying. Wants to be held. Drawing in muscles, then sudden snap. Jerking of single parts. Internal trembling. ....Sees visions. Carphology. Moisture at edge of hair. Fanning of alae nasi, with snoring. Yellow, thick nasal discharge. Flushed face; center of cheeks purple. Moist tongue, with red tip or a dark red spot back of tip; red papillae. Throat dark. **Thick, gray membrane**; on tonsil (left). Fetor. Wants cold air down throat or craves cold drinks. **Diphtheria**; prophylactic; **painless**; relapsing. Post-diphtheric paralysis. Obstinate tonsilitis. Faintness at stomach, > sips of milk. Dry, hot palms; they feel withered. Dry skin. Talks in sleep, with open eyes. Low temperature. Chilly, then hot.

Related to: Carb-ac.

DROSERA ROTUNDIFOLIA

SPHERE OF ACTION
RESPIRATORY ORGANS.
Bones
- Long (Still.).
- Joints.
Larynx.
Chest.
Lungs.
Glands.

AGGRAVATION
After midnight.
On lying down.
Warmth.
Talking.
Cold foods.
Laughing.
After measles.
AMELIORATION
Pressure.

Spasmodic, catarrhal and hemorrhagic effects. Tuberculosis; of bones......................Easily angered. Desire to drown himself. Sensitive to sour odors. Painful sneezing. Putrid taste. PROLONGED, PERIODICAL FITS OF RAPID, INCESSANT, DEEP BARKING OR CHOKING COUGH; as if from abdomen; taking away the breath; compel holding the sides and ending in retching, vomiting (first of ingesta, then of mucus), nosebleed or cold sweat; followed by loquacity. Typical whooping cough. Tickling like a feather or crumb in larynx. Bloody, purulent expectoration. Hoarse, toneless voice. Constriction of chest. Stitches below axillae. Writers' cramp.

Complementary: Sulph.

Related to: Coc-c., Cor-r.

DULCAMARA

SPHERE OF ACTION

MUCOUS MEMBRANE
- Bronchi.
- Bladder.
- Eyes.

BACK.
- **Muscles.**
- LOINS.

SKIN.

Umbilicus.

Lymphatics.

AGGRAVATION

BEING CHILLED
- WHILE HOT.
- **Sudden change of temperature.**
- **Uncovering**
- COLD WET; Feet, ground, cellars, beds, etc.

Suppressed discharges, sweat, eruptions, etc.

Autumn.

Night.

Rest.

Injuries.

Mercury.

Before storms.

Excessive secretion of mucus. Catarrhal—rheumatic—herpetic tendency. Stiff, numb, achy and sore from every exposure to damp cold. Tearing. **Paralytic effects.** Griping in bowels, testes, etc...................... **Confusion. Depression. Scolding.** Difficult speech. Easily becomes delirious. Occiput feels large. Ringworm of scalp. Aching in nose. Coryza; stuffed; **summer colds,** with diarrhea. Nose obstructed by the least fresh air. Nosebleed; replaces menses. Thick, brown-yellow crusts on face. Swelled tongue. Tenacious, soapy saliva. Cutting at navel; then painful, green, **slimy stools.** Sour, watery stools, < night. **Every cold settles in eyes, throat or affects bladder** (Puls.), bowels or respiration (Sulph.). Frequent urination. **Cloudy, slimy or foul urine.** Cystitis. Dropsy. Enlarged testes, with griping pains. Watery menses. Cough : caused by tickling in back of throat; in prolonged fits; with much loose, easy expectoration. **Eruptions;** scaly, thick, crusty, moist, bleeding or herpetic; < before menses. **Urticaria.** Pruritus. Large, smooth, fleshy, flat warts. **Coldness;** in occiput; lumbar region; in bowels; **icy, of paralyzed part.** Chilliness starts from back; not > warmth; < evening. Chill with urging to stool and urinate. Foul sweat.

Complementary: Bar-c., Nat-s.

Related to: Rhus-t.

ECHINACEA ANGUSTIFOLIA

SPHERE OF ACTION
Blood.
Circulation.
Gums.
Lymphatics.
Left side.

AGGRAVATION
Eating.
Injury.
Operations.
AMELIORATION
Rest.

Weak, tired and achy. Slow speech, gait, replies, etc. **Weakness,** in stomach; in bowels; **of heart;** in knees; with vertigo. Sepsis.

Lymphangitis. Rheumatism. .... Depressed or cross and
out of sorts. Can't exert mind. Sharp pain deep in brain, it seems too
large. Throbbing through temples. Hot, burning forehead. Twitching
brows. Bluish face. Teeth sensitive to drafts of air. Mucus, frothy in
mouth; hawks from throat. Tongue numb. Peppery taste. Aphthae.
Nauseated and chilly. Sour, bloody vomitus; like coffee grounds. As
of a load in posterior liver. Blood follows stool. Seminal emissions.
As of a lump under sternum. Burning under left scapula. Hands,
numb alternately or restless; on awaking. Dreams of difficulties;
laborious or quarrelsome. **Irregular chills, heats and sweats.** Chill in
left occiput. Sweat on upper parts; on forehead. Increasing, but
variable pulse.

Related to: Arn., Pyrog., Rhus-t.

ELAPS CORALLINUS

SPHERE OF ACTION	AGGRAVATION
Blood.	**Approach of storms.**
Nose.	Cold; Drink or food.
Ears.	Dampness.
Throat.	Night.
Right side.	In room.

Black discharges; hemorrhages, etc. Internal **coldness;** in chest;
< drinking. Adynamic sepsis. Oscillatory motions. Twisting spasm,
then paralysis; esophageal. Right side feels paralyzed, weak or
insensible. Wrinkled mucous membranes (Ars.). ....Fear causes
chattering teeth and trembling. Fears rain. Black rings before left
eye. Deafness; at night. Stuffed feeling in naso-pharynx. Green-yellow
crusts in nose. Ozena. Nosebleed. Red spots on face. Drinks feel like
ice in stomach. Stools of black, frothy blood. Air hunger. Painful
cough. Pain at apex of right lung. Weak arms. Peeling palms and
fingertips. Rushes of blood to head. Icy cold feet. General cold sweat.

Antidotes: Cedr.
Related to: Crot-h., Helo.

EPIPHEGUS VIRGINIANA

SPHERE OF ACTION
Nerves.
Stomach.
Liver.

AGGRAVATION
Fatigue; Nervous; of Shopping.
Eyestrain.

AMELIORATION
Sleep.

Confusion. Like fingertips pressing into temples. Compressive (right) headache, going backward; < until 4 P. M. then >; **with spitting of viscid saliva** and nausea. Weekly headaches. Neurasthenia. Tartar on teeth.

Related to: Ign., Iris.

EQUISETUM HYEMALE

SPHERE OF ACTION
GENITO-URINARY TRACT.

AGGRAVATION
At close of urination.
Pressure.

Aching, full, tender bladder. Cystitis. Prickling, burning, or cutting in urethra. Dysuria. NOCTURNAL ENURESIS; with irritable bladder. Dribbling urine. **Mucus in urine.**

Complementary: Sil.

Related to: Canth.

ERIGERON CANADENSE

SPHERE OF ACTION
Genito-urinary tract.
Joints.

AGGRAVATION
Rainy weather.

Hemorrhage; bright, gushing; vomits and purges pure blood. **Congestion. Smarting-burning.** Hard aching. .... Burning in stomach and abdomen (Ars.). Tympanites. Anus seems torn. **Vesico-rectal tenesmus** (Canth., Merc-c.). Aching in bladder. Retained urine. **Dysuria.** Sticky sweat on genitals. Ecchymoses.

Related to: Canth., Ter.

EUCALYPTUS

SPHERE OF ACTION	AGGRAVATION
Mucous membranes.	
Blood.	Periodically
Muscles.	Night.
Respiration.	

Aching, stiff and weary, as from taking cold. Grippe. Malaria. Migraine. Sticking, jerking pains at night. **Profuse catarrhal discharges; acrid; foul.** Rheumatic-hydrogenoid constitution. Exhausted, toxemic and hemorrhagic. .... **Mental exhilaration.** Burning eyes. Tinnitus. Tension across nose. Watery coryza. Pasty tongue. Throbbing in stomach. Weight in bowels. Slow digestion, with putrid gas. Diarrhea; dysenteric; typhoid. Diuresis. Cough of influenza. **Bronchial asthma.** Bronchorrhea; senile. Limbs prickle, then ache. Chill, then nausea and vomiting. Fever with aching. Vertigo in all stages. Old malarias.

Related to: Chin., Dulc., **Echi.**

EUONYMUS

SPHERE OF ACTION	AGGRAVATION
Liver.	Eating.
Kidneys.	
Left to right.	

Crawling; < back. .... **Vertigo;** in forehead; as if drawn up and pitched forward (Calc.). Pressure over brows; compressing eyes. Engorged liver. Gall-stones. Pain about navel. Profuse stools; varying or of several colors. Albuminuria.

Related to: Rheum.

EUPATORIUM PERFOLIATUM

SPHERE OF ACTION
BONES.

Stomach.

Liver.

Occiput.

Bronchi.

Muscles

- **Chest.**

- **Back.**

- Limbs.

AGGRAVATION
COLD AIR.

Motion.

PERIODICALLY

- 7-9 A.M.

- 3rd or 7th day.

Lying on part.

Coughing.

Smell or sight of food.

AMELIORATION
Vomiting bile.

Sweating.

Lying on face.

VIOLENT, ACHING, BONE-BREAKING PAINS (Cocc., Pyrog., Ruta). **Bruised, sore ache, < back.** Restless, chilly and nauseated. Colds. **Grippe;** and catarrhal sequelae. **Bilious effects;** yellow eyes, face, vomit, etc. **Weakness.** ....**Vertigo;** sways to left; < lying on right side; > vomiting. Sore throbbing head pains, < occiput; alternating with gouty pains. Sensation as of a metal cap on head. Migraine. Vomits bile at height of head pains, then >. Sore, aching eye-balls. Sneezing. Thirst, but drinks excite **bitter vomiting** or chill. Whitish stools. Urine now profuse, now scanty. Hoarse in A. M. Painful cough, from a laryngeal tickle; it hurts head; **must hold chest.** Raw, hot, **sore** chest and **bronchi.** Intense backache; as if beaten; ascending. Aching lower limbs. Bruised pain in calves. Dropsy of legs. Painful, gouty nodes. **Thirst or nausea, then violent shaking chill**; begins in small of back. **Bitter vomiting, after chill** or during heat. Burning heat. Scanty sweat. Malaria. Catarrhal fevers.

Complementary: Nat-m., Sep.

Related to: Bry., Nux-v.

EUPATORIUM PURPURIUM

Bone-breaking pains. Urinary stream smaller.

EUPHORBIUM

SPHERE OF ACTION	AGGRAVATION
Mucous membranes.	**Sitting.**
Bones.	Rest.
Skin.	Beginning motion.
Teeth.	Mercury.

Internal burning; in bones at night. Caries. Much secretion, with a sense of dryness. Paralytic weakness; in joints. Slow inflammation................ Much abortive sneezing. Coryza, with swelling. Ozena; acrid. Mouth feels coated with rancid grease (Iris). Brittle, crumbling teeth. Stitches from epigastrium into sides of chest on coughing. **Erysipelas; bullosum;** right side: of mucous membranes. **High fever.**

Related to: Nit-ac., Sulph.

EUPHRASIA OFFICINALIS

SPHERE OF ACTION
MUCOUS MEMBRANES
- EYES.
- **Nose.**
- Chest.

AGGRAVATION
SUNLIGHT.
WIND.
Warmth.
Room.
Evening.

AMELIORATION
Open air.
Winking.
Wiping eyes.

Free, acrid, watery secretions. Acute catarrhs. Acrid pus.
.... WATERY EYES; swimming in tears; as of a hair before them, wants to wipe them. ABUNDANT, ACRID OR HOT, SMARTING TEARS, with bland coryza; < open air, lying or coughing (Chel.); leaving a varnish-like mark. Photophobia; with spasm of lids. Pressive, cutting eye-pains. Sticky eye-gum. Red, burning-itching tarsi. Violent injection. Conjunctivitis; of measles. Thick yellow or acrid discharge from eyes. Chemosis. Chronic sore eyes. Gushes of fluent coryza. Loose cough. Easy expectoration, in day time only, less on lying down at night; (reverse—Thuj.).

Related to: All-c.

FAGOPYRUM

SPHERE OF ACTION
Digestive organs.
Skin.

AGGRAVATION
Scratching.
Sun-light.

AMELIORATION
Cold bathing.
Coffee.

Itching; eyes; ears; posterior nares; anus; deep in hands; legs, etc. Pain along lachrymal duct. Scalding, hot, sour eructations. Cardiac pain to shoulder and left arm; > lying on back. Pruritus vulvae; with yellow leucorrhea, < rest. As if neck could not support head. Pains along fingers.

Related to: Puls.

FERRUM METALLICUM

SPHERE OF ACTION

VASOMOTORS

- CIRCULATION.

- **Blood-vessels.**

Blood.

Spleen.

Digestion.

Left deltoid.

AGGRAVATION

NIGHT.
Emotions.
Violent exertion.
Eating.
Drinking.
Vital losses.
Sweats.
Quinine.
Eggs.
Heat and cold.
Sudden motions.
Raising arms.

AMELIORATION
Gentle motion.
Slight bleeding (Calad.,
    Card-m., Lach.).
Leaning head on something.

Pale mucous membranes. False erethism or plethora; weak; lies down. **Excited, irregular surgings.** Wandering orgasms; head, face, chest, etc. **Pulsations. Hemorrhages** (bright or with small clots); in rapidly growing youths. Relaxed blood-vessels; dilated veins, < during menses, etc. **Red faced** old men. Exophthalmos. Pressure on chest, stomach, etc. Nightly pains that **compel motion of part. Dry;** food seems; vagina, etc. Rapid emaciation. **Anemia.** Cachexy. Irritable mind and body................................ Always in the right; excited by the least opposition. Weeps and laughs immoderately. **Sensitive** and excitable, < least opposition. Brain-tire. **Throbbing, hammering headache,** starts in the temple; < cough or stooping; > letting hair down; with vertigo. Pain over left eye. Blind attacks. Puffy eye-lids. **Nose-bleed.** **Face flushes** and pales or **reddens** from the least thing; florid; feels bloated. Erethistic chlorosis. Toothache, > ice water. Stomach won't tolerate any food. Averse to meat. **Spits up his food.** Nausea at midnight. Easy vomiting. Diarrhea; painless lientery; < while eating; nightly gushing; spluttering; alternating with constipation; < if nervous or tired. Chronic nephritis. Enuresis by day only. Emissions; nightly, with backache; after over-exertion. Raw vagina, < coition. Menses pale; intermit. Leucorrhea; acrid, milky, watery, at puberty. Changeable voice. Dry, tickling cough. Blood-spitting (streaked). Constriction of or flying stitches in chest. **Dyspnea** or palpitation, > motion. Sudden cramps or tearing boring in limbs. Cracking joints. Omodynia. Swelled hands and feet. Heels pain, if lies on back. Sleepless. Chill, with red face and thirst. Heat, with distended veins. Sweats, clammy, yellow, cold, acrid or debilitating. Soft pulse.

Complementary: Chin.

Related to: Arn., Mang-met.

FERRUM PHOSPHORICUM

SPHERE OF ACTION

Vasomotors.

Venous circulation.

- LUNGS
- **Ears.**
- **Nose (root).**
- **Eustachian tube.**

AGGRAVATION

Night (4-6 A.M.). Motion.
Noise.
Jar.
Cold air.
Checked sweat.

AMELIORATION

Cold.
Bleedings.
Lying down.

Anemic blondes. FULL, SOFT, FLOWING PULSE.
Hyperemia. Acute exacerbations, phthisis, rheumatism, etc. **Passive
congestion** and weakness. **Bloody** (streaked or meat water) **discharges.**
Bruised **soreness; chest, shoulder,** muscles. Inflamed soft parts.
Burning rawness. .... Keeps quiet. Anger. **Excited** and
talkative. Cerebral irritation. Throbbing headaches, with sensitive
scalp. Headache; shooting pains, aching from vertex down over sides
of head; with **earache** (Puls.), > nosebleed. Suffused eyes. **Violent
earache.** Acute otitis; media. Colds cause deafness. Tinnitus, < lying.
Face pales and reddens alternately. Vomits ingesta. **Frequent stools
of bloody water.** Diarrhea. Impending hydrocephalus. Nephritis.
Enuresis. Urinates after every drink (Sars.). Menses early, with heavy
pain on vertex. Laryngitis; **of singers** (Arum-t). Cough; hacking; <
morning and evening. Cough, tormenting, spasmodic. **Chest** heavy,
sore or **congested.** Omodynia. Jerking limbs. Drowsiness. Chill, with
desire to stretch. Heat with sweaty hands. Sweatiness. **Fevers;**
continued; infectious; **pneumonia;** intercurrent. Measles;
hemorrhagic.

Complementary: Kali-m.

Related to: Gels.

FLUORICUM ACIDUM

SPHERE OF ACTION

FIBROUS TISSUES

- VEINS.

- **Skin.**

Bones.

Mastoid.

AGGRAVATION

HEAT; of room.

Night.

Alcohol.

Sour foods.

AMELIORATION

COOL BATHING.

Rapid motion.

Short sleep.

Bending head back.

Eating.

Always too hot; wants to bathe in cold water. Pale, miserable, cachectic, flabby and broken down. Slow, deeply destructive effects. Puffy, indurated or fistulous tissues. Palmar abscess. Felon. Caries. Bed-sores. Ulcers. Edema. Secondary syphilis. Thin, foul, acrid or salty discharges; that cause itching........................Necessity to be always in the move. Impulse to walk fast. Melancholy. Lecherousness. Stunning headache; > urinating. Brittle, tousy hair. As of a cold wind in eye. Lachrymal stricture. Deafness, > bending head back. Puffy glabella. Thin enamel. Teeth decay rapidly; < at roots. Fissured tongue. Gnawing hunger; for pungent or cold things. Stale eructations. Itching or burning at anus. Upward drawing in urethra (down—Merc.). Profuse, acrid leucorrhea. Sexual erethism. Edema of scrotum. Distorted nails. Varicose veins; varicocele. Dry, harsh, itching or cracked skin; seeming to emit a hot vapor. Scars surrounded by pimples. Keloid. Ebullitions of heat; with pains in bones. Acrid, eroding sweat; excites itching. Oily, pungent sweat on genitals, Sweat on hands and feet.

Complementary: Sil.

Related to: Calc-s., Puls., Sul-ac.

FORMICA RUFA

SPHERE OF ACTION	AGGRAVATION
Joints.	**Cold;** Wet.
Spine.	Motion.
Liver.	Before snow-storms.
Kidneys.	**AMELIORATION**
Right side.	Pressure.

Sudden rheumatic or gouty pains. Takes cold easily. Tuberculosis. Hyperplasia. .... Light, foaming stools. Hydrops ovary. Nervous asthma. Hives, in flat plaques. **Profuse sweat,** without relief.

Related to: Rhus-t., Urt-u.

FRAXINUS

SPHERE OF ACTION	AGGRAVATION
Uterus.	Injury.
	Sprains.
Nerves.	Lifting.

Nervous females with enlarged or **prolapsed wombs.** ....
Must talk. **Hot spot** or dryness **on vertex.** Throbbing in occiput.
Heavy abdomen with bearing down or falling out sensation. Sensitive
left ovary. Profuse menses or leucorrhea. Cramps in feet. Hot flushes.

Related to: Sep., Vib.

GAMBOGIA

SPHERE OF ACTION	AGGRAVATION
Stomach and BOWELS.	AFTER STOOL.
	Motion in open air.
Liver.	

Burnings. .... Burning pains. Itching eye-lids;
he rubs them (Ign.). Sneezing. **Gurgling, pinching in bowels, then
sudden yellow or green,** THIN STOOLS COMING OUT IN
PROLONGED GUSHES, **with burning at anus and much relief.**

Related to: Crot-t.

GELSEMIUM

SPHERE OF ACTION	AGGRAVATION
CIRCULATION.	EMOTIONS; DREAD.
BRAIN CORD	Surprise.
- OCCIPUT.	**Shock.**
	Ordeals.
- **Base.**	Motion.
- **Neck.**	

MOTOR NERVES
- EYES.
  - LIDS.
- VISION.
- MUSCLES.
- Knees.

MUCOUS MEMBRANES
- Nose.
- Gall-ducts.

Right side.

Weather
- SPRING.
- **Foggy.**
- HUMID.
- **Muggy.**

Heat of summer.
Periodically.
Dentition.
Tobacco.
Gas.

AMELIORATION
Profuse urination.
Sweating.
Shaking.
Alcoholic drinks.
Mental effort.

ACHING, TIRED, HEAVY, WEAK AND SORE; < limbs. Grippe. **Overpowering aching.** Heavy single parts, heart, liver, etc. Lies quietly, half reclining. Nerve exhaustion. **Dull, drowsy and dizzy.** TREMOR; or twitches of single muscles, face, **chin,** tongue, etc.; **wants to be held.** Chorea, of pregnancy. **Paretic** effects; eyes, **throat,** anus, bladder, etc. Inco-ordination. **Fulness. Passive congestion. Symptoms accompanied by vertigo, eye or visual effects, drowsiness or polyuria.** ....
CONFUSED, dazed, apathetic, torpid, **dull, drowsy** and **dizzy,** or indifferent; answers slowly. DREAD **of falling;** of ordeals, death, pains, etc. VERTIGO; drunken; in occiput. Headache; dull, HEAVY, band-like, **occipital,** to over eyes; < tight hat; swelled feeling; **basilar.** Meningitis. Apoplexy. Suffused, sore, **aching eyes.** HEAVY, DROOPING EYELIDS. VISION; double; swimming; blind spells; affected, then migraine. **Face full, dusky-red;** heavy, expressionless; **besotted.** Ciliary neuralgia; pains into ears on swallowing. Pains **to occiput.** Nose stuffed. **Sneezing; thin, acrid coryza.** Sensation as of hot water flowing from the nostrils. Heavy tongue; **thick speech.** THIRSTLESS. Griping in gall-bladder. Copious, yellow stools. Painless, nervous diarrhea. Rectal pains after labor. Clear, watery urine, > headache. Alternate pelvic and head symptoms. Atonic seminal losses. **Heavy, sore uterus;** it feels grasped. Dysmenorrhea. La-

bor pains go up, backward or down thighs. Rigid os. Deep yellow leucorrhea. Hoarse, during menses. Tiresome breathing. Chest; as of a lump
behind sternum; congestion. Heart sore; threatens to stop, must move.
Spine, **dull pains up and down, >** walking; with occipital pain. **Pains
under scapulae.** Hard ache in right humerus. Wants hands in cool water.
Heavy lower limbs. **Weak knees, <** descending. **Tottering gait**; can't
direct his legs. **Moist, yellow skin.** DROWSINESS; starts on dropping to
sleep. Heavy, stupid sleep. **Full, round, soft pulse.** Blood rushes from
occiput to forehead. Visual disturbances, then chill. **Chilly and achy;
with languor** (Sil.); **mingled or alternating with heat; up and down
back.** Cold hands and feet. **Heat with sopor.** ABSENCE OF THIRST, or
trembling. Cold sweat on genitals. Fevers; bilious-remittent; malarial;
cerebro-spinal. **Measles.** Ebullitions and heats. Sluggish fever. Shuddering chill.

Complementary: Arg-n., Sep.

Related to: Con., Ign., Mur-ac., Nat-m., Sep., Verat-v.

GLONOINUM

SPHERE OF ACTION

BRAIN.

VASOMOTORS

- CIRCULATION.

- HEAD (Forehead).

- HEART.

Mastoids.

Respiration.

AGGRAVATION

HEAT

- ON HEAD.
- Overheating.
- OF SUN, **lamp, etc.**
- HOT WEATHER

MOTION

- SHAKING.
- JAR.
- Bending head.
- Back.

Injury.

Wine.

Suppressed menses.

Fruits

Weight of hat.

Hair cut.

Open air.
Elevating head
Cool things.
Cold application, bathing, etc.

A tempestuous remedy, full of VIOLENT PULSATIONS. EBULLITIONS **or irregular congestion;** general pulsations; with numbness. UPWARD RUSHES OF BLOOD. **As if enlarged, distended** or being smaller. Bursting, expansion or enlarged feeling of eyes, head, tongue, etc. Pains that come long after injuries..........
...............Confused, bewildered; loses himself. Sinks down unconscious. Sun-stroke. Apoplexy. Congestion to head in suppressed menses, eclampsia, albuminuria, etc. WAVES; OF TERRIBLE BURSTING, POUNDING HEADACHE, as if standing on head; expanding and contracting or blood **surging** back and forth from head, < carotids to heart; alternating between temples; < sunshine; < damp days. Cracking, snapping, shocks, explosions or soreness deep in brain. Head lies too heavy on pillow. Pains in malar bones, ending in a headache. Numb, sore vertex. Sharp, shooting behind ears. **Red lower eyeballs** or lids. Staring, dry, protruding or sunken eyes; lids stick to balls (Guaj.). Blind spells. **Bluish face.** Veins of temples swelled. Heavy tongue. Thick saliva in A. M. Throat feels swelled. Heavy breathing. As of a load on chest. Heart seems full, quivers; strong pulsation, and into (left) neck. **Violent palpitation.** Cardiac pains; radiate to all parts; toward arms. Cardiac pains, < leaning backward or wine. Neck feels full and stiff. Trembling hands. Awakes fearing apoplexy. Full, tense pulse. Venous pulse. **Heat on crown of head** and along spine. Burning in small areas or single parts. Heat, with hot sweat. Horrible sinking in epigastrium.

Complementary: Bell.

Related to: Amyl-ns., Bell.

GNAPHALIUM

SPHERE OF ACTION
NERVES
- SCIATIC.
- **Crural.**
- Abdominal.

AGGRAVATION
Walking.
Lying.
Cold; Damp.

AMELIORATION
Flexing limbs.
Sitting.

Intense sciatic pains; alternating with or followed by numbness or formication. Offensive diarrhea with colic, < morning.

Related to: Coloc.

GOSSYPIUM

SPHERE OF ACTION
Uterus.
Ovaries.
Kidneys.

AGGRAVATION
Motion.

Uterine reflexes...................Flow of saliva. Nausea on awaking. Vomits on motion or raising up. Hyperemesis. Sensitive stomach, with much gas. Ovarian pains extend toward uterus. **Uterine torpor.** Cervical pain. Sensitive womb. Menses late, scanty and watery.

Related to: Senec., Ust.

GRAPHITES

SPHERE OF ACTION
NUTRITION.
Circulation.
SKIN
- Folds.
- Behind
- Ears.
- Angles.
- Flexures.
- Orifices.
- Nails.
Mind.
Mucous membranes.
Glands.
Eyes.

AGGRAVATION
COLD.
Draft.
Light.
During menses.
Suppression of eruptions
Empty swallowing.
Fats.
Hot drinks.
Warmth of bed.
Scratching.
Night.
Wet feet.

AMELIORATION
Open air; After walking in.
Eating.
Touch.

LUMPY, THICK OR HARD (Chin. , Thuj.); skin, glands, tarsi, nails, scars, callosities, stools, crusts, etc. Infiltrations. EXCORIATIONS, CRACKS OR FISSURES; in angles; at margins of mucous membranes; of eyes, nostrils, mouth, finger-tips, nipples, anus, etc. Emaciation; of affected part. Scanty, foul, thin, sticky, corrosive secretions. Watery hemorrhages. Sense of burning, numbness or deadness. Pains go to part not lain on. Fat, relaxed, chilly and costive. ....Impulse to groan. Sad, fearsome and irresolute. Music brings tears. Brain feels numb. Burning spot on vertex. Heavy occiput. Wens. Matted, brittle or falling hair; < vertex and sides. Milk crust. Sore or cracked outer canthi. Scrophula of eyes. Pale tarsi. Ingrown lashes. Photophobia. Inflamed or dry, scaly tarsi. Scales from ears. Briny otorrhea. Tinnitus. Hears > in a noise. Moist eruption behind ears. Dryness in ears and nose. Nose; stuffed coryza; bleeding, < before menses. Acute smell. Sensation as of a cobweb on face. Acne before menses. Barbers' itch. Lumpy goitre. Rotten taste. **Dots of thick, white fur on tongue.** Choking; on swallowing, from goitre, etc. Sour : taste, eructation, blood about teeth, stool, urine, odor from mouth, sweat, etc. Hunger. Averse to meats and sweets. Alternate digestive and skin symptoms. Gastric pains—burning—necessitate eating. Morning sickness during menses. Can't bear pressure about waist. Foul belching. **Flatulence.** Stomach > heat, hot food, eating and lying. **Abdomen distended,** as from incarcerated flatus. **Intestinal torpor. Large, knotty, difficult, stringy, slimy coated stools**; or loose, brown, lienteric and very foul. Constipation; for days (Sep.). Fissures of anus bleed and ulcerate. Stool of masses of mucus. Slender stool and urinary stream. Priapism. Sexual exhaustion. Itching of anus and pudendum; before menses. Averse to coition. Swelled (left) ovary. Cramps in various places or burnings. Indurations; ovaries, mammae, etc. Menses irregular; **late,** scanty, painful, etc.; cold taking, morning sickness or sweats during. Gushes of irritating, white leucorrhea; instead of menses. Suffocation, after mid-night, > eating. Voice lacks control, > using it. Circulation irregular. Flushings. Rushes of blood to head. Bunions, < fire, heat > pressure. Can't stretch enough. Paralysed feeling in limbs. Arms and legs go to sleep. Rawness in folds of skin. Eruptions, cracked, moist and bleed easily; < on head and behind ears. **Foul, acrid foot-sweat; chafes toes.** Crippled, crumbling nails. IRRITABLE, DRY, **rough skin, that breaks easily and exudes** A GLUEY MOISTURE; < in folds—and is **slow to heal.** MOIST, CRUSTY ERUPTIONS. Eczema; anal, crural, palmar, etc. Wandering or **recurrent erysipelas** (Hydr., Rhus-t.). Eruptions, < from heat. **Supersensitive to cold;** it < bone-pains, coryza and stomach. Cold, wet feet. Burning coldness.

Complementary: Sulph.

Related to: Ars., Calc-f., Carbons, Ferr., Kali-bi., Puls.

GRATIOLA OFFICINALIS

SPHERE OF ACTION

Gastro-intestinal tract.

Mind.

Sexual organs.

AGGRAVATION

Eating.

Drinking too much water.

Summer.

Motion.

Coffee.

Dinner.

Atony. Paralytic pains. **Coldness.** .... Weak will. Hypochondriasis. Emptiness after eating. As of cold water or a **loose, heavy load in stomach.** Profuse, gushing, watery or frothy, yellow-green, exhausting stools, then **relief** (Gamb.). Nightly emissions, then erections. Nymphomania. Coccygeal pain. Limb gives way, with sciatic pain.

Related to: Mag-c.

GRINDELIA ROBUSTA

SPHERE OF ACTION

Pneumo-gastric nerves.

Bronchi.

Respiration.

AGGRAVATION

Falling to sleep.

Profuse secretions.......................**Suffocates on falling to sleep** or on awaking. Asthma. Battling breathing. Tenacious expectoration. Bronchorrhea. Cutting soreness about spleen.

Related to: Lach.

GUAJACUM OFFICINALE

SPHERE OF ACTION	AGGRAVATION
Secretion	HEAT.
- **Glands.**	**Touch.**
- **TONSILS.**	**Motion.**
Ovaries	Exertion.
- **Skin.**	Rapid growth.
Fibrous tissue	Mercury.
- Ligaments.	**AMELIORATION**
- Joints.	Cold (Locally).
Chest.	Apples.

Rigid, painfully swelled joints. **Arthritic symptoms.** FREE, FOUL SECRETIONS, expectoration, sweats, etc. **Impending suppuration,** quinsy, old bronchitis, etc. **Burning heat;** in affected parts. Gnawing or sticking pains; < chest. **Muscles seem too short;** eye-lids, back, thigh, etc.; **sore. Growing pains. Contraction;** between scapulae; palmar; distorting. Fixed, short tendons. Nodes....................... **Forgetful.** Pain from head into neck. Eye-balls seem too big for lids. Exophthalmos. **Throat; burning; dry;** painful to touch; **tonsillitis** (right), recurrent (Phyt.), then rheumatism. Averse to milk. Stoppage in epigastrium causes cough, dyspnea, etc. Dry cough, with hot face and burning fever. Sticking in apex of (left) lung. Phthisis. Recurrent pleurisy. Aching, sore neck; one side stiff. Tense, short thigh muscles. Arthritis deformans. Yawning and stretching. Wakes as if falling. Sweats, profuse; on single parts, face, etc. Night-sweats.

Related to: Ferr., Kali-bi., Kreos., Ph-ac., **Phyt.**

GYMNOCLADUS

SPHERE OF ACTION
    Urinary organs.

    Circulation.

    Sensations.

AGGRAVATION
    Cold.
    Walking.

AMELIORATION
    Rest.
    Leaning against something.

Lividity. Numbness. ....Slow grasp. Head feels bound.
Pain under brows and into nose. Outpushing in eyes; wants to rub them.
Crawling on (left) face. Teeth sensitive to cold air. BLUISH TONGUE.
Hot, sour belchings. Burning spot in stomach.

Related to: Op.

HAMAMELIS

SPHERE OF ACTION
    VEINS
    - **Rectum.**
    - Genitals.
    - Limbs.
    - Throat.
    Liver.
    Abdominal and chest walls.

AGGRAVATION
    Injury.
    Bruises.
    Pressure.
    Air
    - **Open.**
    - **Humid.**
    - Cold.
    Jar.
    Motion.
    Touch.

SORENESS, **bruised**; in blood-vessels; localized; abdominal,
etc. Tense, bursting feeling; in piles, joints, or lower limbs. Congestive
fulness. Veins, **sore**; cutting; swelled; inflamed. **Painful varicoses.**
Hemorrhage; capillary; dark, fluid; relieves or **causes undue
weakness.** .... **Irritable and chilly. Hammering headache,
< left temple. Blood-shot eyes. Taste of blood. Pain and heaviness

back of stomach. Piles. Pain up along spermatic cord. Neuralgia of
testes. Orchitis; < touch. Varicocele. Breaking backache. Profuse, dark
menses. Scapular pains. Dull ache about kidneys. Phlebitis.
Ecchymoses. Varicose ulcers with bloody bases.

Complementary: Ferr., Fl-ac.

Related to: Arn., Puls., Vip-t.

HELLEBORUS NIGER

SPHERE OF ACTION
MIND. BRAIN; Sensorium.
Nerves; Motor; Sensory.
Membranes
- **Serous.**
- **Mucous.**
Kidneys.
Muscles.
Exudations.

AGGRAVATION
Cold air.
Puberty.
Dentition.
Suppressions.
Exertion.
Evening (4-8 P.M.).

AMELIORATION
Strong attention.

A dark, dusky remedy; dark face; sooty nostrils; dark lips, hands,
etc. Serous effusions. Gradual onset, with advancing weakness.
Blunted senses and sluggish responses; drops things, staggers, etc.
Automatic acts. Lies on back with knees drawn up. Muscle pains,
spasm or **paralysis.** Feeble and delicate. .... Inattention. **Stupid,
obtuse or apathetic.** Brain symptoms, with anorexia. Blank, **somber
despair.** Won't eat or speak. Fixed ideas. Things look new. Heavy,
numbing headache. **Rolls head or bores it into pillow for relief.**
Congestion. Hydrocephalus. **Stupid, staring or tired look. Eyes half
open. Pale face.** Chewing motions. **Fetor oris.** Numb, dry, trembling
tongue or covered with yellow ulcers. Ptyalism. Averse to vegetables.
Distended abdomen. Watery or **gelatinous** stool. **Urine, scanty,** with
dark flecks or sediment; retained. Nephritis. Uremia. Dropsy.

Amenorrhea from cold. **Small, soft pulse.** Sopor; with **cries or starts.**
Coldness. Chill, with fever or heat; with sweat.

Complementary: Zinc.

Related to: Bry., Op., Zinc.

HELONIAS DIOICA

SPHERE OF ACTION	AGGRAVATION
FEMALE ORGANS.	**Fatigue.**
	- Labor.
Kidneys.	- Abortion.
	- Stooping.
Mind.	**Pregnancy.**
	Pressure of clothes.
Muscles.	**AMELIORATION**
	If busy.
	Diversion.
	Holding abdomen.

Unduly exhausted females. Uterine reflexes. Heavy, sore,
aching-burning; kidneys; in muscles; in back .... Deep gloom.
Melancholy. **Irritable;** wants to be let alone. Heat or upward pressure
in vertex. Aphthae. **Dull ache and heat in region of kidneys.** Excessive
urine. Nephritis of pregnancy. Sugar and albumen in urine. **Heavy,
sore, tender, ulcerated or prolapsed womb.** Dark, foul blood from
uterus; hemorrhage from atony. Foul, **lumpy or curdled leucorrhea.**
Inflamed, **itching,** aphthous vulva. **Heavy dragging in pelvis.
Squeezing in chest.** Swelled, painful mammae. Tender nipples. Aching
between scapulae. Sore pain in outer side of thighs. Anemia. Hot,
when tired.

Related to: Senec., **Sep., Tril-p.**

HEPAR SULPHURIS

SPHERE OF ACTION
NERVES.
CONNECTIVE TISSUE.
RESPIRATORY MEM-
  BRANES.
Flexures.
GLANDS.
Kidneys.
Skin.
Bridge of nose (Kali-bi.).

AGGRAVATION
COLD, **dry**
- AIR.
- WINTER.
- DRAFTS.
- WIND.
- PART BECOMING.
LEAST
- UNCOVERING.
- TOUCH.
- Noise.
- Exertion.
Lying on painful part.
Mercury.
Night.

AMELIORATION
HEAT
- WARM WRAPS.
- TO HEAD.
- Moist.
DAMP WEATHER.

Lax. CHILLY AND OVERSENSITIVE; **to cold; to pain;** or
to touch; faints easily, etc. **Profuse secretions;** foul; **like old cheese.**
Sour, stools, smell of body, sweat, etc. SWEATS EASILY, but dare
not uncover; **and profusely,** without relief. **As of a wind blowing on**
part. Wears overcoat in hot weather. Takes cold from damp exposure.
Sore STICKING, **like sharp splinters.** EVERY HURT FESTERS.
SUPPURATION; threatens, or **much thick pus.** Abscess. Mastoiditis.
Yellow, sclerotic, expectoration, sweat, etc. .... Bad temper.
Sudden weak memory. Touchy, mentally and physically; to pain, cold;
easily becomes cross and violent. **Hasty,** violent, **irritable** or
dissatisfied. Hair falls in spots; sore to touch. Corneal ulcer or
maculae. Photophobia. Chronic otorrhea. Boring at root of nose.

F- 10

Stuffed, painful nose. Ripened colds and old catarrhs. Sneezes from every cold wind. Hawks mucus. Rough sticking like a splinter, fishbone, etc., in throat. Quinsy. The upper jaw projects. Goitre (right); pains into head. **Stomach weak**; easily upset. **Craves** acids, **condiments** or stimulants. Eating refreshes, but causes heaviness. Foul mucus from anus. Stool difficult, although soft. Must wait to urinate; passes blood and pus afterwards. Nephritis; after scarlatina. Very foul, hot, membranous or pussy leucorrhea. Painful larynx. Cough from least uncovering. Whistling, choking breathing; must bend head back. Croup. Hoarseness; chronic; of singers. Aphonia. Asthma; after suppressions. **Cough, choking,** barking; < cold drinks or in A. M.; hacking, as from a feather; LOOSE, **but can't expectorate,** tightens up in cold air. WEAKNESS AND MUCH RATTLING IN CHEST. **Much expectoration;** thick, yellow. Recurrent bronchitis; from every cold. Skin sensitive to cool air (Agar.). Foul, moist eruptions in folds. Torpid, pulsating ulcers; encircled by smaller ones, pimples or boils. Impetigo. Poor granulation. Sweaty and rattles with every cold or cough. Night-sweats. Low fevers. Hectic. Body exhales a foul odor.

Antidotes: Bell., Cham., Kali-i., Merc-s.

Complementary: Iod., Sil.

Follows: Phos., Sil.

Related to: Merc.

HYDRASTIS CANADENSIS

SPHERE OF ACTION	AGGRAVATION
MUCOUS GLANDS	AIR
- **Nasal cavities.**	- **Inhaling, cold.**
- STOMACH.	- Dry winds.
- Gall-ducts.	- Open.
- **Intestines**	Slight bleedings.
Muscles.	Washing.
Uterus.	**Old age.**

A mucus remedy; hawks up much mucus; mucus in stools, urine, etc. Atonic, cachectic or degenerative conditions. Shallow ulcers. Hemorrhagic or CATARRHAL processes. Thick, yellow, acrid (Sanic.), ropy secretions. Sense of raw-burning. Weak, dyscrasic and emaciated...............Neuralgia of scalp and neck. Thin, yellow, sunken face. Nose; sore; bleeds; bloody crusts. Post-nasal dripping. Dirty, yellow, slimy, flabby, indented tongue (Nat-p., Yuc.). Taste bitter; burnt. Aphthae. Loathing. Goneness or as of sharp lumps in stomach. Cutting from liver to right scapula, < lying on back or right side. Lumpy stool; coated or mixed with mucus. Constipation; of pregnancy; after purgatives. Mucus in urine. Thick, acrid leucorrhea. Ulcer of cervix. Loose cough; bloody expectoration. Raises quantities of mucus. Senile bronchitis. Palpitation, with weakness. Heat alternating with chilliness; profuse sweating.

Related to: Ars., Kali-bi., Puls.

HYDROCYANICUM ACIDUM

SPHERE OF ACTION
Brain.
Heart
- Circulation.
- Respiration.
Epigastrium.

AGGRAVATION
Full moon.
Suppressions.
Storms.

Sudden effects; collapse; spasms; apoplexy. Lacks reaction. Cramps everywhere. Evacuations ceases. Lightning-like jerks from head to feet...............Fear of death. Loud, involuntary cries. Sinks down unconscious. Intense cerebral congestion. Prolonged faints. Pale or bluish face. Cramps in masseters; in nape. Mouth dry. Taste pussy; metallic; astringent. Noisy swallowing. Gasping, irregular, slow breathing. Asphyxia. Cholera. Dry, tickling, night cough. Heart: failure; compression at. Contracted dorsal muscles. Blue exanthema,

Pulse, failing; unequal; with occasional strong beats. Distended blood-vessels; writhing in them. Icy coldness; < hands.

Related to: Agar., Cupr., Laur.

HYOSCYAMUS NIGER

SPHERE OF ACTION
  MIND.
  Brain.
  Nerves.
  Muscles
  - Face.
  - Eyes.
  Blood.

AGGRAVATION
  EMOTIONS
  - **Fright.**
  - Jealousy.
  TOUCH.
  Lying.
  Cold.
  Sleep.

AMELIORATION
  Sitting up.

Congested nerve centers; with pale face. **Spasm, tremor, jerks,** cramps, etc., or **active mania**; alternating with or **ending in depressive narcosis**, with angular or **clutching motions**, CARPHOLOGY, **subsultus**, etc. Picks fingers. Zymoses. Eclampsia. ....
Many bewildering aberrations. Confusion. **Delirium.** MANIA, **erotic**, exposes genitals; riotous; laughing, singing, **talking**, babbling, quarreling, etc.; **silly**, with comical acts; plays with fingers. **Fumbles the genitals.** Lascivious (females). **Jealousy. Suspicious;** fears being alone, being pursued, water, etc.; **wants to escape.** Speaks each word louder. First, can't think, then can **barely be aroused**, then relaxation; with **muttering**, the lower jaw drops, he slides down in bed, has involuntary stools— bloody or yellow **watery.** Typhoid states. Vertigo, then spasm. Waves of pulsation in head. Pulsating headaches. Head shakes to and fro; < bending forward. Squint. Averse to light. Spasmodic closure of eyelids. Grimaces. Sordes on teeth. Stiff, dark, red, cracked tongue. Elongated uvula. **Stools involuntary**, although

hard. Frequent, scanty, painful, nightly urination or **retained urine.**
Spasms of dry, hacking, night **cough;** from a dry spot in larynx; <
lying, eating or talking. **Nervous wakefulness.** Starts out of sleep.
Low fever; with hot, pale skin. Warm sweat. Sexuality excited by
Hyoscine is antidoted by Platina.

Related to: Bell., Phos., Stram.

HYPERICUM PERFOLIATUM

SPHERE OF ACTION
SPINAL NERVES
- COCCYX.
- **Inter-scapular.**
- Meninges.

Vertex.

AGGRAVATION
INJURY
- JAR.
- Concussion.
- Penetrating.
- **Shock.**
- Bruises.
Exertion.
Touch.
Change of weather.
Fogs.
Cold.
Damp.
Motion.

AMELIORATION
Lying on face.
Bending back.

LACERATED, **injured or inflamed nerves; mashed fingers,**
etc. Injury to or reflected from brain or **cord. Very painful, sore parts;**
occiput, **coccyx,** etc. Coccygodynia. **Intolerably violent, shooting,**
lancinating along nerves; toward trunk; **down sides of head** or chest;
in epigastrium; interscapular spine; fingertips, etc., with crawling
and numbness. Neuritis, as an outcome of injury. Neuralgia of stump.
Shuddering. Spasms. Tetanus. .... Heaviness **or**

formication in brain. **Head feels drawn to a point.** Bubbling at navel. Dry rectum. Heart seems to drop. Painfully sensitive spine. Commotio spinalis. Pains in hips and small of back after labor. Limbs feel detached. Aching in left sciatic, after long sitting. Feet seem furry or bones ache. Gaping wounds. Laborious dreams.

Related to: Arn., Led., Rhus-t.

IGNATIA AMARA

SPHERE OF ACTION	AGGRAVATION
	EMOTIONS
	- GRIEF.
MIND.	- **Chargin.**
	- WORRY.
NERVOUS SYSTEM.	- **Fright.**
	Shock.
Cerebro-spinal axis.	Air
	- Open.
	- Cold.
	Odors.
	Touch.
	Coffee.
	Tobacco.
	AMELIORATION
	Position
	- Change of.
	- **Lying on part.**
	Urination.
	If alone.
	Pressure.

ERRATIC, CONTRADICTORY OR SPASMODIC EFFECTS; **often violent; with rigidity, twitchings,** tremor, etc.; during pain. Jerks run through whole body. SENSE OF A LUMP, foreign body or sharp pressure. Globus. Clavus. Hysteria. Pain in a spot, < close attention. Symptoms pass off with a profuse flow of urine. Oversensitive to pain. Tonic spasm of single parts, with frothing at mouth. Neurotic inheritance. Spasms from punishment (Agar.). .... **Brooding grief. Silent and sad;** inward weeping. Intolerant of contradiction; of reprimands (Coloc., Staph.). Angry with himself. Delicately conscientious. Everything irks her. Weak and excitable. ALERT, OVERSENSITIVE AND NERVOUS. **Highly emotional.** Capricious. **Moody. Changeful.** Faints easily. SIGHS, **weeps** or laughs by turns. **Unhappy;** love. Enjoys being **sad.** GRIEF; **brooding.** Alternate headache and backache (Meli.). Headache ends in yawning and vomiting. Eyelids seem dry. Flashes of light, from violent coughing. Nose sensitive to inspired air. Pain over root of nose. Sneezing attacks. **One cheek red.** Jaws snap shut; bites inside of cheek, tongue, etc. Masseters stiff and hard. Indurated tonsils; with little ulcers. Cramp in gullet. **Swallows over a lump,** > solids. **Hiccough;** with eructations, empty or bitter. Nausea or vomiting, > indigestible foods. Hunger, with nausea. Craves raw foods. **Empty sinking or spasmodic ache in stomach;** not > eating. Stool painful; difficult although soft, then constriction of rectum. Constipation of neurasthenics. **Pain shoots up rectum.** Piles, > sitting. **Prolapsus recti.** Irregular menses. TAKES DEEP BREATHS; for relief. **Choking.** Spasm of glottis. Hacking cough. Cough violent, it shuts off the breath; dry, as from dust or sulphur fumes; < coughing. Constriction of thorax. Goitre. Tension in nape. Cramp in calf. Heavy feet. Painful skin, > pressure. **Violent, spasmodic yawning.** Light sleep, every sound wakes. Dreams same horrid dreams, over and over. Chill with a red face. **Chill, shaking; nervous;** with thirst; < pain. Heat, with aversion to uncover, but no thirst.

Complementary: Aur., **Nat-m.,** Ph-ac., Sep.

Related to: Cimic., Nux-v., Sep.

IODIUM

SPHERE OF ACTION
GLANDS
- THYROID.
- Testes.
- **Mesenteric.**
- Mammae.
MUCOUS MEMBRANES
LARYNX
- Lungs (right apex or base).
HEART.
Blood-vessels.
Skin.
Nerves.
Connective tissue.

AGGRAVATION
HEAT
- ROOM.
- **Air.**
- Wraps.
Exertion
- Ascending.
- Talking.
Fasting.
Night.
Rest.

AMELIORATION
COLD
- AIR.
- **Bathing.**
Motion.
Eating.

Intensely rapid action. ALWAYS TOO HOT. **Hot, acrid or watery discharges.** Persistent or salty secretions. Infiltration. GLANDS, SWELLED, HARD or heavy; later dwindling. Lean, hungry and hot. **Weak and rapidly losing flesh; can't talk.** Vascular degeneration. Scrofula. Acute exacerbations (Ferr-p.). Local torpidity; little pus. Internal tickling. General pulsation or local throbbings. Burnings. .... **Dejected or intolerably** CROSS and RESTLESS. **Excited.** Sudden dreadful impulses, > if busy, but motion < and exhausts. Thinks he is well. Reverberations in head. Prominent eyes. Pain at root of nose. Subject to head colds, < open air. Catarrh. Nose red and swelled; much sneezing; it drips hot water. Miserable, withered, **brownish,** sallow or dusky look. Increased saliva; soapy; foul. Metallic taste. **Always hungry, yet emaciates, or variable appetite.** Frothy, wheyey, fatty, cheesy or lienteric stools. Sediment in urine like red pepper. Sarcocele. Atrophied testes. Impotency. Menses brown; with weakness; after every stool. **Leucorrhea erodes**

thighs and linen. **Painful, choking hoarseness**; grasps the larynx. Laryngitis. Diphtheria; expectorates cast of larynx (Kali-bi.). Rough voice. **Dry, tickling, croupy cough. Short breath.** Raw bronchi. Violent pulmonary congestion. Pneumonia; rapid extension. Heart feels squeezed. Palpitation. Heavy mammae. **Hard goitre.** Foot-sweat on backs of feet. Skin dry, rough, dirty; **brown** spots on. Restlessness in bed prevents sleep. Hyperpyrexia, or external coldness with anxiety or stupor. Hectic. Heat waves to head. Sweats easily. Early morning sweats, with >.

Antidotes: Ars., Bell., Hep., Op., **Phos.**

Complementary: Lyc., Sil.

Related to: Ars., **Fl-ac.**, Phos., Spong.

IPECACUANHA

SPHERE OF ACTION
MUCOUS MEMBRANES
- DIGESTIVE.
- **Stomach.**
- RESPIRATORY.
- Lungs.
Nerves
- **Pneumo-gastric.**
- Spinal.
- Cutaneous.
Umbilicus.

AGGRAVATION
WARMTH; **Damp;** Room.
Overeating
- Ices.
- Pork.
- Veal.
- Mixed or **rich foods.**
Periodically.
Quinine.
Heat and cold.
Recessions.

AMELIORATION
Open air.

Profuse secretions. Foamy discharges, stool, etc. CONTINUOUS NAUSEA, **gastric disturbances.** BRIGHT RED, GUSHING HEMORRHAGE (rapidly clotting), or **shortness of breath** accompany most complaints. Infantile convulsions..................

Cries, screams and is hard to please. Downward crushing in head, to
root of tongue. Migraine. Occipital pain, < vomiting, during chill,
etc. Gushes of tears. Conjunctivitis. Cold (right), ear. Nosebleed.
Sneezing. Face pale; blue about eyes or lips; white linea nasalis. **Clean
or red, pointed tongue.** NO THIRST. Sudden faintness. HORRID
NAUSEA; **not > vomiting.** Vomiting; bilious; < stooping.
Repugnance to food. Miserable sinking or **hanging loose feeling at
stomach.** Griping, clawing or **cutting at navel;** toward uterus. Brown,
grass or yellow-green, molasses-like or **bloody stools.** Balls of mucus
in stools. Dysentery. **Urging to urinate;** bloody urine. Cutting in
uterus (left to right). Uterine hemorrhage; gasps with each gush of
blood. Painless hoarseness. Larynx and chest tight, < least motion.
Spasm of vocal cords. **Gasps for breath.** Asthma. **Paroxysms of
retching, incessant or** SUFFOCATIVE **cough;** with every breath;
stiffens out, turns red or blue and finally is nauseated, gags or vomits;
< stepping into open air; > warmth and repose. Pertussis. LOOSE
(coarse) RATTLE IN CHEST, WITHOUT EXPECTORATION.
Broncho-pneumonia. Hemoptysis. Pains from kidneys into thighs.
Short chill; alternates with heat or with external heat (Apis). One
hand cold, other hot. Long heat; without thirst. Hands and feet drip
cold sweat. Suppressed or mixed intermittents; **nausea in all stages.**
Catarrhal or gastric fevers.

Complementary: Ars., **Cupr.**

Related to: Ant-t., Lob.

IRIS VERSICOLOR

SPHERE OF ACTION
GLANDS
- DIGESTIVE TRACT.
- LIVER.
- **Pancreas.**
Right side.
Nerves.

AGGRAVATION
Periodically
- **Weekly.**
- **2-3 A.M.**
- Spring and fall.
- After midnight.
Mental exhaustion.
Hot weather.
AMELIORATION
Gentle motion.

Affections accompanied by rapid elimination. **Sour, acrid,** BURNING **excretions. Oily nose, greasy taste and fatty stool** .... Headache, with diarrhea. Mouth feels greasy, burnt or scalded. Tongue feels cold. **Sweet taste. Profuse ropy saliva.** Sour-bitter belching (Nux-v.). Continuous **nausea, bitter, acrid vomiting,** urging to stool and profuse urine, with **periodic visual disturbances,** blindness, hemiopia, etc., accompany ophthalmic **migraine** (right); involving teeth. BILIOUS, WATERY, SOUR OR ACRID VOMITUS, WITH BURNING. **Burning; < along whole digestive tract;** not > by cold drinks. Sore over liver. BILIOUS, ACRID, WATERY STOOLS; BURN LIKE FIRE. **Painless cholera morbus.** Diabetes. Goitre. Zoster (right). The hip feels wrenched out. Shooting laming pains along limb. Sciatica (left.).

Related to: Ars., Merc., Phos.

JABORANDI

SPHERE OF ACTION
GLANDS.
Eyes.
Nerves.

AGGRAVATION
Start of menses.
Cold.
Exhaustion.

Dryness, then hypersecretion of upper respiratory tract and salivary glands. **Colliquative states. Tendency to sweat and take cold.** ....Very nervous and tremulous. Visual disturbances. Eyestrain. Asthenopia. Nervous deafness, > noise. Tension in salivary glands. **Salivation.** Mumps. Nausea on using eyes or looking at moving objects. Stubborn vomiting of pregnancy. Violent ebullitions to heart and chest. Menses start with coldness, throbbing in head and pelvis and backache. Red skin. **Sweats**, with palpitation, general pulsation and tremor. Nervous sweats. Exophthalmos.

Related to: Agar., Ant-t., Ip.

JALAPA

SPHERE OF ACTION	AGGRAVATION
Intestines.	**Night.**
Stomach.	Eructations.

Child is good all day, but screams and tosses about all night. Colic. **Stools watery,** muddy or sour; bloody.

Related to: Coloc.

JATROPHA

SPHERE OF ACTION	AGGRAVATION
Stomach.	Covering.
Intestines.	Morning.
	Summer.

AMELIORATION
Hands in cold water.

Icy coldness; of lower limbs. .... Vomiting; albuminous; **easy. Loud gurgle, like water from a bung-hole, in abdomen; then profuse gushing stools.** Rice water stools. Violent cramps, that draw the calves flat.

Related to: Crot-t.

JUSTICIA ADHATODA

SPHERE OF ACTION
Nerves
- Cerebro-spinal.
Respiratory membranes.

AGGRAVATION
Close room.
Dust.
Noise.
Eating

Sensitive. .... Generalized dry catarrh. Fits of sneezing, with lachrymation and **loss of smell and taste.** Coryza; fluent; acrid; with violent sneezing, coughing or asthmatic attacks. Long paroxysms of violent retching cough; as if chest would burst; with a **bronchial rattle; obstructing the breath;** with sneezing, stiffening out (Ip.), trembling or convulsions; with fever. Whooping cough. Tough expectoration. Puffy hands and feet in A. M. Chilliness.

Related to: Ip., Dros., Puls.

KALIUM ARSENICOSUM

SPHERE OF ACTION

Cardio-vascular system

AGGRAVATION
Touch.
Noise.
Cold feet.
1-3 A.M.

AMELIORATION
Rainy days.

Nights are filled with suffering. Aversion to open air. Palpitation; with nephritis. **Burning,** in throat, aching in stomach, etc. Passes much gas, then diarrhea. Black leg ulcer, running bloody, foul water; with cutting, burning, itching and dyspnea. Chilly and sensitive to cold. Can't get too warm, even in summer.

KALIUM BICHROMICUM

SPHERE OF ACTION

MUCOUS MEMBRANES
- **Air passages.**
- **NOSE.**
- **Pharynx.**
- **Stomach.**
- Duodenum.

Fibrous tissue.

Ligaments.

JOINTS.

Skin.

Circulation.

Kidneys.

Root of nose, tongue, or penis, etc.

AGGRAVATION

COLD
- **Damp.**
- Open air.
- Spring.
- **Undressing.**

MORNING; After sleep.

2-3 A.M.

Protruding tongue (Cist.).

Hot weather.

Alcohol.

Beer.

Suppressed catarrh.

AMELIORATION

Heat.

Motion.

Slow, deep **processes**; little fever, but **great weakness.** Sickly, chilly and cachectic. Fair, fat and sluggish. Bitings, like bugs. ADHESIVE SECRETIONS; STICKY taste, expectoration, leucorrhea, foot-sweat, etc. STRINGY, TOUGH, **lumpy or thick discharges.** Fibrous exudates going downward. **Yellow,** eyes, vision, tongue, etc. Slow reaction. Heaviness. Crusts in nose, on skin, etc. **Pains in small spots; jump about** and finally attack stomach. Sharp stitches. Ascending; gastric pains, chills, heats, etc. Furred membranes. **Old catarrhs.** Ulcers; with dark dots, deep, perforating, round; look punched out; septal; peptic; with overhanging edges or thick crusts. Like a solid block on forehead. As of a hair on tongue, in nostril, etc. Internal itching; vagina, lungs, etc. **Cracking joints.** ....
Indifferent. Indolent. Pains outward along (right) brow. Bristling hair. **Blindness, then pain over one eye,** < cold. > pressing on root of nose. Migraine. Vision seems crossed, > looking with one eye. Eye-

lids red, itching, swelled, granular. **Nose** pains at bridge or root; **pressure or stuffed at root**; retains foul secretions. Abscess. Ozaena. **Nasal discharges, acrid**; profuse; green clinkers. **Nasal diphtheria.** Snuffles. Radiating toothache; with swelled glands. **Tongue**, glistens; cracked, smooth or heavy, lemon yellow cast; **pains when protruded.** **Sticky month.** Sweet, metallic taste. **Hawks thick mucus; must wipe it away.** (edema of uvula. Fissured pharynx. Throat; dry; burning in; something sticks in; with pains into neck and shoulders. Craves beer. Regurgitates liquids. Vomits bright yellow water. Sore spot in stomach, or food lies like a load. Constriction from liver to shoulder. Gelatinous stools or **gushes of brown, frothy water,** then burning and tenesmus, < after rising. Heavy kidneys. A drop remains after urinating. Constriction at root of penis, **Acrid leucorrhea.** Milk is stringy. Hoarseness. Laryngitis. Tickling cough, after eating; with eructations; > heat; then vertigo. Under sternum : rawness; **pains through to back.** As of a bar across chest. Asthma. Deep cough with stringy expectoration. Heart weak; feels cold. Paralytic weakness of hands. Sciatica, > flexing leg. Sore heels. Pains along border of foot. Stubborn suppuration. Pustules with black apices. Skin, > in cool air. Hot flushes, then **sticky** sweat, then chill. Cold sweat on hands and feet. Chill with sweat.

Complementary: Ars., Phos., **Psor.**

Related to: Kali-c., Merc., Phyt., Puls.

KALIUM BROMATUM

SPHERE OF ACTION	AGGRAVATION
MIND.	**Mental exertion.**
NERVES	Emotions.
- **Brain.**	Periodically
- **Spine.**	- Night.
- Genitals.	- Summer.
Larynx.	- New moon.
Skin.	

Sexual excesses.

Puberty.

AMELIORATION

When busy.

Slow onset. **No pain.** General numbness; < occiput.
.... **Depressive delusions.** Nervous. Suspicion; fears
people, yet can't be alone, in the dark, etc.; looks on all sides; fidgety,
busy hands, fumbles. Moves arms about wildly. Mania. Night terrors.
Melancholy; remorse, **wrings hands,** bursts into tears, etc. Slow,
hesitates; omits or mixes up words. Indifference. Hebetude. **Poor
memory.** Brain-fag. Vertigo, as if ground gave way. Catarrh descends
to larynx (Am-br.). Cutting colic. Green, watery stool; with rapid
collapse. Cholera infantum. Depressed sexual power. Flooding of
young women. Croupy cough. Cool skin. Acne. Sleepy.

Related to: Calc., Con., Op., Stram.

Antidotes: Zinc-p.

KALIUM CARBONICUM

SPHERE OF ACTION	AGGRAVATION
Muscles; Ligaments	**Cold**
- HEART.	- AIR.
- **Uterus.**	- Water.
- LUMBAR.	- Drafts.
SEROUS and **Mucous**	- Changes after
membranes	- Overheating.
- CHEST (right lower).	- Exertion.
- Joints.	Time
Eyes.	- 2-3 A.M.
Blood.	- **Winter.**
Left side.	- Before menses.
	- Lying.
	- **On painful** or left side.

Loss of fluids.

After labor.

AMELIORATION

Warmth.

Sitting with elbows on knees.

Open air.

WEAKENING, **intellect; muscles, heart, back,** limbs, etc. **Gives out,** leans on something or **lies down;** with **backache,** profuse secretions, sweat, etc. **Soft, thin blooded and cold.** Old, fleshy, **dropsical** or paralytic. SHARP STITCHINGS, stabbings or catches in joints, muscles, **chest,** head, epigastrium, **back,** etc. **Throbbing, numb or cold single parts,** abdomen, fingers, etc. Acrid discharges. Sub-acute conditions. Parts lain on are painful and go to sleep. Peevish. Easily startled; < touch; on dropping to sleep. **Anxious aversion to solitude.** Headaches, into eyes; wake from sleep. Eyes weak. Vision, spotted; like drops before. **Puffs over,** inner angle of eyes or baggy upper lids. Stitches out of ears. Head colds; go to chest. Nose stuffed, > open air; swelled; yellow-green or crusty discharge. Puffy face. Slimy mouth. Gray tongue. Itching gums. Hawks up tough mucus in A. M. DIFFICULT SWALLOWING. Salty regurgitation. Vomits sour mucus. **Sensitive, distended stomach and abdomen. Fulness;** from little, even after drinks; **as if full of water.** Anxious at epigastrium. **Throbbing** back of stomach; at navel. Gastric pains going to back, chest, limbs, etc. Flatulence. **Hard tympanites. Stool difficult; of large, hard lumps,** then burning or torn feeling. Piles inflamed, bleeding; descend when urinating or coughing, > riding horseback; stick like fine needles, > cool bathing. Burning in left kidney. Nocturnal enuresis of adults. **Urine foamy,** with thick, tough, red sediment. Delayed first menses. Amenorrhea. **Colic, then irritating menses;** > washing. Inefficient labor pains. Catarrhal aphonia. Respiration short, < least motion or walking; **asthmatic** alternating with diarrhea; with vertigo. Incessant, hard retching or **choking,** futile cough; then vomiting. Pertussis. Lungs seem to stick to ribs. Pleurisy.

Stabbing chest pains. Heart seems to hang by a thread; pains toward left scapula. Palpitation; then weakness; in valvular disease. Arrhythmia. Cardiac degeneration. Fine stitches in mammae. Everything affects the small of the back or pains start there. **Back and legs give out;** feel heavy. Lumbago. Arms weak; numb pinching in left. Painful tips of fingers and toes. Edema of left foot. **Sensitive soles;** skin. Dry hair and skin. General itching or hives; during menses. Talks in sleep. **Pulse small, soft, variable, intermittent or dicrotic.** Chilly; with hot hands; and sleepiness; in open air. Internal burning. Sweat scanty, foul on feet.

Complementary: Carb-v., Nit-ac., Phos.

Related to: Calc-hyp., Lyc., Phos.

KALIUM CHLORICUM

SPHERE OF ACTION	AGGRAVATION
Blood.	Cold.
Nerve sheaths.	Mercury.
Mouth.	
Rectum.	
Kidneys.	

Profound prostration. Coldness; and easy **hemorrhage;** nosebleed, bloody stools, etc. Scurvy. **Fetid** mouth, lochia, etc. Gray, white, plastic exudates. .... Swelled face, in morning, ankles in evening. Mercurial salivation. Aphthae. Noma. Sudden vomiting. Gas colic. Continuous rectal pain; in diarrhea. Nephritis. Albuminuria. Constricted chest. Right pulse full, left small. **Coldness;** in blood; tongue, throat, precordium, arms, feet, skin, etc.

KALIUM IODATUM

SPHERE OF ACTION
Glands.

Frontal sinus.

Nose.

Eyes.

Lungs.

- Upper lobe.

Periosteum.

AGGRAVATION
Heat.

Pressure.

Touch.

Night.

Damp.

Mercury.

Changing weather.

Jolting.

Cold foods.

AMELIORATION
Motion.

Cool air.

Open air.

Incipient organic changes; gouty-rheumatic, syphilitic, rickety, etc. Many and diverse symptoms. Feels used up. Cachexy. **Stubborn chronicity.** Arterio-sclerosis. **Craves motion in open air.** Various symptoms. Crushing or sharp stitching pains. **Weakness.** COPIOUS, **watery, acrid, salty**, thick, **green** or foul discharges. Catarrh. Pains long after trauma. **Diffuse soreness;** of affected part. Edematous swelling ....Irritable, harsh tempered and cruel. Can't think. Despondent. Bad temper. Harsh. Head bone pains, lightning like, < warmth or lying on part. Big head and small jaws; rickets. Tender spots on head. Bilateral headache. Scalp sore; fissured. Burning, **watery, puffy eyes.** Chemosis. **Tinnitus.** Acrid coryza with dyspnea and salivation. Burning throb in nasal and accessory cavities. Colds from every damp day. Red, swelled **nose; tight pain at root**, zygoma and root of tongue. Takes cold. Violent sneezing. **Acrid**, watery coryza, < cool air. Ozena. Glutinous mucus on lips in A. M. (Zinc-c.). Nagging toothache. Taste salty; bitter on waking. Salivation. Sorethroat of speakers (Arum-t.). Flatulence; squeaking. Early diarrhea of phthisis. Frequent stools and urine. Leucorrhea, corrosive; like meat washings. **Air hunger;** with flatulency, in A. M.; awakens strangling. Whistling, asthmatic breathing. **Raw air-passages.** Croupy hoarseness. Dry bronchitis. Frothy expectoration. Backward chest pains. Pneumonia. Pain, sternum to back. Painful lumps; in scalp. Giant urticaria. Chilly in bones; in painful parts. Heat in evening; uncovers, then chills. Alternate heat and chill. Heat with shudders. Hot and dry, then drenching sweat. Profuse night sweats, which >. Actinomycosis.

Antidotes: Merc., Nit-ac.

Related to: Iod., Sulph., Syph.

KALIUM MURIATICUM

SPHERE OF ACTION

EPITHELIUM

- **Throat.**
- **Eustachian tube.**
- Middle ear.

Mucous glands.
Occiput (left).
Muscles.
Joints.
Shoulder (left).
One side, < left.
Crosswise.

AGGRAVATION

Open air.
Cold drinks; Drafts.
Heat of bed.
Lying.
Night.
Dampness.
Motion.
Sprains.
Fats.
Rich foods.
During menses.

AMELIORATION

Cold drinks.
Rubbing.
Letting hair down.

WHITENESS. MILKY WHITE, viscid, sticky, **thick,** slimy or lumpy secretions. **Catarrhs. Toughness. Tough,** plastic or **fibrinous exudates. Hard deposits.** Stubborn infiltrations. Swelled **glands. Sore, cutting** (outward—Asaf.) or **stitching, shifting pains.** Crawling. Numbness. Slow reaction............ **Irritable or angry;** at trifles. Discontent, discouraged; fears evil. Sits in silence. Stunning shock in or a leaden load holds occiput down; < binding hair, > wraps. Brain feels loose. Copious, white dandruff. **Head sweats.** Pustular cornea. Cloudy lens. Scintillations on coughing. Snapping, itching or as of a plug in ears. **Deafness. Eustachian occlusion** or soreness. Face bluish; sunken. Eruption around mouth. **Tongue** mapped; gray or **white at base.** Aphthae. Scorbutic gums. Salty taste. Throat grayish-white; ulcerated; chronic sorethroat. Tonsils swelled; inflamed. **Hawks out thick white mucus.** Loathes fat or rich foods. Nausea; with shivers. Stomach heavy; at night. Vomits food. **Fulness in abdomen after eating. Pale,** hard or flocculent **stools. Anus, sore,** < walking or stools; itching or crawling, after stool. Piles. Dribbling urination. Nephritis. **Difficult or oppressed breathing.** Bronchitis. Expectoration sticky or flies from mouth. Dark, clotted or tarry menses. Rawness in chest. Flushes of heat in chest. Coldness at heart. Painful breasts before or at menses. Heaviness under right shoulder. Buzzing under left scapula. Backache, > lying. Lightning pains from small of back to feet. **Cold hands** and feet. Cramps in limbs; in legs. Twitching thighs. Tension in legs alternates with tension in arm (left). Cold foot-sweat. Cutting in bones (Sabad.). Branny skin. Anxious dreams.

Complementary: Calc-s.

Follows: Ferr-p.

Related to: Bry., Puls.

KALIUM NITRICUM

SPHERE OF ACTION
Cavities
- Blood-vessels.
- Heart.
- **Kidneys.**
Vasomotors.
Respiratory organs.

AGGRAVATION
Walking.
Cold.
Damp.
Taking cold.
Veal.
Lying with head low.

AMELIORATION
Gentle motion.

Increased secretion into cavities. Very weak. **Hemorrhage.** Sudden edema. Throbbing. **Dull stitches. Numb,** as if wooden. ....Faintness. External angle of right eye twitches, < chewing. Nausea. Epigastric or sub-sternal pains go toward axillae. Dark, fluid stools. Dull kidney pains. **Diuresis.** Profuse, inky menses. Rapid, gasping breathing; sits upright. VIOLENT DYSPNEA; **can only drink in sips.** Congestion of right lung. Asthma. Free, sour expectoration >. Relapses of phthisis. Palpitation, < lying. Pain from back into chest. Hands and fingers feel swelled. **External coldness;** chin; skin. **Internal burning.**

Related to: Camph., Glon.

KALIUM PHOSPHORICUM

SPHERE OF ACTION

Nerves

- Brain.

- Cord.

Excretions.

One side.

AGGRAVATION

Slight
- Excitement.
- **Worry.**
- **Mental fatigue.**
Touch.
- Pain.
- Cold.
- Dry air.
- Puberty.

AMELIORATION

Sleep.
Eating.
Gentle motion (Ferr., Puls.).

NERVOUS, SENSITIVE, WEAK AND EASILY FAGGED, especially **by pain,** etc. Neurasthenia. Paralysis. PUTRID, or goldenyellow excretions; coat on tongue, stool, etc. Foul odor of body. Carrion odor of secretions. **Irregular menses,** pulse, etc. Stitches. Little pain. Paralytic weakness...................... Shyness. Nervous and sensitive. Dread. Gloom. Averse to her own. Angry. Vertigo on facing sun. Eyes; burn, sting and swim in tears; yellow-gray, milky secretion;

left lid droops. Retinitis. Reflex eye symptoms. **Itching in posterior nares. Sneezing;** at 2 A.M. Hay fever; prophylactic. **Sad, care-worn look.** Brown stripe at edge of hair. Palate feels greasy. Tongue yellow, like liquid mustard. Aphthae. Craves ice water, vinegar and sweets. **Craving hunger;** soon **after eating;** and weakness follow painless, watery stools. Entero-colitis. Empty gnawing in stomach, > eating, Cutting in abdomen. Golden yellow, putrid, hot stools. Milky urine. Enuresis nocturna. Sexual erethism, with prostration after coition or nightly emissions. Horribly foul leucorrhea. Aphonia. Nervous asthma. Axillary sweat smells of onions. Spinal irritation. Prickling hands and feet. Numb fingertips. Foot feels frostbitten. Pains in soles. Drowsy. **Yawning.** Inactive skin.

Related to: Caust., Cocc., Pic-ac., Zinc.

KALIUM SULPHURICUM

SPHERE OF ACTION
EPITHELIUM
- Respiratory organs.
- **Skin.**
Glands.

AGGRAVATION
Warmth; Room; AIR.
Noise.
Consolation.
Evening.

AMELIORATION
Cool air.
Walking.
Fasting.

Torpid processes. PROFUSE, DEEP YELLOW DISCHARGES; **thin** or sticky. **Suppuration. Stitching,** tearing, festering **pains, that shift about.................Hurried.** Irritable. **Yellow, slimy tongue.** As of a heavy load on stomach, Oxaluria. Pyelitis. Croupy hoarseness. **Coarse rattle in chest.** Arthritic nodes. Rheumatism, < heat. Dry skin. **Desquamation.** Ulcers ooze thin, **yellow water. Profuse, easy sweat.**

Related to: Puls.

KALMIA LATIFOLIA

SPHERE OF ACTION
NERVES
- SPINAL.
- Eyes.
- Face (right).
HEART.
Circulation.
Joints.
Skin.
Right; Head; Deltoid.
Left; Chest; Arm.

AGGRAVATION
MOTION
- Lying on left side.
- Bending forward.
- Looking down.
Heat.
Becoming cold.
With the sun.
AMELIORATION
Eating.
Cloudy weather.
Continued motion.

Aching, bruised, stiff feeling. Tingling, numbness, trembling or paralytic weakness. Changing pains; shoot outward along nerves; or dull tearing, crushing, **moving** downward, **then suddenly, to heart** or alternating with cardiac symptoms, or between upper and lower limbs. Neuralgia. Rheumatism...................... Vertigo. Cracking noise in head. Shooting from nape to vertex and face. Maddening supraorbital (right) pain. HEART; irritable; **pains, sharp,** burning; formication; numbness; **weak;** radiating to left scapula or arm; **taking away the breath;** fluttering; palpitation, visible; paralysis. **Pulse very slow;** weak, tremulous. Brachialgia. Stiff, eyelids, lips, skin, etc.

Complementary: Benz-ac., Spig.

Related to: Acon., Dig., Rhus-t., Spig.

KREOSOTUM

SPHERE OF ACTION
MUCOUS MEMBRANES
- DIGESTIVE TRACT.
- **Gums.**
- **Stomach.**
- **Abdomen.**
- **Female genitals.**
- Uterus.
- BLOOD.
- **Teeth.**

AGGRAVATION
DENTITION.
Pregnancy,
Rest.
Cold.
Eating.
Lying.
Summer.
During menses.
6 P.M. to 6 A.M.

AMELIORATION
Warmth.
Hot food.
Motion.

Miserable and weak. **Profuse, FOUL, HOT, ACRID discharges;** sputum, eructations, etc.; **redden the part. Rawness. Burning like fire. Pulsation;** general. **Hemorrhage;** passive; brown, dark. **Lumpy** discharges, menses, etc. Ulceration. Heaviness. Fulness. Tumefaction. Scurvy. Marasmus. **Black,** teeth, leucorrhea, lochia, etc......................... **Dissatisfied** with every thing; wants things, then throws them away and wants something else. Screams at night. **Cross, wilful and obstinate.** Longs for death. Stupid. Buzzing in head. Yellow pallor, with red blotches (Iod.); during chill or heat. TEETH SOON DECAY; black spots on; intolerable ache, < pregnancy; painful dentition. **Puffy, bluish, bleeding, painful gums.** Aphthae or salivation, of pregnancy. Taste bitter, low down in throat. Icy cold epigastrium. Frothy eructations. Nausea. Vomiting; long after meals (Aeth., **Ferr.,** Plat.); undigested food, sweetish; of pregnancy; of uterine ulcer. As of a lump pressing down on bladder. Brown, watery, lienteric stools. **Urination** hurried; **involuntary when lying. Diuresis.** Profuse, lumpy, intermittent menses, < lying. **Leucorrhea; gushing;** like bloody water; with itching. Tormenting cough, with little expectoration; with sore larynx and chest. Senile bronchitis. Neglected phthisis. Hectic, chest; deep pain take her breath; anxious heaviness. Dragging from back to genitals; as if to come out. Violently itching, moist or scurfy eczema on eyelids, face, joints, back of hands. Ulcers break out and heal repeatedly; bleed after coitus. Cold sweat.

Complementary: Sulph.

Related to: Arum-t., Ars., Carb-ac., Graph., Nit-ac., Psor.

LAC CANINUM

SPHERE OF ACTION
NERVES.

THROAT; **Right to left, then back again or reverse.**

Female generative organs.

AGGRAVATION
TOUCH.
Jar.
During menses.
Cold air, or wind, or drinks.
Morning of one day and evening of the next (Eup-per.).

AMELIORATION
Open air.

SYMPTOMS ALTERNATE SIDES, throat, ovaries, etc., or wander about. **Glistening parts.** Glistening, throat, ulcers, etc. Over sensitive; can't have parts, fingers, etc., touch each other-................................. **Full of imaginations**; horrid, of snake vermin, **as if floating,** etc. Every symptom seems a settled disease. Hysteria at height of sexual orgasm. THROAT SORE; has glistening **patches of china whiteness;** or red glistening; gives out from exertion; < at start and close of menses. Diphtheria; paralysis after. Menses green, gushing or ammoniacal; hoarseness, during. Breasts sore and swelled, before menses. Galactorrhea. DRIES UP THE MILK. Scanty milk. Cold creepings down back. Sore heels.

Related to: Lach., Lyss., Puls.

LAC DEFLORATUM

SPHERE OF ACTION
NUTRITION.
BLOOD.

Heart

Head (left).

Thigh (outer).

AGGRAVATION
COLD
- **Least draft.**
Wet.
- Hands in cold water.
Milk.
Loss of sleep.
Weekly.

AMELIORATION
Rest.
Pressure of bandage.

Exhaustion. Despondency. Vertigo, < lying on left side. Blind then throbbing frontal headache, with much pale urine. Migraine. Photophobia. Painless swelling of face. Pale, sickly look. Anemia. **Averse to milk. Nausea. Soar vomiting. Dry, large, painful stools.** Amenorrhea. Boring, sore pain in kidneys. Polyuria, < during pain. Scanty flow of milk. **Always chilly.** Cold finger-tips. Skin is supersensitive to cold. Given to restore milk.

Related to: Nat-m.

LACHESIS MUTUS

SPHERE OF ACTION
Mind.
Throat.
NERVES
- CUTANEOUS.
- VASOMOTOR.
- **Sympathetic.**
- PNEUMO-GASTRIC.
BLOOD; HEART.
CIRCULATION.
LEFT SIDE; **Then right**

AGGRAVATION
SLEEP; AFTER.
MORNING.
HEAT
- SPRING.
- SUMMER.
- SUN.
- ROOM.
- DRINKS.
SWALLOWING; EMPTY;
Liquids.

- THROAT   SENSITIVE TO
- OVARIES   - SLIGHT TOUCH OR
FEMALES.   PRESSURE OF CLOTHES;
Vertex.   < NECK, **Waist** (Apis, Brom.,
                                  Graph.), Noise.
                                  RETARDED DISCHARGES.
                                  Start and close of menses.
                                  CLIMAXIS.
                                  ALCOHOL.
                                  Cloudy weather.

AMELIORATION

OPEN AIR.

FREE SECRETIONS.

Hard pressure.

Bathing part.

COLD DRINKS.

Rapid onset, intensity, prostration or malignancy. LEFT-SIDED COMPLAINTS, OR MOVING FROM LEFT TO RIGHT. Sepsis. Disintegration. Gangrene; diabetic. Carbuncle. Erysipelas. Blueness; hands. FETOR; of acrid, discharges; oris; stools, etc. HEMORRHAGE, thin; dark particles; nose-bleed; vicarious; bloody urine, etc. Purpura. ASCENDING SENSATIONS, in throat; from eyes over vertex; from nape; from ovary to heart; chills; FLUSHES OF HEAT; **rushes of blood.** A LUMP; ascends throat and is swallowed back again; in liver, abdomen, rectum; rolls about in bladder, etc. EXCESSIVE PAINFULNESS; **of throat;** ulcers; spots over body. **Constriction; of throat,** > eating; as of a skull cap; of anus. **Drawing;** vertex to jaws; in **rectum,** etc. Tremor; of tongue; hands, etc. Hard throbbing or **hammering** (Ferr.). Congestion. Apoplexy. Epilepsy.............................Nervous, excitable. LOQUACITY; **rambling;** then sadness or repeats same thing. **Compelling delusions.** Persistent, erotic ideas, without ability. Depression; on awaking. **Insane jealousy. Suspicion.** Feels full of poison. Fears, going to sleep, lying down, or that heart will stop.

Indolence. Vertigo, < turning to right. Headache; heavy; bursting; down nose side (right) feels cut off. Eyes feel small. Nose; **stopped coryza**; discharges with every cough; bloody pus from; rum blossom (**Agar.**, Led.). Face purple, mottled; netted veinlets; dusky during heat. Faceache. Lower jaw drops. Septic mumps. Aphthae. Much thick, pasty saliva. Tongue catches on teeth. Thick, blundering speech. Peppery taste. Can't bear anything before mouth or nose. THROAT; PAINFUL, into ears; as of a soft body in; **choking**; MUST LOOSEN COLLAR; hot lump in; pit feels swelled or sore spots back of pit. SWALLOWING; the wrong way; **painful**; returns through nose. Diphtheria; laryngeal. Tonsillitis. Quinsy. Hawks foul pellets from throat. Thirsty, but fears to drink. Dipsomania. **Soreness or cramp in epigastrium.** Sore festering throb, deep in liver. Septic gall-bladder. Pain from anus to navel. Constipation of pregnancy. Piles; < coughing. Pain in left ovary; must lift covers. **Dark, scanty menses. Suffocates on dropping to sleep.** Must take deep breaths. Air hunger. Tickling, choking cough, < **touching neck** or auditory canal, > retching out a little expectorate. Larynx, as of a skin hanging in, or a valve. **Heart weak;** turns over or too big, as if. Carditis; metastatic. Axilla; swelled glands. Numb, left arm; finger-tips. Cracks in skin, at corner of nails. Cold knees, or cold, foul foot-sweat. Toes feel broken. **Mottled** or livid skin; dark marks. Eating **ulcers**, on legs; with dark areolae; fungoid; **varicose.** Sleepless from cerebral irritation; tipplers. Frightful dreams; of snakes. Dilated capillaries. Chill, < drinking; with sweat. HEAT; **on vertex;** IN FLUSHES, **on waking or falling to sleep.** Sweat; about neck, during sleep; in axillae; bloody; staining blackish; garlicky.

Complementary: Lyc., Phos., Zinc-i.

Related to: Caust., Sep., Zinc.

LAPPA ARCTIUM

SPHERE OF ACTION
Secretions.
Skin.
Liver.
Joints.

AGGRAVATION
Cold wet.
Shaking.
Lying on right side.
Violent exertion.

AMELIORATION
Cloudy weather.

Heavy, sore aching as if lying uncomfortably. **Numbness;** lumbar region. Numb, aching calves. Constriction. .... Vertigo, with nausea and vomiting. Weight on vertex. Red about eyes and across nose. Face, < touch. SOURNESS; sour taste of meat; all food turns sour, vomits it. Trembling in chest. Bruised, sore uterus. Front of thighs weak. Sores about joints. **Eruptions;** sticky; on head, face, etc. Moist, foul eczema. Many small boils. AXILLARY SWEAT; COLD, **runs down chest;** foul.

Complementary: Mag-c.

LATRODECTUS

SPHERE OF ACTION
HEART.
Vaso-motors.
Blood.

AGGRAVATION
Least motion; Even of hands.
Exertion.

Nausea, then abdominal pain. Transfixation of pain or sinking at epigastrium..........................**Gasps, fears to lose breath and die. Restless; with cardiac pains; and prostrated.** Precordial anxiety. Apnea. CARDIAC PAIN; **violent;** sharp to shoulder or **both arms** (left) (Kalm.), with **numbness. Angina pectoris.** Quick, feeble, thready pulse. Skin cold as marble. Dreams of flying. Hard ache in axillae.

Related to: Tarent.

LAUROCERASUS

SPHERE OF ACTION	AGGRAVATION
MIND.	**Sitting up.**
BRAIN.	Exertion.
	Cold.
Nerves.	**AMELIORATION**
Gullet.	**Lying with head low.**
Chest.	Eating.
Respiration.	Sleep.
Heart.	Open air.

Symptoms accompanied by SUDDEN DEBILITY, **lack of reaction, blunted senses, coldness** or **cyanosis. Weak sphincters.** Sinkings. Long faints. Falling down; sensation; in brain; in abdomen, heart, etc. Nervous collapse. Apoplexy. Internal burning. Hemorrhage; of thin blood. Twitchings; facial...................... SUDDEN LOSS OF MEMORY, from pain, fright, etc. Head, < 11 A. M.—1 P. M. Speechlessness. Nightly tearing in vertex. Eyes open, protrude, staring. Objects look large. **Livid face.** Blue babies. NOISY SWALLOWING, then **gurgling flatulence.** Spasm of gullet. Persistent hiccough. Low voice. Raw larynx and trachea. **Suffocation, gasps for breath; on sitting up.** Shallow breathing. Can't raise the chest walls. **Cough, tickling;** spasmodic night cough of phthisis; short or dry; of cardiac origin. Blood flecked or gelatinous sputum. **Holds hand over heart.** Chest pains in cardiac region. Fearful anxiety and restlessness; can't fall to sleep. Coma vigil. Weak, variable, slow or irregular pulse. Cool, livid skin.

Related to: Am-c., Gels., Hydr-ac., Prun-s.

LEDUM PALUSTRE

SPHERE OF ACTION

Fibrous tissue
- JOINTS (Small).
- **Tendons.**
- Eyes.
- Heels.
- **Ankles.**

Capillary circulation
- Skin.
- Lungs.

Periosteum.

Blood.

Nerves.

Left side.

AGGRAVATION

Warm
- **Covers.**
- Stove.
- Air.

Injury.

Motion.

Night.

Eggs.

Wine.

AMELIORATION

Cool
- **Bathing.**
- Air.

Purple, puffy and chilly, yet averse to external warmth. Ascending effects; from feet. Shifting, tearing pain. Painful, cold, edematous joints. Parts become weak, numb, cold and wither. Torpidity. Gouty-rheumatic-hemorrhagic persons. Tipsters. Dropsy. Rushes of blood. **Hemorrhage;** bright, frothy. Petechiae. ....
Raging, pulsating headache; < covers. Scalp, < dampness. **Blood-shot or bruised eyes.** Persistent nose-bleed. Mottled or red (pimply) face. Sub-mental gland swelled. Much uric acid sand in urine. Bleeding fibroids. Cough; tormenting; from tickling in larynx; with epistaxis; then sobbing respiration; < receding eruptions. Double inspirations. Hemoptysis: alternating with rheumatism. Stiff, **crampy back; < rising from sitting.** Lumbago. **Hip-joint;** cramps over. Swelled, blotchy, ecchymotic legs and feet. Larval gout. **Sprained ankles.** Feet (dorsae) itch by night and are stiff in A. M. Sore heels. Tender soles. **Wounds, punctured;** twitches in; from nails, stings, etc.; foul pus. **Coldness** of part, < limbs; with the pain; during fever; as if in cold water. Foul sweat. Profuse night-sweat.

Related to: Arn., Bry., Rhus-t., Sec.

LEPTANDRA

SPHERE OF ACTION

Liver.

Right side.

AGGRAVATION
Cold drinks.
Motion.
Periodically.

AMELIORATION
Lying on stomach or side.

Hepato-hemorrhagic diathesis. **Burnings; in hepatic region.** .... Hopeless, weak and drowsy. Craves iced drinks. Bilious vomitus. **Sore or dull bursting ache over gall-bladder, or liver, down over bowels to navel or toward left scapula,** or along spine. Liver swelled transversely. Acute liver conditions. **Gall-stones.** Muddy, watery, morning stool. STOOLS TARRY OR BLACK, FOUL; **stringy,** waxy; spurting; with pain at navel. Dysentery; after diarrhea. Prolapsing piles; **with hemorrhage** (Lach.). Leucorrhea; warm, watery; runs down limbs. Pain in (left) sciatic nerve on sitting. **Nails very thin;** soft and splitting. Jaundice.

Complementary: Phos.

Related to: Bapt., Card-m., Chion.

LILIUM TIGRINUM

SPHERE OF ACTION

VENOUS CIRCULATION
- FEMALE ORGANS.
- **Uterus.**
- **Ovaries.**
- HEART (RIGHT).
- **Rectum.**
- **Bladder.**
Left side.
Nerves.

AGGRAVATION
WARMTH; of room
Motion.
Miscarriages.
Walking.
Standing.
Consolation.

AMELIORATION
Cool, fresh air.
When busy.
Lying on left side.

F- 12

Sunset (Coca, Med., Sel.).
Pressure.
Crossing legs.

FULL, HEAVY or forced out feeling; uterus; heart; eyelids; ovary (left). **Utero-ovarian sagging.** Marked nervo-hysterical reflexes (Con.), especially mental or cardiac. **Nervous tremor;** in hypogastrium, in spine, knees, etc. **Pulsation,** ebullition, gurglings and burnings. **Backward pains;** about eyes; to occiput; from nipples through chest; **from** heart to left scapula. Venous congestion. Acrid discharges. .... **Hurried, nervous, snappish and erotic or depressed.** Fruitless activity. **Wild,** crazy feeling. **Dread;** of insanity; being incurable, etc. Desires finery. Burning headache, < before and after menses; ache over (left), eye; with vertigo and visual effects. Eyes, feel sprained; bite and **burn, < reading.** Yellowish, patchy tongue. Sweet taste—back of mouth. Craves meat. Hunger, as if from spine. Stiff, tense abdomen. Can't bear weight of covers. Sharp pains, < doubling up. Early, morning diarrhea; frequent, small stools; with tenesmus; < after rising. **Heavy dragging or outward urging in pelvis;** must hold parts (Sanic.); **with dysuria.** Ovarian pain, (left); into limb; with pain below (left) breast. Menses free, while moving only. Thin, brown, leucorrhea; acrid. Oppressive load on chest; air hunger; takes long breaths. As of a rivet or ball under (left) mamma. HEART, **feels clutched,** overful, **cold,** weak, hangs by a thread, etc.; pains into (left) arm; < stooping; < lying on (right) side; nervous. **Palpitation.** Neckache, < tire. Broken feeling between scapulae. Pain from hip to hip. Can't walk on uneven ground. Chilly, > open air. Burning palms and soles.

Related to: Aloe, Plat., Puls., Spig.

LITHIUM CARBONICUM

SPHERE OF ACTION
Heart.
Small joints.
Lungs.
Urine.

AGGRAVATION
Night.
Menses; After; Suppressed.

AMELIORATION
Eating.
Urinating.
Motion.

SORE and heavy. Acidity. Outward pressure or as of a dull point. Gout. Rheumatism......................Headache, > eating. Eyes dry from using them. Vertical hemiopia (right). **Red nose.** Lumps of mucus drop into throat. Gnawing in stomach, with pain in left temple (Ars.), > eating. Urine scanty, with much thirst; with red-brown sediment. **Heart pains; sore;** with eye symptoms; going to head; < bending over, > **urinating;** from mammae to arms. Soreness of fingers, > grasping. Dry, harsh skin. Eczema.

Related to: Lyc., Nat-p., Sul-ac.

LOBELIA INFLATA

SPHERE OF ACTION
RESPIRATION.
Vasomotor nerves.
Secretions.
Heart.
Epigastrium.

AGGRAVATION
Cold bathing.
Suppressions.
Sleep; After.
Tobacco.

AMELIORATION
Rapid motion.
Eating a little.

RELAXATION; **with increased secretions and weakness; with** sweat; with deathly sickness all over; with oppressed, **rattling respiration.** Sits with elbows on knees. Prickles all over............ **Flow of saliva;** with retching, hiccough, nausea, dyspnea, etc. **As of a lump** in throat or stomach. **Deathly nausea**; with vertigo; < night and early A. M., > eating or drinking. **Vomiting**; with sweat (cold on face). **Nausea and vomiting, with** profuse sweat; with respiratory symptoms. **Weak, sinking at stomach.** Deep red urine, with red sediment. Urine suppressed or infrequent. **Dyspnea**; nervous; with labor pains; as from a wedge in larynx; > rapid motion; with general prickling. Asthma. Spasmodic cough; with sneezing, belching or gastric pain. **Rattle in chest, but don't expectorate. Constriction or oppressive** fulness in chest. **Pulse** weak, or soft; flowing. Plaques of edema (figurata); with ecchymoses.

Related to: Ant-t., Ip., Tab.

LYCOPODIUM

SPHERE OF ACTION

NUTRITION
- DIGESTIVE TRACT.
- **Portal system.**
- Skin.
URINARY ORGANS.
RIGHT SIDE **to left**
- THROAT.
- **Chest.**
- Ovary.
Brain.
Lungs.

AGGRAVATION

PRESSURE OF CLOTHES.
WARMTH.
Awaking.
Wind.
Eating; to Satiety; Oysters.
Indigestion.
4-8 P.M.

AMELIORATION

WARM DRINKS, food, etc.
Cold applications.
Motion.
Eructations.
Urinating.

Weak from disgestive disturbances. **Repeating or alternating symptoms;** flexion, then extension; automatic acts; flushing then paling, chill after chill, etc. Progressive affections. **Relapses.** Sudden symptoms. Throbbing. Pains cause anger, jerking, etc. ACIDITY; soar taste, eructations, vomitus, etc. Calculi; gall-stones, gravel, tophi. Gout. Thin, withered and FULL OF GAS. Poor circulation; it seems to stand still; limbs feel dead; numb spots. Descending symptoms; emaciation, etc. Early senility. Dropsy. .... Confused over daily affairs. Mentally active, but grows weaker. Can't think. Miscalls or omits words, etc. Paralysis of brain. AWAKES ANGRY, sad or anxious. Sensitive and fearsome. Averse to being alone. Hateful, cranky, domineering, exacting, reserved or despairing. Headache; pain goes to other side, where it is worse; pulsating in occiput at night; < if hot. Hair falls; comes in gray. Dandruff. Eyes half open. Hemiopia. Sees sparks. FANNING OF WINGS OF NOSE. Nose stuffy; dry posteriorly. Acrid ozena. Face yellowish; pale, gray; wrinkled forehead; frowning; twitching. Hydrocephalus. Meningitis; tubercular. Mouth hangs open. (Merc-c., Mur-ac.). Sore lips. Yellow teeth. Tongue; puts it in and out rapidly; trembling; swelled; heavy; lolling; stiff; cracked; painful vesicle on tip. A ball rises and sticks in throat. Sorethroat (right); < cold drinks. Diphtheria. Hunger, but quick satiety; A LITTLE FOOD OVERFILLS. Averse to soups. Incomplete eructations. Epigastric anxiety, pressure, etc. Gnawing in stomach. As of a band about waist. Sensitive, congested liver. MUCH, NOISY FLATULENCE, < lower bowels. Meteorism. Flatulence, pressing out. Abdomen; sore, < lower; alternating sides; brown spots on chest. Colicky babies, < in evening. Stool, most seems to remain, after; contains sand. Alternate diarrhea and constipation. Piles, > hot bathing. Frequent urging to urinate, > riding in cars, etc. Acrid urine. Urine scanty; cries before urinating; red sand in; suppressed. Sexual exhaustion. Pollutions. Violent dysmenorrhea, with fainting. Menses of clots and serum; < stool. Acrid or periodical leucorrhea. Painful coitus. Gas from vagina. Craves air, but is chilled by it. Short, rattling breathing. Salty, green-yellow, lumpy or foul expectoration. Unresolved pneumonia. Dry, teasing cough, with emaciation. Mammae, achy; sore; nodes in (left). Axillary abscess (right). Bubbling at scapulae. Stiff back. Hands numb; cramps in,

and in feet. Fingers twitch during sleep; sticky sweat on. Pains jerk
legs upward. As of a stone under heel. Feet asleep, < heels; acrid
sweat on. DRYNESS; palms, vagina, skin, etc. **Rawness** in folds,
nipples, anus, etc. Suppurating eruptions. Receding boils, erysipelas,
etc. Vascular swellings. Erectile tumors; < before menses. Aneurism.
Rapid pulse, < eating; evening. **Coldness**; icy; head, throat, stomach;
of one foot; < coughing. Chill, then vomits; after first sleep. Burning,
between scapulae. Foul viscid axillary or foot-sweat; like onions.

Complementary: Calc., Iod., Kali-c., Lach.

Follows: Chel. or Graph.

Related to: Carb-v., Sil.

LYCOPUS VIRGINICUS

SPHERE OF ACTION
   HEART.
Circulation.
   Left Side.

AGGRAVATION
Excitement.
Exertion.
Heat.
After sleep.
Lying on (Right) side.
Abuse of heart remedies.
Suppressions.
Thinking of it.

   Irritable weakness. Heart, with many side-symptoms
concimitants). Symptoms vary with heart action or associated with a
RAPID TUMULTUOUS HEART BEAT. **Cardio-hemorrhagic
cases.** HEMORRHAGE, from nose, piles, lungs, etc. Shifting
pains...................... Nervous, hurried and **tremulous. Slow
comprehension. Protruding eyes.** Tawny, expressionless, bloated face.
Polyuria. Choking on lying down. **Heart cough.** HEART; **violent,
excessively rapid** (Phos.), stormy action; heavy beat, at night;
oppression at; pains, sore, aching constriction. **Pulse,** large, full, soft;

don't synchronize with heart. Hot ache beneath (right) scapula. Coldness.

Related to: Cact., Coll., Crat.

LYSSINUM

SPHERE OF ACTION

Nerves.
Cord.
Throat.
Sexual organs.

AGGRAVATION

Running water (Canth., **Stram.**).
Heat of sun.
Glistening objects.
Drafts.

AMELIORATION

Bending backward.
Gentle rubbing.

Spasm. **Overacute senses.** .... Fear. Anger. Rapid speech. Impatience and **violent temper.** Roams about. **Constant spitting**; ropy, frothy saliva. Spasm of gullet. Can't urinate unless he hears water run. Sexual excitement. Sensitive womb. Barking cough. Pain in neck. Blueness. Convulsions.

Related to: Lac-c., Lach.

MAGNESIUM CARBONICUM

SPHERE OF ACTION

Malar bones.
DIGESTIVE TRACT
- **Stomach.**
- Bowels.
- Liver.
NERVES
- Facial.
- Dental.

AGGRAVATION

NIGHT.
Rest.
Noise.
Cold
- **Changes of weather.**
- Wind; Drafts.
Food; Starchy; Milk.

Slight causes, **touch,** etc.
Children.
Nurselings.
AMELIORATION
Motion; Walking about.
Open air.

Ailing, worn out, **nervous, flatulent** and **flabby. Sour;** all over (Rheum); regurgitation; foamy vomitus; **stool,** etc. **Emaciation.** Marasmus. **Sharp shoots along nerves; must walk about.** Numb, distended feeling. Can't bear hands covered, yet chilled by uncovering. ....Heavy brain. Tearing, digging, boring face or toothache; < pregnancy; > cold. **Sudden deafness.** Waxy pallor. Hawks cheesy masses from throat. Sorethroat at menses. Nibbling appetite. Vomits undigested milk or bitter water. **Cutting colic. Stool, frothy;** GREENISH, LIKE WATER AND SCUM OF A POND; lienteric, with gelatinous or fatty masses; grass green. Menses like thick, dark molasses; **tarry;** viscid; < **night** and on rising; leave a fast stain. Craves open air. Paroxysmal cough; difficult, thin, salty or bloody sputum. Heavy, weary feet. Chilly; takes cold, with coryza, toothache, sorethroat, etc.; before menses; and dry. Sour, greasy, indelible sweat.

Antidodes: Cham., Nux-v., Puls.

Related to: Rheum.

MAGNESIUM MURIATICUM

SPHERE OF ACTION
NERVES.
LIVER.
Digestion.
Pelvic organs
- **Uterus.**
- **Rectum.**
Women.

AGGRAVATION
LYING ON RIGHT SIDE.
Night.
Noise.
Sea bathing.
Eating; Salt foods.
MILK.

AMELIORATION
HARD PRESSURE.
Lying bent
Hanging down.
Gentle motion.
Cool, open air.

Nervous; with hepato-uterine or cardiac symptoms. Globus.
Hysteria. Crampings. Dryness. **Burning.** Darting. Dinner causes
faintness, dyspnea, etc. Chronicity........................... Irritable. Yellow
sclera. Tinea ciliaris. Acrid, crusty ozena. **Broad, yellow, scalloped**
tongue; feels burnt. Loss of taste and smell. Craves sweets. Pain from
liver to spine or epigastrium. **Sore, enlarged liver;** drags if lies on
(left) side. Cramp in gall-bladder, > eating. Flatulence. STOOLS DRY;
KNOTTY; of little balls, like sheep dung; gray; crumbling at anus.
Must press on bladder to urinate. **Profuse, dark, lumpy menses;** like
pitch; with cramps, backache and pains in thighs. **Gushes of**
leucorrhea, follow each cramp or stool. Palpitation; > motion or
lying on (left) side. Throb below (left) scapula. Bruised or burning
feeling in hips and back. Cramps in back, < walking; in thighs, <
sitting. Dead fingertips. Tense thighs and calves; must move limbs.
Ankles cold or nervous, < night. Cutting in heels. Yellow, thin, foul
pus. Jaundice. Sweat on head and feet.

Related to: Nat-m., Puls., Sep.

MAGNESIUM PHOSPHORICUM

SPHERE OF ACTION
NERVES
- **Face.**
- Head.

Muscles.
Right side.

AGGRAVATION
COLD
- AIR.
- Uncovering.
- Drafts.
- Water (Calc.).
Lying on right side.
Touch.

Periodicity.
NIGHT.
Milk.
Exhaustion.
AMELIORATION
WARMTH.
HOT BATHING.
Pressure.
Doubling up.
Rubbing.

Tall, slender, dark and neurotic. **Nervous, tense and subject to sudden, violent neuralgias, colics, cramps, etc.** SUDDEN **paroxysms of pain;** sharp **shooting like lightning, suddenly** changing place; in waves; radiating, boring or constricting; **extorting cries; causing restlessness, prostration, etc. Twitchings.** Tic-convulsif. Spasmodic effects; hiccough, yawning, chorea, writer's cramp, etc. Much pain. ....**Always talking of her pains.** Hot, aching eyes. Photophobia. Faceache, < if body gets cold. Cracks in angles of lips. Nervous angina. **Cutting,** from bowels into thighs. Flatulent colic. Contracted abdomen. Diarrhea ceases, spasms set in. Cough, > cool air. One vertebra seems absent. Tightness of skin of fingers. Pains in lower limbs, alternating sides. Irritable pulse. Tarry menses leaving a fast stain; flowing at night.

Related to: Coloc., Dios.

MAGNESIUM SULPHURICUM

SPHERE OF ACTION
Intestines.
Urine.
Female sexual organs.

AGGRAVATION
Morning on awaking.
AMELIORATION
Rubbing.
Walking.

Diarrhea, with diuresis. Greenish urine; with red sediment.
Profuse, dark, intermittent menses. Much, thick leucorrhea. As of a
lump between shoulders. Back feels broken. Left arm and foot fall
asleep. Crawling in fingertips (left). Warts.

Related to: Nat-s.

MANCINELLA

SPHERE OF ACTION	AGGRAVATION
Surfaces	Cold
- Mucous.	- Feet.
- Throat.	- **Drinks.**
- **Skin.**	Dampness.
	Touch.
Mind.	Puberty.
	Climacteric.

Irritation. Acridity. Burning.....................Depressed, with sexual erethism. Thoughts vanish. Forgets her errand. **Terror of insanity.**
Emptiness in head. Pain in vertex, < lying. **Eyes, smart, < closing lids;
lids** heavy and sore; dull ache behind. Photophobia. **Face swelled**; spotted; herpes on lips. **Profuse, foul saliva. Throat;** cutting pains; < **cold
drinks.** Diphtheria. **Cookings,** ascend throat. Craves cold water. Swelled
epigastrium. Bowels sore and burn. Colics or cough, < cold drinks. Ache
behind sternum. **Soles; biting vesicles on;** desquamation; **dry.** Acrid,
sticky foot-sweat (Sil.). Vesicles. Bullae. Brown crusts. Scarlet fever. Pulse
slow; very large and soft.

Related to: Arum-t., Canth., Rhus-t.

MANGANUM

SPHERE OF ACTION	AGGRAVATION
INNER EAR.	Varies with the weather.
Larynx and trachea.	**Touch.**
LOWER LIMBS.	**Cold.**
Periosteum	**Damp.**

- **Joints.**	**Night.**
- **Ankles.**	**Speaking.**
- **Shins.**	**Feather bed.**
Heels.	**AMELIORATION**
Skin.	**Lying down.**
	Open air.

Very sensitive bones. **Painful, deep soreness;** ears; **bones;** joints; **skin. Diagonal pains.** Pains extend to ears from other parts. Yellow-green, lumpy or bloody discharges. Catarrh. Infiltrated, glistening joints. **Festination.** Motor paralysis. .... Weak and nervous. Headache, < straining at stool, etc. **Everything affects his ears** (Canns., Gels., Plan.). Blowing nose is painful. Pale, sickly, mask-like face. Anemia. **Flow of saliva,** with colic, paralysis, etc. Late or pale first menses. Raw, dry, larynx. Rough, hoarse voice; chronic, < A. M.; > expectorating a lump of mucus. Cough, < reading or laughing; > lying; with aphonia; laryngeal; of phthisis. Weak, uncertain legs. Inflamed ankles. Digging in shin bones. Rough, cracked (flexures) or bluish skin. Dry, hard ulcers. Sudden hot flushes. Pruritus of diabetes. Skin festers about joints.

Related to: Chin., Psor.

MEDORRHINUM

SPHERE OF ACTION	**AGGRAVATION**
Mind.	**Damp;** Cold.
Nerves.	**Daytime.**
Mucous membranes.	3-4 A.M.
Lymphatics.	After urinating.
Cellular tissue	Touch.
- Lungs.	Close room.
- Pelvis.	Before storms.
- Small joints.	**AMELIORATION**
Spine.	LYING ON ABDOMEN.
Kidneys.	Bending backward.
Left ovary.	

Stretching out.
Fresh air.
Being fanned.
Uncovering.
Hard rubbing.
Seaside.
Dampness.
Sunset (Coca, Lil-t., Sel.).

Stiff, puffy, achy, sore and rheumatic. Dwarfish. **Many pains.**
SYCOTIC TAINT, poor reaction. Joints feel loose. **Profuse, acrid discharges; causing itching** (Tell.). Fishy odors. Nephritis. Small, very sore aphthae, blisters, etc. **Burnings.** Burning at root of tongue. Formication; internal. **Numbness.** Tremor. Emaciation. Sour children. Offensiveness. Tumors. Loss of power in joints.................. Memory weak, can't concentrate; forgets words, names; can't finish sentences. Mental confusion. Wild feeling. Meanness. Cruelty. **Things seem strange.** Tells it over again. **Hurried;** and anxious; and irritable; and sensitive. Forgetful; of names; of her errand. Suicidal. Fearsome. Apprehensive; anticipates events. Persistent ideas or alternating states, or erratic. Impulsive, abrupt or rude. Many ideas; but uncertain of execution; non-commital. **Sensitive, nervous and hurried. Feels far off,** unreal; some one behind her. **Sad,** tearful and **fearful.** Dismal out-look (Cimic.); > weeping. Vertigo; < in vertex. Head tight; tense pains; pulls hair. Occiput pains to behind eyes. **Tousled heads.** Coryza with loss of taste and smell. Post-nasal discharge. Face, grayish, greasy, greenish; **yellow at edge of hair.** Red spiderlets on face (right). Acne on face; < after menses. Water tastes like perfume. Exhaled breath feels hot. Craves stimulants. Morning nausea. **Vomiting of pregnancy.** Heavy lower abdomen or **prostate.** Grinding colic; must brace feet. Dysmenorrhea. Leans back to force a stool; then shivers. Cholera infantum. **Fiery red, moist, violently itching anus.** Scalding ammoniacal urine. Air hunger. **Cough, > lying on face.** Sore, oozing or icy nipples. Cutting, crawling, burning above (left) scapula. Fingertips burn and crack. Heavy legs. **Tender, itching ball and soles. Sleeps in knee-chest position.** A short nap seems a long one, but >

(Nux-v.). Cold skin, but blood feels hot (Sec.). Burning heat, with
sweat; wants to uncover, but is chilled thereby. Burning feet. Sweat
easy; toward morning. Hay fever. Body smells badly to her; can't
wash it off (Lac-c.). Teeth soft, crumbly. Aphthae under tongue.
Burning in epigastrium. Flatulence with numbness. Dark fluid from
rectum. Drawing in ovaries, > pressure. Sycotic sterility.
Dysmenorrhea. Profuse, dark, clotted, foul menses (Psor.). Blistering
leucorrhea (Am-c., Kreos.). Pruritus, > rubbing. Lungs feel stuffed
with cotton. Can't exhale. Asthma; sycotic; infantile. Sensation as of
a cavity in chest or heart. Heat in spine. Spine sore and tender. Arms
hairy. Hot palms. Bites nails. Leg cramps, > stretching leg. Itching
soreness. Condylomata. Sycotic red node. Deep red spots.

Follows: Rhus-t.

Related to: Bar-c., Nat-m., Psor., Thuj.

MELILOTUS ALBA

SPHERE OF ACTION
HEAD.
Vasomotor nerves.

Circulation.

AGGRAVATION
Climacteric.
Walking.
Weather
- **Changing.**
- Stormy.
- Rainy.

AMELIORATION
Bleeding.
Profuse urine.
Vinegar.

Raw feeling. **Congestions.** Bright red hemorrhage; which >
.... Desires to escape. Rushes of blood to head.
VIOLENT, THROBBING HEADACHE; threatens his reason; >
nosebleed. FIERY RED FACE. Profuse nosebleed. Dry skin.

Related to: Bell., Glon.

MENYANTHES

SPHERE OF ACTION
Circulation.

Motor nerves.
Vertex.

AGGRAVATION
Walking.
Rest.
Malaria.
Ascending.
Quinine.

AMELIORATION
Hard pressure.
Twilight.
Laying on hands.

Icy coldness is prominent, **single or** affected parts; nose (Apis, Med.), ears, fingers, knees, abdomen, etc.; at night (Phos.). Visible jerks or twitches. **Vertex; heavy pressure on;** pains, < stooping; or as of a weight in nape. **Bursting headache. Pain ascends from nape.** Misty vision. Frequent, scant urine. Boring at left scapula. Cramp in posterior thighs, < sitting, or from ankles to calves (right). Skin feels tight. Vivid dreams. Shivering, with yawning. Quartan malaria.

Related to: Verat.

MEPHITIS

SPHERE OF ACTION

Nerves.

AGGRAVATION
Lying.
Night.
After menses.

AMELIORATION
Cold bath or weather.

Spasmodic effects. Foul breath and expectoration. Debility after severe illness. Trembling and twitching of exophthalmos.............. Excitable. Loquacious. Vivid fancies. Violent vertigo. As of a finger pressing on occiput. Food goes the wrong way. **Chokes easily.** Can't exhale. Asthma. Asthma of consumptives or drunkards. Cough; violent; spasmodic; nervous; suffocative; whooping; < talking or drinking. Choking cough.

Related to: Coral., Mosch.

MERCURIUS

SPHERE OF ACTION

BLOOD.
Mucous membranes.
GLANDS
- Buccal.
- SALIVARY.
- TONSILS.
- THROAT.
- LYMPHATICS.
- **Liver.**
- Kidneys.
- MUCOUS.
GENITALS.
Cellular tissues.
Joints.
Right side.
Bones.
Skin.

AGGRAVATION

NIGHT; Night air.
SWEATING.
LYING; ON RIGHT SIDE.
HEATED, IF; < **Bed** or fire.
SENSITIVE TO
- DRAFT, to head.
- **Changing,** cloudy or **cold damp weather.**
- Taking cold.
- **Heat and cold.**
- Wet feet.
- Firelight.

AMELIORATION

Moderate temperature.

Great variety of symptoms. Uncertain, **tremulous,** weak and **sweaty.** Swelling, redness; livid congestion. Continued exudation. **Rawness.** FREE SECRETIONS, **thin, slimy, acrid,** burning, foul or thick, **green-yellow.** Salty, lips, taste, expectoration, etc. **Suppuration;** bloody. **Ulceration;** of mucous membranes. Catarrhs. **Glandular activity.** Biliousness. **Yellowness;** eyes, teeth, nasal discharge. Jaundice. Pains stick to one point. Syphilis. Everything seems too short. Rheumatism. Sycosis. Scrofula. **Weak, exhausted**

and ready to sink down .... **Hurried;** nervous. Stammering. Violent impulses (homicidal), etc. Restless and sweaty. Filthy in mind and body. Senses impending evil. Forgetful. As of a band about head. Headache with ear and toothache. Swelled, scurfy tarsi. Eyes draw together. Photophobia, < lamplight (Glon.). Musca volitantes. Arcus senilis. **Pains into ears, from teeth,** throat, etc. Deaf on becoming heated. **Colds travel upward** or attack eyes. Coryza; acrid; purulent; every autumn. Heavy nose. Red, raw, **dirty** nosed children. Face yellow; puffy under eyes. **Swelled cheeks.** Aching jaws. Mumps. Lips salty; cracked in right angle. Painful, ragged, swelled, **bleeding gums.** Gumboil. Loose, hollow, black or aching teeth, < heat and cold; < night. MUCH SALIVA; **flows during sleep;** yellow; bloody; bad tasting. Aphthae. METALLIC TASTE. Broad, flabby, INDENTED TONGUE. Itching palate. Enlarged tonsils. THROAT; SORE; as of an apple core, choke pear, or something hanging in; ulcer, pharyngeal, behind lingual tonsil; hawks large lumps from. **Sore liver.** Weak bowels; holds them. Swelled inguinals. STOOLS; painful; scanty; bloody; **green slime;** ashen white; acrid; then tenesmus or chill. Tenesmus recti, with tenesmus vesicse. Urine causes itching. Urinates more than he drinks. Frequent, scanty urine; then burning. Swelled glans or foreskin. Red meatus. **Genitals, inflamed;** pulls at. Bloody emissions. Gonorrhea. Collapse and fainting at start of menses. Thick, white leucorrhea, when urinating. Cough; in double bouts; dry at night; **yellow-green sputum,** by day. Right lower chest. Mammae; pain below right through to scapula; milk, instead of menses, spoiled. Awakes with cardiac tremor. Respiration < lying on left side, but cough < lying on right side. **Neck stiff;** cervicals enlarged. Trembling limbs. Numb fingers. Cold sweat on feet in A. M. in bed. Phlegmasia dolens. Pain forward from right scapula. Cool heels. **Skin yellow;** tender; excoriated, like raw meat. Moist, crusty eruptions. **Ulcers,** irregular, spreading, shallow, bleeding; with cutting and proud flesh. **Jaundice.** Measles. Nightly bone pains; deep or near surface. **Orgasms** (to head and chest). **Erethism and restlessness, < least exertion.** Easily chilled or **overheated.** Alternate chill and heat.

F- 13

Creeping chills. Chilly within abscesses. Catarrhal fevers; after
suppressions. EASY, PROFUSE SWEAT; **without relief,** with the
pains; oily; **foul;** sour; stains an indelible yellow; on head; on chest;
at night. Must get up and walk about at night.

Antidotes: Aur., Carb-v., Hep., **Nit-ac.,** Sulph., Thuj.

Complementary: Bell., Sil.

Related to: Kali-i.

MERCURIUS CORROSIVUS

SPHERE OF ACTION	AGGRAVATION
RECTUM.	AFTER
Bladder.	- URINATING.
Eyes.	- STOOL.
Throat	- **Swallowing.**
- Uvula.	**Night.**
	Cold autumn.
- **Fauces.**	Hot days; Cool nights.
- Palate.	Acids.
Kidneys.	
Bones (Flat).	

Violent effects. Burning, internal; throat, stomach, **rectum,
neck of bladder,** kidneys, etc. Inflammation, with swelling and
constriction. **Constriction** of throat, rectum, bladder, etc. **Cracks,**
on palms, soles, angles of mouth, etc. **Erosive discharges;** acrid, fluent
coryza, lachrymation, etc. Phagedena. Syphilis. ....
Anxious and restless; **rocks hard.** Difficult thinking. Disturbed speech.
Stupid. Aching temples, < looking sidewise. Photophobia. Iritis.
Keratitis. Gluey nasal discharge. Swelled nose. **Pale about month.**
Patchy tongue. Nightly toothache. Red, swollen uvula. **Astringent,**
taste, regurgitation, etc. Sore, painful swelling in left throat, < heat;
sharp pains into ears, < pressure. DYSPHAGIA. Insatiable thirst.

Vomits slime and blood. Cramp in epigastrium. Distended, sensitive stomach. Gastritis. **Cutting colic.** Painful flatulence. **Continuous urging to stool and urine (Canth.,** Lil-t., Sabin.). A NEVER GET DONE FEELING. SCANTY, BLOODY, SHREDDY OR SLIMY STOOLS, WITH TORMENTING TENESMUS. Passes pure blood or bloody water. Bleeding kidneys. Dysentery. Spasm of rectum, during coition. HOT URINE, PASSED DROP BY DROP, or scanty, frequent, dribbling; < sitting. Urethra bleeds after urinating. Nephritis; slow; of pregnancy. Cystitis. Gonorrhea. Phimosis. Chordee. Hard chancres. Breathes as through a metallic tube. Cold skin. Chilly, after stool. **Sweats from every motion;** partial; < forehead and lower parts; foul, at night.

Related to: Ars., Canth., Merc-pr-r.

MERCURIUS CYANATUS

SPHERE OF ACTION	**AGGRAVATION**
MOUTH.	Swallowing.
THROAT.	Speaking.
Larynx.	
Glands.	
Capillaries.	
Nerves	

Early, rapid and **extreme prostration**; with tremor, coldness and cyanosis. **Putridity.** Rapid, local destruction. .... **Cutting** pains in **throat or larynx.** Much thick, or grayish membrane in throat. Septic diphtheria; of soft parts; has prophylactic value. Enlarged tonsils. Early and complete anorexia. Croupy cough. Cough causes suffocation. **Weak heart. Sweatiness.**

Related to: Lach.

MERCURIUS DULCIS

SPHERE OF ACTION
Ears.
Eustachian tube.
Tonsils.
Liver.
Duodenum.
Bowels.
Mucous membranes.
Pleura.

AGGRAVATION
Acids.
AMELIORATION
Cold drinks.

Pallid, flabby, catarrhal and bilious. Pale mucous membranes. Deficient oxidation. Reabsorbent action. .... **Painful** scalp. Meningitis. Rapid winking. Obstructed Eustachian tube (Kali-m., Petr.) or larchrymal duct (Fag.). Deafness from every cold. Blows lumps from nose. Indurated tongue. Increased saliva. Fetor oris. **Tonsil,** (right); inflamed; > **cold drinks** (Apis, Merc-i-f., Phyt.). Biliary stasis. Acrid, grass-green diarrhea; of infants. Slimy, pussy expectoration. Inflamed pleura. Sweatiness.

Related to: Kali-m.

MERCURIUS IODATUS FLAVUS

SPHERE OF ACTION
THROAT; **Right.**

Right side.

Glands.

AGGRAVATION
Odors.
Raising up.
Warm drinks.
Lying on left side.
AMELIORATION
Open air.

Faint or dizzy on rising. Forehead aches. Cornea looks scratched or chipped. Dark circles under eyes. Swelling below right eye (Arn.). Jaws tired from clenching during sleep. Teeth on edge, < heat, cold and sweets. Pyorrhea. **Moist, filmy coat on tongue or** YELLOW AT BASE. **Sorethroat** (right then left); swelled tonsils; > cold drinks. **Tonsillitis.** Hawks lumps from posterior nares. Yellow leucorrhea; of children. Heart, then head pains. Palpitation, with dyspnea, < lying on back. Numb knees. Swollen glands; cervicals. Syphilis. Flat warts.

Related to: Lyc., Merc.

MERCURIUS IODATUS RUBER

SPHERE OF ACTION	AGGRAVATION
THROAT.	Empty swallowing.
Glands.	After sleep.
Left side.	
Cellular tissue.	

Swellings....................... Painfully heavy occiput. Granulated eyelids. **Aching, sore malar bones.** Slimy, sticky lips on waking. **Dark, red fauces.** Wrinkled tongue. SORETHROAT (left to right); tonsils or glands greatly swelled, yet little exudate. As of a lump in throat. Stiff throat, root of tongue and neck (Phyt.). Indurations in urethra. Hard chancre. Profuse, acrid, green leucorrhea. Stubborn, suppurating bubo. Right lower chest. Asthma. **Hard, glandular** swelling; cervical adenitis. Moist cracks on palms. Wandering pains.

Related to: Lach.

MERCURIUS PRAECIPITATUS RUBER

SPHERE OF ACTION
Mucous membranes.
Heart.
Skin.
Right side.

AGGRAVATION
Falling to sleep.
Lying.

Burning. Fissures. Syphilis; of pregnancy.........................Patchy tongue. Coat like old cheese on mouth and throat. Mucous patches. Suffocation on lying or falling to sleep. Asthma.

Related to: Ars., Lach.

MEZEREUM

SPHERE OF ACTION
SKIN.
Nerves; **Bones**
- **Head.**
- **Face.**
- Jaws
Mucous membranes
- **Mouth.**
- **Stomach.**
One side.

AGGRAVATION
NIGHT.
Suppressions.
WARMTH OF BED,
　　Fire, etc.
Cold air; Drafts; Damp.
Motion.
Touch.
Mercury.
Vaccination.

AMELIORATION
Wrapping up (Nerves, Bones).
Eating.
Open air.

Acrid secretions, pus, leucorrhea, etc. **Violent, Irritative burning itching,** burning smarting, burning boring, etc. with **coldness of part affected.** Neuralgia; after shingles. Ulcers. Effects of suppressed eczema capitis. As of a cool breeze. **Sudden pains,** then chilly, sore or numb. Emaciation of part. Gouty-rheumatic-syphilitic dyscrasia. **One-sided** symptoms, whole or partial; numbness of one side of scalp. Head pain (left), into eyes, malar bones, neck, etc., with lachrymation. Painful skull. Pains outward along brows. Eyes seem dry. Ears feel open to cool wind. Deafness. Facial neuralgias. Cracks in angles of mouth. Dry, dark red mouth. Blunt teeth. Toothache into temples; > cool air. Tongue coated along one side only. Sorethroat in winter. Gastric pain, > milk. Contracted, prolapsed rectum. Glistening particles in stool. Stubborn, leucorrhea. Dry, tickling cough; unto vomiting; < hot things. Aching, itching in popliteae. Internal burning with external violent itching in small areas or single parts. Intolerable itching; changes place on scratching. Pruritis senilis. Eruptions ooze acrid, gluey moisture, form thick crusts, with pus beneath, or are chalky white. Milk crust. Deep, hard, painful ulcers; acrid pus, drying into crusts; < touch and warmth. Bones seem enlarged. Periostitis. Chilly; limbs feel cold. Heat of one hand.

Complementary: Merc.

Related to: Ars., Guaj., Kali-i., Merc.

MILLEFOLIUM

SPHERE OF ACTION	AGGRAVATION
CAPILLARIES	Injury.
- LUNGS.	Violent exertion.
- Nose.	**AMELIORATION**
- Uterus.	Bleeding.
	Discharges.

Bruised soreness. Congestion. Profuse, painless, bright red, fluid hemorrhage; nosebleed, hemoptysis (Acon., Led.), etc. Spasms after suppressed secretions, menses, etc.................................. Flatulent colic. Oppression of chest, with palpitation.

Related to: Arn., Led.

MOSCHUS

SPHERE OF ACTION
NERVES
- SENSORY.
- **Genital.**
Respiration.
Circulation.

AGGRAVATION
Excitement.
Cold.
Suppressions; Menses, etc.

AMELIORATION
Open air.

Poor reaction. Spasmodic, nervous effects; laughter, hiccough, shuddering, etc. **Twitchings. Chokings. FAINTS. Hysteria.** Buzzing, squeezing or plug-like sensations. Globus. .... Hurried, tremulous and **awkward.** Anger; talks excitedly or scolds until she **faints. Fears noise,** dying, etc. **Imaginary sufferings.** Nervous shuddering. Headache, with coldness, faintness and polyuria. One cheek red, but cold (Ferr.), other pale and hot. Blue lips. Violent eructations. Tympany. **Sudden nervous suffocation or anxious palpitation;** wants a deep breath; < becoming cold (Act-sp.); >belching. Cramp in lungs. Sleepy by day; sleepless at night; wakes every minute. **So sensitive, cold air** makes him shudder. Shivering on scalp. **Cold skin.** Burning heat, with restlessness.

Related to: Carb-v., Castm., Ign., Nux-m., Valer.

MUREX

SPHERE OF ACTION
˙FEMALE SEXUAL
ORGANS.

AGGRAVATION ·
Touch.
In sun.
Sitting.
Abortion.

AMELIORATION
Before menses.
Eating.

Sensitive. Very tired and weak. .... Fearful and anxious. Cold nose. Violent hunger, even after eating. **Sinking at stomach.** Urging in bladder. Urine smells like valerian. Pains in genitals; up through abdomen; into breasts; stitches. **Painfully sore uterus.** Bearing down pains; **must cross limbs. Nervous, frantic desire.** Nymphomania. Copious menses. Leucorrhea; thick; yellow, bloody; alternating with mental symptoms. Lumbar pain impels walking, which <. Hives.

MURIATICUM ACIDUM

SPHERE OF ACTION

BLOOD.

MUSCLES

- HEART.

- ANUS.

MUCOUS MEMBRANES

- **Digestive tract.**

- MOUTH.

TONGUE.

Brain.

AGGRAVATION

Touch.

Wet weather.

Walking.

Cold drinks.

Bathing.

Sitting.

Human voice.

AMELIORATION

Motion.

Warmth.

Lying on left side.

Sore, RESTLESS AND ERETHISTIC, **but soon grows weak** and **very debilitated;** wants to lie down; slides down in bed, eyes fall shut; lower jaw drops, etc. Muscle exhaustion. **Bluish parts;** tongue, piles, ulcers, etc. Tearing in limbs. BURNINGS. Dry, bleeding, cracked or **deeply ulcerated parts.** Thin, acrid, foul **discharges.** Decomposition. Violent hemorrhage. Bloody mucous membranes. Typhoid or scorbutic states. .... Introverted. **Sad and taciturn.** Irritable. **Muttering. Persistent, loud moaning.** Vertigo if lies on right side. Brain feels bruised. Periodical pain over left eye. Occipital pains; **leaden** heaviness. Cutting from mastoid to nape, < touch. Deafness. Nosebleed. **Dark or glowing red face;** with cold hands, but no thirst. **Lips, sore, cracked and scabby. Dry, mouth and throat.** Tongue heavy, stiff, shrunken or burnt looking (Ars.). Aphthae. Teeth, < acids or sweets. Sordes. **Averse to meat.** Ascites. Profuse, **involuntary stool** or prolapsing bowel, **on urinating, or passing flatus. Very sore piles,** > heat. Atony of bladder; must press until rectum comes down. Can't urinate without also stooling. Red, swelled, burning fingers and toes. Weak thighs. Scurfy eruption on dorsum of hands. Ulcers throb on walking. Pulsations in single parts. Sparse scarlatina, mixed with petechiae. Large, full and soft pulse. Pulse drops every third beat. Cold in bed, in early morning. **Intense, burning heat, with aversion to covers.** Adynamic fevers; typhoid, septic, etc.

Related to: Bapt., Bry.

MYGALE LASIODORA

SPHERE OF ACTION
Nerves.

Chorea of upper parts, ... Twitching facial muscles and head (Cic.).

MYRICA CERIFERA

SPHERE OF ACTION
Liver.
Heart.

AMELIORATION
Open air.

Discouraged. Dull headache, in the early morning. Yellow sclera. **Very red eyelids. Combined liver and heart symptoms.** Liver affections, with dull pain; with pain under either scapula; with urticaria; with **jaundice.** Jaundice of infants. Fulness and burning in gall-bladder. Foul, adhesive mucus in mouth, throat, or stool. Slow pulse.

Complementary: Dig., Kali-bi.

Related to: Chel.

NAJA TRIPUDIANS

SPHERE OF ACTION
 Cerebellum; Medulla.
 NERVES
 - HEART (Mitral valve).
 - **Respiration.**
 - **Throat.**
 Left side
 - **Ovary.**
 - Temple.
 - Arm.

AGGRAVATION
 Lying on left side.
 After
 - Sleep.
 - Menses.
 Air
 - **Cold.**
 - **Drafts.**
 Pressure of clothes.
 Alcohol.

AMELIORATION
 Riding in open air.
 Sneezing.
 Smoking.

 Nervous, excited and tremulous; with cardiac effects; often reflex. Collapse. Sepsis. Many pains. Parts seem drawn together. **Constrictions,** throat, chest, etc. Insensible right side.................... Suicidal brooding. Shootings in head. As of a blow on occiput and neck. Vertex sensitive to cold. As of a lump in throat. PAIN FROM LEFT OVARY TO HEART. Suffocative **choking;** grasps the throat. Puffing breathing. Cardiac asthma or cough. HEART; **weakness at;** violent pain; shooting to left scapula, **shoulder** or neck; cramp ascends into neck; holds hand over it; excited, tremendous action; palpitation, visible; hypertrophy; endocarditis, septic. Dry or empty in left lung.

Ribs feel broken. Cramps in shoulder, nape or thigh. Numb left arm. Terrifying racking in marrow of thigh. Puffy or sweating hands and feet. Itching cicatrices. Pulse changes force. Internal heat, < chest. Sweat on lumbar back and ankles.

Related to: Cimic., Lach., Laur., Spig.

NATRIUM CARBONICUM

SPHERE OF ACTION
DIGESTION.

Nerves.

Skin.

Hands (dorsum).
Heels.

AGGRAVATION
HEAT
- Sun weather (Head).
- Sultry air.
- Gas-light.

Periodically; Winter (Body).
5 A.M.
Music.
Mental exertion.
Onanism.
Dietetic errors.
Milk.
Drafts.
Thunder-storms.

AMELIORATION
Motion.
Rubbing.
Eating.
Sweating.

Irritable weakness. Puffy, relaxed, easily exhausted. Easy dislocation. Oversensitive; to open air, music, noise, dietetic errors, etc. Pains cause tremor, cold sweat, anxiety, etc. .... Cross and irritable. Gloomy. Lively, yet fearful; < thunderstorms. Averse to company. Vertigo, from wine. Hot weather headache. Head bent backward; pains out through eyes. Dazzling flashes or stars before vision. Swelled or peeling nose. Coryza, < least draft; < alternate days. Violent sneezing. **Post-nasal discharge.** Pale, wilted face. Mouth open. Must drink to swallow solids. **Acidity,** flatulence and rheumatism. **Weak digestion.** Averse to milk. Greedy, always nibbling. Gastric pain, > eating. Abdomen pouts here and there. Diarrhea, from starches. Stools like orange pulp. Pollutions. Cough; loose; hollow; 9-11 A. M.; < entering warm room. Purulent, salty sputum. Cough from continuous tickle in throat, < going from a cold into a warm room. Boring at tip of left scapula. Painful popliteae. Heavy legs. **Weak ankles.** Cramps from ankles into toes. Sleepy after meals. Blisters on small joints; tips of toes or fingers. Milky, watery or dry, rough skin; pustular eruptions. Cold between scapulae. Burning wrists and ankles. **Sweats easily.**

Complementary: Sep.

Related to: Lyc., Nat-m.

NATRIUM MURIATICUM

SPHERE OF ACTION

NUTRITION
- **Digestive tract.**
- BRAIN.
- BLOOD.
- MUSCLES.

MIND.

HEART.

GLANDS
- MUCUS.
- Spleen.
- Liver.

Skin.

AGGRAVATION

PERIODICALLY
- 9-11 A.M.
- **With the sun.**
- After menses.
- Alternate days (Ars., Chin.)

HEAT
- **Sun.**
- Summer.
- Dampness.

Exertion; Eyes, mental.

Violent emotions.

Sympathy.

Puberty.

Quinine.

Old malaria.

Silver salts.

AMELIORATION
Open air.
Cool bathing.
Sweating.
Rest.
Before breakfast.
Deep breathing.

Thin, thirsty, hopeless and poorly nourished. Emaciation; descending; < **neck** or abdomen. Anemia. DRYNESS; skin, mouth, **throat,** rectum, vagina, etc. Numbness; of one side; parts lain on; fingers. **Tremulous.** Easy exhaustion. **Parts seem short,** hamstrings, nape, etc. Not very sensitive to pain. Takes cold. Nervous erethism. **Thick white or clear acrid discharges. Exact periodicity.** Malarial cachexia. .... Hateful; detests consolation or a fuss. Inconsolable. Easily angered; < if consoled. **Sad, reserved;** company distresses. Hypochondria. Weeps bitterly. Boisterous grief. Scattered thoughts, or an idea clings, prevents sleep, inspires revenge, etc. Anxiety. Apprehension. Fears or **dreams of robbers.** Vertigo; as if falling, on closing eyes. Nodding motions. HEADACHES; **hammering;** heavy; bursting; maddening; **over eyes;** on vertex, **on awaking;** with partial numbness or disturbed vision; < reading; < motion, even of eyes; > pressure on eyes. Migraine. Falling hair. Eyes feel drawn together. **Lachrymation** on affected side (Spig.); on sneezing, coughing, etc. Ptosis, on lying down. Vision blurred, wavering. Letters run together. Hemiopia, then headache. Can't read by artificial light. **Nose** stopped, high up; sneezing early in A. M.; alternate fluent and dry coryza; gushes of fluid; little ulcers in. Face; pale, muddy or greasy. HERPES ABOUT LIPS; or at edge of hair; pearly. Throbbing in lower jaw, < biting, < heat and cold. Exophthalmic goitre. Hawks much mucus; bitter. TONGUE MAPPED; **beaded or striped along edge.** Blunted taste and smell. Uvula hangs to one side. **Throat; a spot** is dry, sore, tickles, causes cough, etc.; glistens. **Thirst; drinks large quantities.** Hunger great, yet emaciates; without appetite. CRAVES SALT. **Averse to bread.**

Burning eructations; after eating. Waterbrash. Epigastric pulsation. Anxiety in stomach, rises to head. Tense abdomen; < groins. Dry, **hard, crumbling stool,** tears anus or causes burning; coated with glassy mucus; on alternate days. Chronic diarrhea. Constricted rectum. Herpes ani. Red urinary sediment. **Coition**; painful; averse to; then backache, weak legs, depression, etc. Suppressed gonorrhea. Debilitating leucorrhea, replaces menses. Cough; from tickling in epigastrium; with asthma or palpitation; < winter. Respiratory catarrhs, after suppressed sweats. **Heart; palpitation,** shaking body or alternates with beating in head; fluttering; weak; sore; < emotions, lying on (left) side, or motion. Sore neck muscles. Bruised backache, early in A. M.; < coughing, > lying on back, or pressure. Cracked finger-tips. Catch in knees. Hamstrings seem short or drawing in. Sobs during sleep. **Awakes feeling weak. Skin, oily;** dry, harsh, dirty, unhealthy or yellow; chaps or **herpetic eruptions,** < flexures or about knuckles. Coldness of many parts; hands, feet; heart. Morning chill, with thirst. Chilly, but < in sun. Sweat, cold, scanty; at edge of hair; on nose, on face, while eating (Cham.).

Complementary: Ign., Sep.

Related to: Puls.

NATRIUM PHOSPHORICUM

SPHERE OF ACTION
Occiput.
Mucous glands.
Duodenum.
Bile-ducts.
Mesentery.
Genitals.

AGGRAVATION
Sugar.
Children.
Milk.
Mental exertion.
Thunder-storms.
Gas-light.

AMELIORATION
Cold.

SOURNESS, **eructations,** vomitus, stomach, stools, leucorrhea, expectoration, sweats, etc. **Acidity. Deep yellow discharges;** from

eyes, etc. **Debility. Overfed children, with acidity.** ....
Mental weakness. Fear, < night. **Itching; nose; about mouth and
anus. Child picks nose.** Worms. One ear red and hot. **Pale face** or
red on alternate sides. YELLOW CREAMY COAT ON BASE OF
TONGUE; on tonsils. As of a hair on tongue or a lump in throat.
Cheesy vomitus. Noisy flatulence. Gastro-duodenal catarrh. Fulness
in abdomen, < standing or < eating a little. Hacked stool. Eruptions
about joints, < ankles; itching. Alternate joint and heart pains.
Rheumatism.

Related to: Cina, Kali-s., Kreos.

NATRIUM SULPHURICUM

SPHERE OF ACTION
OCCIPUT.
Glands
- LIVER; Bile.
- Pancreas.
- Intestinal.
- Descending colon.
Chest
- Left (Lower).
- Lower.
Left side.

AGGRAVATION
DAMP
- Weather.
- **Night air.**
- Cellars.
Lying on left side.
Injuries; Head.
Lifting.
Touch.
Pressure.
Late evening.
Wind.
Light.

AMELIORATION
Open air.
Change of position.

Sudden violent effects; in ailing patients. **Piercing pains,** at left
short ribs; in left hip, < rising or sitting down; in heels. **Yellow, watery**
secretions, stool, **skin,** vesicles, etc. Thick, yellow-green pus. **Fulness.**

Sour, bilious and lithemic. Rheumatic-hydrogenoid constitution. Sycosis............ Sensitive and suspicious. Sadness, < music or subdued light. Melancholia. Dire (suicidal) impulses. Vertigo; > head sweat. Crushing or gnawing in **occiput**. Meningitis. PHOTOPHOBIA. Nose runs water at night. Epistaxis, during menses. Thick, tenacious, white slime in mouth. **Dirty** brown or **greenish-yellow, thick, pasty tongue**, < at base; tip feels burnt. Bitter taste. Thirst at start of fever only. Slow digestion. Concomitants to nausea. **Green**, bilious **vomit**. Sore, heavy liver; < **lying on left side**. As of a lump below liver. Crawling in gall-bladder. Colic, > rubbing abdomen. Cramp at umbilicus. FLATULENCE; **painful;** pushes here and there, < left abdomen. RUMBLING, GURGLING IN BOWELS, THEN SUDDEN GUSHING, NOISY, SPLUTTERING STOOL; **after rising in A. M.**, or drives from bed. Foamy or yellow diarrhea, mixed with green slime. White sand in urine. Dyspnea. Sycotic asthma. Loose, but violent cough; must hold chest or sides. **Run rounds.** Hang nails. Retracted nipples. Sharp cutting back pains, spreading upward like a fan. Throbbing in heels. Vesicles on soles. Chilly, can't get warm, even in bed. Heat with aversion to uncover. Burning below knees. Foul axillary sweat. Warty nodules.

Complementary: Ars., Thuj.

Related to: Coloc., Glon., Med., Puls.

NITRICUM ACIDUM

SPHERE OF ACTION
MARGINS OF OUTLETS
- Throat.
- Anus.
- Mouth.
GLANDS.
- **Liver.**
- Prostate.

AGGRAVATION
Slight CAUSES
- TOUCH, JARRING
- **Noise.**
- **Rattling.**
Motion.
Mercury
Milk, after eating.

F- 14

- Salivary.
Tubular organs.
Blood.
Skin.
Bones.
Joints.
Right side.

COLD; **Air; Dampness.**
Night.
Evening.
Changing weather.
Heat of bed.
Mental exertion, or shock.
AMELIORATION
Guiding motions.
Riding.
Mild weather.
Steady pressure.

Exhausted, shivery, sensitive and **sore.** STICKINGS LIKE A SPLINTER, **or ulcerative gnawing.** DISCHARGES, ACRID; thin, dirty or brown; cause redness or destroy hair. FOUL; ozena, foot, or night sweats, etc. Malignancy. Phagedena. HEMORRHAGE; easy; bright; of bloody water. Red, swelled or cracked orifices. Hard, gristly exudates. Dark, smooth mucous membranes. **As of a band about** or a weight hanging to **part. Sore or stiff,** during pains. Cracking joints. Yellow **brunettes,** of spare habit. .... Hateful. Profane. So angry, he trembles. Quarrelsome delirium; talks to spirits, in other tongues. Confusion. Thoughts vanish. **Crushing head pains,** < pressure of hat. Sore in skull. Puffs on scalp. Warm flowing over eyes. Conjunctiva pouts in spots. Spots on cornea. Deafness, > noise. **Nose;** red, scurfy tip; dark lumpy epistaxis; dripping, diphtheria of; cutting pains; caries of bones. Coryza, with shortness of breath. **Yellow, sickly face.** Peeling lips; raw, cracked or scabby **in angles.** Loose teeth. Gums flabby; sore; bleeding inner. Moist, fissured or mapped tongue (Fl-ac., Psor.). Salivation. Sore palate. As of a stick in throat. Craves fats. Stools tear anus, even if soft; then prolonged pain. **Painful piles.** Itching, eczematous anus, or oozes moisture. URINE, **strong as horse's;** cold; alternately profuse and scanty. Cramp from kidney to bladder. As of a **hot wire** in urethra. Infective nephritis. Itching, burning fore-skin. Phagedenic chancre. Edematous prepuce. Bloody water from vagina. Weak, irregular menses. **Shattering cough;** from a spot in larynx; with lumbar stitch, > cold. Expectoration smeary, pussy, etc. Cavernous phthisis. Cutting in larynx. Orgasms to chest; with palpitation and fear. Swelled finger joints. **Warts;** on back of hands. Weak ankles. **Skin,** dry; **eroded;** cracks in every angle; coppery spots, on shin bones; itches on undressing. Crusts form and fall. **Ulcers;** rapid; raw; ragged; with proud flesh or plugs of pus. Stubborn suppuration. Burrowing pus. Fistulae. Cancer. Syphilis. Painful, broken chilblains. Painfully **sore bones,** < tibia; caries. Pulse drops each 4th beat. Jagged or soft warts (Staph., Thuj.). Condylomata. **Icy coldness;** soles. SWEAT; easy, then takes cold; exhausting (urinous), mornings; in axillae; on feet.

Complementary: Calc., Thuj.

Follows: Kali-c.

Related to: Ars., Kali-c., **Kreos.,** Merc.

NUX MOSCHATA

SPHERE OF ACTION	AGGRAVATION
SENSORIUM	**Cold**
Mind.	- **Bath.**
	- **Damp.**
NERVES.	- Drafts.
	- **Wind.**
FEMALE ORGANS.	- Fogs.
	- Feet.
Digestion.	**Pregnancy.**
	Change of season.
Children and old women.	EMOTIONS.
	Excitement.
	MENSTRUATION.
	Jar.
	Bruises.
	Slight causes.
	Mental **exertion** or shock.

AMELIORATION
Moist heat.
Warm room.
Dry weather.

Narcotic effects and **dryness**. Little pain. OVERPOWERING
DROWSINESS, with or caused by almost every condition; by day;
< exertion; **during menses; when flatulent; with dryness, yet NO
THIRST; with coldness. Fleeting pains. Heaviness;** of eyes, tongue,
etc. **Dark, hemorrhages.** Scrawny women, **who faint easily;** < at stool
or menses; **laugh or cry by turns;** have small breasts, etc. As of hard
lumps in stomach, liver, throat, etc. Hysteria.
Automatism............................ Dreamy, clairvoyant state. Dazed;
objects seem changed or to grow larger. Slow ideation. Thoughts
suddenly vanish. Uses wrong words. Brain exhaustion. Talks loud.
Mockery. Laughing. Jesting. **Vertigo.** Sense of levitation. Headache;
in **temples;** > hard pressure. Cerebral congestion. Pale face. Retracted
lips. Teeth feel pulled. **Dry month and throat, without thirst;** < sleep.
Tongue sticks to palate. Thick, cottony saliva. Chalky taste. Loathing,
when eating or thinking of food. Weak digestion. Enormous bloating;
all food turns to gas. **Flatulent colic.** As of a board across
hypogastrium. **Stool difficult, although soft;** putrid, bright yellow
and lienteric; < night. Inactive rectum. Strangury from alcohol.
Thick, dark, irregular menses. Flatus from vagina. Leucorrhea;
replaces menses. Deficient, irregular labor pains. Cough, > heat of
bed. **Hoarse; when walking against wind. Palpitation,** > walking.
Acute pain now in spine, now in lumbar region. Dry palms. Dry,
cold skin. **Sleepy attacks.** Sudden; with vertigo. Weak, irregular pulse.
Alternate chill and heat. Chills with sopor. Red sweat, or sweat absent.

Complementary: Calc., Lyc.

Related to: Cann-s., Croc., Gels., Mosch., Op., Rhus-t.

NUX VOMICA

SPHERE OF ACTION

Cerebro-spinal axis.
NERVES.

DIGESTIVE ORGANS
- STOMACH.
- LIVER.
- Bowels.

RESPIRATORY ORGANS.

Male brunettes.

AGGRAVATION

EARLY MORNING.
COLD
- OPEN AIR (dry).
- **Drafts.**
- Seats .
- Wind.
- UNCOVERING.
HIGH LIVING
- COFFEE.
- Condiments.
- **Liquor.**
- Drugs.
- **Debauchery.**
- **Purgatives.**
Sedentary habits.
Overeating.
Mental
- **Exertion.**
- **Fatigue.**
- Vexation.
Disturbed sleep.
SLIGHT CAUSES
- **Anger.**
- **Noise.**
- **Odors.**
- Light.
- **Touch.**
- PRESSURE; **of clothes,** <
                    waist.

AMELIORATION

FREE DISCHARGES.
Naps (Kali-bi.).
Wrapping head.
Resting.
Hot drinks.
Milk.
Moist air.

VIOLENT ACTION; often irregularly fitful or inefficient. Increased reflexes. Irritable and hypersensitive, mentally and physically. Firm fibred brunette. **Twistings. Jerks.** Spasms; with consciousness. Tense, contracted feeling. Lightning-like pains. Neuralgia; prodromal. Sensation as of a rough body internally. **Bruised soreness;** OF ABDOMEN, brain, etc. INTERNAL scrapy RAWNESS; throat, larynx, etc. **Takes colds.** Biliousness. **Faintings** after vomiting, after stool, after labor pains, etc................ Sensitive and critical. **Active, ANGRY AND IMPATIENT; can't stand pain;** so mad, he cries. **Zealous, nervous and excitable.** Nagging. Spiteful. Irritable hypochondriasis. Sullen. Fears poverty. **Violent,** ugly (suicidal) impulses. **Vertigo;** on an empty stomach; with blank spells. Sensitive scalp. Swelled forehead. Lachrymation; on affected side. Migraine. Blood-shot eyes. Sore nostrils. Nose stopped, but runs water; on one side. **Sneezing;** violent; **abortive;** from intense crawling in (left) nostril. **Coryza;** fluent by day and in open air, dry at night. Epistaxis on coughing. Acute smell. **Red, turgid** or yellowish **face,** < about nose and mouth. Left angle of mouth droops. **Jaws snap shut;** stiff. Teeth chatter. Fetor oris. TASTE, **bitter**—sour; **bad in A. M.** Itching palate; Eustachian tube. **Rough, scratchy throat;** putrid taste in, on coughing. Craves piquant foods or stimulants. HICCOUGH. Violent retching, < hawking. **Eructations;** sour. Heartburn. **Waterbrash. Nausea; > if he can only vomit.** VIOLENT VOMITING; bilious-sour. **Food lies like a heavy knot in stomach.** Gastric pains, into back; chest; > vomiting, etc. As of a band about waist; **clothes oppress it.** Indigestion. Liver sore; sticking; enlarged. Gall-stone colic. Bowels gripe here and there. SORE BOWELS, < COUGHING OR STEPPING. Hernia; infantile. Flatulent colic. UNEASY, **fitful and FRUITLESS URGING FOR BOWELS TO ACT, > STOOL.** Strains hard at stool. Inactive peristalsis. **In rectum;** retained flatus; as if more stool remained; spasm of. Constipation. PILES; itching; > cool bathing. Sexual erethism. Onanism. Premature ejaculation. **Menses profuse, early and prolonged** or intermittent; of dark, lumpy blood. Dysmenorrheal cramps; spread over whole body. **Cough violent,** throwing the patient down; paroxysmal; whooping. Painfully stiff neck; pains down (right) shoulder. Lumbar ache, as if breaking; **must raise up to turn over.** Acute lumbago. Crawling along spine. Shooting from toes to thighs, < after stool. Tense cramps in calves and soles. Feet feel clubby and raw. Goose-skin. Jaundice. **Yawning.** Sleepy in evening or sleepless from rush of ideas. **Awakes too early; can't sleep again.** Finally sleeps, but on waking feels miserable. Nightmare. Chill with thirst and heat without thirst. EASILY CHILLED; CAN'T UNCOVER, < **motion;** < drinking even during the heat. Sour sweat.

Complementary: Kali-c., **Phos.,** Sulph.

Related to: Ign., Lyc.

OCIMUM CANUM

SPHERE OF ACTION

Ureters (Right).

AGGRAVATION

Scanty urine.

Sore pains in ureters. Renal colic with hematuria and violent vomiting. Red sand in the urine. Swelled inguinal and mammary glands.

Related to: Canth., Lyc., Urt-u.

OENANTHE CROCATA

SPHERE OF ACTION

CEREBRO-SPINAL AXIS.

Heart.

AGGRAVATION

Injury.
Menstrual and sexual disturbances.

Mania. Swelled, twitching face. Rosy red blotches on face and chest. Burning heat, < head and throat. **Epilepsy;** with priapism. Status epilepticus (Absin., Acon.). As of a bug creeping under skin about waist; < touch of clothes.

Related to: Bell., Cic.

OLEANDER

SPHERE OF ACTION
Digestive tract.
Skin.
Scalp.
Nerves
- **Cerebro spinal.**
- Motor.

AGGRAVATION
After suckling.
Rubbing.
Undressing.

AMELIORATION
Looking sidewise.

Numbing, paretic effects; on limbs and skin. Sopor. Tremulous **weakness.** Sense of vibration. Emptiness in stomach and chest; after eating; > brandy. ....Sadness with lack of confidence and power. Distraction. Slow comprehension. Vertigo. Numb tongue. Thin, lienteric stool escapes with the flatus; passes food eaten the day before. Crampy contraction of upper limbs. Sensitive skin; **chafes** and **oozes** or bleeds. Eruptions with itching biting, as of lice. Moist milk crust, < occiput. **Heat from mental exertion.** Paresis after infantile paralysis. General crampings. Numb-skin.

Related to: Anac., Chin.

OLEUM ANIMALE

SPHERE OF ACTION
NERVES; Pneumo-gastric.
Digestive organs.
Here and there; in single spot
    or parts.
Excretions.

AGGRAVATION
Cold.
Eating.
Suppressions.

AMELIORATION
Rubbing.
Pressure.
Open air.

Soreness. Weak, tremulous; hands, knees, feet, etc Pain in spots. Neurasthenia. Nervous irritability. **Shuffling gait. Urinous,** eructations, leucorrhea, etc. **Icy coldness;** from tips of teeth, in throat, stomach, etc. .... Sad. Introverted. Vanishing thoughts. Speaks in whispers. Faintness or vertigo; of gastric origin; > bending head back. Sees glistening bodies. A skin seems to overhang the eye. Lachrymation, on eating. White of egg seems dried on lips. Malar bones feel pulled up. Twitching lips. Mouth feels greasy. Snowy saliva. Toothache, > biting. Hawks out brown, gluey lumps. Acrid vapor or raw streak in throat, < cough. **Waterbrash,** > chewing tobacco. Pulsation or as of water in stomach. Meteorism. PROFUSE, **pale urine; fish-brine** odor; < hysteria, migraine, etc. Frequent scanty urine, then headache. Seminal losses; on straining at stool. **Testes, swell alternately; feel pulled up.** Anxious palpitation. Sore mammae, before menses. Outward dartings in nipples. Aching (right), scapula, > pressure. Raw flexures. Flesh feels torn from bones. Slow pulse. Alternate chill and heat. Cold, foul foot-sweat; fishy on heels.

Related to: Sulph., Tell.

OLEUM JECORIS

SPHERE OF ACTION	AGGRAVATION
Chest.	Milk.
Liver.	**Cold damp.**
Tendons.	

Rigid tendons. Faulty nutrition. **Atrophic infants.** Intolerance, of milk. .... Yellow tongue, leucorrhrea, sputum, skin, etc. Hoarseness. Cough, with palpitation. Early phthisis. **Soreness or stitches in chest.** Burning spots. Milk crust. Ringworm. Always taking cold. Chilly up back. Heat in palms, toward evening. Hectic.

Related to: Phos.

ONOSMODIUM

SPHERE OF ACTION

MUSCLES AND **Nerves**
- **Eyes.**
- **Occiput.**
- FEMALE PELVIC
  ORGANS.

Spine.

AGGRAVATION

Sprains
- EYE STRAIN.
- **Sexual excesses.**
Darkness.
Tight clothes.
Warm, humid air.

AMELIORATION
Rest.
Sleep.
Eating.

Aching, sore and stiff; after the pain. Incoordination....................
Irresolute. Confused. Forgetful. Slow thinking. Aphasia. Nervous
exhaustion. Vertigo; with the headache; < lying on (left), side.
Headache; occipital; **screwed in,** as if; < eye strain and lying on back.
Pains up and down from (left), **occiput** to shoulder, < exertion.
Migraine. Dull, heavy oppressing in occiput. **Aching, heavy, tired,
stiff eyes.** Eye, combined with ovarian symptoms. **Misjudges
distances.** Mushy, yellow stool. Aromatic urine. **Sexual desire gone.**
Sexual neurasthenia. Pains alternate between ovaries. **Sore ovaries
and rectum. Acrid leucorrhea.** Sticky white expectoration. Swelled,
tender mammae. Itching nipples. **Tired,** numb legs and popliteae.
Seems to tread on cotton. Staggering.

Related to: Cimic., Hyper., Lil-t., Rhus-t.

OPIUM

SPHERE OF ACTION
MIND.
SENSES.
NERVES
- **Brain.**
- Cerebro-spinal.
- Sympathetic.

Lungs.
Respiration.
Digestive tract.

AGGRAVATION
EMOTIONS.
FEAR.
Fright.
Joy.
Odors.
ALCOHOL.
Sleep.
Suppressed discharges.
Receding eruptions.
If heated.

AMELIORATION
Cold.
Uncovering.

Negative, torpid states; but little pain, secretion or reaction. Paralysis; painless; of brain, tongue, **bowels**, lungs, etc. Tremor. **Twitchings**; during sleep. Convulsions. Epilepsy, in sleep. **Internal dryness.** Hot, head; sweat; bed seems, hunts a cold place, etc. **Stupid sleep**, spasms, violent chills, etc., during. .... PLACID; says nothing ails him. **Dreamy.** Sluggish. Dull. Stupid. No will power. Lying. **Fears**; after fright. Delirium; with terror; alcoholic. Wants to go home. Carphology. Cerebral congestion; intercurrent; apoplectic. Heavy occiput. Visual hallucinations. Inactive pupils. Red, bulging, staring eyes. Dark, turgid, sweaty or hot red face or red and pale alternately. **Old look;** after cholera infantum. Mouth twitches or hangs open. Cravings; without appetite. Vomiting; in peritonitis. As of a weight in abdomen. Bowels feel obstructed. **Paralytic atony of bowels and bladder;** after laparotomy. Hard tympany. Colic; lead. **Stools of hard, black balls.** Constipation. Bloody mucus oozes from open anus. Retained urine. Lively fetal motions. Rattling, **unequal breathing.** Sighing. Snoring. **Stertor.** Tickling cough. Pneumonia. Weak heart. Crawlings here and there. **General itching.** Skin rough and dirty. Painless ulcers. Tired and sleepless; drunkards. SOMNOLENCY.

Heavy, stupid sleep; of the aged. **Full, slow pulse** (Dig.). **Hot, sweaty** (Samb.) **and drowsy;** with cold limbs. Sweaty, without relief.

Complementary: Alum., Bar-c., Bry., Phos., Plb.

Related to: Arn., Nux-m.

OSMIUM

SPHERE OF ACTION	**AGGRAVATION**
Respiratory tract.	Coughing.
Trachea.	Talking.

Foul secretions. Pains go up and down. Crawlings. ....
Greenish, rainbow colors about light. Snuffling. Fluent coryza, with a sense of stoppage. Stomach feels full of broken stones or lumps. Spasmodic cough; with torn loose feeling and tenacious sputum. Sensitive air passages. Foul axillary sweat.

Related to: Ars., Iod., Phos.

OXALICUM ACIDUM

SPHERE OF ACTION	**AGGRAVATION**
Digestive tract.	**Thinking of it.**
Navel.	**Cold.**
Nerves	**Touch.**
- **Cord.**	**Shaving.**
- Heart.	Mental exertion.
Left side; Lung.	**AMELIORATION**
	After stool.

Weak, cold, livid and numb all over; < lower limbs. **Violent pains;** in streaks, like lightning, **in spots,** burning, etc. Neuralgia. .... Nervous and sleepless. Swimming vertigo. Band-like sensation about head. Numb pricking in occiput and back. **Sour taste.** Gnawing emptiness. Colicky urging about navel or **involuntary, muddy-brown stools, < lying.** Oxaluria. Testes throb or feel crushed. Low voice. Paroxysmal, jerking breathing. Nightly dyspnea. Pain extent from lower (left) chest to epigastrium. Palpitation, < lying. Fixed chest. Angina pectoris. **Back feels too weak to hold body.** Cold creeps up spine. **Weak trembling hands and feet.**

Related to: Ars., Pic-ac.

PAEONIA OFFICINALIS

SPHERE OF ACTION	AGGRAVATION
Anus.	STOOL.
Veins.	**Touch.**
Skin.	Night.
	Motion.

Sensitiveness. Shooting or splinter-like pains. .... Moisture (foul) at anus. **Excessive pains at anus,** continue long after stool; must rise and walk about. Fissure or fistula ani. Anus covered with crusts. Large, inflamed, ulcerated piles. Bunions. **Swelled veins.** Terrifying nightmare.

Related to: Rat.

PALLADIUM

SPHERE OF ACTION	AGGRAVATION
Uterus.	**Emotions**
Right ovary.	- **Lively.**
Mind.	- Chagrin.
	Social functions.
	Standing.
	AMELIORATION
	Touch.
	Pressure.
	Diversion.
	Rubbing. ,

Fleeting pains. .... Loves praise. Easily offended Headache from ear to ear, across vertex. **Glairy** mucus from throat, or leucorrhea. Shooting from navel into breasts or pelvis. Hollowness in flanks. Bearing down, > rubbing. Cutting in uterus and bladder, > stool. Menses flow when nursing. Glairy leucorrhea, before and after menses. Leaden heaviness in pelvis.

Related to: Asaf., Plat.

PAREIRA BRAVA

SPHERE OF ACTION	AMELIORATION
Genito-urinary organs.	Sitting on hands and knees.
Left side.	

Must get on hands and knees to urinate; pains go into **glans** and thighs. Bursting feeling in bladder or glans. Dysuria. Urine contains thick, stringy, white mucus or **red sand.** Renal colic. Enlarged prostate.

Related to: Berb., Med.

PARIS QUADRIFOLIA

SPHERE OF ACTION	AGGRAVATION
Head.	Thinking.
Spine.	Eyestrain.
Eyes.	Touch.
One side.	**AMELIORATION**
	Pressure.

Heaviness. Numbness (left). Joints feel broken. **Parts feel too big** or drawn together. **Garrulous loquacity.** Weight in nape. **Eyeballs seem pulled back** (Puls.) or **feel too large.** Face seems drawn into root of nose. Imaginary bad smells. Hawks up **tough, green mucus.** As of a ball in throat. **Periodical** painless **hoarseness. Painful skin;** objects feel rough. Unilateral coldness or heat.

Related to: Bell., Nux-v.

PETROLEUM

SPHERE OF ACTION

OCCIPUT.

SKIN
- **Folds.**
- Scalp.
- Genitals.
- Face.

Mucous membranes.

Stomach; bowels.

AGGRAVATION

MOTION
- CARS.
- CARRIAGE.
- BOAT.

Weather
- **Cold; Winter.**
- Changing.
- **Thunderstorms.**

Eating.

Vexation.

Cabbage.

AMELIORATION

Warm air.

Weak and tremulous; feels sick internally. **Internal itching.** Emaciation, < chest. Dreads open air. ....Excitable and quick temper. Death seems near. Irresolute. Sense of duality; **loses himself.** Worries but don't know why. VERTIGO; **in occiput.** **Occiput; aching; heavy.** Inflamed tarsi. Deafness. Moist spots behind ears. **Dryness** in ears, nose, throat, etc. Foul mucus in throat. Hunger, causing nausea; after stool. Aversion to meat. Gastric symptoms, > eating. **Nausea; sea and train sickness.** Abdomen inflated; coldness in. **Diarrhea by day only** (Phyt.); < cabbage; then miserable emptiness. Involuntary urine on rising. Cough at night only or < then; shatters the head, > pressing temples. Cold air oppresses chest. Coldness at heart. Stiff or cracking joints. Limbs go to sleep. Ragged, **chapped hands and fingers;** bleeding; in house-maids. SKIN, **fragile; cracks deeply,** < **in angles,** nipples, finger-tips or palms. Psoriasis palmaris. DIRTY, HARD, ROUGH, THICKENED SKIN; like parchment; **it gets raw, festers or won't heal,** < in folds. Brown spots. Eruptions having thick, hard, moist or yellow-green crusts; on occiput or genitals, < cold. Eczema. Herpes. Vesicles. **Itching;** orifices; with burning. Cold spots. Chilly, with dry mouth. Hot palms and soles. Sweat in spots; foul on feet or in axillae.

Complementary: Sep.

Related to: Graph., Sep.

PHELLANDRIUM

SPHERE OF ACTION
Mucous membranes.
Right side
- Chest.
- **Mammae.**
Nerves.

AGGRAVATION
Air; Cold; Open.
Using eyes.

AMELIORATION
While nursing.

Catarrhal symptoms. Phthisis........................**Clang, like striking on metal, in brain.** Everything tastes sweet. **Expectoration; terribly foul;** loose; profuse; smeary; causing dyspnea. Pain in milk-ducts, into abdomen; on nursing. Pain from (left), border of (right) mamma, to between shoulders. Pains going backward through (right) chest. Sleepy.

Related to: Asaf.

PHOSPHORICUM ACIDUM

SPHERE OF ACTION
MIND.
Nerves.
Metabolism.
Sexual system.
Spine
- **Sensory nerves.**
- Muscles.
Bones.

AGGRAVATION
DEBILITY from
- LOSS OF FLUIDS.
- **Sexual excesses.**
- **Fatigue.**
- Fevers.
- Convalescence.
EMOTIONS (Chronic)
- **Grief.**
- Chagrin.
- Mental shock.
- Unhappy love.
- Homesickness.
Drafts.
Cold.
Music.

Talking.

AMELIORATION

Warmth.

Short sleep.

Stooling.

WEAK OR DEBILITATED, **with free secretion. Slowness.** Pains go to part lain on. Bruised soreness; like growing pains. Sense of pressure. Formication; at roots of hair; **along spine,** limbs, etc. Loose joints. Grows too fast .... **Quiet. Indifferent,** APATHETIC, obtuse or torpid; with tendency to diarrhea or sweating. Slow grasp. Can't collect his ideas; hunts for words. Poor memory. Dull despair. Averse to talking. Brain-fag. Mild delirium; easily aroused. Crushing weight on vertex. Early grayness. Falling hair. **Dull, sunken eyes with blue circles;** they feel pressed out. Eye-balls feel large. Pale, sickly face; white of egg seems **dried on it.** Bleeding gums. Slimy tongue. Craves juices. Sour stomach. PROFUSE, PAINLESS, DIRTY WHITE, WATERY or LIENTERIC STOOL; BUT LITTLE DEBILITY. THICK, MILKY URINE. **Polyuria.** Diabetes. Weak, relaxed genitals; suddenly during coitus. Pollutions. Takes colds; < draft on chest. Shaking cough. Twisting under xiphoid. Paralytic **weakness along spine.** Heavy forearms. Scraping bone-pains, at night. Clammy wrinkled skin. SLEEPY BY DAY; but wakeful at night. Cold parts; one side of face, abdomen, etc. Burning along spine; below waist; kidney region. Heat with sweat. **Profuse sweats;** < night; as a sequel. **Sluggish, painless fevers.**

Complementary: Chin.

Related to: Gels.

PHOSPHORUS

SPHERE OF ACTION

CAVITIES
- **Head.**
- LUNGS.
- **Heart.**

CIRCULATION
- **Blood.**
- BLOOD VESSELS.
- **Arteries.**

MUCOUS MEMBRANES
- STOMACH.
- BOWELS.
- Lungs (Lower).

NERVES
- **Brain.**
- Cord.

Bones
- Jaw; upper.
- Shin.
- Spine.

Liver.

AGGRAVATION

LYING ON
- LEFT or painful **side.**
- BACK.

SLIGHT CAUSES
- EMOTIONS.
- Talking.
- Touch.
- Odors.
- Light.

COLD
- HANDS (in water).
- Open air.

WARM INGESTA.

Salt.

Puberty.

Sexual excesses.

Weather
- **Sudden changes.**
- Windy.
- Cold.
- Thunderstorms.

Morning and evening.

Mental fatigue.

AMELIORATION

Eating; Sleep; Cold.
- Food.
- Water; to Face.

Rubbing (Magnetic).

Sitting up.

Active metabolism. Rapid growth. Insidious onset, gradually **increasing debility,** ending in severe or rapid disease (Tarent.). Recurring effects, colds, croup, bleedings, etc. HEMORRHAGE; vicarious; blood-streaked discharges of ulcers, etc. Decomposition.

Polypi. Symptoms due to heart and lung affections. **Tall, gracile, nervous and delicate.** Phthisical habit. Acidosis. Weak spells; in joints; < exertion. **Emptiness;** in chest, stomach, etc. Acute senses. Erethistic exhaustion. TIGHTNESS; **chest** (left), cough, etc. **Spots;** pains or soreness in. Internal paralysis; throat, rectum, etc. Internal itching, tickling. Throbbings, here and there. Numbness. Jerkings, localised; subsultus. Joints stiff, with little pain. **Human barometer** .... **Amative,** but excitable and easily irritated. **Anxious;** fears being alone, twilight, ghosts, **thunderstorms,** etc. Quickly **prostrated** by unpleasant impressions. Timid and irresolute. VERTIGO; accompanies many symptoms; floating; on waking; whirling; > stool. Head, heavy, **aches over one eye;** with hunger; < children; < lying on right side; > cold. Burning in temple. Cold occiput. Vertex throbs. Dandruff. Bald spots. Lachrymation, in wind. **Vision; flashes;** halos; **red;** green; black; > shade; narrow field of; colored, then migraine. Choroiditis. Retinitis albuminurica. Glaucoma. Ears; echoes or reverberations in; deaf to human voice. Otitis; media. Mastoiditis. **Nose; nervous motion of alae;** coryza, flows and stops; on alternate sides; swelled; caries; ulcer, etc. **Epistaxis;** of youths; then pneumonia; with cough,   etc. **Sneezing;** < odors, smoke, etc.; with dyspnea. **Descending nose colds.** Sensitive to smell. **Pale about nose and mouth.** Changing, sickly face; hollow eyes, with blue rings. Numb teeth. Gum sore **behind central incisors.** Palate itches. Abscess of hard palate. Sour taste and eructations. As of cotton or something hanging in throat. CRAVES COLD DRINKS WHICH >, but are VOMITED IN A LITTLE WHILE; after chloroform. **Regurgitates ingesta.** Waterbrash. **Ravenous hunger;** nightly; precedes attacks. **Craves salt;** what is refused when offered. Burning in gullet and stomach, < eating. Pressure above epigastrium. **Stomach;** EMPTY, HOLLOW FEELING IN; as if hanging down; < emotions; tremor, flutter or rolling over in. Sore spot in epigastrium. Rubs abdomen for >. **Stool,** like cooked sago; granular; **slender;** tough; diarrheic, gray, bluish, **watery, pouring out,** painless, nervous, involuntary, **exhausting.** Anus open; prolapsed. Dysentery. Urinates, then weak. Pellicle on urine. Periodical albuminuria. **Sexually erethistic,** but impotent. Prolonged menses; replaced by smarting leucorrhea. **Oppressed for breath;** < least motion. Tight, suffocating breathing, < cough. **Larynx,** raw, sore, furry; pains on speaking. **Voice, low, hoarse,** < evening; croupy, then bronchitis. **Cough;** hard, wheezing; dry; violent; **painful; tickling;** hacking; exhausting; with retching, burning in air-passages or trembling; < change of temperature, before strangers, laughing, exertion or singing. Expectoration; easy, bluish, rusty, salty, foamy or cold. Pneumonia; **left lower lung;** secondary, with sopor. **Chest** full, heavy; stitches (left upper); **pains into throat** or right arm or alternating sides; rattling, < cold drinks. Dry, burnt feeling in chest with cough, at first dry then loose. **Heart;** pains into right arm; violent palpitation from least thing; during goitre, etc.; weak; fatty; orgasms to. Left infra-mammary pain. Mammary abscess. **Between scapulae;** cramp; **burning.** Spinal irritation, < heat. Pain forward from left **scapula.** Tearing in left shoulder at night. Burning spot in lumbar region. **Numb fingers** and toes. Palms burn. Paralyzing stitches in hips; then up back. Pains in tibiae; periostitis. Ankles, as if to break. Suppressed foot-sweat. **Tottery;** stumbles easily. Icy cold feet. Toes cramp. Blood red spots. Thin, foul, bloody pus. Pyemia. Yellow spots on abdomen. Jaundice; as a concomitant. Skin burns on shaving. Fatty cysts. Sleepless; eyes won't stay shut; from internal heat. Sleepy by day, sleepless before midnight. Sleeps in cat naps. Dreams, of fire; lewd. Somnambulism. Congestion to head, **lungs,** etc. Soft pulse. Coldness in cerebellum; of knees, in bed. Chilly in a warm room; down back. Craves ices, during the chill. **Burning heat; local; up back.** Hectic. Sweaty; early morning; sticky; without relief. Painless fevers.

Complementary: Lyc., Sang., Sep.

Antidotes: Coff., **Nux-v.**

Related to: Caust., Con., Sil.

PHYSOSTIGMA

SPHERE OF ACTION
Spinal motor nerves.
Eyes.
Muscles.
Left side.

AGGRAVATION
Change of temperature.
Eyestrain.
Injury.
Bathing.
Heat and **cold.**
Descending.
Motion.

AMELIORATION
Lying with head low (Verat-v.).
Exerting the will.

Weakness; muscles won't respond or draw into knots; < cold. Weakness in lower limbs; coming from a spot between hips. Cramp in left calf at night in bed. Shuddering, < every draft. **Horror of cold water.** Averse to bathing. .... Active mind, even during sleep. Floating sensation. Nothing seems right. Brain falls to side lain on. Pains from forehead down nose. Sensation as of a tight cap on head. Vertigo; stumbles on ascending or descending steps. Sensation as of a band about head. **Twitching of eye muscles or of nose.** Can't bear to raise eyelids. Accommodation affected. Seems to have swallowed a lump. Torpid bowels. Numb womb. Flushes of heat, < in palms. Sore, bloated, red navel; hypogastrium, < standing. Tremor; in head, eyes, vision, nose, teeth, muscles, etc. Dartings, here and there. Tense eye-lids, can't open or close them. Blood-shot eyes. Creeping numbness from occiput down spine. Licks lips. Teeth feel rough. Tongue feels oily; scalded. Loose skin feeling in roof of mouth. Thick, leathery saliva. Hiccough with short breath. Gripe in right hypochondrium. Groins pain alternately. Abdomen, >extending legs. Numbness at womb. Offensive odor from hands. Sweat in excitement. Heart seems to flutter in throat or over body. **Sensitive spine.** Jerking limbs. Shudders from every draft of air. **Attacks of overpowering sleepiness,** with feeling as if to lose consciousness.

Related to: Agar., Gels., Nux-v.

PHYTOLACCA DECANDRA

SPHERE OF ACTION

Glands
- MAMMAE.
- Naso-pharynx.
- Throat.
- Tonsils.

Fibrous tissue
- NECK.
- Back.
- Tendons.
- Joints

Periosteum.
Kidneys.
Tongue (Root).
Digestive tract.
Right side.

AGGRAVATION

Raising up.

Motion.

Swallowing.

Hot drinks.

Heat.

Cold.
- Damp.
- Night.

Change of weather.

AMELIORATION

Lying on abdomen.

Cold drinks.

A remedy of long and deep action. SORE, HARD ACHE, all over; sudden; < eyeballs, kidneys, neck, shoulders, back, forearms and below knees. Restlessness. Bluish-red parts, fauces, glands, etc. Spreading pains. Rheumatism; after tonsillitis. Shreddy, stringy secretions; stools, menses, etc. Hard mammary glands. Obesity. .... Faint on rising. Frontal headache. Head feels beaten sore; < brain. Hot tears. Green vision. Nose seems heavy. Nostrils close alternately. Acrid coryza. Yellowish sickly face. Aching, malar bones. Glands swelled at angle of jaw. Jaws ache, as in mumps. Everted lips. Clenches teeth. Tongue, fiery red at tip; feels burnt or pains at root and into ear on swallowing. Much stringy saliva. White-gray spots on fauces. Mucous patches. THROAT; very sore; very painful swallowing; dark, puffy; burning, as of a stick, hot ball or lump in. Like dark wash leather on tonsil. Tonsillitis. Diphtheria. Hard throb in right tonsil. Quinsy. Violent retching and vomiting; he would rather die. Continuous urging to stool; even during sleep. Dysentery. Hard ache in kidneys. Dark, red urine; chalky sediment. Albuminuria.

Sore spermatic cords. Menstruation, with flow of saliva and tears.
Chronic aphonia. Dry, tickling cough. STONY HARD, HEAVY,
SWELLED (< left) OR TENDER MAMMAE, **paining during
suckling,** spreading over whole body; **hard nodes in.** Mastitis. Nipples
cracked; inverted. Heart symptoms go to right arm. Fatty heart. **Neck
stiff. Right arm numb** and fuzzy. Hips and thighs pain on change of
weather. Aching tibiae, Syphilis. Aching heels, > elevating feet. Bone
pains. Dry, harsh skin.

Complementary: Sil.

Related to: Bry., Kali-bi., **Kali-i., Merc.,** Rhus-t.

PICRICUM ACIDUM

SPHERE OF ACTION	AGGRAVATION
Nerves	**Exertion; Mental** or physical.
- **Brain.**	Seminal losses.
- Occiput.	**Heat.**
- **Cord.**	**AMELIORATION**
- **Lumbar region.**	Rest.
Kidneys.	Cold.
Sexual organs.	**Bandaging.**
	In sun.

Weak, tired and heavy, in mind and body. Profound anemia.
Easily prostrated. **Burning,** in many parts; **along spine;** in legs, etc.
Numbness. Formication. .... Weak will. **Heavy occiput;**
down spine and in **lower limbs.** Brain-fag. Headache, < mental
exertion, > nose-bleed (Ferr-p.). Neurasthenia. Oily burning stool.
Ammoniacal, dribbling urine. Priapism, or sexual erethism. Backache
with languor; from mental exertion. Writers' cramp. Aching, legs.
Small, painful boils, < nape. Sleepiness.

Related to: Gels., Ox-ac., Phos., Ph-ac.

PLANTAGO MAJOR

SPHERE OF ACTION
Nerves
- **Ears.**
- **Teeth.**
Kidneys and bladder.

AGGRAVATION
Night.
Warm room.

AMELIORATION
Sleep.
Eating.

Sharp, shifting pains. Soreness. Neuralgia. As of a body between ears; in groins, etc. .... As if brain turned over. As of a hair before (left) eye. **Pains center in ears and teeth** or alternate between them. Earache. **Saliva flows with the pains.** Toothache. **Dirty taste.** Bowels seem cold. Brown, frothy stools. **Polyuria.** Enuresis. Throbbing between scapulae. Cold sweat on sacrum. Numb, tremulous legs. Sensitive skin. Gloomy dreams, exciting tears

Related to: Arn., Ferr-p., Puls.

PLATINUM METALLICUM

SPHERE OF ACTION
FEMALE ORGANS.

Nerves
- Vagus.
- Sensory.
- Trifacial.

AGGRAVATION
EMOTIONS
- **Sexual.**
- Coition.
- Chagrin.
TOUCH.
Nerve exhaustion.

AMELIORATION
Walking in cool air.
Sunshine.

A remedy of pains. **For prim old maids.** Oversensitive **mind and nerves. Violent cramping,** squeezing, thrusting or **numbing pains,** and then spasms. Neuralgia. Many and various ovarian or uterine reflexes. **Irregular,** spasm, congestion of blood or coldness of

single parts, eyes, ears, etc. Tremor. **Alternate mental** and physical or **sexual symptoms. Numbness;** scalp, face, coccyx, calves, etc. **Bandaged feeling. Sticky;** tears, stool, menses, etc. ....
Laughs at wrong time. Unkind, abrupt and quarrelsome. **Disordered sense of proportion; objects seem smaller,** strange, frightful, etc. Hysteria. Horrors; fears death. CONTEMPT. **Hauteur. Proud and erotic** (Aur.). Alone, deserted feeling. Mentally < in twilight. Bad humor, yet weeps. Gradually increasing, then slowly lessening headache. Clavus. Tense scalp. Cramp at root of nose. Grimaces. Boring in jaws. Congestion to abdomen. Colic. **Hard, black, scant or soft, difficult stools;** of travellers; of pregnancy. Crawling itching anus in evening. **Painfully sensitive genitals,** with itching, tickling or crawling. Dark, thick, profuse menses, with dragging. Heat in ovaries. Ovarian irritation. Vaginismus. Dysmenorrhea, with shrieks and jerks. **Eroticism.** Onanism. Spasmodic yawning. Bruised backache, < pressure or bending backward. Knees drawn up and spread apart. Cramp in calves. In sleep wants to uncover entirely.

Related to: Cupr., Ign., Plb., Stann.

PLUMBUM METALLICUM

SPHERE OF ACTION

CORD AND NERVES
- **MUSCLES.**
- ABDOMEN.
- **Kidneys.**
- Navel.

Blood-vessels.
Blood.

AGGRAVATION

Clear weather.
Open air.
Exertion.
Motion.
Company.
Grasping smooth objects.
Touch.

AMELIORATION

Hard pressure.
Rubbing.

Slow, insidious processes, having violent side symptoms; often of a very changeable or incoherent character; coming in **single parts,**

etc. Paralysis. Atrophied limbs with plump body; paralysed parts <
touch. Sensitive to open air. Impulse to stretch. Exaggerates her
condition. **Retraction; anus, testes,** navel, etc. Increasing slowness
and apathy. Deep, bluish red sclerotic. Abdomen is drawn into uneven
lumps (Ars., Ign.). Abdominal distress that impels her to stretch.
Urination slow, yet profuse. VIOLENT CONTRACTION.
Retraction. Lightning pains that extort cries. Boring. Cramps
(periodical), **convulsions** or (flaccid) paralysis; with hemorrhage or
hyperesthesia. Chronic epilepsy, with marked aura. Wasting of single
(upper) parts, or of paralysed parts. Sclerosis. Gout. ....
Taciturn. Timid, restless and anxious. Fears assassins. Physical labor
exhausts the mind. Stupidity. Melancholy. Delirium; nocturnal;
alternating with colic or pains in limbs. Twitching of right face. Yellow
sclerotic and inside of mouth. Trembling tongue. Sticky saliva. Sweet
taste. Aphthae. Dysphagia. Foul or fecal eructations. NAVEL FEELS
RETRACTED. **Colic;** accompanies many symptoms. **Radiating**
abdominal pains, or **boring,** or as if forced through a narrow place.
Tense abdomen. Hernia at narml. **Anus feels drawn up, or painfully**
contracted. Stool, granular; **of hard, black balls, like sheep dung;**
passed with an urging cramp. **Stubborn constipation or colics of**
infants. Retracted testes. Pollutions. Bluish, red spots. **Dry**
oversensitive skin. Dry, burning ulcers. Takes odd positions during
sleep. Wiry pulse. Coldness from exertion. General cold sweat during
stool. Feet cold, when walking only.

Complementary: Rhus-t., Thal.

Related to: Op.

PODOPHYLLUM PELTATUM

SPHERE OF ACTION

Liver
- **Duodenum.**
- Intestines.
RECTUM.
Right side
- Ovary.
- Scapula.
- Throat.

AGGRAVATION

EARLY MORNING.
Eating.
Hot weather.
Dentition.
Drinking.
Motion.
Mercury.

AMELIORATION

Stroking liver.
Lying on abdomen.

Biliousness...................... Whining. Rolls head. Eyes half open. Bad breath. Burning, rough or flabby, indented tongue. **Bites gums together**; grinds teeth. Bitter taste. As of a lump in esophagus. Craves acids which <. Vomits hot froth. **Constant gagging. Sore, painful liver. Weak, empty sinking or sick feeling in abdomen.** Rubs abdomen for >. GURGLING THROUGH BOWELS, THEN PROFUSE, PUTRID STOOLS GUSH OUT PAINLESSLY. Summer diarrhea. **White stools; like dirty water; foaming; with meal-like sediment**; runs right through diaper; then weakness. Cholera morbus. Diarrhea, alternating with other symptoms, head, etc. Pale, hard, chalky stools. **Rectum**; raw, sore; weak; **prolapsed,** before stool. Moist, foul piles. Numb ache in ovaries; radiating to right crural nerve, etc.; < stretching legs. Ischias antica. Generative organs threaten to prolapse, during stool. Rectum, prolapsed after confinement. Burning in small of back. Jaundice, < face and eyes. Moaning and whining during sleep. Loquacity during the fever (Pyrog.). Sleepy after the paroxysm (malaria).

Complementary: Nat-m.

Related to: Aloe, Chin., Merc.

POLYGONUM SAGITTATUM

SPHERE OF ACTION
 Genito-urinary organs.
 Intestines.

AGGRAVATION
Cold.
Dampness.

CUTTING; along ureters; along fallopian tubes, with bearing down; up spine. **Pulsative pain**; wandering; in prostate. Smarting discharges......................... Puff under right eye. Itching, burning palate; wants to scratch it. Tongue feels swelled. Nausea in abdomen. Painful affections of urinary tract. **Grinding, griping, catting bellyache**, with kidney symptoms. Nephritic colic. Urine scanty; dribbling; dark or calcareous, adherent sediment. Nephritis; suppurative. Cystitis. Excoriated scrotum. Itching pimples within anus. Hips feel drawn together. Aching lower limbs. Sore pains in heels. Urticaria.

Related to: Calc.

PRUNUS SPINOSA

SPHERE OF ACTION
 Nerves
 - **Respiratory.**
 - Orbital.
 Bladder.

AGGRAVATION
Stooping.
Ascending.

Pains causing SHORT BREATH, shooting or pressing **outward**; lightning like; wandering. Neuralgia. Cramp. Nerve paralysis. Compensatory effects......................Pains from forehead (right), to occiput. **Bursting in eyeballs.** Eyes feel pressed apart. Teeth feel pulled out. Cramp in bladder; he doubles up to urinate (reverse— Alum.); urine reaches glans and then goes back again. Strangury. Glans pains on urinating. Pulsating pudendum. Leucorrhea; watery, purulent and acrid. **Dropsy;** cardiac; of feet. Air hunger. As of a lump below left scapula. Heart disease. Night-sweat.
Related to: Laur.

PSORINUM

SPHERE OF ACTION

SKIN
- FOLDS OF.
- Sebaceous glands.

EARS.
BOWELS.
Respiration.
Right side.

AGGRAVATION

COLD
- Open air.
- Washing.

Weather; Stormy; Changing.
Winter.
Heat
- Of bed.
- Exertion.
- Woollens.

SUPPRESSIONS.
Yearly.
Contact of his own limbs.

AMELIORATION

Lying with head low, or
    quietly.
Eating.
Washing.
Nosebleed.
Hard pressure.
Profuse sweating.

Feels sick all over. **Lack of reaction,** in chronic diseases. Aftereffects of infectious diseases, lasting for years. Enfeebled. RECURRENCE. Clears up confused cases. Migraine. Quinsy. FOUL; **discharges;** stools; eruptions; sweat; stubborn foot-sweat; **odor of body.** Thick secretions. **Weak, tender** and thin, **easily chilled; takes cold;** clothing seems large or he feels pushed down. Joints seem loose. HUNGRY or unusually well BEFORE AN ATTACK; **but debilitated and reacts badly, and chronicity threatens. Wants to wash parts..................** ANXIETY. Forebodings. **Despair,** of recovery. **Gloomy.** Feels good and bad by turns. Horrid thoughts. Averse to work. Feels himself poor (reverse — Sulph.). Mind dull, clouded, difficult thinking. Head feels separated from body. **Headache, follows visual disturbances;** alternates with other troubles. Twitching in temples. **Sensitive to drafts about head; wants it**

covered, in hot weather. Dull, dry, tangled hair. Gummy, everted eyelids. Humid sores behind ears. **Putrid otorrhea.** Hay fever. **Face** pale, sickly, **dirty,** fuzzy or puffy. Loose teeth. Tip of tongue feels burnt (Ign.). Hawks out foul, cheesy masses. **Filthy taste.** Anorexia; with great thirst. Flatus like bad eggs. DARK, GUSHING, HORRIBLY PUTRID STOOLS; **of penetrating odor,** going through whole house (Podo.); < at night. Cholera infantum. Stool soft, but difficult. Bed-wetting; at full moon. Offensive genitals. Griping in testes. Chronic gonorrhea. Breathes > lying down or spreading arms apart. Breathing; < open air. Cough, < lying. Gurgling at heart. Panaris. Lumbar ache, < standing or walking. Hot, itching soles. **Skin breaks out;** < flexures; **is dirty,** rough or scabby, greasy. Condylomata, on edges of skin. **Intolerable itching;** < heat (of bed); he scratches it raw or until it bleeds. Heat, with steaming sweat. **Sweat;** profuse; < night; on palms; cold; **easy.**

Complementary: Sep., Sulph., Tub.

Related to: Graph., Mang., **Phos.,** Sulph.

PULSATILLA

SPHERE OF ACTION	AGGRAVATION
MIND.	WARMTH
VEINS.	- AIR.
	- ROOM.
MUCOUS MEMBRANES	- **Clothes.**
- TONGUE.	- BED.
- STOMACH.	**Getting feet wet.**
- BOWELS.	SUPPRESSIONS.
- FEMALE AND GENITO-	EVENING.
URINARY ORGANS.	REST.
Respiration.	BEGINNING MOTION.
One side.	LYING; **One side (Left).**
Right heart.	EATING
	- RICH FOOD.
	- **Long after.**

- FATS.
- Ices.
- Eggs.
PUBERTY.
PREGNANCY.
Before menses.
Iron.
Quinine.
AMELIORATION
COLD; FRESH, OPEN AIR.
Uncovering.
ERECT POSTURE.
Gentle motion.
Continued motion.
After a good cry.

CHANGING SHIFTING SYMPTOMS; **rising to a certain pitch, then suddenly ceasing; going to part lain on**; unilateral. THIRSTLESS, SHORT OF BREATH AND CHILLY; with digestive or menstrual disorders. SUPPRESSIONS; otorrhea, menses, lochia, milk, etc. Metastases. Alternations. Phlegmasia. Venosity. Hemorrhage; passive; vicarious. Anemia. PROFUSE, BLAND, THICK, YELLOW-GREEN DISCHARGES: bitter mucus. Jerking, tearing or ulcerative pain. **Numbness;** part lain on; hands, feet, etc. Pale, chilly blondes. .... MILD, TIMID, EMOTIONAL, WEEPY. Discouraged. Whining. Easily offended. Craves sympathy. **Can't lie with head low.** Headache starts in vertex. Occipital ache, < coughing. Profuse sweat on scalp. **Eyes;** fill with tears (acrid) or seem covered; < wind; sticky lids; colds affect the; ophthalmia, gonorrheal. Blepharitis. Styes. Blind attacks; < menses. Nightly earache. Foul discharge or bad odor before nose. Coryza; stopped on lying or in room. Anosmia. Pale face. Peeling cracked lips. **Licks lips. Crack in center of lower lip. Bad breath.** Drawing toothache, > cold. **Taste bad; in A. M.;** bloody; greasy. **Slimy month** or **dry, without thirst.** Tongue feels scalded. Alternate sides of throat or neck. Food leaves an after-taste or **lodges in throat. Averse to water or fats.** Craves acids or what disagrees. Sudden loathing, < eating. Heartburn. Nausea. Epigastrium; cutting; pulsation. HEAVY OR DERANGED STOMACH. Abdomen; as of a heavy stone; aching; numb; pains into groins. Stools; changeable; green mucus, < after midnight; bilious. Piles, < lying. Urination; involuntary on lying; followed by blood. Heavy pressure on or cramp in bladder. Sensation as of a stone rolling in bladder. Nocturnal enuresis. Burning down the left spermatic cord. Enlarged prostate. Orchitis; gonorrhea. Bloody emissions. Feels like menstruating. MENSES DARK; LATE, at puberty; SCANTY, < bathing; irregular; vicarious; absent. Dysmenorrhea. Weak labor pains. Bearing down, < lying. After-pains. Retained placenta. Leucorrhea; milky; acrid. AIR HUNGER; < lying on left side; as if from abdomen; if heated. Loose cough in morning, then dry evening cough; from tickling in epigastrium; must sit up. Expectoration thick; purulent (Cetrar), slimy, sweet, salt, etc. Asthma from suppressions. Cough; dry hacking; expectorates bitter or salty as it loosens up. Chest oppressed; as by a load. Sore stitch beneath clavicles. Palpitation. Mammae; milk in virgin; sore, aching lump (right); scanty milk. Swelled joints; backs of feet. Numb elbows. Lower limbs; pains down, alternate sides; heavy legs. Sticking in tibia, < lying, > cool air and motion. Acute periostitis. Cold sweat on legs. Foul foot-sweat. Swelled glands. Veins full; varicose; painful. Ulcers, with hard, glistening areolae; varicose. Skin itches on being heated. Measles. Day sleepiness. Lies with hands over head. Disturbed dreams. Awakes confused or tired. Chilly, yet averse to heat; IN A WARM ROOM; with the pain; on lying down at night. One hand cold. Partial sweat.

Complementary: Ars., Kali-bi., Sep., Sil., Zinc.

Related to: Apis, Cimic., Graph., Ham., Kali-bi., Nat-s.

PYROGENIUM

SPHERE OF ACTION

BLOOD.

Heart.

Circulation.

Muscles.

AGGRAVATION

Cold damp.

Motion

- Constant change of position.
- Hard rocking.

AMELIORATION

Heat.

Hot bath.

Pressure.

Aching, BRUISED, SORE **and prostrate;** yet restless. Bed seems hard. **Bone pains. Foul,** taste, **secretions,** odor of body, etc. **Rosy, red streaks.** Decomposition or sepsis...................... Rapid ideation. **Loquacious. Excited.** Feels as if he covered the whole bed. Anxious and **sensitive.** Confused. Sense of duality. Hallucinations. Violent, throbbing headache. Pains are > during hot stage. Throbbings, < neck (Bell., Spig.). Sudden pulsation, with fever and intense restlessness. Rolls head side to side. Throbbing headache, > tight band. Sensation as of a cap on the head. Disgust at his own body odor. Fiery red, smooth tongue. Sweet taste. Nausea, > very hot drinks. Adhesive urinary sediment. Purring at heart. Feels heart; as if tired, big or **full.** PULSE QUICK, OUT OF ALL PROPORTION TO TEMPERATURE (Lil-t., Thyr.) **or the reverse. Quickly oscillating temperature.** The nails threaten to fly off. Chilly, wants to breathe heat of fire. **Chills** start between scapulae; **felt in bones;** with sweat; at night. Fever, at menses. Puerperal sepsis. Slowly advancing hectic. Sweat, without relief; cold. Wants to inhale heat of fire.

Follows: Lach.

Related to: Anthraci., Ars., Bapt., Echi.

RADIUM BROMATUM

SPHERE OF ACTION
Skin.
Nerves.
Lymphoid tissue.
Bones.
Muscles and joints
- Lumbago-sacral.
- Great toe.
Shifting sides.

AGGRAVATION
Motion.
Shaving.
Washing.
AMELIORATION
Open air.
Hot bath (Rhus-v.).
Eating.
Cold drinks.
Continued motion.

Dry, **burning heat** as if afire; craves cool air. **Sudden shifting** or electric pains; must lie down. **Dull, hard ache; deep in joints. Constriction,** chest, heart, etc.; with air hunger. Numbness, < stretching part. Rheumatism. Gout. Weak muscles. Necrotic changes. .... Pain over eyes (left), backward. Red, smarting eyes, < reading. Rushing in ears, > lying on face. Raw throat. Craves pork. Averse to sweets. Abdominal, alternating with ear or chest pains. Sore, prolapsed rectum. Dysuria, then erections. **Itching genitals.** Cough, < smoking; > open air and exertion. Tightness at heart. Weak between scapulae. Ascending **lumbar pain. Irritable, thick, burning, itching skin;** moist if scratched; < face and genitals. Branny scales. Scabby; on ears. Eczema. Psoriasis. Scleroderma. Callosities. Vivid dreams; of fire; awakes panting, with pounding of heart; seeming true. Rheumatism of hands.

Related to: Phos., Puls., Rhus-r.

RANUNCULUS BULBOSUS

SPHERE OF ACTION	AGGRAVATION
NERVES.	AIR
Muscles.	- **Damp.**
	- **Cold.**
Eyes.	- Open.
Scrous surface.	- Drafts.
THORAX.	**Changing**
SKIN.	- Weather.
	- Temperature.
Fingers and toes.	- Position.
Left side.	**Alcohol.**
	Evening.
	Motion: of Arms.
	Breathing.
	Touch.

PAINS; **stitching;** stabbing; **shooting;** extort tears; with shuddering; can't rest. Burning, biting, **bruised soreness** or as of **deep ulceration. Sore spots.** Neuralgia. Trembling. Distended feeling. .... Quarrelsome. Smarting eyes. Tick (right), to ear (Puls.). Crawling on palate; wants to scratch it. Increased saliva. Scraping-burning down throat. Bruised hypochondria. Tender abdomen. Pinching colic; alternates with chest pains. Anxious, oppressed breathing. SHARP, CUTTING, STITCHING CHEST PAINS; bilateral. Chest is sensitive to air. Pleurodynia. Pleurisy. Pain along inner edge of scapulae (left). Itching palms. BLUISH VESICLES. Shingles. Pemphigus. Corrosive ichor. Horny scabs. Herpes. **Chilliness.**

Related to: Canth., Rhus-t.

RANUNCULUS SCLERATUS

SPHERE OF ACTION
CHEST.
SKIN.
Vertex.
Right side.

AGGRAVATION
Evening.
Motion.
Deep breathing.

AMELIORATION
After midnight.

Acridity, rawness or **burning-smarting. Eating, gnawing or boring** pains; causing faintness, or short breath. ....
Sneezing coryza, with burning urine. Blunt teeth. Mapped tongue. Nausea after 12 P. M. **Stitches in chest muscles;** it is sensitive externally. As of a **plug forced between ribs,** under navel, in heart, etc. Gout of small joints. Gnawing in knees. **Yellow vesicles. Bullae;** with acrid contents. Pemphigus.

Related to: Ars., Arum-t.

RAPHANUS SATIVUS

Numbness, changing place. Retained flatulence. Hysterical meteorism. Coldness of a foot.

RATANHIA

SPHERE OF ACTION
Rectum.
Anus.
Nipples.
Teeth.

AGGRAVATION
Night.
Anxiety.
Heat.
Exertion.
Touch.

AMELIORATION
Cool bathing.
Walking in open air.

Pains here and there. **Hemorrhage. Sense of constriction. Fissure.** Dark, thin, scrawny and irritable.................. As if brain would fall out of forehead. Bursting headache when straining at stool. As if cool air came from teeth. Nightly toothache, < lying; must walk about. Griping in stomach, > eructations. Violent, painful hiccough. Sharp **cutting,** in stomach, **rectum,** etc. **Constriction or as of sharp splinters** (of glass) in rectum; stool is forced out with great straining and followed by **prolonged aching-burning,** > hot water. Dry or itching anus. Ascarides. Fissure ani. Cracked nipples.

Related to: Nit-ac., Paeon.

RHEUM

<table>
<tr><td>**SPHERE OF ACTION**</td><td>**AGGRAVATION**</td></tr>
<tr><td>Muscles of</td><td>**Dentition.**</td></tr>
<tr><td>- **Bile ducts.**</td><td>Eating.</td></tr>
<tr><td>- Duodenum.</td><td>Summer.</td></tr>
<tr><td>- **Intestines.**</td><td>Nursing women.</td></tr>
<tr><td>Liver.</td><td>**AMELIORATION**</td></tr>
<tr><td></td><td>Warmth.</td></tr>
<tr><td></td><td>Wrapping up.</td></tr>
</table>

Sour, impatient, colicky children, who are always **screaming** and crying. Sour taste, vomitus, stools, sweat, etc...................... Offensive mucus in mouth, after sleep. Difficult teething. Loathing after first bite. Colic with cries; > doubling up, < uncovering any part; then **pappy, sour, brown, green, fermented, slimy or acrid stools;** with shivering; < eating unripe fruit; < evening. Burning in bladder. Sleep, restless; with whining, cries and twitching of face, fingers, etc. **Sopping, wet hair.** Sweat on scalp, about nose, mouth or on upper lip.

Complementary: Mag-c.

Related to: Cham.

RHODODENDRON

SPHERE OF ACTION
FIBROUS TISSUES
- Forearm.
- Lower legs.
- Small joints.

Bones.
Genitals.
Nerves.
Vascular system.
Single parts.

AGGRAVATION
Weather
- BEFORE STORMS.
- **Rough; Windy.**
- COLD DAMP.
- Changing.
- Cloudy.

Night.
Midsummer.
Wine.
Rest.

AMELIORATION
Heat.
In sun.
Motion (At once).
Wrapping head.

Gouty-rheumatic subjects. SENSITIVE TO WINDY OR STORMY, WET WEATHER. Sensitive to windy weather, even if he is in house. **Tearing, zigzag,** boring, rapidly changing, descending, **paralytic pains** .... Confused and stupid; forgets his subject (Bar-c.). Headache, < early in bed, > eating. Throbbing in right head. Deafness long after rising. Nostrils obstructed alternately. Tearing, jerking faceache or toothache; > food or warmth. Cool drinks lie heavy. Colic at navel. Pain from rectum to genitals. Diarrhea, < fruit. Profuse, foul urine. **Drawing from spermatic cord into abdomen and thighs.** Testes and glans feel crushed. Testes hard; pain alternately. Orchitis. Itching, sweaty, wrinkled scrotum. Hydrocele (of boys). Menses with fever. Bruised, sprained feeling in chest and wrists. Strong heart-beat. As of a weight hanging to feet. Wants to cross legs. Drawing, tearing in periosteum of long bones and under scalp. Rheumatism of hot weather (reverse—Rhus-t.). Formication; with sweat. Must cross legs to sleep.

Related to: Rhus-t.

RHUS TOXICODENDRON

SPHERE OF ACTION

SKIN
- **Face**.
- Scalp.
- **Genitals**.

Blood.

Tissues
- **Cellular**.
- **Ligaments**.
- **Fibrous**.
- Joints.

Mucous membranes.

GLANDS
- **Payer's**.
- Parotid.

NERVES
- **CORD**.
- **Sciatic**.

Left side or left to right.

AGGRAVATION

EXPOSURE TO
- **WET; COLD air**.
- **WASHING**.
- **Chill or draft**.
- When hot or sweaty.

Uncovering; Hands, etc.

BEGINNING MOTION.

REST.

Before storms.

SPRAINS.

Over-exertion.

AFTER MIDNIGHT.

AMELIORATION

Continued motion.

HEAT
- Wraps.
- Bath.
- If heated.

Rubbing.

Nose-bleed.

Holding abdomen.

An infectious irritant, exciting TYPHOID, RHEUMATIC OR PARETIC EFFECTS. NIGHTLY SHOOTING, STITCHING, TEARING PAINS; CAN'T REST IN ANY POSITION. Grippe. Variola. **Sore, bruised or STIFF. Flesh feels beaten or torn loose.** Dislocative sensation. Twitching muscles. **Crawling**. Numbness. Trembling. **Burning, swelling and lividity.** Cellulitis. **Acrid, rusty-red, meat water or musty secretions**; causing eruptions. Scraping, gnawing or tearing loose in periosteum .... **Sad, anxious, depressed or beclouded.** Slow answers. Low delirium. Whirling vertigo; then headache. Shattering or loose feeling in brain; < jar. Board-like pressure in forehead. Painfully stiff scalp, > lying on it. **Pain behind eyes**; < motion. **Eyelids, stiff**; adherent; dry; firmly closed. Profuse, hot, gushing tears. Photophobia. Vertical diplopia. Saccular conjunctivitis. Red, sensitive tip of nose; it drips water.

Roseola. Nose-bleed; at night. Violent aching in bones of nose. Face-ache. Maxillae crack; easily dislocated; pains in. Red spot on left cheek. **Swelled, stiff face.** Dry, cracked, crusty lips; herpes on. Sordes. Bloody saliva runs during sleep. Teeth feel loose. TONGUE; RED TRIANGLE AT TIP; **coated diagonally** or on one side only; dry red center; cracked, stiff, sore. Coppery or straw-like taste. Red, puffy, itching fauces. As of chamois skin stuck on tonsils. Sore throat (left) in A. M.; **with swelled glands.** Craves cold drinks, although they < cough, chill, etc. Vomits from coughing, lying on back, etc.; **fecal.** Abdomen sore; swashing in; as of a lump in. **Ileo-caecal symptoms.** Stools watery, frothy or bloody; foul; **brick red**; slimy; gelatinous; involuntary or with tenesmus, < drinking. Piles, < lifting. **Genitals, edema,** < prepuce; **Itching;** swelled. Nephritis. Metritis; septic. Chest pains on using arms. Dry, hoarse, tearing, tormenting cough, from tickling behind upper sternum; with bloody taste. Sudden hypostasis or edema of lungs. Palpitation; > motion. Heart; feels tired; hypertrophy; pains going down left arm. Shingles. Stiff neck. **Inter-scapular pain,** < swallowing. Contractive or breaking backache, > hard pressure, walking about or bending backward. Lumbago. Coccyx aches into thighs. **Numb,** prickling limbs. Arms nervous and shaky, (left). Paralytic pain in elbows. Rhagades on backs of hands. Palms, dry, hot, cracked and sore; washing causes burning. **Pains down back of thighs;** < stool. Sciatica. **Legs** feel dead, wooden; cramp in calves; gangrenous ulcer, runs bloody water; itching. SKIN; **stiff; thick;** dry; hot; itching; burning; < warmth; **painful to cold air, Fine** VESICULAR, **crusty, eczematous, moist or** ERYSIPELATOUS ERUPTIONS, < genitals; alternating with dysentery. Pus erodes the hair. Rhus poisoning. Milk-crust. Barber's itch. Vesicles over abscess. Weeping ulcers. **Dreams, laborious;** of blood; awakes tired or nervous. Weak, rapid, sharp, tremulous or irregular pulse. **Easily chilled;** < **least uncovering; with pains in limbs;** < cough, etc. Chill as if dashed with cold water or cold water in veins; preceded by cough; alternating with heat; in single parts. Heat with busy delirium. Sweat, < during pain; with sleepiness.

Complementary: Bry., Calc., **Mag-c.,** Med., Phyt.

Related to: Arn., Bry., Dulc.

ROBINIA

SPHERE OF ACTION	AGGRAVATION
Secretions.	**Eating.**
Stomach.	**Night.**
	Fats.

Acridity; sour taste; **sour stomach;** acid belching; **vomitus so sour it sets the teeth on edge** or dulls them. Acid dyspepsia. Waterbrash. Burning in stomach and between scapulae. Squeezing in stomach. Sick headache.

Related to: Iris, Mag-c.

RUMEX CRISPUS

SPHERE OF ACTION	AGGRAVATION
Mucous membranes	COOL AIR
- **Larynx.**	- INHALING.
- Trachea.	- Open air.
- THROAT-PIT.	- Raw changes.
- Bowels.	Uncovering.
Nerves.	Night.
Skin.	Pressure; on trachea.
Left side; Chest.	**AMELIORATION**
Joints.	**Covering mouth.**
Ankles.	Wrapping up.

Dry, sensitive mucous membranes. Stickiness, with burning. Every cold affects the joints. **Sharp pains;** neuralgias, etc. Obesity. .... Eyes burn, indoors; puffed in A. M. Dry posterior nares. Sneezing attacks. Sodden complexion. Hawks out much tenacious mucus. Throat feels hollow. Ravenous appetite. Borborygmi. **Sudden, profuse, foul, early morning diarrhea** (5-9 A. M.); after catarrh; in phthisis. Respiration < wind. Suffocative choking. Dyspnea, on retiring. EVERY BREATH OF COLD AIR CAUSES TICKLING, as from a feather or dust, IN THROAT-PIT, AND CONTINUOUS COUGH; > **closing or covering mouth or head.** Profuse, frothy expectoration. Pain from right ovary to back. **Pain,** rawness or burning **under clavicle** (left); as if the air penetrated there. Chest sore. **Pain under sternum;** under left nipple. Heart seems impeded, then heavy pulsation through chest. Pain in left shoulder on coughing or raising arm, **right scapula.** Spasmodic cramps in ankles and feet. Skin itches if exposed to air. Acne vulgaris on back. Sudden sleepiness.

Related to: Caust., Seneg.

RUTA

SPHERE OF ACTION
Fibrous tissues
- EYES.
- **Flexor tendons.**
- **Joints; Wrists and ankles.**
- Back (Lumbar).

Cartilages.
Periosteum.
Uterus.
Skin.

AGGRAVATION
Over-exertion
- EYE-STRAIN.
- Injury.
- **Sprains.**

COLD
- **Air.**
- Wind.
- **Damp.**
- Wet.

LYING.
SITTING.
Pressure on an edge.

AMELIORATION
Lying on back.
Warmth.
Motion.

BRUISED, SORE ACHING AND RESTLESSNESS. **Painful weariness.** Heaviness; as of a weight in forehead or hanging to feet; of lower limbs. **As of a rough, blunt plug in part;** head, nose, etc. Nodes. **Paralytic rigidity.** Distortions. Rheumatism. **Gnawing-burning.** Neuralgia .... **Dissatisfied.** Fretful. Itching inner

canthi. Eyes burn. Lachrymation. **Dim vision.** Woody taste. Swelled
spleen. Urging to stool, but only **rectum prolapses;** < after labor,
stooping, etc. Corrosive leucorrhea. Weak, bruised feeling in small
of back, hips or lower limbs in A. M. Nodes in palms. Stumbles
easily. Lumbago. Deep pains. **Thighs feel broken.** Pains as if deep in
long bones; must walk about. **Bursae.** Erosive itching. **Chafing.** Flat
warts. Contractions. Brittle bones. Cracking joints, < walking in open
air. Ganglion. Glowing heat of face, skin, etc.

Complementary: Calc-p.

Related to: Arn., Phyt., Ran-s., Symph.

SABADILLA

SPHERE OF ACTION

MUCOUS MEMBRANES
- NOSE.
- ANUS.
- Digestive tract.
NERVES.
Lachrymal glands.
Throat.

AGGRAVATION

COLD; Air; Drinks.
PERIODICALLY
- **Same hour.**
- Forenoon.
- New and full moon.
Odors.
Undeveloped exanthema.

AMELIORATION
Open air.
Heat.
Eating.
Swallowing.

Weak; nervous; easily startled. Alternate nerve and bodily
symptoms. **Formication.** Twitches. Trembling. Worms..................,......
Miserable. Anger. Erroneous (fixed), personal ideas. Pain in alternate
sides of forehead. Unilateral head pains. Itching scalp. Red, itching
tarsi. **Lachrymation;** when in pain; < open air. **Nose;** ITCHES; rubs
or picks it; very-dry; tickling in, spreads over whole body, then dyspnea
follows. **Persistent** VIOLENT or ABORTIVE SNEEZING. Hay

fever. Influenza. **Sensitive smell.** Itching soft palate. Tongue feels burnt. Sorethroat; left to right; < empty swallowing; > hot drinks. As of a **lump,** morsel, thread or skin hanging in throat. Canine hunger. Thirstless. Craves hot things, sweets or milk. Bowels feel knotted. Burning, frothy, floating stools. **Crawling, itching at anus;** alternating with tickling in nose or ears. Pinworms. Violent coughing attacks; muffled; < anger. Upward jerking of arms. Cracks under toes. Cutting in bones. Itching skin — in nose and anus — with asthmatic breathing. Shivers; as a concomitant. Thirst, after chill only.

Related to: Ars., Puls., Urt-u.

SABAL SERRULATA

SPHERE OF ACTION
Genito-urinary organs.
- **Prostate.**
- **Ovaries**
- Mammae.
- **Bladder.**
- Urethra.
Mucous membranes.

AGGRAVATION
Women and **old men.**
Weather
- Cold, damp.
- Cloudy.
Sympathy.

Sharp, **stinging pains** in urethra. **Debility.** .... Voices seem distant. Abdominal pains into thighs. Irritable bladder and urethra. Strangury. Enuresis. Limy urinary sediment. Testes drawn up. **Enlarged** or congested **prostate;** senile. Painful erection or emission of semen. Ovarian pains. Vulva feels open. **Coldness in genitals.** Absent sexual passion; with nervous irritability. Mammae sore, tender and full, or small; < cold bath. Backache from coition.

Related to: Sep., Sil.

SABINA

SPHERE OF ACTION

FEMALE PELVIC ORGANS
- UTERUS.
- Rectum.
- **Nerves.**
Fibrous and serous **tissues.**
- **Small joints.**
- Heels.

AGGRAVATION

Nightly.
HEAT
- Bed.
- Room.
- Exercise.
Pregnancy.
Climacteric.
Foggy weather.

AMELIORATION

Cold.
Cool.
Open air.

Hot, full-blooded females; with rheumatic or gouty-
hemorrhagic tendency, epistaxis, hematuria, etc. Violent pulsations.
Fulness. Red, shiny swelling. Acutely inflamed arthritic nodes.
.... Music is unbearable. **Bursting toothache.** Craves
lemonade. Abdomen plethoric; quivering, as if alive in. Piles, alternate
with pains in limbs. **Itching, excited genitals.** PAIN FROM
LUMBAR REGION FORWARD TO PUBES or reverse; or **shooting
up vagina. Gushes of fluid, hot or watery blood,** mixed with (dark)
clots, from uterus; < motion; with joint pains. Abortion; habitual; at
3rd. month. Bleeding between periods. Foul, acrid leucorrhea.
Pruritus of pregnancy. Crawling in nipples. Gout in right big toe.
Foul itching, burning, moist, figwarts. Intolerable, burning heat.

Complementary: Thuj.

Related to: Caul., Puls.

SAMBUCUS NIGRA

SPHERE OF ACTION
Respiratory organs.
Respiration.
Kidneys.
Skin.

AGGRAVATION
Dry, cold air.
Cold drinks.
While heated.
Head low.

AMELIORATION
Pressure over a sharp edge.
Motion.
Wrapping up.

Sweats or gets short of breath; with many symptoms. Nephritis. Dropsy. .... Fretful. Half open eyes. Snuffles. Bluish, puffy face; < coughing. SUDDEN SUFFOCATION, or **strangling cough,** on falling to sleep or **waking him after midnight; with violent sweat;** < fright. Whistling breathing. Spasm of glottis. Screeching voice. Croup. Icy cold feet. **Dry, burning heat during sleep, but copious sweating on waking;** < cough. Debilitating sweats; at night.

Related to: Bell., Brom.

SANGUINARIA CANADENSIS

SPHERE OF ACTION
RIGHT SIDE
- **Head.**
- LIVER.
- Chest.
- Deltoid.
VASOMOTORS.
Capillaries.
Mucous membranes.
Stomach.

AGGRAVATION
Periodically
- WITH SUN.
- Weekly.
- Night.
Climaxis.
Odors.
Jar.
Light.
Raising arms.
Looking up.

AMELIORATION
SLEEP.

Lying on back.
Vomiting.
Cool air.
Passing flatus.

Redness; abdominal; tongue, etc. BURNING HEAT AND
EBULLITIONS. Dry mucous membranes. Burnt feeling; tongue.
Burning; in throat; under sternum; spot or stitches in chest; **palms
and soles**, etc. **General pulsation. Congestion**; to head, abdomen,
chest, etc. **Symptoms ascend, or end in bilious vomiting.** Migraine.
Internal rawness. **Acrid, blood-streaked** or foul **discharges.** Lies on
back with head elevated. .... Irritable and bilious. Grumbling.
Borrows trouble. **Pain over right eye** or ASCENDS FROM
OCCIPUT TO OVER RIGHT EYE, > free urination. Sun pains.
Swelled temporal veins. **Pain at root of nose.** Coryza; stopped, then
diarrhea. Sensitive to odors. **Red, burning cheeks.** Hectic spot. Full
and tender behind angle of jaw. Anteriorly tongue looks red, like raw
beef. Palate feels scalded. Sorethroat (right); pains to ear and chest.
Craves spices. Averse to butter. Nausea, < sneezing or blowing nose,
> eating. Tension in epigastrium. Stomach pains to right shoulder.
Bilious or gushing stools. Acrid leucorrhea. Larynx full and dry; in
singers. Coughs; raises foul air, tough, bloody plugs or purulent
sputum, or passes flatus; dry, tickling—behind sternum, in evening.
Pneumonia. Phthisis. Itching axillae, < before menses. Cutting, stiff
right deltoid, < raising or turning arm. Omodynia; < night. Wrinkled
palms. Dry skin; of jaundice. Polypi. Pain in bones near surface.
Flushes of heat, rising into face and head; with headache. Burning,
scanty sweat. General pulsation. Heat of palms and soles, < covers.

Complementary: Ant-t., Phos.

Related to: Bell., Phos.

SANICULA AQUA

SPHERE OF ACTION
Nutrition.
Female Organs.
Neck.
Rectum.
Skin.

AGGRAVATION
Motion
- Downward.
- **Of hands behind him.**
Cold wind on.
- Occiput or neck.

Looks old and thin. **Marasmus.** Body smells like old cheese. Child kicks off covers at night. Enlarged feeling in throat, vagina, etc. Thick, yellow, acrid pus .... Stubborn and touchy. Can't bear cold air on occiput and neck. Eyelids stick to balls. Fluent coryza, < eating. Water smells like old, musty rain water. Aphthae. Craves bacon, or ice cold milk. **Stool of one, large, heavy mass;** impacted. Briny urine or leucorrhea, < stool. **Backache, < putting hands behind** him or raising arms. Cold lumbar spine. Lumbago. Cold clammy hands and feet. Cramps in feet. Burning soles. Dry, brownish skin, < neck. Profuse sweat on occiput and neck. Foul foot sweat; chafes toes, destroys shoes or stiffens the hose; sticky:

Related to: Lyc., Psor., Sulph.

SARSAPARILLA

SPHERE OF ACTION
Genito-urinary organs.

Skin.

Right side; Lower.

AGGRAVATION
At close of micturition.
Spring.
Cold wet.
Mercury.
Night.
Suppressed gonorrhea.
Yawning.

AMELIORATION
Uncovering neck or chest.
Standing.

Thin frail, shrivelled and old looking. Marasmus. Tendency to gravel and **itching eruptions.** Parts feel screwed together. Nightly bone pains. Rheumatism. **Very sore, gouty nodes.** Sycosis. .... Pain depresses him. Pain from occiput to eyes or root of nose, which is swelled. **Painful urination, extorts screams,** > standing; < before menses; passes drops of blood or white, acrid material at close. Urine dribbles while sitting. Renal colic (right). Gassy urine. **Crusty urinary sediment.** Sand in the stools. Moist, foul genitals. Bloody semen. Retracted or cracked nipples. Backache with colic. **Deep cracks** on fingers and toes, < sides. Cutting under nails. Ulcerated finger-tips. **Blotchy,** hard or shrivelled skin, < about neck. Itching, scaly spots. Irritating pus. Chill starts from region of bladder; to back.

Antidotes: Bell., Merc.

Complementary: Sep.

Related to: Calc., Petr.

SCOPARIUS GENISTA

SPHERE OF ACTION	AGGRAVATION
Heart.	Turning on left side.
Kidneys.	**AMELIORATION**
Cord.	Cool air.
Muscles.	Rapid motion.
Left side.	Passing flatus.

Heavy ache; stomach and bowels seem filled with stones or a firm mass. **Flatulency.** Colic, then bright, acrid, foamy stools followed by burning at anus. **Very profuse,** bright, foaming urine, then burning pudendum. **Intercurrent congestion of kidneys.** Anxious oppression at heart, radiating to left shoulder and neck. Palpitation, with congestion to head. Deadness of right arm and fingers. Barber's itch.

Related to: Phos.

F- 17

SCUTELLARIA LATERIFOLIA

High strung neurotic women. Sleepless from nervous excitement.

SECALE CORNUTUM

SPHERE OF ACTION

Muscles
- BLOOD-VESSELS.
- UTERUS.
BLOOD.
Nerves.
Cord.
Limbs.

AGGRAVATION
WARMTH.
During menses.
Pregnancy.
Loss of fluids.
COVERS.
AMELIORATION
Cold; Bathing.
Uncovering.
Rocking.
Forcible extension.

hemorrhagic. Numbness, insufferable tingling, crawling, twitching, gnawing or **cramping;** with stiffness; in single parts; starting in face or back; in limbs; in finger-tips; after the pains, etc. **Burnings;** here and there, like fire. **Dark, thin, foul or exhausting discharges.** Decomposition. Petechiae. Varicoses. Passive bleedings or discharges. Contracted arterioles. Tonic spasm .... Mental weakess after spasms. **Fear,** depressed by; **maniacal.** Sparks before eyes. Distorted or sunken countenance; blue rings under eyes. Wild look. **Thirst;** craves acids. Empty retching. Empty feeling in hypogastrium. **Wants abdomen uncovered.** Gushing, painless, watery, olive-green or bloody stools; with collapse. Bloody urine. Everything seems loose and open. Senile enuresis. Inert uterus, or **bearing down with coldness.** Contracted uterus; hourglass contraction. Miscarriage. Green lochia. Septic placenta. Metritis. Gangrene of female organs. Leucorrhea; brown, foul; continuous. Pains through chest on pressing spine. Cold limbs. Bluish fingers and toes. **Cramps** in hands, **legs** and feet. **Fingers spread apart;** bent backward or clenched; look water soaked. Boils with green pus. Blood blisters. **Cold, dry,** wrinkled or **bluish skin, <** over affected part. Raynaud's disease. Foul, indolent ulcers. Twitching tremor or quiver in skin. EXTERNALLY, ICY COLD, YET BURNING HOT INTERNALLY OBJECTS TO BEING COVERED, < ABDOMEN. Heat, as of sparks on skin. Erysipelas. Cold or foul sweat; destroying shoes.

Antidotes: Sol-ni.

Related to: Nux-m., Ust.

SELENIUM

SPHERE OF ACTION

Nerves
- GENITO-URINARY
      ORGANS.
- Supra-orbital (Left).
LARYNX.
Liver.

AGGRAVATION

Debilitating causes
- **Hot days.**
- Sexual excesses.
- Loss of sleep.

Singing.
Drafts.
After sleep.
Tea.
Lemonade.

AMELIORATION

After sunset.
Inhaling cool air.

Easily debilitated; by heat of sun; a little mental or physical exertion makes him sleepy. Senility. **Emaciation;** of single parts, face, hands, etc. Cramp, then stiffness. Bitings..............Loquacity. Sadness. Frets when awake and dreams of it as he falls asleep. Nervous headaches. Scalp feels gathered together. Falling hair, < eyebrows; don't want hair touched. Ache over left eye; < tea. Coryza, ending in diarrhea. Thirstless. Craves stimulants, tea, etc. Sharp stitches in or rash over liver. Abdominal pulsation; hinders sleep. Very large stools. Coarse sand in urine. **Lascivious,** but impotent. Urine and semen dribble. **Easy loss of semen;** at stool, etc. Watery semen. Chronic gleet. VOICE HOARSE, as soon as he sings; affected by every cold; rattles. Nodes in vocal cords. Hawks up clear mucus. Sudden sciatic

pains (left), leave soreness behind. Oily skin; itches in folds or about
ankles. Skin remains moist after scratching. Burning spots. Acne.
Imagines drafts of air. **Sweat, profuse, yellow; leaves a salty deposit,**
stiffens the linen or makes the hair stiff and wiry; < genitals.

Related to: Nat-m., Sulph.

SENECIO AUREUS

SPHERE OF ACTION
  FEMALE
  - GENITO-URINARY
      ORGANS.
  - **Bladder.**
  MUCOUS GLANDS.
  Nose.
  Lungs.
  Lumbar spine.

AGGRAVATION
  Puberty.
  Sexual excitement.
  Dampness.
  Cold.
  Open air.

AMELIORATION
  Menstruation.

Lack of reaction in genito-urinary sphere. Passive congestion,
w ith **irritation,** profuse catarrhs, **debilitating** or vicarious **discharges.**
Muscles draw into knots. Tightness, in nose, throat, etc. Globus.
.... **Nervous, pale, weak, and sleepless women.** Whining and
irritable. Self-centered. Elated and sad alternately.   Sharp pain
backward over left eye. Burning in nostrils. **Sneezing.** Itching; caused
by tears; in Eustachian tube. Twitching about mouth. Averse to sweets.
Nausea or vomiting of renal origin. Uremia. Griping at navel. Bloody
stool or urine. Heat in neck of bladder; with renal pain. **Dysuria;**
with dysmenorrhea. Pains from ovaries into breasts. Functional
amenorrhea. Sexual irritations; excite discharges. Thick, yellow
leucorrhea; **flows down thighs.** Feels as if menses would come. Cough;
tickling, with blood-streaked sputum; > menstruation. Burning in
left nipple. **Lumbar backache,** as if to break; < **amenorrhea,** renal
disease, etc. Periodical, wandering rheumatism. Many dreams; erotic.
Feet cold in bed. Brittle nails. Hay fever, with anorexia. Sleepless
with anemia.

SENEGA

SPHERE OF ACTION
MUCOUS **and serous**
   membranes
- CHEST.
- **Eyes.**
- Nose.
- Bladder.
Muscles.
Left side.

AGGRAVATION
Air
- Open.
- Wind.
- Inhaling cold.
Rest.
Pressure.
Touch.
Looking fixedly.
AMELIORATION
Motion; In open air.
Bending head back.

Sub-acute, catarrhal or paretic states; of old people or fat, chubby children. Lax tissues. Profuse, albuminous secretions. **Burning in air-passages** .... Headache, into eyes, > cool air. Eye-balls feel distended. Bends head backward for > diplopia, ptosis, etc. Eye-balls feel like balls of ice. **Sneezes,** until dizzy. Coppery taste. **Dry scraping in month, throat and chest;** < talking. Nausea. Shreddy urine. Hoarse, unsteady voice; < sexual losses. Wheezing. Emphysema. Cough, incessant; strangling, choking, ends in sneezing; < lying on right side or evening. **Loose rattle in chest, but the profuse, clear expectoration is tough and slips back.** Blood-tinged or albuminous expectoration. **Chest sore** (in spots), as if bruised; shifting pains on stooping. As of a crushing weight on or weakness starting from chest. Pleuro-pneumonia.

Related to: Caust., Hep.

SEPIA

SPHERE OF ACTION
Venous circulation
- Digestive tract.
- **Portal system.**
- FEMALE PELVIC
    ORGANS
Nerves.
Skin.

AGGRAVATION
COLD
- AIR; North wind.
- Wet.
- Snowy.

Sexual excesses.
Before menses.
Pregnancy.
Abortion.
Morning and evening.
After first sleep.

AMELIORATION
VIOLENT MOTION.
Warmth.
Cold drinks.

Draggy, relaxed females—lithemic, **plethoric**, —subject to prolapses or easy dislocations. Uterine reflexes. **Symptoms settle in back;** shoot up, < rectum, vagina, etc.; backward, towards head (left), ileo-caecal region, ovary, etc., or cause shuddering. AS OF A LUMP or a **rolling over internally. Weak, empty,** hollow feeling; in epigastrium, chest, muscles, lumbar back, hips, knees, etc., or fulness. Milky discharges. Bleedings . ... Angry, sensitive and irritable and miserable. Sensitive to pain. Anxious fear; **over trifles.** Averse, to one's own; to sympathy; **to company;** yet dreads solitude. Stifled affections. **Poor memory.** Sad irritability, **alternating with indifference or** sulkiness. Sexually minded. Sad over her health and domestic affairs. **Indifference. Stupid,** wants to go away. **Headache;** over left eye; alternate sides of occiput; < lying on it; heavy on vertex; sho· ∪ings; bursting. Hemicrania. Jerks head back and forth. **Drooping eyelids.** Red, itching tarsi. Falling out feeling in eyes. Sees motes, flashes, zigzags, photopsies; then collapse. **Odors are repulsive.** NOSE; BROWN STRIPE ACROSS (Menis.); pressive pain at root; foul plugs or green crusts from. Dark circles under eyes. Changing color of face. Chloasma. Numb malar bones. Swollen, cracked lower lip. Mouth feels burnt. Hawks mucus or foul, cheesy grains in A. M. Taste cheesy, fishy or bitter-sour. Ascending throat colds. Eructates tough, foamy mucus. **Nausea** at thought or **smell of food**; in A. M. **Vomits**; solids only; milky. Gnawing hanger. Craves acids. FAINT SINKING AT EPIGASTRIUM, not > eating, or a lump in. Griping in gall-bladder, < stooping. Falling out or heavy **bearing down feeling in hypogastrium**; holds it or crosses legs. Pot belly. Stool, then gelatinous mucus. **Diarrhea,** from boiled milk. Rectum constricted and powerless; no urging for days. Constipation. **As of a ball in anus.** Piles, prolapsing; sticking; of pregnancy. Oozing from anus. Slow urination; cutting before. Enuresis, during first sleep; < coughing, sneezing, etc. THICK, FOUL URINE; ADHERENT, RED, SANDY SEDIMENT, or white, gritty. Menses absent; at puberty; after weaning, etc. Grasping, burning or sticking in uterus (os). Sub-involution. WEAK, DRAGGING OR BEARING DOWN FEELING; must sit close or hold parts. Tends to abort. Labia swelled; abscessed. Leucorrhea; in large lumps; foul; gonorrheal. Stomach cough; < rapid change of temperature; with foul sputum. **Circulation, irregular**; seems to stagnate. Palpitation; visible; ascends to occiput. General pulsation. Ebullitions at night. Overful blood-vessels. Collar feels tight. **Aching;** inter-scapular; LUMBAR—paralytic—wants it pressed. Purple hands. Cold knees or heels. **Skin blotched**; raw, rough, hard or cracked, < flexures. Herpes. Ringworm. Itching vesicles. Boils in axillae. Thick crust on elbows. Ulcers, on small joints. Epithelioma of eyelids, lips, etc. Skin; wine colored. Spots on the skin. Loud talking in sleep. Dreams if lies on left side. Easily chilled, Chilly, with air-hunger. **Cold; in spots; on vertex; between scapulae; feet, in bed.** Sudden weakness; then anxious, hot flushes. Hot hands, with cold feet or vice versa. Sweat, **easy;** with orgasms; on genitals, **axillae** or back. Irregular fevers.

Complementary: Nat-m., Phos.

Related to: Caust., Gels., Lil-t., Nat-m., Puls.

SILICEA TERRA

SPHERE OF ACTION
NUTRITION.
Children.
Tissues
- **Elastic.**
- **Cellular.**
NERVES.
GLANDS.
Tubes
- Eustachian.
- Tear ducts, etc.
- Fistulae.
Bones.
Cartilage.
Mucous membranes.
Skin.

AGGRAVATION
COLD CHANGES
- AIR.
- DRAFTS.
- **Damp.**
- Uncovering.
- Bathing.
- Checked sweat, < **feet.**

Sensitive to
- Nervous excitement.
- Light.
- Noise.
- Jarring.
- Spine.
Change of moon.
Night.
Mental exertion.
Alcohol.

AMELIORATION
WARM
- WRAPS; to head.
- Becoming.
Profuse urination.

Cachectic or senile patients. Large head, with wasted body. Fair, clear complexion. KEENLY SENSITIVE; **to noise, pain or cold**; hugs the stove. **Violent sticking pains**; localized; in ears, throat, ulcers, etc. Exaggerated reflexes. Contracted sphincters. Spasms. Tendency to easy exhaustion, abnormal sweats and suppuration. Cerebral softening (Phos.). **Slow, incomplete processes, then induration.** EVERY HURT FESTERS; **stubborn suppuration**; fistulas; abscess; proud flesh; **induration**; cicatrices, etc. Torpid cellular tissue. Malnutrition. Arrested development. Late learning to walk. Swelled, diseased glands. Emaciation. Scrophulo-rachitic diathesis. Parts lain on go to sleep. Edema in A. M. Extrudes foreign bodies. ....

Mental acuteness, with physical weakness or torpidity. Fidgety. **Lacks grit.** Slouchy gait. Sullen and stubborn. ASCENDING EFFECTS; violent vertigo; OCCIPITAL PAINS, etc.; > pressure. Headache, then blindness. Migraine. Vertex throbs. Open fontanels, with distended abdomen. Lumps on scalp. Inflamed eyes. Spotted vision. Cataract. Deafness; hears again with a snap. Frothy nasal discharge. Coryza; with epistaxis. Waxy pallor. Enlarged parotids. As of a hair on tongue, in throat, etc. Bitter taste in throat. Abscess at roots of teeth. Hawks down foul lumps. Averse to hot food. Averse to mother's milk; vomits it. **Big, hard or hot belly; with thin legs. Rectum;** cutting; cramping; paining into testes; <coition. Stools; **receding;** < menses; retained, for fear of pain. Fissure ani. Foul urethral discharge. Itching, moist spots on scrotum. Hydrocele. Cutting upward in vagina, < urinating. Nursing < uterine flow. Biting, gushing leucorrhea. Itching vulva. Retching, shaking, gagging cough; < cold drinks. Respiration difficult from draft on neck. Profuse, foul, lumpy sputum. Rattling in chest. Sore, retracted nipples. Nodes or fistulae in mammae. Sharp pains in breasts and uterus. Axillary glands swelled. Fingertips painful; dry, Panaris. Weak ankles. FOOT-SWEAT; FOUL; itching; **acrid,** destroying shoes; **suppressed.** Sore ache in arch of foot. Distorted, ingrown nails. Bunions. Soggy, wilted skin. Acuminate eruptions. Carbuncle. Ulcers; painfully sensitive; foul; spongy; on feet, toes; at nails; > heat. Osteitis. Somnambulism. Frightful dreams, wake him on falling to sleep. CHILLY; < lying in bed, exertion, etc. **Coldness of painful part. Icy chills.** Hectic. SWEAT; **profuse; on upper parts; head, or affected parts; at night;** foul; easy; acrid.

Complementary: Fl-ac., Phos., Thuj.

Follows: Calc. or Hep.

Related to: Calc., Hep., Kali-p.

SOLIDAGO

SPHERE OF ACTION
KIDNEYS.
Digestive tract.
Lower limbs.
Blood.

AGGRAVATION
Pressure.

AMELIORATION
Profuse urine.

Weak; easily takes cold. Hemorrhage. Kidney disfunctions; chronic nephritis; uremic asthma .... Bitter taste. Profuse, involuntary, mucous stools. Difficult, **dark and scanty** or clear, sinking **urine**. KIDNEYS **sore or tender over; ache;** feel distended. Nephritis; chronic. Cystitis. Prostatitis. Lumbar ache; makes her sick all over. **Petechiae on lower limbs (Agave);** with edema, Gangrene; diabetic. Eczema; < suppressed urine.

SPIGELIA ANTHELMIA

SPHERE OF ACTION
NERVES
- TRIFACIAL.
- HEART.
- **Neck.**
Fibrous tissue.
EYES.
Teeth.
LEFT SIDE.

AGGRAVATION
TOUCH.
MOTION.
Jar.
Periodically; **With the sun.**
Tobacco.
Coition.
Raising arms.

AMELIORATION
Lying on right side, with head high.

Combined heart and eye symptoms, or the latter as an accompaniment. PAIN; **in violent attacks; radiating;** from left occiput to over left eye; < stooping. Neuralgia. Sun pains. Vertigo; **feet feel higher than the head. Shudders;** if touched or bruised........ Stammering. Fears pointed things. Left supra-orbital or occipital pain; boring. EYES; **sore,** drawing ache; sunken; **feel large;** red; flowing tears on affected side; squinting; yellow rings about. Post-nasal dropping. **Fetor oris.** Toothache. Ravenous hunger. Pain about navel; in children. Mucus lumps in stools. Worms. Dyspnea, < moving arms. HEART; **violent, audible** PALPITATION, attending other symptoms; **violent sticking** or compressive pain radiating to throat, arm or scapula, < least motion; or bending double; soreness; purring; crackling. Cardiac angina, etc. Neck stiff; pains into left temple or from left shoulder into neck. Cutting about left scapula. Numb left arm. Weak, tremulous or irregular pulse. Pulsation in patellae.

Complementary: Spong.

Follows: Acon.

Related to: Cact.

SPONGIA TOSTA

SPHERE OF ACTION
HEART; Valves.
Larynx.
Trachea.
Glands.

AGGRAVATION
DRY<. COLD wind.
Roused from sleep.
Exertion.
Raising arm.
Before 12 P.M.

AMELIORATION
Lying with head low.
Eating a little.

FLABBY. **Weak and heavy.** Feels stuffed up. Orgasms. Hard swellings; glands (ductless). ....Terrified, anxious look. Eyes seem to protrude. Sorethroat, < sweets. Painfully swelled spermatic cord and testes; stitches in; squeezing in. Hard testes. Noisy, whistling inspiration on falling to sleep. SUFFOCATION; as from a plug, leaf or valve in larynx; **waking him;** with **violent, painful palpitation** and blue lips; with heavy sweat. Anxious, **gasping breathing.** HOLLOW, BARKING, CROWING, SAWING OR TIGHT CROUPY COUGH; **wakes child;** then burning in chest; < cold drinks or excitement; > eating. Voice gives out. **Croup;** sudden. HOARSENESS. Larynx pains, < touch, singing, talking or swallowing; he grasps it. Diphtheria. Neck; as if a cord about. Choking on falling to sleep. Goitre. **Fulness in chest.** Apical phthisis. HEART; **surgings mount up to neck, head and face;** with closure of eyelids and tears. **Palpitation.** Goitre-heart. Valvular disease. Numb fingertips or lower half of body. Awakes in anxiety. **Heat;** in spells, with anxiety and cardiac pain, would rather die; and sudden weakness after walking in open air, he must lie down; with cold, moist thighs; < thinking of it.

Follows: Cact.

Related to: Iod., Led.

SQUILLA MARITIMA

SPHERE OF ACTION	AGGRAVATION
MEMBRANES	**Early morning.**
- MUCOUS.	Motion.
- **Serous.**	Uncovering.
Kidneys.	Old people.
Heart.	
Spleen.	

Exudations and profuse secretions. Dropsy; with **profuse urine.** Cardio-urinary effects. Gurglings. ....**Rubs eyes,** sneezes. Acrid coryza. Black spots on teeth. **Sweet taste;** of food, expectoration, etc. Stomach pains, > lying on left side. Aching hypochondria. Dark brown, frothy stools. Sudden urging; passes much urine. Bloody urine. Erotic pollutions. COUGH; stubborn, **rattling with sneezing, coryza, watery eyes, spurting urine,** or heat; ends in gagging; < cold drinks and inspiration. Easy, heavy expectoration; < morning and evening. Stitches in chest (left). Pleurisy. Broncho-pneumonia. Heat, with aversion to uncover. Absence of sweat.

Complementary: Ant-c.

Related to: Ars.

STANNUM METALLICUM

SPHERE OF ACTION

NERVES.

MUCOUS MEMBRANES.

CHEST.

FEMALE ORGANS.

AGGRAVATION

Using voice.

Cold.

10 A.M.

MOTION

- **After.**
- Gentle.
- **Lying on right side.**

Ascending steps.

AMELIORATION

Rapid motion.

Hard pressure; Over an edge.

Expectoration.

Repeated short attacks. EXTREME WEAKNESS; < IN CHEST; **in throat,** stomach, upper arms and thighs; drops into a chair; can't even talk; trembles on moving. **Paralytic heaviness. Profuse, muco-purulent secretions.** Emaciation. PAINS INCREASE GRADUALLY, THEN SLOWLY SUBSIDE. **Pressive drawing.** Neuralgias. Cramps. Spasms. Hysteria .... **Anxious, nervous and sad;** < before menses. **Weak and miserable, and discouraged.** Pressive, stupefying headache. Pale face, with sunken eyes. Malar neuralgia. Faceache. Tickling at root of tongue. Vomiting; violent; early morning, with odor of ingesta. Burning in liver. Painful, pinching colic, > hard pressure and stool, which exhausts. Child wants to be carried over shoulder. Worms. Atony of bladder. Easy sexual orgasms. Pollutions. Before menses, mania erotica. During menses, strong odor of body. Gushes of debilitating leucorrhea. Prolapse, of vagina or uterus, < stool. Much mucus in trachea. Deep, hollow voice. **Short breath, from every effort;** must loosen clothes. **Cough; easily expectorates quantities of sweet** or bright yellow pus or balls of mucus. Catarrhal phthisis. **Chest feels** raw or **hollow.** Tremulous knees. Swelled hands and ankles. Chill at 10 A. M.; with numb fingertips. **Burning palms and soles.** Hectic, debilitating, musty sweat at 4 A. M. Night-sweats.

Antidotes: Hep., Puls.
Related to: Lach., Nat-m.

STAPHYSAGRIA

SPHERE OF ACTION

NERVES.

TEETH.

Genito-urinary organs.

Fibrous tissues
- Eyelids.
- Tarsi.
- Skin.

Glands.

Right deltoid.

AGGRAVATION

Emotions
- Chagrin.
- Vexation.
- Indigestion.
- Quarrels.

Sexual excesses; Onanism.

Touch.

Cold drinks.

Lacerations.

Stretching parts.

Mercury.

Night.

AMELIORATION

Warmth.

Rest.

Breakfast.

Nervous trembling. Squeezing or stinging smarting, as if cut. Pains that move into teeth. ....Morbidly sensitive; easily offended. Always angry. Gloomy and petulant; throws things. Poor memory. Hypochondriasis. Sexually minded; unsatisfied urge; widows. Sheepish; sensitive mentally and physically. Imagines insults. Irritable, nervous, excitable and violent. Brain feels torn. Compressive, stupefying headache. As of a heavy load in forehead. Moist, foul, eroding milk-crust; < occiput. Dryness in eyes. Nodes in lids. Styes. Blepharitis. Sickly, peaked and hollow-eyed. Neuralgia, from caries; pains go to eyes. Coryza, now thick, now thin; ulcerating. Swelled sub-mental gland; abscess. Pale, bleeding gums. Loose, aching, black, crumbling teeth; < eating and during menses; > hard pressure and heat. Pyorrhea. Musty taste. Hungry; craves milk. Colic; flatulent; ovarian; < coition. Dysentery. Irritable bladder. Urinates a slender stream. Trickling or burning along posterior urethra; < after walking or riding, > urinating. Priapism. Prostatitis. Dysuria; of brides; in pregnancy (Pop-t.). Itching or sensitive vulva. Pains from ovaries into thighs. Salpingitis. Crural neuralgia. Tight chest, at close of coition. Cough, <cleaning teeth or alternating with sciatica. Violent yawning; brings tears; after headache. Pains that precede shingles. Backache; in bed in A. M. Fine tearing in or numb fingertips. **Nodes on finger joints.** Skin symptoms, alternate with joints pains. Weak knees. Biting itching; as of vermin; changing place on scratching. LACERATED WOUNDS; < **sphincters**; perineum, etc.; stitch pains. Amorous dreams, with pollutions. Sweat and flatus smell like bad eggs.

Complementary: Coloc.

Related to: Cham., Merc.

STICTA PULMONARIA

SPHERE OF ACTION	AGGRAVATION
Nerves.	**Night.**
Membranes	Lying down.
- **Nose.**	Motion.
- Chest.	Change of temperature.
Bronchi	**AMELIORATION**
- Joints.	Free discharges.
Shoulder (Right).	Open air.

Nervous, stiff and rheumatic; develops catarrhs. Painful, dry mucous membranes. Diagonal pains. .... Must talk. Seems to be floating. Burning eyelids. **Pressure or stuffy fulness at root of nose**; blows it without relief. Coryza; that dries up again. Hay fever. Tickling high up in pharynx. **Incessant, dry, hacking cough; prevents sleep;** < **coughing** and inspiration; croupy; < if tired; after measles. Numbness in air-passages. Bronchitis. Sore, stiff neck; pains to shoulder. Restless hands and feet. **Rheumatism**. Red spot on affected joint. Bursitis. Cold, moist limbs. Profuse sweat on hands.

Related to: Cetr., Elaps, Guaj., Sang., Thuj.

STRAMONIUM

SPHERE OF ACTION	**AGGRAVATION**
BRAIN.	**Glistening objects.**
Circulation	**Fright.**
- Throat.	AFTER SLEEP.
- Skin.	Dark, cloudy days.
Spinal nerves	**Suppression.**
- Arms.	Intemperance.
- Hip (Left)	**AMELIORATION**
- Genitals.	LIGHT.
	Company.
	Warmth.

A remedy of TERRORS, BUT LACKING IN PAIN; **with
suppressed excretions** (Verat.), passing neither urine nor stool (Led.).
Very mobile states. Tremor; nervous. **Disorderly, graceful** or rhythmic
motions (Elaps), < head or arms. Chorea. Spasms, < night.
.... DREADS DARKNESS, and has a horror of glistening
objects. **Fearful,** desires company or wants to escape. **Active, variable
delirium**; talks incessantly; sees many, vividly brilliant or hideous
phantoms, more to one side. **Wildly excited,** as in **night terrors** or
delirium tremens, or does all sorts of crazy things. Raving **mania,**
with cold sweat;, cursing and praying. Religious insanity. The talk
of others is intolerable. Self accusation. **Loss of reason** or speech.
Stupid. Imbecile. Vertigo, < in dark. Jerks head up and drops it again.
Fixed, sparkling **stare.** Squint. Diplopia. Night blindness. Green
vision. Crowding, visual hallucinations. **Sees black.** Delusions as to
size and distance. **Red, bloated** or rapidly changing **face;** now flushed,
now pale; a sardonic grin, then expresses **terror.** Frowning. **Fine red
dots on tongue.** Stammering. Constantly spits saliva. Dry throat,
with great thirst, yet **dreads water;** it chokes him. Hydrophobia.
Putrid, dark, painless, involuntary **diarrhea.** Sexual excitement (in
males). Excessive menses, preceded by sexual excitement. Grasps the
genitals. Nymphomania. Spasmodic cough. Spasm of larynx. Voice

suddenly fails, in higher tones. Nervous asthma. Drawing in back. Sensitive spine. Violent pain in hip. Unilateral paralysis, with twitchings. Crawlings, as of many bugs. Non-appearing exanthema. Fiery scarlatinous rash. Sopor. Weeping, in dreams. **Awakes in fear or screaming.** Frightful visions.

Antidotes: Coff., Nux-v.

Related to: Bell., Hyos., Op.

STRONTIUM CARBONICUM

SPHERE OF ACTION
Vasomotors
- **Circulation.**
- Heart.
- Kidneys.
Marrow.
Ankles.
Right side.

AGGRAVATION
COLD; Changes.
Uncovering.
Walking.
Sprains.
Bleedings.
Evening

AMELIORATION
Heat and light
- Sun.
- Wraps.
- **Baths.**
Itching.

Congestive tension. **Fleeting pains**; seemingly in bones. Rheumatism. Burning. **Gnawing.** Pains increase and decrease gradually or make him faint and sick all over. Violent starts. **Immobility**; of one side. Edema. Sense of **paralytic weakness.** Emaciation. Prostration after operations. Formication in limbs. Arterio-sclerosis. .... **Headaches;** into upper jaw; with vertigo and nausea. Violent pain in nape, > wraps, Very pale or violently red face. **Numb mouth.** Pressure in stomach during digestion. Cramp about navel. Hard, knotty, difficult stool, then burning at anus. Exhausting, nightly diarrhea, of yellow water;

periodically. Pale, ammoniacal urine. As of a load on chest. **Heart feels smothered.** Heart block. Numb hands. **Sprained or puffed ankles.** Cramp in calves and soles. Surgical shock. **Flushes of heat;** in face; **yet averse to uncovering.** Night-sweats. Climacteric.

Related to: Calc., Rhus-t.

STROPHANTHUS

SPHERE OF ACTION	AGGRAVATION
HEART; Circulation.	**Exertion.**
Stomach.	Alcohol.
Kidneys.	Tobacco.
	Tea.

Stitches, Twitchings. Increased secretions. **Alternations;** rapid, with slow pulse; surgings to head and heart; dilated, with contracted pupils, etc. **Undulations.** Throbbing. .... **Fear of ordeals.** Feels lifted up, during siesta. Vertigo, with swimming vision. Faintness. Very mobile pupils. Glimmering vision. Red spots on face. Throat seems constricted. Craves coffee. Anorexia. Vomiting. Rumbling, colicky diarrhea; with burning at anus. HEART; **sense of lively action; aching;** anguish at; weak. Palpitation; chronic, especially nervous. Cardiac dyspnea. Atheroma. Small, weak, rapid or irregular pulse. Heavy forearms and fingers. Itching feet. **Hives;** receding.

Related to: Apoc., **Glon., Ign.,** Spig.

SULPHUR

SPHERE OF ACTION	AGGRAVATION
CIRCULATION	SUPPRESSIONS.
- VENOUS.	BATHING.
- **Portal.**	Milk.
- **Abdomen.**	HEATED.
NUTRITIVE ORGANS.	- EXERTION.

MEMBRANES
- Mucous.
- Serous.
Rectum.
Chest.
SKIN; Folds.
VERTEX.
SOLES.
Joints.
GLANDS.

- IN BED, by woollens, etc.
Atmospheric changes.
Speaking.
Periodically.
- **11 A.M.**
- **Climacteric.**
- Full moon (Cina, Sil.).
AMELIORATION
Open air.
Motion.
Warm applications.
Sweating.
Dry heat.

STOOPED, LANK, UNCURED, UNTIDY AND
UNWASHED. **Emaciation;** with good appetite. Atrophy of children.
Psora. Scrofula. Rheumatism. DEFICIENT REACTION; effusion;
deposits; slow reabsorption. CHRONICITY. RED ORIFICES, or
single parts; **lips,** tarsi, ears, etc. (Aloe). LOCAL THROBBING,
BURNING OR CONGESTION; SOLES; VERTEX; bones; painful
spots, etc. ITCHING; parts; discharges cause, etc. **Foul, acrid or
blood-streaked discharges. Weak, faint spells. Empty,** overful, rough
or asleep feeling. ASCENDING EFFECTS; heats, orgasms, vertigo,
etc............... **Slow, lazy, hungry and always tired. Hopeful dreamers;**
ecstatic, religious, philosophic, etc. Peevish, mean, prying or easily
excited. Melancholic. Tired of life. Vertigo; in forehead. VERTEX,
throbs, hot, heavy, sore, etc. **Nape to vertex;** pain, chills, pressure,
etc. As of a band about or pain deep in brain. Sunday headache;
preceded by photopsies. Hot head, with cold feet. Sweaty scalp. Dry,
cold hair. **Eyes;** burn; cutting, as from sand; bursting in balls;
quivering. **Halo about light.** As of floating soot before. Photophobia.
Ophthalmia. Swashing in ears. **Nose,** obstructed on alternate sides;
drips; swelled; **red,** < cold. Catarrhal colds. Epistaxis, < night or lying
on right side. Sensitive smell. Imaginary odors. Swelled veins of
forehead. OLD LOOK. Spotted face. Dry, tremulous tongue; red
edges and tip. Sensitive dental fangs. Grinds teeth. Nursing sore
mouth. **Throat;** as of a swelling or a **vapor** rising in; external redness.

Eructations, like bad eggs, > eating. **Drinks much, eats little.** Averse
to meat. SUDDEN HUNGRY AND WEAKNESS; < 11 A. M.; **at
epigastrium.** ABDOMEN SORE, > pressure; **heavy,** as of a lump;
stitches; bearing down, against rectum; congested. Borborygmi.
Colicky babies. RECTUM pains; itches; urging in; **hemorrhoidal
habitus.** Holds stool back from pain. DIARRHEA; HURRIED,
EARLY MORNING (Tub.), changing; mushy; stinking; **painless;
watery;** gray froth; < milk; alternating with constipation. Burning,
itching urethra. Hurried or nightly urination. Bed wetting. Testes
hang low. Cutting in uterus; < menses. Burning, itching, sore vulva;
< sitting. Puerperal sepsis. Acrid, foul menses. SUFFOCATIVE AIR
HUNGER. Irregular breathing. **Cough;** violent, in 2 or 3 incomplete
bouts. Deep, hoarse voice; early. **Chest;** rattling and heat at 11 A.
M.; as of a band about or a load on; red; brown spots on. **Pain
backward from left nipple.** Pneumonia. Heart seems too big.
Palpitation, < lying. Nipples crack at base. Sharp burning in mammae.
Neck weak; boils on. Heavy shoulders. Aching between scapulae.
Lumbar pains; to stomach; **walks bent;** supports weight on hands,
when sitting. Coccyx, pains during stool. Numb left arm, < lying.
Palms crack and peel; eczema on; warts on. Numb fingers (right).
Tense hamstrings (left). Cramp in calfs (left). SOLES BURN;
STICKS FEET OUT OF BED, AT NIGHT or are cold in bed; dry.
Jerks one limb, on dropping to sleep. SKIN; **dry : rough, wrinkled,
scaly;** ITCHING, violently at night; BREAKS OUT; **festers, and
won't heal;** burning, when scratched; painfully sensitive to air, wind,
washing, etc. **Eruptions alternate with other complaints,** asthma,
etc. Crops of boils. Itch. Creeping erysipelas. Rhagades. Eczema.
Ulcers. Skin under-nourished. Suppuration with air bubbles.
Localised congestions. Hot vertex and soles. Inclined to uncover single
parts. Craves fresh air. Drowsy, then migraine. Sleeps in cat naps.
Sleepy by day, wakeful at night. Sleep; unrefreshing; sings during.
Chills up back. Heat; **feels too hot; flushes of;** with general throbbing;
between scapulae. Sweat; in axillae; on hands or feet.

Antidotes: Merc., Puls., Sil.

Complementary: Aloe, Calc., Sul-i.

Related to: Psor., Sel., Syph.

SULPHURICUM ACIDUM

SPHERE OF ACTION
DIGESTIVE TRACT.

Blood.

Blood-vessels.

Left side.

AGGRAVATION
Open air.
Cold.
Spirits.
Injuries.
ODOR OF COFFEE.
Climacteric.
Towards evening.
Excessive heat or cold.

AMELIORATION
Hot drinks.
Hands near head.
Moderate temperature.

Suited to **topers**, old age, etc. Disproportionate weakness. TREMOR; INTERNAL; wants to be held. **Sourness.** Erosion. **Profuse, acrid or stringy discharges.** Hemorrhage; violent; black, thin. Parts feel stiff and tight. **Pain increases slowly, then** suddenly ceases. Gnawing. **Great painfnlness. As of a blunt plug being driven in.** ....Hurried, irascible, vacillating and morose. Brain feels loose. **Deathly pale** or wrinkled face; white of egg seems dried on it. Congestion to head. Aphthae. Throat sore; looks white-washed. Pyrosis. Hiccough; of drunkards. Sour belching; sets teeth on edge. **Nausea.** Vomiting; < lying on left side. Weak, sinking at stomach, < after stool. Drinks chill the stomach. Very foul, green, black or **hacked diarrhea.** Oozing piles. Coughs, then belches; bloody expectoration. Fingers jerk when writing. Weak knees. Black and blue spots. Petechiae. HOT **flushes,** then trembling or cold sweat; < after warm ingesta; < upper parts; > motion. Drenching sweats.

Complementary: Puls.

Related to: Ars., Lach., Sep.

SULPHUR IODATUM

SPHERE OF ACTION
Tissues.
Skin.
Glands.
Right side.

AGGRAVATION
Exertion; Slight.
Heat.
Lying on right side.
Before storms.
Night.

AMELIORATION
Cool air.
Standing.

Grippy feeling. Weak; and sensitive to everything. Faint and sick. **Raw, burning heat, internally, with external coldness.** Acrid discharges. Single parts, fingers, etc., turn white and insensible. Suppuration. Infiltration. **Favors reabsorption**............... Headache, > sundown. Hair seems erect. Zigzags before vision. Teeth feel soft. **Glazed tongue.** Raw, dry mouth and throat; painful swallowing; wants to moisten it. Tremor in epigastrium on exertion. Mesenteric disease. Bright yellow stools. Stubborn constipation. Foul anal discharge. Urine scanty; purulent; brown sand in. Soft testes. Deficient erections. Cracked prepuce. Aching soreness below knees. **Itching.** Ulcers. Moist eczema. Acne. Barber's itch.

Follows: Sulphur.

SUMBUL

SPHERE OF ACTION
Nerves.
Heart
Left side.

AGGRAVATION
Motion.
Inspiration.
Climacteric.
Music.

AMELIORATION
Gentle motion.

Nervous, irritable and sleepless. As of hot water flowing through part. Yellow, tenacious discharges. Early senility...................... Laughs and weeps by turns. As of a hair or cobweb on face. **Choking constriction in throat.** Hysteria. Burning pyrosis. Oppressive tightness in left chest. Dyspnea. Asthma; **cardiac.** Sexual excitability. Trickling along spine. Pale, cold skin. Internal itching. Dreams of falling.

Complementary: Lact.

Related to: Mosch.

SYMPHYTUM OFFICINALE

SPHERE OF ACTION	AGGRAVATION
CARTILAGE.	INJURIES.
PERIOSTEUM.	Blows from.
Flat bones.	Blunt; instruments.
	FRACTURES.

Excessively painful (old) **injuries;** to periosteum or cartilage. Comminuted fractures. **Prickling,** stitching pains. **Eye and face injuries.** Non-union. **Deficient callus.** Coldness.

Related to: Calc-p.

SYPHILINUM

SPHERE OF ACTION	AGGRAVATION
	NIGHT; Damp.
	Sundown to sunrise.
Mucous membranes.	Gradual < then slow >.
	Protruding tongue.
Nerves.	Extreme heat or cold.
Bones.	Every alternate full moon.
	During thunderstorms.

AMELIORATION

Changing position.
Continued or slow motion.
High altitudes.
Applied heat.

Poor reaction or it does not hold. Chronicity. Great weakness,
with but few symptoms. Multiphase symptoms. SYPHILITIC
TAINT. Weakness; on waking. Ulceration. Bald head, pouting lips
and big belly. Dwarfish. Marasmic. Foul odor of body. Violent or
linear pains. Knots in muscles. .... Antisocial. Horrid
depression or despair. Cross. Feels like going crazy. Impulse to wash
hands. Syphilitic insanity. Poor memory. Nightly delirium. Cerebral
softening. Deep, crushing head pains; across base. Beats head against
wall. Linear headaches. Head feels pulled back. Slowly advancing
hemiplegia. Hair falls profusely. Inflamed cornea; > cool bathing.
Ophthalmia. Glimmering vision. Vertical diplopia. Ptosis. Abscess
of middle ear. Nose painful to inhaled air; in sinuses. Ozena. Snuffles.
Face wrinkled; looks old. Pain over right eye, < protruding tongue.
Teeth feel sticky; as of a worm in; decay at edge of gums. Salivation;
at night. Putrid taste. Crack along center of tongue. Green lumps
from posterior nares. Sore throat; right to left; < cold drinks.
Capricious appetite. Craves alcoholic liquors. Rectal fissure or
stricture. Frothy urine. Nocturnal enuresis. Voids urine > standing.
Menses have odor of rotten meat. Profuse, acrid leucorrhea; runs to
heels; with itching. Cough, < lying on right side. Pain from base to
apex of heart. Neck feels short. Backache, < urinating. Deltoid pains
extends to middle fingers. Itching eruption about elbow. Cold pain
in legs. Festination. Bones pain as if sawed. Bilateral exostoses. Skin;
biting as from bugs; swelled and blotched, > hot bathing. Pains in
shins, > heat. Wandering erysipelas. Succession of abscesses. Foul or
green pus. Conical crusts. Bullae. White cicatrices. Distorted nails.
Sleeplessness. Large, soft pulse. As of hot water in veins.

Related to: Merc.

TABACUM

SPHERE OF ACTION
 Nerves
 - Cerebro-spinal.
 - Vagus.
 - Sympathetic.
 - Ganglia.
 - HEART.
 GLANDS.
 SECRETIONS.

AGGRAVATION
 MOTION; **of riding.**
 Lying on left side.

AMELIORATION
 Cold; Fresh air.
 Twilight.
 Uncovering abdomen.

Relaxing irritant; causing prostration, free secretions and exciting muscles of hollow organs. Cramp, then paralysis; of bowels, heart, etc. Paroxysmal or jerky effects. Stormy, dangerous cases, with rapid changes. Pains, < from heat. Faintness slides down. Tremor. .... Morose, despairing and wretched or **indifferent.** Confusion. Mental fag. **Excessive vertigo;** with copious sweat (cold), < opening eyes. Retina retains images too long. **Deathly pale, pinched look.** Retracted lips. Spasm of lower jaw. Tetanus. **Much spitting;** with complaints. Clutching about throat. **Deathly nausea and violent vomiting; < least motion;** with much spitting. Retching. Pregnancy. Seasickness. Acidity. **Sinking at epigastrium. Wants abdomen uncovered.** Heaviness in right abdomen. Colic; with weakness. Involuntary choleraic or thick, **curdled,** watery **stool;** like sour milk. Ileus. Dribbling urine. Renal colic. Emissions. Impotency. Constricted chest. Asthma. Twisting about heart. Angina pectoris; with nausea, cold sweat and collapse. Unsteady heart beat. Backache, < lying > walking. Fuzzy fingertips. Nightmare. **Icy cold skin.** Thready, intermittent pulse. Cold legs. Heat; of one cheek; down spine; internal. Sudden **cold sweats;** with chills; in renal colic, angina pectoris, etc.

Complementary: Op.

Related to: Ars., Gels., Verat.

TARAXACUM

SPHERE OF ACTION	AGGRAVATION
Liver.	**Rest.**
	Sitting.
Stomach.	Standing.
	AMELIORATION
	Walking.
	Touch.

Bilious, sick feeling. Stitches. .... Depression. Coated tongue, with **raw patches; mapped.** Sour taste or hawks sour mucus. White stools. Bilious diarrhea. Jaundice. Restless limbs, with tearing pains. Chilly after eating. Cold fingertips. Burning toes. Night sweats.

Related to: Nux-v.

TARENTULA HISPANICA

SPHERE OF ACTION	AGGRAVATION
NERVES.	TOUCH.
HEART.	**Cold.**
Spine.	**Noise.**
RESPIRATION.	**Damp.**
Generative sphere.	Periodically
Right side.	- Same hour.
	- Yearly.
	After menses.
	Evening.
	AMELIORATION
	Relaxation
	- **Rubbing.**
	- **Sweating.**
	- Smoking.
	Open air.
	Music.
	Riding horseback.
	In the sun.

VIOLENCE; sudden. **Restless, fidgety, hurried**; in incessant motion, but walking <. **Rolls from side to side** (Am-c., Ars., Lach.); < head, and rubs it. Quivering. Numb prickling. **Jerking. Twitching.** Chorea. **Synalgias; sexual** (Apis). Violent pain. Sepsis; deep. Emaciation; < face. ....Averse to green colors. Dances up and down. Sensitive and nervous. Nervous laughter, then screams. **Lacks control. Erratic.** Impulsive. Selfish. **Suddenly** changing moods, fancies or strength. Hysteria. Hateful, adroit, crafty, **cunning and destructive** or depraved (Bufo). Throws things. Malingering. Kleptomania. Angry despair. Death agony. Vertigo, then spasms. As of needles pricking brain. Heavy, left parietal ache to face and neck, with impatience and nausea. **Sleepless;** from excitement. Violent, crushing **headache,** as an accompaniment. Meningitis. Thick tears. Expression of terror. Face fiery red; bloated. Craves raw foods. Heaviness in pelvis. Stool; oily; excited by washing head. Foul urine, with sandy sediment. **Sensitive genitals.** Sexual erethism. Hot semen. Dry, hot, **raw, itching vulva and vagina,** < scratching. Motions or burning in uterus. Cancer of cervix. Leucorrhea of clear, acrid, sticky lumps. SUFFOCATION; must have fresh air; < coughing. Cough, > smoking, < noise. Heart, twists around; takes sudden jump. Chorea cordis, with arm symptoms; < hands in cold water. **Painfully sensitive spine;** touch excites pains in heart, chest, etc. (Bell.). Restless arms; **keeps hands busy;** picks fingers. Restless legs; impulse to walk. Festination. Cold, moist feet and hands. Itching soles. Sawing bone pains. **Skin, purplish** (Sol-n.); ecchymotic; cold spots or as of cold water flowing or dropping on part. Suppuration; deep; evacuates pus rapidly. Noma. **Alternate chill and heat.** General heat, with cold feet. Fever; septic. Sweat, profuse; excoriating.

Complementary: Ars.

Related to: Agar., Ars., Mygal.

TARENTULA CUBENSIS

SPHERE OF ACTION
Cellular tissue.

AGGRAVATION
Cold drinks.
Exertion.

Spasmodic difficulty of breathing. Shattering cough; pertussis. Slow incubation, then **rapid onset, with alarming prostration, atrocious burning or sharp stinging pains, board like** HARDNESS OF PART **and copious sweat.** Intense diphtheritic fever. Malignancy. Sepsis. Carbuncle. **Felon. Bluish abscess.** Painful abscesses. **Death agony.** Paralysis, then convulsions .... Nervous restlessness. Fulness in head. Tendency to vomit. Pruritus vulvae. Trembling hands. **Fidgety feet. Purple discoloration.** Gangrene. **Pungent heat of surface.** Drowsy. Unsteady gait.

Related to: Anthraci., Lat-m.

TELLURIUM METALLICUM

SPHERE OF ACTION
Spine.
Nerves.
Ears.
Eyes.
Skin.
Right to left.

AGGRAVATION
Touch.
Lying on part.
Cold.
Empty swallowing.
Spinal injuries.
Weekly.

Offensive; like putrid **fish brine** or garlic. **Salty;** taste; mucus from throat; pus, etc. **Acrid discharges;** excites itching, vesicles, etc. Periostitis. **Numbness.** Sharp, quick pains, then soreness. Sense of retention......................... **Vertigo;** < falling to sleep. Linear head pains. Thick tarsi. **Inflamed, bluish, puffy ears.** Otitis. Fluent coryza, hoarseness and watery eyes. Twitching face; pains jerk angle (left) of mouth up. Rancid belching. Retching, ends in yawning. Stomach feels hollow. Sprained pain in chest muscles, over heart, < raising *arms.* **Very sensitive or sore spine.** Deep sciatic pain, < coughing, sneezing, straining or lying. Itching, pricking, as from bugs. Circular eruptions. Ringworm. Burning in an old scar. Chills down spine, < lying on back.

Related to: All-c., Sel.

TEREBINTHINIAE OLEUM

SPHERE OF ACTION	AGGRAVATION
Mucous MembranesM	**Dampness.**
- KIDNEYS	Cold.
- Bladder	**Night.**
Bronchi.	Lying.
Respiration.	Pressure.
Heart.	**AMELIORATION**
Blood.	Motion.

Kidneys affected, with rheumatism. Sudden, grippy **aching.**
Stiff, sore muscles. Pain; **excites urination;** along larger nerves.
Burning; tip of tongue, epigastrium; small of back; **kidney; uterus,**
etc. Congestion. HEMORRHAGE; **passive;** oozing mucous surfaces.
...................Exhausted and **sensitive.** Smooth, sore, glossy tongue.
Bruised, sore abdomen and bladder. Flatulence. Tympanites. Ascites.
Profuse mucous stools. **Burning** or pains along ureters. Strangury.
Urine; **smoky;** with coffee grounds or thick, yellow, slimy, muddy
sediment; odor of violets; **bloody.** Nephritis; early; scarlatinal; with
violent **bronchitis.** Cystitis. Bleeding bladder. Pains alternate between
bladder and navel. Metritis. Bronchial asthma. Hands feel swelled.
Cramp in knees. Advancing purpuric spots. **Drowsiness.** Rapid pulse.
Heat under skin. Cold sweat on legs.

Antidotes: Canth.

Related to: Canth., Erig., Phos.

TEUCRIUM MARUM VERUM

SPHERE OF ACTION
NOSE.

Lungs.

RECTUM.

Finger-tips.

Toe-joints.

AGGRAVATION
Weather
- Changing; Damp.
- **Cold**
In bed.

AMELIORATION
Open air.
Sweat.

Over-sensitive and excitable. Delicate and sensitive. Internal tremor; < excitement......................Sleepless, after excitement. Crawling in nose; must pick it; side lain on closes; lumpy discharge. Polypi. Anosmia. Atrophic catarrh. Mouldy taste in throat, on hawking or coughing. Itching of palate and ears. Solid lumps from posterior nares. Follicular pharyngitis. Itching anus; prevents sleep. Pinworms. Cough, < coughing. Ingrown nails.
Complementary: Calc.
Related to: Cina, Sil.

THERIDION

SPHERE OF ACTION
NERVES.

Spine.

Bones.

Left side; Head; Chest.

AGGRAVATION
NOISE.

Touch.

CLOSING EYES.

Least motion.

Riding.

Jar.

AMELIORATION
Rest.
Warmth.

Hypersensitive. NOISE IS INSUFFERABLY PENETRAT-ING; affects the teeth; causes nausea, chills, and pains all over; strikes painful spots, etc. Water feels too cold. Bounding internally.

.... Startled by the least thing. Fruitless activity. Sense of duality. Hysteria. **Vertigo with nausea, on closing eyes.** Headache felt during sleep, < jarring. Migraine. Glittering vision on stooping. Luminosities, then blurred vision. Pain over root of nose. Yellow-green, thick, foul nasal discharge. Ozena. Post-nasal catarrh. Nausea, < least motion. Sea-sickness. Burning in liver. **Pains at end of left floating ribs.** Gonorrhea. Cough; jerks body together. Too much air seems to enter chest. Stitch back through apex of left lung. Phthisis florida. Cardiac anxiety. Spine is sensitive to pressure or jar. Burning in upper arms. Restless feeling in hands; wrings them. Bones seem broken. Necrosis. Scrofula. **Stinging thrusts in skin.** Internal coldness. Cold sweat is easily excited.

Related to: Asar., Sil.

THLASPI BURSA PASTORIS

SPHERE OF ACTION	AGGRAVATION
Vascular system.	Every other month.
	AMELIORATION
	Bathing.
Female organs.	Dampness.
	Rapid motion.

History of hemorrhage or suppressed vaginal discharges. .... Impulse to walk far. **Pain from above eyes up over head to nape.** Taste like bad eggs. Craves butter-milk. Flatulence (right). Kidney stone. **Menses or leucorrhea leaves a fast stain.** Leucorrhea excites itching. Milky water runs from right nipple. Weakness between scapulae.

Complementary: Sep.

THUJA OCCIDENTALIS

SPHERE OF ACTION
Mucous membranes
- GENITO-URINARY.
- Intestines.

Mind.
Nerves.

Occiput

Glands.
SKIN.

Left side; Ovary.

AGGRAVATION
COLD DAMP.
Heat; of bed.
Periodically
- 3 A.M.
- Yearly.
- Increasing moon.
- During menses.
Urinating.
Gonorrhea.
Syphilis.
Mercury.
Vaccination.
Tea.
Onions.

AMELIORATION
Warm
- Wind.
- Air.
- Wrapping head.
Free secretions.
Sneezing.
Motion.
Crossing legs.
Touch.

Exhausted and soft. Great prostration. Rapid emaciation. **Soft, exuberant, fungoid tissue;** polypi; condylomata; warts, pediculated, black, suppressed, etc. Sycotic, hydrogenoid or lymphatic-constitution. Foul, acrid, **musty, rancid** or **sweetish odors.** Oily stool, skin or sweat. **Trickling;** in urethra. Burning, sticking, numbing, drawing or **wandering pains,** < warmth. Rheumatism. Jerkings, of spinal origin. Parts look dead...................... Ill-humored; sad; loathes life. **Illusions,** then **fixed ideas;** of fragility; **of a live thing internally;** of some one at his side; of being in hands of a stronger power, etc.

Hasty and anxious; over trifles. Can't concentrate. Neurasthenia; prostatic. Vertigo; as if in a swing. Tearing or like a nail in left head. Neuralgia. Dry, split hair. Eyes blood red; full of tears; stand open. Sclerotitis. Jagged iris. Photopsies, beyond visual field. Bloody scabs or briny odor in nose. Epistaxis. Face, pale, waxy, shiny; dark under eyes; spiderlets on. Boring in zygomae. Teeth decay at edge of gums; gnawing pains, < cold. Ranula. Mucus in choanae. Noisy swallowing or belching. Rancid or greasy eructations. Pushings in abdomen. Cutting squeezing in lower bowels, groins, bladder or urethra. Ileus. Gurgling in bowels; then painless, watery, grass green stools. Stools gurgle or pop out; < breakfast. Stools, of hard, black lumps mixed with gushing water; hurried; explosive; spraying; gassy. Moist anus or perineum. Urine burns; dribbles; foul; copious; frequent; must wait. Pain from left kidney to epigastrium, < motion. Forward, cutting in urethra on urinating. Lithemia. Offensive genitals. Testes seem bruised. Prepuce puffed; sloughing. Gonorrhea. Chordee. Tearing in ovaries (left). Itching, sensitive vagina. Short, difficult breathing. Asthma. Cough by day only. Expectorates easier lying. Cheesy sputum. Anxious palpitation. Retracted nipples. Chest pains take various directions. Back; throbs; pressure over kidneys; atrophy of long muscles. Cracking joints. Numb fingers, on waking at night (Nat-m.). Crawling or inflamed finger, or toe tips. Hips give way; limbs feel paralyzed. Restless knees. Painful soles. Foul, acrid foot-sweat. Skin brown; spotted; dirty; hairy. Eruptions itch or burn violently from cold bathing. Moist, foul polypi. Prurigo. Nevi. Bluish white ulcers. Stinging, jumping out feeling. Itch. Blood-boils on back. Foul pustules, with sunken apices. Nails ribbed, soft, brittle, crumbling, discolored or distorted. Sleepless when on left side. Dreams of the dead. Shaking chill, with yawning; < urinating; not > heat. Heat rises into chest; with icy hands, nosebleed or cough. Sweat on bare parts; with dry heat on covered ones; with cold hands, > washing; profuse on genitals; gushing, < company; foul; pungent; staining.

Complementary: Nat-m., Nit-ac., Sabin., Sil.

Related to: Merc., Nit-ac., Sabin.

F- 19

THYREOIDINUM

SPHERE OF ACTION
HEART.
Central nervous system.

Right side.
Skin.

AGGRAVATION
Least
- Cold.
- Exertion.

AMELIORATION
Lying on abdomen.

Splitting sensation; chest; ensiform appendix; spine. Clutchings. Choking. Wants to lie down. Nervousness. Faintness. Rapid emaciation. .... Tired and **irritable**. Heavy ache over eyes. Falling hair. Nose dry, indoors, moist in open air (Nux-v.). Dry, red lips. Metallic taste, at tip of tongue. Dry throat and larynx. As of a splinter stuck across throat. Cutting in liver, < deep breathing. Rolling flatulence with gurgling, then a loose, gassy stool. Bearing or aching down through pelvis, into anterior thighs. Gnawing in uterus. Cough on entering a warm room from cool air. **Heart; palpitation,** hammering; beat felt in ears; pains, radiating into axillae; clutching, causing short breath. As if blood were rushing downward through body. Hypertrophy; after hard labor. Numb left finger, then right leg. Large veins on arms and hands. Very dry skin. As of a cold wind blowing on body. Icy cold left hand. Cold clammy hands. Hot flushes, then chills, or drenching sweats (Aml-ns.). Oily, musty sweat.

Related to: Calc., Glon.

TILIA EUROPAEA

SPHERE OF ACTION
Muscles.
Female genitals.
Urinary organs.

AGGRAVATION
SWEATING.
Drafts.
After sleep.

Dragging pains. Edema. Sore; **uterus**, abdomen, etc.; bed feels too hard. Rheumatism. Neuralgia.............................Heavy drag in urethra. Scanty urine. Cough from tickle in left throat (Hep.). **Sleepy;** < during pain. Profuse sweat, without relief; THE MORE HE SWEATS THE GREATER THE PAIN (Cham.).

Related to: Apis, Calc., Lil-t.

TRILLIUM PENDULUM

SPHERE OF ACTION
FEMALE SEXUAL
ORGANS.

AGGRAVATION
Motion.
Climaxis.

AMELIORATION
Exertion in open air.
Tight bandage.
Bending.
Forward.

Hemorrhage; gushing. ....As if eyes would fall out, the **bones of hips, back or thighs be forced apart,** etc.; with **faintness and sinking** at stomach. Menses every two weeks. Bleeding fibroids. Menorrhagia. Varices of pregnancy.

Complementary: Calc-p.

Related to: Sabin.

TUBERCULINUM

SPHERE OF ACTION
LUNGS.
Mind.
Head; Occiput.

Glands.

Larynx.

AGGRAVATION
CLOSE ROOM.
Motion.
Exertion.
Weather: DAMP (cold).
Changing.
Draft.
Awaking.
Noise.
Mental excitement.
Thinking of it.
Pressure of waistband.

AMELIORATION
Cool wind; Open air.

Obscure, changeful indications. Susceptible, given to relapse, increasing exhaustion and **lowered vitality.** Rapid breakdown (Lyc.).

Takes cold easily; ends in diarrhea. TUBERCULAR TAINT.
Scrofula. Quiverings. .... SENSITIVE; **every trifle irritates;**
< awaking. Fits of violent temper. **Dissatisfied;** always wants a change;
reckless. **Fear;** of dogs. Confusion. Shooting from over eyes to occiput.
Head pains; deep; violent; tears hair or beats head, < motion. Brain
feels loose. Sensitive scalp. Eczema tarsi. Sweat on nose. Old, dingy
look. Aching malar bones. Teeth; feel jammed; sensitive to air. **Delayed
dentition.** Dryness in mouth; in choanae. Sticky mouth. Hawks
mucus after eating. Adenoids. **Craves cold milk,** or sweets. Drum
belly. Brown, **foul,** watery, explosive stools. Tearing in rectum on
coughing. Bed-wetting. Sticky urinary sediment. Menses soon after
child bearing. Frightful dysmenorrhea. AIR HUNGER. Hoarseness,
> talking. Dyspnea, < cough. **Cough;** fits of; with chill and red face;
< **evening;** < raising arms. Mucus rattle in chest, without
expectoration. Pneumonia; of grippe. Asthma. Sore spot in chest.
Heaviness at heart. Tension in nape. **Skin: dry, harsh;** sensitive, easily
tanned; itching in cool air. Brown fingertips. Branny scales. Many
enlarged glands. Dreams, frightful, vivid; of shame; awakes in horror.
Chilly; yet wants fresh air. Cold feet; < left; in bed. Heat; on cheek of
affected side; flushes of; in spots; burning; on genitals; < eating. **Sweat;**
easy; cold; clammy; in upper parts; on hands; < coughing. **Clothes**
feel damp. Wants covers in all stages.

Complementary: Calc., Kali-s., Sep.

Related to: Phos., Puls., Sep.

URTICA URENS

SPHERE OF ACTION	AGGRAVATION
MAMMAE.	**Cool**
Genito-urinary organs.	- Moist air.
	- Bathing.
Liver.	Yearly.
Spleen.	**Burns.**
	Stings.
	Snow air (Sep.).

Stinging or **stinging-burning.** Urinous odor of body. Uric acid
diathesis. Hemorrhage. .... White stool. Pinworms. Acrid
urine, causing itching. Lithiasis. Swelled mammae. **Absence of milk.**
Fever at night; with vertigo and general pulsation. Acute gout.
Itching-burning; on genitals. **Uric acid intoxication. Pruritus.**
Nettlerash. Prickly heat. **Hives;** elevated; with rheumatism; after shell
fish; with pinworms. Angio-neurotic edema. Sweatiness. Vesicles.

Related to: Form., Nat-m., Oci.

USTILAGO MAYDIS

SPHERE OF ACTION	AGGRAVATION
Epithelium.	Climacteric.
- Skin.	Touch.
- Hair.	
- Nails.	Motion.
Female sexual organs.	

Tumid tissues, tending to **bleed slowly. Dark hemorrhage. As**
of a knot; in throat, bowels, uterus, etc. ....Depression.
Loss of hair and nails. Sticky secretion matting the hair. Milk crust.
Masturbation. Menses half liquid, half clots or stringy; vicarious.
The uterus seeps dark, clotted blood. Spongy cervix. Metrorrhagia.
Acute ovarian pain. Burning in right ovary; soreness in left ovary and
of uterus; pains shoot down thighs. Foul, yellow or brown leucorrhea.
Pain under left breast. Dry, hot skin.

Related to: Asaf., Bov., Sec.

VALERIANA OFFICINALIS

SPHERE OF ACTION	AGGRAVATION
NERVES	REST.
- **Spinal.**	STANDING.
- Genito-urinary.	**Excitement.**
Mind.	Evening.
Muscles, etc.	**AMELIORATION**
- Calf.	**Changing position.**
- Heels.	Walking about.
- Tendo Achilles.	Rubbing.

Suddenly changeable disposition and symptoms. Alternations and want of reaction. Pains move outward; are here and there or come and go. Illusions; of smell, taste or hearing. Sense of floating; of a ball or plug. Globus. Impulse to move. Jerks. Weak single parts; eyes, arms, wrists, popliteae, etc. .... NERVOUS, excitable and weak; wriggles or squirms about; inclined to faint. Anger. Very mobile ideas, going from one extreme to another. Hysteria. Luminosities, before eyes in dark. Objects seem too near eyes. Greasy or rancid taste. As of a thread in throat. Eructations, like bad eggs. Hunger, with nausea; as if from navel. Gastric cramp. Flatulence. Colic. Polyuria. Strangling on dropping to sleep. Crampy pain in left humerus, wakes from sleep. Heels pain when sitting. Coldness in upper head. Chills start and go down back from occiput. Fever composed of disagreeable heat only. Sudden gushes of sweat.

Related to: Asaf., Ign., Puls.

VARIOLINUM

SPHERE OF ACTION
BLOOD.
Spine.
Muscles.
Metabolism.

AGGRAVATION
Motion.
Vaccination.

General aching, < in back, occiput and legs. Calcareous deposits in the blood-vessels, spinal cord, etc. .... Green vision on rising. Every odor nauseates. Putrid, coppery taste. Tongue protrudes during sleep. Food seems to want to regurgitate. Tympanites, pouting upward; she looks pregnant. **Breaking backache.** As of bugs crawling under skin. Eczema of palms. **Pustular eruptions**; foul. Smallpox. Shingles and pains that follow. Ulcers look scooped out. As of cold water trickling down back. Violent chill. Intense burning fever. Foul sweat.

Related to: Ant-t., Cimic., Maland.

VERATRUM ALBUM

SPHERE OF ACTION
NERVES
- ABDOMINAL.
- Heart.
- Blood-vessels.
Vertex.
Blood.
Respiratory and digestive
                systems.

AGGRAVATION
EXERTION.
DRINKING.
Cold drinks.
Fright.
During pain.
Wet cold.

AMELIORATION
Hot drinks.
Walking about.
Covering.
Lying.

VIOLENT EFFECTS; PROFOUND PROSTRATION, COLD SWEAT ON FOREHEAD, FAINTNESS OR COLLAPSE. SUDDEN, EXCESSIVE EVACUATIONS. **Cramps;** in chest, bowels, fingers, toes, etc.; with rigidity. Progressive weakness and emaciation; in acute diseases, e.g., whooping cough, ague, etc. .... **Delirium; early;** with violence, loquacity or lewdness; during pain. Prays, curses and howls in turn. Acute manias, insanities, etc. Remorse. Loss of ideation. Sits in silence. Melancholia. Overpowering headache. Hair bristles; painful. Face; deathly pale on rising; **bluish,** pinched or distorted; frowning; terrified look. Red left cheek, as if burnt. Jaws cramp on chewing. Heaviness in teeth. Burning thirst. **Craves ice water or** sour drinks. Vomits or eructates froth. EXCESSIVE VOMITING, WITH PURGING; **violent retching, cutting colic, cramps in limbs and rapid prostration. Cholera;** morbus, infantum, etc. Painful epigastrium. **Watery,** green, odorless or colorless (rice water) **stool,** or in large masses. Nymphomania. The air seems too hot. Dyspnea. Tickling down throat, into lungs. Continuous, violent cough; with retching; < cold drinks. Neglected pertussis, with complications. **Aphonia.** Heart; cuttings at; weak; visible palpitation. Fine burnings, in arms; right to left. **Cramps in calves;** during stool (Apis, Sec.); between scapulae, etc. > motion. Skin feels scorched. Awakes at night trembling. Thready pulse. GENERAL COLDNESS (icy); **on vertex;** of nose; in mouth; of waterbrash; limbs, sweat, etc. Blood seems to run cold or internal heat with cold (wrinkled) surface. Fevers showing external coldness only. Congestive chill.

Complementary: Carb-v.

Related to: Ars., Camph., Cupr., Cyanides, Tab.

VERATRUM VIRIDE

SPHERE OF ACTION
Vasomotors.
- MEDULLA.
- Occiput.
- CHEST.
- **Stomach.**
- Heart.
- Capillaries.

AGGRAVATION
RAISING UP.
Motion.
Cold.
Lying on back.
Puerperal states.
AMELIORATION
Rubbing.
Lying with **head low.**
Eating.

SUDDEN VIOLENT CONGESTION; **cerebellar or thoracic; with nausea and vomiting,** weakness, staggering, etc. Markedly uneasy. Trembling here and there during sleep, as if on the verge of convulsions. **Muscle prostration.** General pulsation. Erratic motions. **Spasms;** with twitchings, shrieks or opisthotonos; before or **after** menses; as a prodrome. Eclampsia. Uremia. **Burnings;** in places; tongue, pharynx, gullet; of skin, which is cold; with prickling. Lies with head low ....Loquacity. Mania; puerperal. Delirium, with wild staring eyes and restless hands. Carphology. Head, thrown back; nodding or rolling motions; throbs on raising up; aches on vertex and between eyes. Pains up occiput, with dim vision and dilated pupils. Vision, of red spots; purple, on closing eyes. Deafness, < quick motion. LIVID, TURGID FACE, BUT BECOMES FAINT ON SITTING UP. Apoplexy. Heat stroke. Tension across malar bones. Chewing motions. **Red or dry streak down center of tongue.** Foul breath. Nausea,. with vomiting and purging. **Vomiting;** violent, without nausea. Hiccough. Esophagitis. Stomach seems to press against spine. Gastritis. Abdomen aches; cutting at navel. **Slow, heavy breathing;** as of a weight on chest. Dyspnea. Violent cough from very start. Pneumonia. Dull, burning ache at heart. Aching neck and shoulders. Vesicles on hands. Cramps in feet, dorsae, soles, etc. Dreams of water. **Full, large, soft pulse** or slow, with strong or violent heart beat. **Hyperpyrexia** or rapidly oscillating temperature; with sweat. Sepsis. Burning in chest. Clothes feel damp. Cold, **clammy sweat.** Cerebro-spinal fever.
Related to: Acon., Gels.

VERBASCUM THAPSUS

SPHERE OF ACTION
Nerves (Facial)
- Orbits.
- Ears.
- Zygomae.
Respiratory tract.
Bladder.
Left side.

AGGRAVATION
Drafts.
Change of temperature.
With every cold.
9 A.M. to 4 P.M.
Twice a day, at same hour.
Talking.

AMELIORATION
Deep inspiration (Osm.).

Spasmodic catarrhal or neuralgic effects. Earache. Coryza; with tears (Euphr.). **Cramping, squeezing, crushing, paralyzing faceache;** in malar bones. As of a lump at navel. Piles. Enuresis; < coughing; nightly. Deep, hollow, bellowing or trumpet toned cough. Cough; without waking; nervous; > deep breathing. **Hoarseness.**

Related to: Acon., Plat., Sep.

VIBURNUM OPULUS

SPHERE OF ACTION
FEMALE ORGANS.

Nerves.

Left side.

AGGRAVATION
Fright.
Before menses.
Cold; Snow air.
Lying on left side.

AMELIORATION
Rest.
Pressure.
Open air.

Violent nervous or spasmodic effects; **in females.** Can't keep still. **Cramping.** Hemorrhage. .... Faint on sitting up. Left parietal pain. Snuffles. **Frequent, profuse urination;** during headache, menses, hemorrhage, etc. Heavy ache or **excruciating** cramps in pelvis; > menses; Dysmenorrhea; with flatulency, loud eructations and nervousness. **Miscarriage.** False labor pains. Violent, persistent after-pains. **Uterine hemorrhage. Suffocation, at night;** < cold damp. Infantile asthma. Pains in back, end in a **cramp in uterus or go down face of thighs.** Cramps in calves before menses. Tettery spots on cheeks, arms, etc.

Related to: Caul., Puls., Sep.

VINCA MINOR

SPHERE OF ACTION
Skin.
Hair.

AGGRAVATION
After swallowing.

Weak and faint, as if to die...................Foul, matted hair. Cutting in lower esophagus. Menorrhagia; blood flows and flows, with weakness. Weeping eczema intermingled with foul, thick crusts.

Related to: Ust.

VIOLA ODORATA

SPHERE OF ACTION
Nerves.
- Eyes.
- Ears.
Wrists (right).
Skin.
Vision.

AGGRAVATION
Cloudy weather.
Cool air.
Music.
Puberty.

Tension. Nervous activity, then sudden exhaustion. Combined **eye, ear and kidney** or worm symptoms...................Pain over brows. Pain left eye to vertex, < cough. Cramp in eyes. Otorrhea. Craves meat. Itching at anus. Milky urine. Enuresis. Weight on chest. **Dry skin, with moist palms.** Cold shoulders,

Related to: Puls., Spig.

VIOLA TRICOLOR

SPHERE OF ACTION
Skin.
Scalp.
Urinary organs.

AGGRAVATION
Pressing on opposite side.
Suppressed eczema.

Cracked, gummy crusts on scalp, exuding profuse, tenacious, yellow fluid, matting hair together; with swelled cervical glands. Milk crust. Eczema. Urine smells like cat's urine; involuntary in bed. Emissions, with vivid dreams.

Related to: Rhus-t.

VIPERA BERUS

SPHERE OF ACTION
VEINS.

Blood.

AGGRAVATION
LETTING LIMB HANG DOWN
Cold.
Yearly.
Touch.

Bursting feeling. Hemorrhagic tendency. ....
Epistaxis. Excruciating pain at epigastrium. Enlarged liver. **Fulness and unbearable pain, as if limb would burst;** must elevate parts; sits with feet high. Cramps in or blue lower limbs. Varicose veins or ulcers. Phlebitis. Goitre.

Related to: Elaps.

VISCUM ALBUM

SPHERE OF ACTION
Female sexual organs.
Nerves.

AGGRAVATION
Becoming chilled while hot.

Vertigo; persists after epileptic attack. Vertex; sudden throbbings in. Sore about waist. Milky urine. Bronchial asthma. Blood won't clot and wounds won't heal.

Related to: Bufo.

XANTHOXYLUM

SPHERE OF ACTION
Nerves.
Respiration.
Female sexual organs.
Left side.

AGGRAVATION
Sleeping.
Dampness.

AMELIORATION
Vomiting.

Grinding, shooting, radiating pains. Numb left side...............
Nervousness. Head threatens to fly to pieces. Throat feels like a hollow cavern. Violent, **agonizing,** grinding dysmenorrheal pains, not > in any position; pains go into thighs or radiate over whole body, even to heart. Leucorrhea replaces menses. Soreness of face of thighs, before menses.

Related to: Ars., Lach.

ZINCUM METALLICUM

SPHERE OF ACTION
BRAIN AND NERVES
- **Occiput.**
- **Spine.**
- Orbital region.
Root of nose.
Blood
Inner canthi.

AGGRAVATION
EXHAUSTION; Mental.
Suppressions.
Noise.
Touch.
Wine.
After being heated.

AMELIORATION
Motion.
Hard pressure.
Warm open air.
FREE DISCHARGES.

Fagged, enervated or depressed; can't throw things off; develop exanthema or discharges, etc. Increasing **weakness;** < eating; **with restlessness. Isolated effects;** one part numb, another sensitive; **formication;** pain in spots; between skin and flesh, etc. Transverse pains. Automatic acts. **Tremor. Jerkings;** nightly. **Spasm.** Shootings. Descending paralysis. Disabling bone pains. Bloody discharges..................Fretful and sensitive; cries if vexed. Easily startled, excited or intoxicated. Muddled. **Forgetful;** repeats the question, then answers. Brain-fag. **Screams;** if moved; during sleep; with pain, etc. Violent vertigo; with stupor. **Headache** of varying intensity; **pressive on vertex or root of nose;** into eyes; with weak vision; < warmth, > hard pressure. Temples; heavy ache in; pain, < biting. Occiput; dragging, down back; as of a blow on, then weak legs; heat in. Crashing in head on falling to sleep. Rolls head and grinds teeth. Brain paralysis. Hair painful; on vertex; bristles. Eyes feel drawn together. Squint. Lachrymation on eating. Pterygium. Swelled nose. Pale, bluish, miserable face. Sticky lips. Bitter mouth. Voracity. As of a lump in liver region or at navel. Hypogastric flatulence. Itching at anus during stool. Piles draw down, > heat < walking; ulcerate. Violent urging but urinates only in certain positions, bending backward, crossing limbs, etc.; blood follows urine. Pressive cutting about kidneys. Grasps genitals; with each cough, etc. Sexual excitement. Onanism; during menses. Profuse, lumpy menses. Pain (boring) in left ovary. Spasmodic dyspnea, < flatulency > expectoration. Bursting, one hard throb or as of a cap over heart. Hard heart beat. Constricted chest. Nape tired; < mental exertion; lame, then stupor. **Spine aching, burning along,** < sitting; **sensitive;** inter-scapular cutting, > eructations; weak lumbar, < standing. **Spasms,** from spinal injuries. Pains in limbs on becoming heated. Hands tremble; eczema on. CAN'T KEEP FEET AND LEGS STILL; cramp when cold. Toes feel swelled; sore; ache in tips. Sensitive soles. Bones of feet feel broken. Sweaty feet, with sore toes. Stumbling. Spastic gait. Varicoses; painful; chronic; on genitals. Broken, unrefreshing sleep.

Antidotes: Tab.

Complementary : Puls.

Related to: Ign., Kali-p., Lach., Pic-ac.

ZINCUM ARSENICOSUM

AGGRAVATION
10 A. M. and 3 P. M.

Light exertion.

Occipital pain. Blue vision. Burning in **bladder.** Numb right arm, then left, > writing. Soles ache when tired, > pressure. **Lumbar pain,** < **exertion,** sitting, jarring, or standing.

ZINCUM CHROMICUM

SPHERE OF ACTION
Ears.
Nose.
Throat.
Left side.

AGGRAVATION
MOTION.
Lying on back.
Washing head.

Gnawing, grinding ache. Wandering, shock-like pains. Catching stitches, that impede motion.........................Averse to work; can't bring herself to it. Inward pressing; in spot on bregma. Throbbing temples; behind ears. Wavering vision. Bad odor within nose. Blows quantities of blood, pus and scabs from nose. Metallic taste. Indefinite cravings. Thoughts of eating are a bugbear. Can't tolerate her hands on abdomen. Dryness in vagina, with a sense of coming unwell; 10-12 A. M. Cough from tickling in throat-pit; expectorate sweet and loose, but had to be swallowed, or tough with spitting spells. Shooting from left larynx up through tonsil into ear. Cutting at apex of heart; at night. Gnawing grinding below and above left scapula. Feet sore. Cramps in toes at night; or grinding gnawing.

Related to: Puls.

ZINCUM IODATUM

SPHERE OF ACTION
Heart.
Nerves.
Valves.

AGGRAVATION
Lying on left side.
Heat.

Jerkings, startings, etc. **Lying on left side** causes vertigo, palpitation, floating sensation, etc. .... Nose, obstructed at night; blows thick, yellow chunks from; hot, dry nares. Goitre; presses inwardly. Myocardial exhaustion. Lower limbs feel as if floating. Cramps in calves, in ankles; must press feet to floor.

Related to: Stict.

ZINCUM PHOSPHORICUM

Mental fatigue, depression and paralysis. Abuse of Bromides. Epilepsy.

ZINCUM VALERIANICUM

SPHERE OF ACTION
Nerves.
Ovaries.
Spine.

AGGRAVATION
Rubbing.

Oversensitive, nervous and sleepless. Spasmodic nervous effects. Yawning. Hiccough. .... Excitable. Ticking over left ear. Sour taste in A. M. Flatulent cramps; hypogastric. Mucous colitis. Smothers on attempting to eat. Ovarian or dysmenorrheal pains, down limbs; during and after menses. Achings up back. Chills after mental excitement or exertion. Cold parts burn as they warm up.

PART TWO

REPERTORY

A Short Repertory Containing:

(a) *The Periods of Aggravation.*

(b) *Conditions of Aggravation and Amelioration.*

(c) *Generalities i.e. Consideration of Drug Affinities for the Entire Organism.*

(d) *Regional Repertory.*

TIME

PERIODICALLY, in general, Agg.: Aran., ARS., Cact., Cedr., CHIN., Chinin-s., Eup-per., Gels., Hep., Ip., Kali-c., Lyc., NAT-M., Nux-v., Puls., Rhus-t., Sulph., Tarent.

daily, Agg.: Aran., Ars., Caps., Ip., Nux-v., Puls.

at same hour, Agg.: Ant-c., Aran., Ars., Bov., Cedr., Chinin-s., Cina, Ign., Lyc., Nat-m., Sabad.

alternate days, on, Agg.: Ars., Canth., Clem., CHIN., Ip., Lyc., Nat-m., Nux-v., Puls., Rhus-t.

every 4th day, Agg.: Ars., Lyc., Puls., Sabad.

every 10th, day, Agg.: Lach., Phos.

weekly, Agg.: Ars., Canth., Chin., Gels., Iris, Lac-d., Lyc., Phos., Sang., Sil., Sulph.

fourteen days, Agg.: Ars., Con., Lach., Nicc., Sang., Sulph.

every 3rd., week, Agg.: Aur., Mag-c.

every 4th, week, Agg.: Nux-v., Sep.

every 6th, week, Agg.: Mag-m.

yearly, Agg.: Am-c., Ars., Crot-h., Echi., Elaps, Lach., Lyc., Naja, Nat-n., Psor., Rhus-t., Tarent-c., Thuj.

MORNING, Agg.: Am-m., Ant-t., Aur., Borx., Bov., Bry., Calc., Cann-s., Carb-v., Castm., Chel., Con., Croc., Echi., Elaps, Hep., Kali-bi., Kali-c., Kali-n., Lach., Naja, Nat-m., Nat-n., Nat-s., Nit-ac., NUX-V., Phos., Podo., Rhod., Rhus-t., Sabad., Sep., Squil., Sulph., Verb.

in bed, Agg.: Aloe, Ambr., Am-m., Bry., Con., Kali-c., Lyc., Nux-v., Phos., Sep., Sulph.

and evening, Agg.: Alum., Bov., Calc., Caust., Coc-c.,

Graph., Kali-c., Lach., Lyc., PHOS., Psor., Rhus-t., Sang., SEP., Stram., Stront-c., Thuj., Verat.

6 A. M.: Aloe, Alum., Arn., Bov., Ferr., Hep., Lyc., Nux-v., Sil., Sulph., VERAT.

7 A. M.: Eup-per., Hep., Nat-c., Nux-v., PODO., Sep.

8 A. M.: Eup-per., Nux-v.

9 A. M.: Bry., Eup-per., Kali-bi., Kali-c., Lac-c., Nat-m., Nux-v., Sep., Sul-ac., Verb.

10 A. M.: Ars., Borx., Chin., Chinin-s., Eup-per., GELS., Iod., Med., NAT-M., Petr., Phos., Rhus-t., Sep., Sil., Stann., Sulph., Thuj.

10 A. M., to 3 P. M.: Tub.

11 A. M.: Ars., Asaf., Bapt., Cact., Chinin-s., Cocc., Gels., Hydr., Hyos., Ip., Lach., Mag-p., Nat-c., NAT-M., Nat-p., Nux-v., Phos., Puls., Rhus-t., Sep., Stann., SULPH., Zinc.

12 Noon: Ant-c., Arg-met., Chel., Chin., Elaps, Eup-per., Gels., Kali-c., Lach., Nat-m., Nux-m., Nux-v., Phos., Polyp., Sil., Spig., Stram., Sulph., Valer., Verb.

AFTERNOON, Agg.: Alum., Ang., Apis, Asaf., BELL.,

Chin., Colch., Dig., Hell., Ign., Kali-n., Lyc., Puls., Rhus-t., Sep., Sil., Sulph., Thuj., Zinc.

1 P. M.: Ars., Cact., Chel., Cina, Grat., Kali-c., Lach., Phos., Puls.

2 P.M.: Ars., Chel., Eup-per., Ferr., Gels., Lach., Mag-p., Nit-ac., Puls.

3 P. M.: Ang., Ant-t., Apis, Ars., Asaf., BELL., Cedr., Chel., Chinin-s., Con., Nat-n., Samb., Sang., Staph., Thuj.

4 P. M.: Aesc., Anac., Apis, Ars., Cact., Caust., Cedr., Chel., Chinin-s., Coloc., Gels., Hep., Ip., LYC., Mang., Nat-m., Nat-s., Nit-ac., Nux-v., Puls., Rhus-t., Sulph., Verb.

4 to 8 P. M.: Coloc., Hell., Lyc., Nux-m., Sabad., Zinc.

5 P. M.: Alum., Bov., Caust., Cedr., Chin., Coloc., Con., Gels., Hep., Hyper., Kali-c., Lyc., Nat-m., Nux-v., Puls., Rhus-t., Sulph., THUJ., Tub., Valer.

EVENING, Agg.: Acon., All-c., Ambr., Am-c., Ant-c., Ant-t., Arg-n., Arn., Ars., Bell., Bry., Caps., Caust., Colch., Cycl., Euphr., Fl-ac., Hell., Hyos., Kali-n., Kali-s., LYC., Mag-c.,

Meny., Merc., Mez., Nit-ac.,
Phos., **Plat.**, Plb., **PULS.**, Ran-
s., Rumx., **Sep.**, Stann.,
Stront-c., **Sulph.**, Sul-ac.,
Syph., Valer., Zinc.

6 P. M.: Ant-t., **Cedr.**, **Hep.**,
Kali-c., Nat-m., **NUX-V.**,
Petr., **Puls.**, **Rhus-t.**, Sep.,
Sil.

7 P. M.: Alum., **Bov.**, **Cedr.**,
Chinin-s., Ferr., Gamb.,
Gels., **Hep.**, Ip., **Lyc.**, Nat-
m., **Nat-s.**, **Nux-v.**, Petr.,
Puls., Pyrog., **Rhus-t.**, Sep.,
Sulph., Tarent.

8 P. M.: Alum., **Bov.**, Caust.,
Coff., Elaps, Hep., Mag-c.,
Merc., Phos., **Rhus-t.**,
SULPH.

NIGHT, **Agg.**: Acon., Arn., **Ars.**,
Bell., **Cham.**, **Chin.**, Cimic.,
Coff., **Colch.**, Con., Dulc.,
Ferr., **Graph.**, **Hep.**, Hyos.,
Iod., Jal., **Kali-i.**, **Mag-c.**, Mag-
m., Mang., Meph., MERC.,
Nit-ac., Phos., **Plb.**, **Psor.**,
Puls., Rhus-t., Sabin., **Sil.**,
Stront-c., **Sulph.**, **Syph.**, Ter.,
Zinc.

9 P.M.: **Ars.**, Bov., BRY., **Gels.**,
Merc.

10 P. M.: Ars., Bov., CHININ-S.,
Graph., Ign., Lach., Petr.

11 P. M.: Aral., Ars., Bell., CACT.,
Calc., Carb-an., Sulph.

12 **Midnight: Acon.**, Arg-n., **Ars.**,
Calc., Calad., Canth., **Caust.**,
Chin., Dig., **Dros.**, **Ferr.**, Kali-
c., Lach., Lyc., Mag-m., Mur-
ac., Nat-m., Nux-m., Nux-v.,
Op., Phos., **Rhus-t.**, **Samb.**,
Stram., Sulph., Verat.

1 A. M.: ARS., Carb-v., Mag-m.,
Puls.

2 A. M.: ARS., Benz-ac., Canth.,
Caust., Com., Dros., Ferr.,
Graph., **Hep.**, Iris, Kali-ar.,
KALI-BI., **Kali-c.**, Kali-p.,
Lach., Lachn., Lyc., Mag-c.,
Mez., Nat-m., Nat-s., **Nit-ac.**,
Ptel., **Puls.**, Rumx., Sars., **Sil.**,
Spig., Sulph.

3 A. M.: Am-c., **Am-m.**, Ant-t.,
Ars., **Bry.**, Calc., Canth.,
Cedr., Chin., Ferr., Iris, KALI-
C., Kali-n., **Mag-c.**, **Nat-m.**,
Nux-v., Podo., **Psor.**, Rhus-t.,
Sel., Sep., Sil., **Sulph.**, Thuj.

4 A. M.: **Alum.**, Am-m., Anac.,
Apis, **Borx.**, **Caust.**, CEDR.,
Chel., Coloc., **Con.**, Ferr.,
Ign., Kali-c., **Lyc.**, **Mur-ac.**,
Nat-c., Nit-ac., NUX-V.,
Podo., **Puls.**, Rad-met., Sep.,
Sil., Stann., **Sulph.**, Verat.

5 A. M.: Aloe, **Apis**, CHIN., Dros.,
Kali-c., Kali-i., **Nat-m.**, Nat-
p., Ph-ac., Rumx., Sep., Sil.,
Sulph.

CONDITIONS OF AGGRAVATION AND AMELIORATION

AIR, cold, dry, Agg., see Dry draft, Agg., see Wind.

inspiring cold, Agg.: Am-c., Aesc., Ars., CAUST., Cimic., Cist., Hep., Hydr., Hyos., Ign., Merc., Nux-v., Psor., Rumx., Sabad., Seneg., Sep., Syph.

night or evening, Agg.: Acon., Am-c., Carb-v., MERC., Nat-s., Nit-ac., Sulph.

open, cool, Agg.: Acon., Am-c., Aran., Calc., Calc-p., Camph., Caps., Caust., Cham., Chin., Cist., Cocc., Coff., Colch., Cycl., Dulc., Guaj., Hep., Ign., Kali-bi., Kali-c., Mag-p., Merc., Nat-c., Nit-ac., Nux-m., NUX-V., Petr., Phos., Rumx., Seneg., SIL., Sulph., Urt-u., Viol-o.

open, cool, Amel.: Bapt., Nit-ac., Plat., Rad-met., Tab., Tarent.

and in house, both Agg.: Ars., Aur., Iod., Mez.

Amel., in Room, Agg., Air Hunger, etc.: Alum., Apis, Arg-n., Ars., Aur., Cann-s., Carb-v., Croc., Ferr., Glon., Iod., Kali-

i., Lach., Lil-t., Lyc., Mag-c., Op., Prun., PULS., Rad-met., Rhus-t., Sabad., Sabin., Sulph., Tub.

ANTICIPATIONS, Agg.: Arg-n., Ars., Carb-v., Gels., Lyc., Med., Plb., Ph-ac., Sil.

ASCENDING, Agg.: Ars., Aur., Bry., CALC., Merc., Nat-m., Nux-v., Phos., Puls., Sep., Spong.

ATTENTION, Agg.: Ign.

BATHING, Cold applications, Amel., see Cold, becoming.

cold, Agg.: Ant-c., Clem., Dulc., Rhus-t., Sil.

Amel.: Apis, Bell-p., Bry., Fl-ac., Hyper., Led., Meph., Phyt., Puls., Sulph.

BED, getting out of, Agg.: Am-m., Bry., Calc., CARB-V., Cimic., Cocc., Con., Ign., Lach., Phos., Puls., Rhus-t., Sulph.

Amel.: Aur., Dulc., Ign., Puls., Sep.

BENDING, Agg., see Stretching.

Amel., see Lying Bent.

backward, Amel.: Med.

Bending or doubling up, Amel.: Acon., Calc., Caps., Caust., Cham., Chin., Cimic., Coloc., Graph., Kali-c., Lil-t., Lyc., Mag-m., Mag-p.,

Merc-c., Pareir., Plat., Puls.,
Rheum, Rhus-t., Sec., Sep.,
Sulph., Thuj.

BITING OR CHEWING, Agg.:
AM-C., Am-m., Bry., Chin.,
Cina, Euph., Hep., Ign., Nit-
ac., Merc., Mez., Nat-m., Nit-
ac., Phos., Podo., Puls.,
RHUS-T., Sep., Staph., Verb.

BLEEDING, Amel.: Ars., Bufo,
Calad., Card-m., Ferr., Ham.,
Lach., Meli-a., Sars.

BLOWING NOSE, Agg.: Arn.,
Aur., Calc., CHEL., Graph.,
HEP., Iod., Kali-bi., Merc.,
Puls., Spig., SULPH., Zinc.

BORING INTO PART, Amel.:
Arum-t., Nat-c.

BREAKFAST, Agg.: Carb-v.,
Cham., Nat-m., Nat-s., Nux-
v., PHOS., Sep., Thuj., Zinc.

BREATHING DEEPLY, Agg.:
Acon., Arn., Borx., BRY.,
Calc., Caust., Coca, Kali-c.,
Phos., Ran-b., Rhus-t.,
Rumx., Sabin., Sang., Spig.,
Squil., Sulph.

out, see Exhalation.

CELLARS, see Dampness.

CHANGE of Position, Amel.:
Agar., Ars., Cham., IGN.,
Meli-a., Nat-s., Ph-ac., Puls.,
RHUS-T., Sep., Valer., Zinc.

of Temperature, weather, sea-
sons, oncoming storms, etc.,
Agg.: Ars., Calc-p., Dulc.,
Gels., Hyper., Lach., Meli-
a., Mez., Nat-c., Nux-m.,
Petr., Phos., Psor., Ran-b.,
Rhod., RHUS-T., Rumx.,
Sep., Sil., Sul-i., Tub., Verb.

wants: Sep., Tub.

CHILLED, becoming, see Cold.

CHLOROFORM, Agg.: Phos.

CLUTCHING, grasping, Agg., see
Fingers.

CLOTHES, pressure of, Agg.:
Bov., Bry., Calc., Carb-v.,
Caust., Con., Glon., Hep.,
LACH., Lil-t., LYC., Nit-ac.,
Nux-v., Psor., Sec., Sep.,
Sulph., Tub.

Amel.: Psor., Sabad.

CLOUDY WEATHER, fogs., etc.,
Agg.: Am-c., Aur., Bar-c.,
Rhus-t., Sabin.

COITION, Agg.: AGAR., Bufo,
Calad., Calc., Chin., Graph.,
KALI-C., Kali-p., Kreos., Lyc.,
Nat-m., Sel., Sep., Sil., Staph.,
Sulph.

Amel.: Staph.

COLD, Agg.; easily chilled, lacks
heat: Agar., Am-c., Ant-t.,
Aran., ARS., Aur., Bar-c.,
CALC., Calc-p., Camph.,

Caps., CAUST., Chin., Cimic., Cist., Cocc., Colch., Dulc., Eup-per., Ferr., Graph., Hell., Hep., Hyper., Kali-bi., KALI-C., Lac-d., Lyc., Mag-c., Mag-p., Merc., Mez., MOSCH., Nit-ac., Nux-m., NUX-V., Phos., Ph-ac., Psor., Pyrog., Ran-b., Rhod., RHUS-T., Rumx., SABAD., Sep., SIL., Spig., Stann., STRONT-C., Sulph., Verat.

Amel.; he feels too hot, etc.: Acon., Aloe, Ant-t., APIS, Arg-n., Bell., Bry., Carb-v., Cham., Coc-c., Cycl., Dros., Euph., Fl-ac., GELS., Glon., Guaj., IOD., Kali-i., Kali-m., LACH., Led., Lil-t., Lyc., Med., Merc., Nat-c., NAT-M., Nat-s., Op., Puls., Sabin., Sang., Sec., Sulph.

becoming, Agg.; uncovering or undressing, Agg.: warmth of beds, wraps or external heat, Amel.: Ars., Bell., BRY., Caust., Cham., Chin., Clem., Cocc., Dros., GRAPH., HEP., Hyos., Kali-bi., KALI-C., Led., Lyc., Mag-c., Mag-p., MERC., Nat-c., Nux-m., NUX-V., Rhod., RHUS-T., Rumx., Samb., Sep., SIL., Squil., STRONT-C.,

SULPH., Zinc.

of single parts; as hands in cold water, of head, feet, etc., Agg.: Agar., Am-c., Bell., Calc., HEP., Ign., Nat-m., Nux-v., Phos., Psor., RHUS-T., Sep., SIL., Tarent., Thuj., Zinc.

Amel., uncovering or cold bathing or applications, Amel.- Heat of bed, wraps, etc. Agg.: Acon., Apis, Arg-n., Asar., Aur., Calc., Camph., Cham., Dros., Ferr., Fl-ac., Gels., Guaj., IOD., Led., LYC., Merc., Mur-ac., Op., Psor., PULS., Rhus-r., Sabin., Sec., SULPH., Syph., Tab.

by entering, Agg.: Ars., Bell., Ip., Nux-v., Ran-b.

by sitting or lying on ground or a moist floor, Agg.: Ars., Calc., Caust., Dulc., Nux-v., Rhod., Sil.

COLD, becoming chilled, etc., Agg.: ACON., Ars., Bell., Bry., Cham., Clem., Coff., Colch., Dulc., Hyos., IP., MERC., NUX-V., PHOS., Puls., RHUS-T., Sep., Sil., Spig., Sulph., Verat.

while hot, sweating, by ices, un-covering a part, as hand, etc.

Agg.: Acon., Ars., Bell., Bell-p., Bry., Dulc., Ferr-p., **Hep.,** Kali-s., Merc-i-f., **Nux-v.,** Phos., Psor., Puls., Rhod., RHUS-T., Sep., SIL., Zinc.

and heat, Agg.: Ant-c., Calc., **Caust.,** Ferr., Fl-ac., Graph., Hell., Kali-c., Lach., Mag-c., MERC., **Nat-m., Ph-ac.,** Sep., Sil., Sulph., Sul-ac., Syph.

nights with hot days, Agg.: Acon., Dulc., Merc-c., Rumx.

wet Agg.: Calc., **Dulc.,** Nat-s., Nux-m., Phos., **Rhus-t.**

COLLAR, **Agg.:** Ant-c., Cench., Lach., Merc-c. See **Clothes.**

COLORS, **bright, Agg.:** Sil.

COMPANY, **crowds, etc., Agg.:** Acon., Ambr., Ant-c., Aur., BAR-C., Bell., Carb-an., Cham., Cic., **Gels.,** IGN., Lyc., **Nat-c.,** Nat-m., Nux-v., SEP., Thuj.

Amel., desire for, etc.: Arg-n., **Ars.,** Bism., Dros., Hep., Hyos., Kali-c., Lac-c., Lyc., **Phos., STRAM.**

CONSOLATION, **Agg.:** Kali-s., Nat-m., Syph.

CONTINENCE, **Agg.:** Calc., **Con.,** Lyc., Pic-ac., **Plat.**

COUGHING, **Agg.:** Acon., Ars., Bell., BRY., Calc., Carb-v., Dros., Ip., NUX-V., **Phos., Puls., Rhus-t.,** Sep., Sulph.

COVERS, **Agg.: Lach.,** Lil-t., Sanic.

wants: Tub.

DAMPNESS, **Agg.;** getting wet, wet weather, bathing, working in water, damp rooms, etc., **Agg.:** Alum., Am-c., Ant-c., Ant-t., Ars., Bry., CALC., Calc-p., Card-m., Cimic., Clem., DULC., Form., Kalm., Lyc., **Nat-s.,** Nux-m., Phyt., **Puls.,** Rhod., RHUS-T., Sabal, Sabin., Seneg., **Sep.,** Sil., Sulph., Ter.

Comp. **Room.**

cellars, vaulted places: Aran., Ars., Calc., Dulc., Nat-s., Puls.

ground: Dulc., Rhus-t.

cold, Agg.: Bar-c., CALC., Carb-v., Cimic., DULC., Lach., **Merc.,** Nat-s., Nux-m., **Rhod., RHUS-T.,** Verat., Zing.

feet to, bathed of or wet feet Agg.: All-c., Cham., Cupr., **Dulc., Merc.,** Nat-c., Nat-m., Nit-ac., Nux-m., **Phos.,** PULS., Rhus-t., **Sep., SIL.**

night, Agg.: Merc., Phyt., Rhus-t.·

DANCING, Amel.: Sep.

DAYBREAK, Amel.: Colch., Syph.

DENTITION, Agg. see Teeth.

DESCENDING, Agg.: Borx., Gels., RUTA, STANN., Phys.

DINNER, Agg.: Mag-m.

DISCHARGES, etc. Amel.: Ars., Bry., Calc., Camph., Ip., LACH., Lyc., Nux-v., Ph-ac., PULS., Rhus-t., Sec., Sep., Sil., SULPH., Verat., Zinc.

loss of vital fluids, etc., Agg.: Acon., Agar., Calc., Carb-v., CHIN., Cimic., Ip., Kali-c., Phos., PH-AC., Staph., Verat.

Amel.: Cupr., Psor., Stict., Stram.

DIVERSION, Amel.: Orig., Pall., Pip-m.

DRINKING, Agg.: Arg-n., Ars., Bell., Calc., Canth., Chin., Cocc., Crot-t., Ferr., Lach., Merc-c., NUX-V., Phos., Phyt., Puls., Rhus-r. (warm), RHUS-T., Sil., Stram., Sul-ac., VERAT.

Amel.: Bism., Bry., CAUST., Cist., Cocc., Cupr., Lob., Nux-v., Phos., Sep., Spong.

rapidly, Agg.: Ars., Nit-ac., Nux-v., Sil.

DRINKS, cold, Agg.: LYC.

DRY, clear or cold weather, Agg.: ACON., Ars-i., Asar., Bry., CAUST., Hep., Ip., Kali-c., Med., NUX-V., Sep., Spong.

DUST, feathers, etc., Agg.: Am-c., Ars., Bell., CALC., Chel., Chin., DROS., Hep., Ign., Lyc., Ph-ac., Puls., Rumx., Sil., Sulph.

Comp., Vapor.

EATING, Agg.: Aloe, Anac., ARS., Bell., Bry., CALC., CARB-AN., CARB-V., CAUST., Chin., Coloc., CON., Ferr., Hep., Ign., KALI-BI., KALI-C., Lach., Lyc., Merc., Nat-c., NAT-M., NIT-AC., NUX-V., Petr., Phos., Puls., Rumx., SEP., SIL., SULPH., Verat., Viol-t., Zinc.

EATING, Amel.: Anac., Bov., Cham., Chel., Con., Fl-ac., Ign., IOD., Kali-bi., NAT-C., Nat-m., PHOS., Plb., Rhod., Sep., Zinc.

before, Agg.: fasting, Agg.: Calc., Croc., Fl-ac., IOD., Laur., Nat-c., Phos., Staph., Sulph.

Amel.: Cham., Con., Nat-m.

breakfast, Agg.: Cham., Nux-v., Phos.

dinner, Agg.: Aloe, Bry., Grat., Sul-ac., Zinc.

a little, **Agg.**: Bry., Carb-an., **Chin.**, Con., **Kali-c.**, **LYC.**, Nat-p., **Nux-v.**, Petr., **Phos.**, Puls., **Sulph.**

long after, **Agg.**: Anac., Carb- v., Ferr., **Kali-bi.**, Nat-m., PHOS., PULS., Sulph., Zinc.

over-eating, **Agg.**: Aeth., ANT-C., Calc., **Carb-v.**, **Lyc.**, NUX-V., Sulph.

EMOTIONS, **mental excitement, etc.**, **Agg.**: ACON., Ambr., Aml-ns., **Arg-n.**, Aur., Bell., Bry., Caust., **Cham.**, Cob., Coff., COLOC., Con., Croc., Ferr., Gels., Hyos., IGN., Kali-c., Lach., **Nat-m.**, NUX-V., Op., Pall., Phos., PH-AC., Plat., Psor., PULS., Sep., Sil., STAPH., **Stram.**, Verat.

Comp. **Nervous effects.**

mortification, chagrin, vexation, etc., **Agg.**: **Acon.**, Alum., Bell., **Bry.**, Cham., **Coloc.**, Ign., Lyc., NAT-M., **Nux-v.**, Op., **Petr.**, Ph-ac., Plat., Staph., Zinc.

ERUCTATIONS, **Agg.**: Bry., Carb-an., CHAM., Nux-v., Phos.

Amel.: Ant-t., **Arg-n.**, CARB-V., **Graph.**, **Ign.**, KALI-C., LYC., **Nux-v.**, Puls., Sang.

EXERTION, **Agg.**: ARN., Ars., Berb., BRY., **Calc.**, Carb-an., **Cocc.**, Con., Dig., Ferr., Nat-m., Nit-ac., RHUS-T., Staph., Stroph-h., Sulph.

Comp., **Sprains.**

Amel.: Fl-ac., **Ign.**, Kali-br., Lil-t., RHUS-T., SEP., Thlasp.

mental, **Agg.**, see **Mental Exertion.**

EXHALATION, **Agg.**: Ant-t., Arg-met., Ars., Caust., CHLOR., Colch., Dros., Kali-i., Med., Meph., **Puls.**, Samb., **Spig.**, Viol-o.

Amel.: Acon., **Bry.**, **Rhus-t.**, Sabin.

EYES, **opening, Amel.**: Bry., Ther.

FANNING, **Amel.**: Ant-t., Apis, Arg-n., Bapt., CARB-V., **Chin.**, Crot-h., Ferr., Kali-n., Lach., Med., Sec.

FANNED, **Amel.**: Xan.

FEATHERED, **Agg.**: Mang.

FEMALES, **Agg.**: Acon., Apis, BELL., Calc., Caps., Cham., Chin., Cimic., Cocc., Con., Croc., Mosch., PULS., SABIN., SEP., Valer., Vip-a.

Comp., **Female organs.**

FINGERS OR HANDS, **using, as in writing, sewing, piano-playing, grasping**, etc., **Agg.**:

Arn. (cramp), **Calc.**, **CAUST.**, **Cham.**, Cimic., Dros. (cramp), Gels., **KALI-C.**, Mag-p. (cramp), **NAT-M.**, Phos., Pic-ac., Plat., Sec., Sep., Sil., **Stann.**, Sul-ac., Valer., **ZINC.**

FLATUS, emission of, Amel.: **CARB-V.**, **Lyc.**, Nat-s., Nux-v., Puls., **Staph.**, **Sulph.**

FOODS, DRINK, alcoholic drinks, Agg.: **Ars.**, Calc., Caps., Carb-v., Cimic., Hyos., Kali-bi., Lach., **NUX-V.**, **Op.**, Phos., Puls., Ran-b., Stram., Sulph., Sul-ac., Zinc.

baked, agg.: Carb-v., **Puls.**

beer, Agg.: Kali-bi., Nux-v.

brea', Agg.: Bry., Nux-v., Puls., Sulph.

   and butter, Agg.: **Puls.**

butter, Agg.: Carb-v., **Puls.**

cabbage, Agg.: **Bry.**, **Lyc.**, Petr.

cakes, Agg.: Ant-c., Ip., **Puls.**

cheese, bad, Agg.: **Bry.**

coffee, Agg.: Ars., Canth., Caust., **Cham.**, Coloc., **IGN.**, Merc., **NUX-V.**, Puls.

   Amel.: Cham., Coloc., **Ign.**

odor of, Agg.: Fl-ac., Lach., Nat-m., Osm., Sul-ac., Tub.

cold, Agg.: **ARS.**, Bell., Calc., **Canth.**, Cham., Chel., Ferr., **Hep.**, **Lyc.**, Merc-i-r., **NUX-V.**, **Rhus-t.**, Sabad., Sep., **Sil.**, Staph., Verat.

   Amel.: Apis, Arg-n., Bell., Bry., Cann-s., **CAUST.**, Cupr., Ign., **LACH.**, Merc-i-f., **Phos.**, Phyt., **Puls.**, Sang., Sep.

condiments, drugs, etc., Agg.: Nux-v.

dry, Agg.: Calad., **Calc.**, Chin., Ferr., Ign., Kali-i., Ox-ac., Raph.

eggs, Agg.: Calc., **Puls.**

farinaceous, Agg.: Lyc., **Nat-s.**

fat, Agg.: Ars., **CARB-V.**, Chin., **CYCL.**, Ferr., **Graph.**, Kali-m., **PULS.**, Tarax.

fish, Agg.: Ars., Plb., Puls.

frozen, ices, etc., Agg.: Arg-n., Ars., Puls.

fruit, Agg.: Ars., **Bry.**, Chin., Coloc., Nat-s., **Puls.**, **VERAT.**

   juicy, Agg.: Ant-c., Calc., Iod., Puls., Sulph.

honey, Agg.: Phos.

hot cakes, Agg.: Puls.

ices, Agg.: Ars., Kali-bi., Puls.

indigestible foods, Agg.: Iod.

legumes, Agg.: Bry., Lyc.

liquid, Agg.: ARS., Chin., Cocc., Coloc., Crot-t., Ferr., Ign., Lach., Nat-m., PHOS., Rhus-t., Sil., Verat.

meat, Agg.: Arg-n., Ars., Caust., Carb-v., Chin., Colch., Ferr., Merc., Puls.

milk, Agg.: AETH., Bry., CALC., Chin., Lac-d., Mag-m., Nit-ac., Ol-j., Phos., Puls., Sep., Sulph.
  Amel.: Acon., Chel., Cina, Ferr., Iod., Merc., Ph-ac., Squil., Staph., Verat.

pork, Agg.: CARB-V., Cycl., Graph., PULS., Sep.

potatoes, Agg.: Alum., Puls., Verat.

raw, Agg.: Puls., Ruta, Verat.

rich, Agg.: Ars., Carb-v., Puls.

salads, cucumbers, etc. Agg.: All-c., Puls.

sausage, Agg.: Ars., Bell., Bry.

sour, Agg.: Ant-c., Carb-v., Puls., Sep.

sourkrant, Agg.: Bry., Petr.

strawberries, Agg.: Sep.

sweets, Agg.: Arg-n., Cina, Ign., Merc., Nat-p.

tea, Agg.: Ars., Ferr., Sel., Thuj.

tobacco, Agg.: Ars., Camph., Gels., Ign., Nux-v., Puls., Sel., Spig., Spong., Staph.
  Amel.: Aran., Hep., Naja, Plat., Sep., Stront-c., Tarent.

unripe, Agg.: Rheum.

veal, Agg.: Ip., Kali-n.

vegetables, Agg.: Ars., Bry., Nat-s.

vinegar, Agg.: Ant-c., Ars., Sulph.
  Amel.: Asar., Puls.

warm, Amel.: Lyc.

warm, Agg.: Phyt.

wine, Agg.: LED., Nux-v., Rhod., Zinc.

FROST, frost air, hoar frost, etc., Agg.: Agar., Calc., Caust, CON., Lyc., Nux-v., Ph-ac., Puls., Rhus-t., SEP., Sil., Sulph., Syph.
  Comp. Frostbite.

GLISTENING objects, Agg.: Bell., Canth., Lyss., Mur-ac., Stram.

GRASPING, see Fingers.
  Amel.: Cimic.

HAIR, combing; or brushing, Agg.: Form., Glon., Tarent., Ust.

cutting, Agg.: Bell., Glon., Phos., Sep.

touching, Agg.: Apis, **Ars.**, Bell., **Chin.**, Ferr., Lach., Nux-v., Puls., SEL., Sep., Verat., Zinc.

HEAT of fire, sun, becoming heated or overheating, etc., Agg.: Acon., Ant-c., BELL., Bry., Carb-v., Gels., GLON., Kali-c., **Lach.**, Lyss., Merc., Nat-c., Op., Puls., Rat., Sel., Ther., Verat-v.

    Amel.: Ars., Borx., Ign.

           Comp. Sun.

    and cold, Agg.: Phys.

    eating, Agg.: Tub.

HEMORRHAGE, Agg. from: Chin., Ferr., Nat-m., Sul-ac.

          Comp. Discharge.

    Amel.: Ars., Ferr-p., Ham., Lach., Meli-a., Sars.

HICCOUGH, Agg.: Am-m.

HOLDING or being held, Amel.: Ars., Bry., Carb-an., Diph., Dros., Eup-per., **Gels.**, Glon., Lach., Lil-t., Murx., Nat-s., Sang., **Sep.**, Sil., Stram., Sul-ac., Sulph.

          Comp. Carried.

HOT APPLICATIONS, Amel.: Anac., **Ars.**, Hep., Kali-c., Mag-p., Rad-met., **Rhus-t.**, Sil.

HOT BATH, Agg.: Apis.

    Amel.: Mag-p., Mez., Pyrog., Rad-met.,

HOT DAYS and cold night, Agg.: Acon.

HOT DRINKS, Amel.: Ars., Nux-v., Sul-ac..

HUMID, warm, damp weather, Agg.: Aloe, **Brom.**, Bry., **Carb-v.**, Carbn-s., **Gels.**, **Ip.**, Kali-bi., LACH., **Nat-s.**, Puls., Rhus-t., Sil., **Verat.**

INATTENTION, Agg.: Gels., Hell.

INSPIRATION, Agg.: Crot-h., Ip., Kali-n., Lob., Mez., Spong.

    Amel.: Colch., Cupr., **Ign.**, Lach., Spig., Stann., Verb.

JARRING, shaking, stepping hard, riding, etc., Agg.: ARN., BELL., Bry., **Chin.**, Cic., Cocc., Coff., Con., GLON., Hep., **Nit-ac.**, Nux-v., RHUS-T., SEP., SIL., Ther.

    Amel: Gels., Nit-ac.

          Comp. Sensitive.

KINDNESS, sympathy, etc., Agg.: Ars., **Bell.**, **Calc.**, IGN., **Nat-m.**, **Plat.**, Sep., **Sil.**

LAINS ON, parts, Agg.: Cimic., Graph., **Nat-m.**, Phys.

LAUGHING, Agg.: Acon., Arg-met., Ars., Aur., Bell., BORX., Cann-s., Carb-v., Chin., Hyos., Kali-c., Mang., PHOS., Plb., STANN., Sulph.

LEAD, effects of, **Agg.**: Alum., Op., Plb.

LEANING on **Agg.**: Cimic., Ther.

Amel.: Kali-c., Nat-m.

LIFTING, **Agg.**, see Sprained.

LIGHT, **Agg.**: Acon., Arg-n., **Ars.**, BELL., CALC., **Con.**, Dros., EUPHR., **Glon.**, **Graph.**, Hep., **Lyc.**, Merc., **Merc-c.**, Nat-s., **Nux-v.**, Phos., Ph-ac., Puls., **Rhus-t.**, Sang., SEP., **Sil.**, Stram., **Sulph.**

Comp., Twilight.

Amel., darkness, **Agg.**: Am-m., Calc., **Cann-s.**, Carb-an., Carb-v., **Gels.**, Lyc., Plb., STRAM., **Stront-c.**, Valer.

artificial, firelight, etc., **Agg.**: Bell, Calc., Con., Dros., **Euphr.**, Glon., **Lyc.**, MERC., Nat-m., Phos., Sep., **Stram.**

Comp. Sensitive.

bright, bright objects, etc., **Agg.**: Bell., Stram.

LOOKING AT running water, or moving objects, **Agg.**: Bell., Con., Ferr.

LYING, **Agg.**: Ambr., Ant-t., **Apis**, ARS., AUR., Caps., **Cham.**, Con., Dros., Dulc., Euph., Ferr., Hyos., Lyc., Meny., Merc., Nat-s., Phos., **Plat.**,

PULS., RHUS-T., Rumx., **Samb.**, Sang., Sep., Stront-c., Tarax., Verb.

Amel.: BRY., Calc., Cham., Coloc., **Form.**, Ign., **Nat-m.**, Sil., Stann., NUX-V., Puls., Rhus-t., Sep.

on abdomen, **Amel.**: BELL., Calc-p., Chel., Cina, COLOC., Elaps, **Eup-per.**, Lach., Lept., MED., Nit-ac., Pareir., **Phos.**, **Podo.**, Psor., Sep., Stann., Stram., Thyr.

on back, **Agg.**: Acon., Am-m., Arg-met., **Ars.**, **Caust.**, **Cham.**, Colch., **Coloc.**, **Cupr.**, IGN., **Iod.**, Kali-n., Nat-s., NUX-V., Op., PHOS., Puls., **Rhus-t.**, Sep., Sil., Spig., Sulph.

on, with head elevated: Gels., Sang.

Amel.: BRY., CALC., Dig., Merc-c., **Puls.**, **Rhus-t.**

in bed, **Agg.**: **Ambr.**, Calc., Chel., Dros., Ferr., Hell., Hep., Iod., Kali-c., **Lach.**, Lyc., Merc., Nit-ac., **Phos.**, PULS., Rumx., Sang., **Sep.**, Sil., **Sulph.**

Amel.: Am-m., BRY., Cic., Cocc., Hep., NUX-V., Squil., Stann.

bent or doubled up, Amel.: see Bending or Doubling up.

Agg., see Stretching.

down, Agg., see Inactive.

on hands and knees, Amel.: Con., Eup-per., Euph., Lach., Lob., Med., Pareir., Petr., Sep., Tarent.

with head low, Agg.: Ant-t., Arg-met., Ars., Bell., Caps., Chin., Colch., Gels., Hep., KALI-N., Lach., Puls., Sang., Spig., Spong.

hard surface on Amel.: Nat-m., Sep.

horizontal position, Amel.: Apis, Arn., Bell., Laur., Psor., Spong., Tab., Verat-v.

on it agg.: Tarent.

on side, Agg.: ACON., ANAC., Arg-n., Bar-c., BRY., Calad., CALC., CARB-AN., Cina, Con., Ferr., Hydr. (r), Ign., Ip., KALI-C., Kreos., Lyc., Merc., Merc-c., Nat-s., Pareir., PHOS., Ph-ac., Ptel.(l), PULS., Rhus-t., Seneg., SIL., STANN., Sulph., Thuj., Tub.(l), Zinc-io. (l).

Amel.: Cocc., Nux-v.

on side, right, Agg.: Alum., Am-m., Benz-ac., Borx., Caust., Iris, Kali-c., Lycps., Mag-m.,

MERC., Nux-v., Phos., Rumx., Spong., Stann.

left, Agg.: Acon., Am-c., Apis, Arg-n., Bar-c., Bry., Cact., Carb-an., Colch., Ip., Lil-t., Lyc., Naja, Nat-c., Nat-m., Nat-s., Pareir., Petr., PHOS., PULS., Sep., Sil., Sulph., Thuj.

pain goes to side lain on: Bry., Phos., Puls.

painful or affected part, see Pressure.

painful side on, Agg.: Cycl., Lach., Laur., Mag-m.

painless, Agg.: BRY., Cham., Chin., Coloc., Fl-ac., Ign., Nat-s., PULS., Rhus-t., Sec., Sep.

on wet surface, floor, etc., see Cold.

pillow, on: Glon.

MENSES, before, Agg.: Calc., Cimic., Cocc., Cupr., KALI-C., LACH., Lyc., Nat-m., PULS., Sep., Stann., SULPH., Verat., Vib., Zinc.

before and after, Agg.: Borx., Calc., Ferr., Kali-m., Graph., Lac-c., Kreos., Lach., Lil-t., Mag-c., Nat-m., Pall., Thuj.

at start of, Agg.: Acon., Hyos., Lach.

during, **Agg.**: AM-C., Arg-n., Castr., Caust., Cham., Cimic., GRAPH., HYOS., Ign., **Mag-c.**, MAG-M., Nux-m., Nux-v., PULS., Pyrog., **Sep.**, Staph., **Sulph.**, **Zinc.**

after, **Agg.**: BORX., GRAPH., Kreos., Lach., Lyc., **Nux-v.**, Sep.

suppressed, **Agg.**: Acon., Bry., Lyc., Puls., Sulph.

MENTAL EXERTION, **Agg.**: Agar., Anac., Arg-n., Aur., CALC., **Ign.**, **Lach.**, **Nat-c.**, Nat-m., NUX-V., Phos., Ph-ac., Pic-ac., Plb., Puls., Rhus-t, Sep., Sil., **Sulph.**

MENTAL SYMPTOMS, **menses**, **before Agg.**: Stann.

MERCURY, **Agg.**: **Aur.**, **Bry.**, Carb-v., Guaj., **HEP.**, **Lach.**, NIT-AC., Phyt., Sars., **Staph.**, **Sulph.**

MESMERISM, see **Rubbing.**

MIND, **Pain**, **Agg.**: Cham., Sars., Verat.

menses, **Agg.**: Nat-m., Stann., Stram.

before, **Agg.**: Stann.

syphilis, **Agg.**: Aur., Asaf., Hep., Lach., Merc., Nit-ac., Phyt.

MOON PHASES, full moon, etc., **Agg.**: ALUM., Bry., Calc., **Cina**, Cupr., **Lyc.**, Nux-v., **Phos.**, SIL., Sulph.

MOONLIGHT, **Agg.**: **Ant-c.**, Sep., **Sulph.**, Thuj.

MOTION, **Agg.**: Arn., **BELL.**, BRY., Calc., Chin., **Colch.**, Kali-c., Led., Nat-m., **Nux-v.**, Pyrog., **Sil.**, **Spig.**, Sulph., Tab., Tarent., Tub., Vib., Zinc., Valer.

after, **Agg**: Spong.

on rough ground, **Agg.**: Hyos., Lil-t.

Amel.: Gels., Helon., Lil-t.

air, open, in **Amel.**: Dios., Iod., Kali-i., Lil-t., Mag-c., Mag-m., Puls.

Amel., activity, walking, Amel., rest, Agg.: Ant-t., Arg-n., **Ars.**, **Aur.**, **Caps.**, **Con.**, **Cycl.**, **Dulc.**, **Euph.**, **Ferr.**, Fl-ac., Iod., Kali-c., Kali-i., Kreos., Lyc., Mag-c., Mag-m., Merc-c., PULS., **Rhod.**, **Rhus-t.**, **Sabad.**, **Samb.**, Sep., Sulph., Tarax., **Valer.**, Zinc.

Comp. Restlessness.

after, **Agg.**: Agar., ARS., **Cann-s.**, Puls., RHUS-T., SEP., Stann., Sul-ac., **Valer.**

arms, of, Agg.: Led., Ran-b., Rhus-t., **Spig.**

behind him, Agg.: Ign., Puls., Sanic., Sep., Teucr.

continued: Anac., Rob.

distant parts, of Agg.: Apis, Bry., Cocc.

gentle, Amel: Sumb., Syph.

raising, Agg., see **Position.**

Beginning, Agg., continued, **Amel.: Ambr., Calc-f.,** Caps., Con., Euph., **Ferr.,** Lyc., Phos., **Puls.,** RHUS-T., Sep., Syph.

rapid, violent, etc., Agg.: **Ars.,** Bry., Sil., Sulph.

Amel., running, dancing, etc.: Ars., Aur-m., Brom., Fl-ac., Graph., Nit-ac., Scopar., **Sep.,** Stann., Sul-ac., Tarent., Thlasp.

slow, gentle, etc., **Amel.:** Agar Alum., Ambr., **Aur.,** Coloc., FERR., Glon., **Kali-p.,** Mag-m., PULS., **Tarent.**

MOUTH, opening the, Agg.: Ang., Arum-t., Bry., Caust., Cocc., **Lach., Merc.,** Merc-c., Nux-v., Phos., Sabad., Spig.

MUSIC, Agg.: Acon., **Calc.,** Croc., Graph., Lyc., Med., **Nat-c.,** NUX-V., **Ph-ac.,** Sabin., SEP., Viol-o.

Amel.: Aur., Tarent.

NARCOTICS, Agg.: Am-c., Bell, Carb-v., **Cham., Coff, Lach.,** Merc., NUX-V., Puls.

NOISE, Agg., see **Sensitive.**

penetrating, Agg.: Asar., Cop., Ferr., Lept., Manc., Tarent., **Ther., Tub.**

rattling, Agg.: Nit-ac.

sudden, Agg., reports, etc.: Borx.

Amel.: Graph.

ODORS, smells, etc., Agg.: Ars., Aur., Bell, Carb-ac., Coff., COLCH., Dros. (sour), Eup-per., Graph., Ign., Lyc., **Merc-i-f., Nux-v.,** Phos., Sang., SEP., Stann., Sulph., Ther., Vario.

Agg.: Carb-ac., Dros. (sour), Ther., Vario.

Comp. **Sensitive.**

ONANISM, Agg.: **Calc., Carb-v., Chin.,** Con, Lyc., Merc., **Nat-m.,** Nux-v., Phos., **PH-AC.,** Plat., Puls., Sep., **Staph., Sulph.,** Ust.

Comp. **Discharges.**

menses, Agg.: Zinc.

ORDEALS, Agg. see **Fearsome.**

PAIN, Agg., during: Ars., Coloc., Ign., Onos., Rhus-t., Sep., Verat.

absence of: Ant-c., Ant-t.

PIANO playing **Agg.**: Nat-c.

POSITION, bending backward see Lying.

crossing limbs, **Agg.**: Agar., Asaf., Bell., **Dig.**, Lyc., Phos., **Rhus-t.**, **Valer.**

Amel.: Ant-t., SEP.

hanging down limb, **Agg.**: Barc., BELL., **Calc.**, CARB-V., Con., M-aust., Puls., **Sabin.**, Vip-t.

Amel.: Acon., **Arn.**, Asar., Berb., CON., Lyc., Mag-c., Magm., Mang., Merc., Phos., Rat., Rhus-t., Teucr.

leaning against a support, **Amel.**: Ferr.

Agg.: Cimic., Ther.

rising from a seat, **Agg.**: Berb., BRY., Caps., Con., Lyc., Nat-s., Phos., Puls., Rhust., Spig., Sulph.

sitting, **Agg.**: Agar, Am-m., Apis, Ars., Asaf., Caps., Cob., Con., Cycl., Dulc., Euph., Ferr., Lyc., Mag-m., Murac., Nux-v., Phos., PLAT., PULS., Rhus-t., Sep., Sulph., Tarax., Valer., Verb., Viol-t., ZINC.

Amel.: BRY., COLCH., Cupr., Nux-v., Sep.

down, **Amel.**: Caps., Con.

erect, **Agg.**: Kali-c., Nat-m.

Amel.: Ant-t., Ars., Dig., Hyos., Kali-bi., Nat-m., Nat-s.

standing, **Agg.**: Aloe, Bry., Cocc., Con., Cycl., Glon., Ign., Lilt., Nat-m., Nat-s., Puls., Rhus-t., Sep., SULPH., Valer.

Amel.: Ars., BELL., Colch., Led., Phos., Ran-b., Squil.

stooping, **Agg.**: Am-c., Bell., BRY., Calc., Caust., Lyc., Mang., Nux-v., Puls., Sep., Sil., Spig., Sulph., Valer.

Amel.: Colch., Hyos., Iris.

stretching, extending limbs, **Agg.**: Calc., CHAM., COLCH., Iod., Merc-c., PLAT., PULS., Ran-b., RHEUM, RHUS-T., Sep., STAPH., Sulph., Thuj.

Amel. see Bending double.

turning head, **Agg.**: Calc., Cic., Kali-c., Puls., Spig., Spong.

over in bed, **Agg.**: Bell., Cact., Calad., Carb-v., Con., NUX-V., Puls., Sang., Staph., SULPH., Zinc.

walking bent forward, **Amel.**: Phos., Sulph.

PRAISE, **Amel.**: Pall.

PRESSURE, Agg.: Lying on painful or affected side, etc., Agg: Acon., **Agar.**, Apis, Arg-n., Ars., **Bar-c.**, Bry., Calad., Calc., **Carb-v.**, **Cina**, Ferr., **Hep.**, IOD., LACH., **Lyc.**, Nux-v., Psor., SIL., Vib., Zinc-chr.

on opposite side: Agg.: Viol-t.

Amel., lying on affected part, etc., Amel.: Am-c., Arg-n., BRY., Castm., Chin., COLOC., Con., Cupr-ar., Dros., IGN., Mag-m., Mag-p., Meny., Nat-c., Plb., **Puls.**, **Rhus-t.**, Sep., STANN.

of clothes, Agg., see Clothes, about neck, Agg.: Agar., Apis, Caust., Chel., Con., Glon., Kali-c., LACH., Merc-c., **Sep.**

over a hard edge, etc. Amel.: Bell., **Chin.**, COLOC., Con., Ign., Lach., Samb., Sang., Stann., Zinc.

spine, on, Agg.: Agar., Arn., Bell., **Chin**, Kali-c., **Phys.**, Sep., SIL., Ther.

PURGATIVES, Agg.: Hydr., **Nux-v.**, Op., Sulph.

QUININE, Agg.: Arn., **Ars.**, Carb-v., Ferr., Ip., **Nat-m.**, Nux-v., **Puls.**, Sulph., Verat.

RAISING ARMS, Agg.: Apis, Arg-n., Bar-c., Berb., Bry., Cocc., CON., Dig., Ferr., Graph., Led., Mag-c., Nit-ac., Ran-b., Rhus-t., Sanic., **Sang.**, Spig., **Sulph.**, Tell.

up, Agg.: Acon., Bell., BRY., Cadm-s., Cham., Cocc., Ferr., Ign., **Merc-i-f.**, Nat-m., Nux-v., Op., Phos., **Phyt.**, Puls., Rhus-t., Sil., Sulph., Verat-v., Vib.

Amel.: **Am-c.**, Ant-t., ARS., Calc., Dig., Glon., **Samb.**, Sep.

RAISING up, Amel.: **Am-c.**, Ant-t., Aral., Kali-c., ARS., **Calc.**, Dig., Glon., **Samb.**, Sep.

READING, Agg. eyestrain, Agg.: Calc., Cina, Con., Croc., Kali-c., Mang., NAT-M., Onos., Phos., Rhus-t., RUTA, Seneg., Sep., Sil., Sulph.

aloud, Agg.: Carb-v., Sel., Verb.

RELAXATION, Amel.: Tarent.

REPRIMANDS, Agg.: Coloc., **Ign.**, Staph.

RIDING ON HORSEBACK, Agg.: Ars., Bell., Borx., Bry., Graph., Lil-t., Mag-m., **Nat-c.**, Ruta, SEP., Sil., Spig., **Sul-ac.**, Valer., Tab.

Comp. **Swaying.**

RISING FROM SITTING, Agg.:
Aesc., Bry., Calc., Caps.,
Caust., Con., Kali-bi., Led.,
Lyc., Nat-s., PHOS., Puls.,
Rhus-t., Sep., Spig., Staph.,
SULPH.

RISING, from bed, Amel.: Ph-ac.,
Puls.

ROCKING, Agg.: Borx., Cocc.
Amel.: Pyrog.

ROOM full of people, Agg.: Lyc.,
Phos., Sep.

ROOM, IN, Agg., see Air, Open,
Amel.

ROTATION, Agg.: Coloc.

RUBBING, stroking, etc., Agg.:
Anac., Con., Puls., Sep.,
Stront-c., Sulph.
Amel.: Calc., Canth., Cina,
Cupr., Dros., Mag-p.,
Merc., NAT-C., Pall.,
PHOS., PLB., Podo., Rhus-
t., Ruta, Sep., Sil., Tarent.,
Thuj., Zinc.
abdomen, Amel.: Nat-s., Pall.,
Podo.

RUNNING, see Motion.

SALT, Agg.: Ars., Nat-m., Phos.,
Sel.

SCRATCHING, Agg.: Anac., Ars.,
Asar., Caps., Kali-c., Lach.,
Olnd., PULS., RHUS-T.,
SULPH.

Amel.: Asaf., Calc., Cycl., Mur-
ac., Nat-c., Phos., Ruta,
Sulph.

SEA, Agg.: Ars., Brom., Mag-m.,
Nat-m., Nat-s., Rhus-t., Sep.

SEA AIR, Amel.: Brom., Med.

SEASONS, spring, melting snow,
etc., Agg.: All-c., Ambr., Bell.,
Bry., Calc., Calc-p., Carb-v.,
Crot-h., Gels., Kali-bi.,
LACH., Rhus-t., Sars., Verat.
summer, hot weather, etc., Agg.:
Aeth., Ant-c., Bell., Bry.,
Carb-v., Dulc., Fl-ac., Gels.,
Hep., Iris, Kali-bi., Lach.,
Mat-c., Nat-m., PODO.,
Sel., Verat-v.
autumn, Agg.: Chin., Colch.,
Dulc., Merc., Merc-c.,
RHUS-T., Verat.
winter, Agg.: Ars., Aur., Dulc.,
Kalm., Nux-v., Petr., Psor.,
RHUS-T.

SEDENTARY LIVING, Agg.:
NUX-V., Sulph.

SHAVING, Agg.: Carb-an., Ox-
ac., Ph-ac., PULS., Rad-met.,
SULPH.

SHUDDERING, shivers, emo-
tions, Agg.: Asar.

SIGHT of knives, Agg.: Alum.,
Plat.

SINGING, Agg.: Arg-met., Arum-
t., Carb-v., Nux-v., PHOS.,
Sel., Stann.

SLEEP, before, Agg.: Ars., BRY., CALC., Carb-v., Lyc., Merc., Phos., PULS., Rhus-t., Sep., Sulph.

Amel.: Med.

during, Agg.: Op.

falling to or first, Agg.: Aral., Ars., Bell., Bry., Carb-v., Grind., LACH., Merc-p-r., Op., Puls., Samb., Sep., Sulph.

half asleep, when, Agg.: Camph., Nit-ac., Sabad., Valer.

during, Agg.: Acon., Ars., Bell., Borx., Bry., Cham., Cina, Con., Hep., Hyos., LACH., Merc., OP., Puls., Sil., Stram., Sulph., Zinc.

Amel., loss of, Agg.: Ars., Carb-v., Cocc., Coff., Colch., Merc., Nux-v., Pall., PHOS., Puls., Sang., Sep., Zinc.

waking from, after, Agg.: Apis, Ars., Bell., Chin., LACH., Lyc., Lycps-v., Nux-v., Op., Phos., Puls., Sel., Spong., Stram., Sulph.

waking from and on falling both 'gg.: Stann.

SMOKE, Agg.: Ars., Chin., Kali-bi., Lyc., Phos., Sep., Spig.

SNEEZING, Agg.: Ars., Bell., Ign., Lyc., Rhus-t., Seneg., Squil., SULPH.

least uncovering Agg.: Nux-v., Pyrog., Rhus-t., Sil.

odors, Agg.: Phos.

Amel.: Chlol., Lach., Mag-m., Naja, Thuj.

SNOW AIR, Agg.: Calc., Con., Form., Lyc., Phos., Ph-ac., Puls., Rhus-t., Sep., Sil., Sulph., Urt-u., Vib.

SOUR KROUT, Agg.: Lyc., Puls.

SPEAKING, talking, etc., Agg.: Acon., Alum., Anac., Arg-met., Arn., Ars., Arum-t., Calc., Cann-s., Chin., COCC., Dros., Ign., Iod., Mang., Nat-c., Nat-m., Nux-v., PHOS., Ph-ac., Rhus-t., Sel., Seneg., Sep., Sil., Spong., Stann., SULPH.

SPOKEN to addressed, Agg.: Cham.

SPRAINED, dislocated, etc., lifting etc., Agg.: ARN., Ars., Bry., Calc., Carb-an., Caust., Chel., Led., Lyc., Nat-c., Onos., Psor., Prun., Puls., RHUS-T., Ruta, Sep., Sil., Stront-c., Sulph., Valer.

Comp. Exertion, Sprains.

STANDING, Agg.: Ars.

STONECUTTERS, see Dust.

STORMS, Agg., see Change of Temperature.

thunderstorms, **Agg.**: Nat-c., **Phos.**

storms after, **Agg.**: Calc-p., Rhus-t.

STOVE heat, **Amel.**: Bov., Hep., Lach.

STRANGERS, **Agg.**: see **Company.**

STRETCHING, bending backwards, etc., **Amel.**: Alet., **Alum., ANT-T.,** Arn., Bell., **Calc., Dios.,** Guaj., Hep., **Ign.,** Lyc., Med., **Nux-v., Puls.,** Rhus-t., Sabin., **Sec.**

Agg.: Rad-met.

SUCKLING, **Agg.**: Calc., Calc-p., Kali-bi., Ph-ac., Puls., Sulph.

SUN, exposure to, **Agg.**, see **Heat.**, **Amel.**: Con., Crot-h., Iod., Kali-m., Plat., **Stront-c.**

light, **Agg.**: Ant-c., Bell., Euph., **Glon., Nat-c.,** Sel.

Amel.: Thuj.

SUNSET, **Agg.**: Merc., Phyt., Syph.

Amel.: Med., Sel.

to sunrise, **Agg.**: Colch., **Syph.**

SUPPORT, **Amel.**: Ferr., Kali-c., Nat-c., Nat-m., Ph-ac., Sep.

SWALLOWING, **Agg.**, also painful: Apis, Bar-c., **Bell.**, Bry., Canth., Caust., Cina, **Gels.,**

Hep., Hydr-ac., Hyos., Kali-c., Lac-c., **LACH.,** Laur., Meph., Merc., **Nit-ac.,** Phyt., **Rhus-t.,** **Stram.,** Sulph., Sul-i.

Comp. Throat.

Amel.: Alum., Ambr., Arn., **Caps., IGN.,** Lach., Led., Mang., Mez., Nux-v., Puls., Rhus-t., Spong., **Zinc.**

empty, **Agg.**: Bar-c., Bell., Bry., Cocc., Hep., **Kali-c.,** LACH., Merc., Merc-c., **Merc-i-r.,** Nux-v., Puls., Sabad., Rhus-t., Sulph.

hasty, **Agg.**: Nit-ac., Sil.

liquids, drinking, etc., **Agg.**: Arg-n., Ars., **Bell.**, Brom., **Canth., Crot-t.,** Ign., LACH., Merc., **Merc-c.,** Nux-v., **Phos.,** Stram., Verat.

Amel.: Alum., Nit-ac., Nux-v.

warm, **Amel.**: Alum., Nux-v.

solids, **Agg.**: Bapt., Sil.

solids, **Amel.**: Brom., Ferr., Hyos., **Ign.,** Lach., Merc-cy., **Rhus-t.**

SWAYING, swinging, **Agg.**: car or seasickness, etc.: Ars., COCC., Colch., Glon., Kreos., PETR., Sel., **Sep.,** **Tab.,** Ther., Thuj.

Comp. Riding.

SWEAT, **Agg.**, also sweats without relief.: Ars., BELL., Benz-ac., Benz-ac., **Caust.**, Cham., Chel., **Chin.**, Dig., Form., Hep., MERC., **Nux-v.**, **Op.**, Phos., Ph-ac., **Pyrog.**, **Rhus-t.**, Sal-ac., **Sep.**, **Stram.**, **Sulph.**, Tarent-c., Til., Tub., Verat.

Amel.: Bapt., Canth., Cupr., Iod., Psor.

Comp. **Discharges.**

TALK, HEARING OTHERS, **Agg.**: Am-c., ARS., Cact., Chin., **Hyos.**, **Mang.**, **Mez.**, Nat-c., **Nux-v.**, Rhus-t., Seneg., **Sep.**, Sil., Stram., **Verat.**, **Zinc.**

THINKING, **Agg.**: Par.

THINKING OF IT, **Agg.**: **Ambr.**, Arg-n., Aur., Bar-c., Caust., Colch., Lycps-v., **Nit-ac.**, Nux-m., **Ox-ac.**, Par., **Sabad.**, Thyr.

Amel.: Cic.

TONGUE, **protruding**, **Agg.**: Cocc., Kali-bi., Phyt.

TOUCH, **Agg.**, see **Sensitive.**

Agg., **hard pressure**, **Amel.**: Bell., **Castr.**, **Chin.**, Ign., **Lach.**, Nux-v., Plb.

Amel.: **Asaf.**, **Bism.**, **Calc.**, **Cycl.**, **Mur-ac.**, Sang., Spig., Staph., **Thuj.**

Comp. **Sensitive.**

slight, **Agg.**: Acon., **Apis**, **Bell.**, Chin., Ign., LACH., Merc., **Nit-ac.**, **Nux-v.**

each other, **Agg.**: Lac-c., Sanic.

TWILIGHT, **Agg.**: Ars., Berb., CALC., Caust., Nat-s., Phos., Plat., PULS., **Rhus-t.**

Amel.: Bry., Meny., **Phos.**, Seneg., Tab.

ULCER, **heat Agg.**: Puls.

Amel.: Ars., Clem., Con., Hep., Lach., Rhus-t., Sil.

UNCOVERING, **Agg.** see **Wind.** **Amel.**, cold applications, **Amel.**, warm wraps., **Agg.**: Acon., **Apis**, Calc., Camph., **Iod.**, Kali-i., Kali-s., Led., LYC., Op., Puls., Sec., Spig., **Sulph.**

least Agg.: Hep., Nux-v., Rhust., Sil.

Comp., **Wind.**

URINATING, **Amel.**: Chinin-s., **Gels.**, **Ign.**, LYC., Ph-ac., Sang., Sil., Verat.

URINATION, **at close of**, **Agg.**: Canth., Equis-h., Merc-c., Mez., Nat-c., **Sars.**

VACCINATION, **Agg.**: **Ars.**, Antt., Hep., Kali-m., Maland., Sulph., Sil., **Thuj.**, **Vario.**

VAULTS, **Agg.** see **Dampness.**

VERTIGO, **during**, **Agg.**: Acon., Calc., GELS., NUX-V., Phos., Puls., Stram.

VOMITING, Agg.: Aeth., Ars., CUPR., Ip., Puls., Sulph.

Amel.: Ant-t., Coc-c., Eup-per., Kali-bi., Nux-v., Sang.

WALKING, Agg. see Motion.

on rough ground, Agg.: Hyos., Lil-t.

WARMTH, in general, Agg.: APIS, Bell., Bry., Carb-v., Gels., IOD., LACH., Led., Lil-t., Lyc., Merc., Nat-m., PULS., Sabin., Sec., Sulph.

WARMTH, covers etc., Amel.: Hep., Ign., Mag-c., NUX-V., Puls., Rhus-t., Samb., Squil., Sil., Stram.

WARMTH, warm applications or poultices, Agg.: Carb-v., Crot-h., Cupr., Fl-ac., Kali-i., Lyc., Sabin., Sec.

WASHING, bathing, wet, etc., Agg., see Dampness.

WATER, running, sound or sight of, Agg.: Bell., Brom., Canth., Lyss., Stram., Sulph.

WEATHER, temperature, etc., change, see Change.

cloudy Agg.: Arn., Rhus-t., Stram., Viol-o.

dry, clear, Agg., see Dry.

frosty, Agg., see Frost.

hot, Agg., see Seasons

humid, heavy, foggy, etc., Agg., see Humid.

wet, Agg., see Dampness. Amel. see Dry.

and warm, Agg., see Humid.

WEEPING, Agg.: Arn., Bell., Hep.

Amel.: Graph., Lach., Puls.

WET: see Dampness.

WIND, draft, etc., Agg.: Acon., Ars., BELL., Calc., Calc-p., Caps., Cham., Chin., Colch., Coloc., Hep., Kali-c., Lach., Lyc., Mag-c., Med., Nux-v., Phos., Ph-ac., Psor., Puls., Rheum, Rhod., Rhus-t., Samb., Sel., SIL., Stront-c., Squil., SULPH., Verb.

Amel.: Ferr., Iod., Sec., Tub.

Comp. Change.

north wind, Agg.: Ars., Asar., Carb-v., Caust., Hep., Nux-v., Sep., Spong., Zinc.

WIPING, Agg.: Aloe, Graph., Mur-ac.

Amel., (Eyes): Calc., Cina, Cycl., Euphr., Nat-c.

WOOLENS, Agg.: Merc., Psor., Puls., Rhus-t., Sulph.

WRITING, Agg.: see Fingers.

YAWNING, Agg.: Cina, IGN., Kreos., NUX-V., Rhus-t., Sars.

GENERALITIES

ABSORBENT ACTION: Arn., Kali-i.

ACHING: Agar., Arn., **Bapt.**, Bry., Carb-v., **Chin.**, Cimic., Dulc., Echi., Erig., Eucal., **Eup-per.**, **Gels.**, Hyos., Ign., Kalm., Lach., Lept., Merc-i-f., Nux-v., **Phyt.**, Pyrog., Rad-met., Rhus-t., Ruta, Verat-v., Ter., Vario.

ACIDOSIS: Phos.

ACRID: Chlor., Cist., Colch., Euphr., Fl-ac., Hydr., Iris, Lilt., Mez., Mur-ac., Prun., Rans., Sabin., Sang., Sul-ac., Sul-i., Tell., Thuj., Tub.

ACRIDITY, excoriations, etc.: Allc., ARS., Ars-i., Arum-t., **Brom.**, **Caust.**, Cham., **Graph.**, Hep., **Iod.**, Kreos., Lyc., MERC., Merc-c., **Nitac.**, Phos., **Rhus-t.**, Sep., Sil., SULPH.

ACTIVE, **agile:** Apis, Lach., Nuxv., Tarent., Valer.

Amel., when: Cycl., Helo., Lil-t.

ACTIVITY, **fruitless:** Apis, Borx., Calc., Stann., Ther.

ACUTE: see **Sensitive.**

AFFECTIONS, **stiffed:** Sep.

ADHESIVE, **adherent, torn loose,** etc.: Berb., Bov., **Bry.**, Calc.,

Coloc., Hep., Ign., Kali-bi., **Kali-i.**, Merc-c., Nux-v., Olan., Osm., **Phos.**, Plb., Puls., Rumx., RHUS-T., SEP., Stann., Ust.

AFFECTIONS, **stifled:** Sep.

AIR, **blowing on,** see **Wind.**

hot, as if: Aster., Bry., Puls., Verat.

hunger: Ferr., Prun., Rad.met.

flatulency with: Kali-i., Zinc.

passages, burning: Ars-i., Sang., Seneg.

plumb: Stict.

sensitive: see **Nose.**

penetrating, too: Calc., Coloc.

smoky, as if: Berb., Brom.

ALBUMINOUS, **glairy discharges:** Alum., Am-m., Berb., BORX., Coc-c., Jatr-c., NAT-M., Pall., Petr., Seneg., Sep., Stann.

Comp. **Gelatinous.**

ALBUMINOUS, **clear:** Calc-p., Phyt., Tarent.

ALCOHOLISM, **acute:** Acon., Bell., **Op.**

later: Carb-v., Nux-v.

recurrent: Anac., Aur., Bell., **Chin.**, Hyos., Nux-v., Op., Stram., Thuj.

ALIVE SENSATION: **Cann-s.,** Cocc., **CROC.,** Cycl., Ign., Op., **Puls., Sabin.,** Sil., **Sulph.,** THUJ.

Comp. **Formication.**

ALL GONE: see **Empty.**

ALTERNATING effects, states, sides, etc.: Agar., Bell., Cimic., Cocc., Croc., Glon., **Ign.,** LAC-C., Lach., LYC., **Phos.,** Puls., Rad-met., SULPH.

Comp. **Periodicity, Waves.**

ALTERNATIONS of: Abrot., Arn., Berb., Croc., Cupr., Psor., Stront-c., Sul-ac., Valer.

contraction and relaxation: Cupr., Lyc., Tab., Tarent.

diarrhea and asthma: Kali-c.

mental: Sep.

rheumatism and hemoptysis: Led.

AMMONIACAL ODOR: Am-c., Asaf., Aur., **Benz-ac.,** Iod., Lac-c., Lach., Mosch., **Nit-ac.,** Phos., Stront-c.

ANASARCA: Ant-c., Apis, Ars., Bell., Bry., Chin., Colch., Dig., Dulc., Ferr., Hell., Kali-c., Led., Lyc., Merc., Phos., Puls., Rhus-t., Sabin., Samb., Sars., Squil., Sulph.

ANEMIA, chlorosis, etc.: Ars., Calc., Calc-p., CHIN.,

FERR., Graph., Kali-c., Lac-d., Nat-c., **Nat-m.,** Nit-ac., Nux-v., **Phos., Puls., Sulph.**

ANEURISM: Aur., Bar-c., Calc-fl., Carb-v., Lach., **Lyc.,** Puls., Sulph., Thuj.

pain of: Gal-ac., Sec.

ANTHRAX: Lach.

APOPLEXY: **Acon.,** Ant-c., Ant-t., **Arn.,** Ars., Aur., Bar-c., **Bell.,** Calc., **Cocc.,** Coff., Ferr., Gels., Glon., Hyos., **Hydr-ac.,** Ip., Kali-m., Lach., Lyc., Nux-v., **Op.,** Ph-ac., Puls., Rhus-t., Samb., Sep., Stram., Thuj., Verat., Verat-v.

with slow, full pulse, red face and small pupils: Op.

weak, small pulse and pale, bluish face: Lach.

very irritable pulse: Acon.

waves of congestion, bursting, throbbing; holds head: Glon.

ARTHRITIC, see Joints.

ARTHRITIS DEFORMANS: **Ars., Aur., Caust.,** Cupr., Guaj., Hep., Merc., **Puls.,** Rad-met., **Sabin.**

ASLEEP (of Limbs) see **Numbness.**

ASSOCIATED effects: Ars., Cham., **Merc., Nux-v.,** Phos., PULS., Sep., Sulph.

ASTHENOPIA: Ferr-p., Jab., Ruta.

ATTACKS, recurrent: Acon., Ars. Bell., Chin., Cupr., Dios., Mag-p., Nat-m., **Psor.**, Valer., Verb.

ATHEROMA., see **Calculi.**

ATHLETES FOOT: Graph., Sanic.

ATONY: Op.

ATTITUDES, bizarre., **Cina,** Cocc., **Coloc.**, Gamb., Lyc., Merc., Nux-v., **Plb.**, Zinc.

AWAKING **Agg.**: Calc., LACH., Lyc., STRAM., Tub., Zinc.

AWKWARD, drops things, etc.: Agar., Bar-c., Hell., Lol., Mosch.

AWKWARDNESS: Apis, Bov., **Caps,** Ign., Nat-m.

BALL, **lump, knot, globus etc.:** **Arn.**, Asaf., Bry., Cham., Chin., Cob., Con., Gels., **Ign.**, Kali-c., Kali-m., Lac-c., LACH., Lil-t., Lyc., Merc-i-r., Mosch., Nat-m., Nat-s., Nit-ac., Nux-m., **Nux-v.**, Phos., Plan., **Puls.**, Rhus-t, Senec., SEP., Teucr., Ust., **Valer.**, Zinc.

Comp. **Plug.**

hot: Carb-ac., Phyt.

BAND, see **Constriction:** Ox-ac.

BANDAGE: Pic-ac., Plat., Tril-p.

BAROMETER: Merc., **Phos.,** **Rhod.**

BEARING DOWN, see **Pressing.**

BEATEN, see **Soreness.**

loose from bones, as if: Apis, Bry., Lach., **Rhus-t.**

BED, heat of: Dros., **Merc.**, Op., Psor., Puls., Sabin., Sec., **Sulph.**

leaves: Cham., Graph., Lac-c., Led., Merc., Verat.

lumps in: Arn., Mag-c.

sliding down in: Apis, Ars., **Bapt.**, Chin., Colch., Hell., **Hyos.**, Mur-ac., Zinc.

BEHIND: Anac., Brom., Med., Sanic.

BENDING, see **Lying bent.**

backward, see **Stretching.**

BILATERAL: Arn., Kali-i.

BILIOUSNESS, see **Yellow.**

BITING, **fleas** as of: Mez., Staph., Tab., Visc.

bugs like: Kali-m.

BITING, see **Rawness.**

BLACK **dark, etc.:** Ant-t., Arn., ARS., Bapt., Carb-ac., Carb-v., **Chin.**, Crot-h., Cycl., Elaps, Gels., Hell., Kreos., **Lach.**, Mag-m., **Merc.**, Merc-c., Nux-v., Op., Phos., Plb., **Sec.**, Staph., Sul-ac., Verat.

BLACK WATER FEVER: Crot-h.

BLACK, dark, etc.: Ant-t., Arn., ARS., Bapt., Carb-ac., Carb-v., Chin., Crot-h., Cycl., Elaps., Gels., Hell., Kreos., Lach., Mag-m., Merc., Merc-c., Nux-v., Op., Phos., Plb., Sec., Staph., Sul-ac., Verat.

and blue: see Petechiae.

BLONDS: Puls.

BLOOD, see Heart, Circulation, etc.

BLOOD VESSELS, see Heart.

BLOWS, shocks, thrusts, crash, explosion, etc.: Aloe, Apis, Arg-met., Bell., CANN-S., Chin., Cic., Croc., Dig., Glon., Naja, Nat-m., Phos., Spig., Stront-c., Sul-ac., Tab., Tarent., Zinc., Zinc-chr.

Comp. Injury.

as of a: Cupr.

BLUISH, purple, etc.: Acon., Arn., Ars., Bapt., Camph., Carb-v., Crot-h., CUPR., DIG., Ferr-p., Kreos., LACH., Mang., Merc-cy., Nux-v., Op., Sil., Sulph., Tarent-c., Thuj., Verat., VERAT-V.

affected parts: Lach.

injury from: Arn., Bell., Con., Lach., Puls., Sul-ac.

spots: Agar., Phos., Sep., Vip-t.

with burning: Anthraci., Ars., Lach.

BOARD-LIKE: Nux-m., Rhus-t., Tarent-c.

BONES: Arg-n., ASAF., Aur., Calc., Calc-f., CALC-P., Chin., Cocc., Cupr., Eup-per., Fl-ac., Hep., Kali-i., Lyc., MERC., Mez., Nit-ac., Phos., PH-AC., Phyt., PULS., Pyrog., Rhod., Rhus-t., Ruta, SIL., Staph., SULPH., Syph.

bare, becomes: Ars., Asaf., Aur., Calc., Chin., Con., Hep., Lach., Lyc., Merc., Mez., Nit-ac., Ph-ac., Puls., Ruta, Sabin., Sep., Sil., Staph., Sulph.

breaking: Ran-b.

breaking, injuries, bruised pains: Arn., Eup-per., Puls., Valer.

brittle: Ruta.

brittle, breaking, fractures, etc.: Asaf., Bufo, Calc., Calc-p., Cupr., Fl-ac., Lyc., Merc., Par., Ph-ac., Ran-b., Ruta, SIL., Sulph., Symph., Thuj.

Comp. Breaking

caries: Ars., Asaf., Aur., Calc., Calc-f., Con., Fl-ac., Hep., Lach., Lyc., Merc., Mez., Nit-ac., Ph-ac., Phos., Puls., Sep., Sil., Staph., Tell.

cartilages: Calc-p., Sulph., Symph.

chilly, cold: Aran., Calc., Eup-per., Kali-i., Pyrog.

condyles, prominences, etc.: Cycl., Rhus-v., Sang.

curvature, soft, etc.: Asaf., Calc., Calc-p., Lyc., Merc., Ph-ac., Phos., Sil., Sulph.

cutting: Anac., Aur., Dig., Kali-m., Lach., Osm., Sabad.

exostoses: Aur., Calc-f., Hecla, Merc., Ph-ac., Phos., Sil., Sul-i., Syph.

syphilitic: Fl-ac., Hep., Merc

gnawing: Bell., Stront.

growth, defective: Agar., Calc., Calc-p., Ferr., Ph-ac., Sil.

heavy: Sulph.

itching: Caust., Cocc., Cycl., Kali-m., Phos., Verat.

jerk in: Chin., Sil.

large, as if: Mez.

marrow: Am-c., Chel., Chin., Kali-c., Lyc., Mag-m., Naja, Ol-an., Op., Stront-c., Sulph.

necrosis: Ther.

night: Lyc., Merc.

non-union: Calc-f.

pains: Eup-per., Merc., Phyt., Pyrog.

periosteum: Asar., Fl-ac., Kali-bi., Kali-i., Mang., Merc., Mez., Phos., Ph-ac., Phyt., Rhod., Ruta, Sil.

periostitis: Ars., Asaf., Aur., Calc., Con., Hep., Lach., Merc., Mez., Nit-ac., Ph-ac., Puls., Sep., Sil., Staph., Sulph., Tell.

pricking: Thuj.

rent asunder, shattered: Chin., Kali-c., Spig.

sawing: Phos., Sulph., Syph., Tarent.

scraping: Chin., Ph-ac., Rhus-t., Thuj.

sensitive: Mang.

skin, near: Sang.

sore: Nit-ac.

torn loose, fresh: Dros., Nat-c., Ol-an., Ph-ac., Ruta.

walk, must: Ruta.

weather changes, Agg.: Am-c.

BORING, grinding: ARG-N., Asaf., Aur., Bell., Bism., Coloc., Dios., Hep., Lach., Mag-p., Med., Merc., Mez., Plat., Plb., Puls., Ran-s., Spig., Xan., Zinc., Zinc-chr.

BOUNDING, internal: Croc., Ther., Thuj.

Comp. Alive

BRANNY: Calc-p., Rad-met., Sanic., Thyr., Tub.

BREAKING, broken, brittle, etc.: Arn., BELL., Calc., Calc-p., Cocc., EUP-PER., Graph., Guaj., Lyc., Merc., Nat-m., Nux-v., Petr. (fragile), Phos., Ran-b., Rhus-t., Ruta, Sil., Sulph., Thuj., Valer.

Comp. Shattered.

BRINY: see Salty.

BROMIDES, abuse of: Zinc-p.

BROWN: Kreos., Lycps-v., Manc., Petr.

spots: Crot-h., Lach., Merc., Sanic.

BROWNISH, rusty, etc.: ARS., Bapt., Berb., Bry., Carb-v., Chel., Hyos., Iod., Lyc., Nit-ac., Op., Phos., Rhus-t., Sec., SEP., Staph., Sulph., Thuj., Verat.

BRUISED, see Soreness.

BUBBLING: Berb.

Comp. Gurgling.

BUNION: Agn., Sil.

BURNING, see Heat: Canth., Merc-c., Merc-i-r., Pic-ac., Ran-s., Thuj.

cold parts in: Sec., Verat-v.

internal, with external coldness: Ars., Verat.

pepper, like: Coc-c., Lach.

painful: Acon., ARS., Canth., Carb-v., Caust., Merc., Phos., Sulph.

prickling: Verat-v.

raw, smarting, biting: Am-c., Arum-t., Berb., Canth., Caps., Carb-v., Erig., Hydr., Lyc., Manc., Ran-s., Sinap., Sulph., Sul-i.

shivering, with: Acon., Ars., Bry., Chin., Ip., Samb., Verat-v.

spot, local: Agar, Glon., Sang., Sulph.

stinging: Ant-c., APIS, Ars., Berb., Con., Dulc., Glon., Iris, Lyc., Mez., Nux-v., Phos., Ph-ac., Rhus-t., Sil., Tarent., Urt-u.

washing, Agg.: Rhus-t., Sulph.

BURNS: Ars., CANTH., Carb-v., Caust., Kreos., Urt-u.

BURNT, scalded, scorched, as if: ARS., Canth., Cycl., Hydr., Hyos., IRIS, Lyc., Mag-m., Phyt., Plat., PULS., Ran-b., Sang., Sep., Verat., Verat-v.

BURR: Aesc. see Rectum,

BURROWING, digging, see Boring.

BURSAE, see Ganglion.

Comp. Cysts.

BURSTING, splitting, etc.: Act-sp., BELL., BRY., Calc., Carb-ac., **Chin.**, Eup-per., **Glon.**, Ham., **Ign.**, Kali-m., Lac-c., Lept., Lil-t., Lyc., Mag-c., Merc., NAT-M., **Nux-v.**, Ran-b., Rat., Ruta, Sep., **Sil.**, Spig., Stann., **Sulph.**, Thyr., **Vip.**

Comp. **Shattered.**

BUTTOCKS, jerking up: Cupr.

CALCULI, atheroma, etc.: **Bell.**, Benz-ac., **Berb.**, Bry., **Calc.**, **Chin.**, Coc-c., **Coloc.**, Dios., Hydr., Lach., LYC., Merc., **Nux-v.**, Oci., Pareir., Podo., **Sars.**

CANCER: **Ars.**, Aur., Calc., **Carb-an.**, Clem., **Con.**, Cund., **Graph.**, Hydr., Iod., **Kreos.**, Nit-ac., Phos., Phyt., **Sec.**, Sep., **Sil.**, **Sulph.**, Symph., Thuj.

sarcoma, see **Fungus.**

scirrhus type: Bell-p., Clem., Con., Petr., Sep., **Sil.**, Sulph.

CAP, see **Compression:** Lach.

CAPILLARIES: see **Heart, Circu-lation, etc.**

CARBUNCLE: Anthraci., Ars., Hep., Lach., Lyc., Sil., Tarent.

bluish red: Lach.

scarlet: Apis, Bell.

CARPHOLOGY, **picks at imagi-nary objects:** Ars., Bell., Hell., **Hyos.**, Lyc., Mur-ac., Op., Ph-ac., Rhus-t., **Stram.**, Tarent., Verat-v.

one spot, lips, fingers, etc.: Ars., **Arum-t.**, Cham., Con., Kali-br., Lach., Tarent., Thuj.

CARRIED, **wants to be:** Ant-t., Benz-ac., **CHAM.**, Cina.

fast: Acon., **Ars.**, **Brom.**, Verat.

over shoulder: Cina, Podo., Stann.

sitting up: Ant-t.

slowly: Puls.

CARSICKNESS see **Swaying.**

CARTILAGE: Ruta.

CELIBACY: **Con.**, Phos.

CELLARS, see **Dampness.**

CELLULAR TISSUE: Apis, Rhus-t., Tarent.

CHANGE, of **temperature; wants:** Sep., Tub.

CHANGING, see **Wandering.**

CHILBLAINS: Abrot., Hep.

CHILDREN, **infants, etc.:** Acon., Ant-c., Ant-t., **Bell.**, Borx., **CALC.**, **Calc-p.**, Cham., Cina, Coff., Ip., **Merc.**, Phyt., Podo., Puls., Rheum, Sep., **SIL.**, SULPH.

CHILL, cold, etc.: Kali-chl., Lac-d., Phys. (water), Thyr.

air, craves: Tub.

anticipates: Apis, Ars., Bry., Chin., Chinin-s., Nat-m., Nux-v.

becoming while hot: Samb., Visc.

congestive: Acon., Verat.

covers, averse to: Calc-s., Camph., Led., Sec.

don't Amel.: Lyc.

cough, Agg.: Apis, Eup-per., Thuj.

drinks, Agg.: Ars., Caps., Chel., Chin., Eup-per., Lach., Nux-v.

Amel.: Manc.

drowsiness, with: Camph., Gels.

exertion, Agg.: Plb., Zinc-val.

head, to: Glon.

heat with: Gels.

heat and, alternate: Nux-m., Arn.

lying, Agg.: Puls., Tell. (on back).

menses, at start: Jab.

motion, least: Nux-v.

motion of arms, Agg.: Rhus-t.

nervous: Gels., Zinc-val.

night, at: Pyrog.

nosebleed, with: Thuj.

pain, Agg.: Agar., Coloc., Mez., Puls., Sep.

partial: Berb., Cist., Dulc., Lyc., Nat-m., Ph-ac., Plat., Rhus-t.

one part, with heat of another: Apis, Bry., Cham.

prominent: Menth.

pressure, Amel.: Bry., Phos.

scratching, Agg.: Petr.

sleepy and: Chel., Gels.

stool, after: Rheum.

sweat, with: Lach.

thro' and thro': Am-c., Aran., Calc., Cinnb., Elaps, Kali-bi., Mosch.

uncovering, least, Agg.: Hep., Nux-v., Rhus-t., Sil.

waves, in: Carb-an.

wet, from: Lap., Led., Rhus-t., Thuj.

wind, in: Sanic.

yawning, with: Carb-an., Kreos., Meny., Thuj.

CHILLY, cold: Acon., Arn., ARS., Bell., Bry., Calc., Camph., Caps., Chin., Eup-per., Ferr., Gels., Hep., Ign., Ip., Lyc., Merc., Nat-m., NUX-V., PULS., RHUS-T., Sabad., Sep., Sil., VERAT.

CHIN, submental gland: Glech., Lach., Led., Staph.

quivers: Agar., Ant-t., Gels.

CHLOASMA: Card-m., Caul.,
Lyc., Rob., Sep.

CHOLERA: Ars., Camph., Cupr.,
Verat.

infantum: Med., Psor.

morbus: Ant-t., Crot-h., Iris,
Podo., Verat.

CHOREA: Agar., Cimic.. Stram.,
Tarant.

CHRONICITY: Alum., Arg-n.,
Ars., Calc., Caust., Con., Kali-
bi., Kali-i., Lyc., Mang., Phos.,
Plb., Psor., Sep., Sulph., Syph.,
Tub.

CICATRICES: Graph., Merc.,
Naja, Petr., Syph.

CLAIRVOYANCE: Acon., Med.,
Nux-m., Op., Phos.

CLEAR, see Dry.

CLIMAXIS: Acon., Aml-ns,
Cimic., Con., Ferr., LACH.,
Mang., Meli-a., Murx., Puls.,
Sang., Sep., Stront-c., Sulph.,
Sul-ac., Ust., Xan.

CLOTHES damp: Calc., Guaj.,
Lyc., Phos., Sanic., Sep., Tub.,
Verat-v.

large, too: Psor., Thuj.

CLUTCHING, see Cramp: Bell.,
Lil-t., Thyr.

COAT, wears in hot weather:
Hep., Merc., Psor.

COATED OR FURRED, as if:
Alum., Caust., Chin., Cocc.,
Colch., Dig., Dros., Iris, Kali-
c., Merc., Nux-m., PHOS.,
Ph-ac., PULS., Rhod., Verat.

COBWEB, hair etc. as if: Graph.
see Formication.

COITION, motions as of: Phos.

COLD, taking: Acon., Ars-i.,
CALC., Calc., Carb-v.,
Cham., Dulc., Hep., Kali-c.,
Nat-m., Nit-ac., NUX-V, Ol-
j., Phos., Psor., Rhus-t., Sep.,
SIL., Solid., Sulph., Tub.

ascending: Arum-t., Brom., Lac-
c., Merc., Sep.

chill of snow, and ice from: Ant-
c., Dros., Iod., Laur., Puls.,
Seneg., Verat., Verb.

descending: Bry., Carb-v., Kali-
c., Phos., Lyc., Sulph., Tub.

menstrual: Bar-c., Graph., Mag-
c., Senec.

painful, is: Cist., Mez., Mosch.

pains: Syph.

COLIC: See Cramp.

weakness, with: Castr., Tab.

COLLAPSE, sudden prostration
etc.: Acon., Aeth., Am-c., Ant-
t., Arn., Ars., Camph., Carb-
v., Colch., Con., Cupr., Hydr-
ac., Ip., Laur., Merc-cy., Naja,
Phos., Sec., Sep., Tab.,
VERAT., Verat-v.

dry: Am-c., Camph., Phys.

Comp. **Faint.**

COMA VIGIL: Laur.

COME and go: see **Fleeting.**

COMPRESSION, **squeezing, pinching, as of a vise, cap, etc.:** Alum., Anac., **Ant-t.,** Asar., Berb., Bry., **Cact.,** Calc., Cimic., **Carb-v., Cocc.,** COLOC., Graph., Ign., Meny., **Merc., Nat-m.,** Nit-ac., Olnd., PLAT., Ruta, Thuj., Valer., Verb., Zinc.

Comp. **Bursting.**

CONCUSSIONS: Arn., Bry., Cic., Con., **Rhus-t.,** Sulph.

CONDYLOMATA., see **Fungoid Growth.**

CONGESTION: **Acon.,** Aml-ns., Apis, **Arn.,** Aur., BELL., Bry., Cact., **Calc.,** Chin., Cupr., **Ferr-p.,** Gels., Glon., Lach., Mill., Nat-s., Nux-v., Op., **Phos., Puls.,** Rhus-t., Sang., Sep., SULPH., Ter., VERAT-V.

sudden: Acon., Bell., Glon., Verat-v.

CONICAL formations: Sil., Syph.

CONJUNCTIVA, pouting: **Nit-ac.**

raw: Kali-i., Lyc.

CONSCIOUSNESS: See **Senses.**

CONSTRICTION, band, gathered together, etc.: Anac., Argn., Ars., BELL., CACT., Carbac., Carb-v., Chel., **Chin.,** Hyos., **Ign., Lach.,** Lyc., NIT-AC., Nux-v., **Plat., Plb., Puls.,** Rad-met., Rat., Rhus-t., Sil., Sulph.

Comp. **Cramp.**

glands, in: Ign., Iod.

joints, in: Anac., Aur., Graph., Nat-m., Nit-ac.

Comp. **Band, Squeezing.**

CONSUMPTION, **tuberculosis:** Ars., **Calc., Calc-p.,** Hep., Iod., **Kali-c.,** Kreos., Lach., **Lyc.,** Nit-ac., Ol-j., Phel., **Phos., Puls.,** Sang., Sep., Sil., Spong., **Stann.,** Sulph., Ther., **Tub.**

incipient: Iod., Tub.

Comp. **Scrofula.**

CONTORTIONS, **distortions, etc.:** Bell., Cic., Hyos., Plat., Stram.

CONTRACTIONS: **Am-m.,** Anac., Calc., Caust., Coloc., Graph., Guaj., **Ign.,** Lyc., Nat-m., **Plb.,** Sec.

sense of general: Am-m., Cact., **Guaj.,** Kali-m., Nux-v., Phos.

CONTRACTURES, stricture, etc.: Cic., **Clem.**, Fl-ac., Guaj., **Merc.**, Nux-v., Rhus-t.

Comp. **Distortions.**

CONTROL, lacks: Caust., Tarent.

CONVULSIONS, see **Spasmodic**, bending backwards: Ang., Ign.

choreiform: Bell., **Caust.**, Cupr., Ign., **Lach.**, Nux-v.

consciousness, with: Cina, **Ign.**, Stram.

unconsciousness, with: Calc., Canth., Cic., **Hyos.**, Plb.

hemorrhage, after: Ars., Bell., Calc., Cina, Con., Ign., Lyc., Nux-v., Puls., Sulph., Verat.

fever, with: Ars., Bell., Camph., Carb-v., Hyos., Op., Sep., Stram., Verat.

internal: Caust., **Cocc.**, **Hyos.**, Ign., Ip., Mag-m., Nux-v., Puls., Stann.

menses, during: Cupr., Plat.

sleeplessness and: Alum., Bell., Bry., Calc., Carb-an., Carb-v., Cupr., Hep., Hyos., Ign., Ip., Kali-c., Merc., Mosch., Nux-v., Phos., Ph-ac., Puls., Rheum, Rhus-t., Sel., Sep., Sil., Stront-c., Thuj.

suppressions, from: Absin., Mill.

tonic: Bell., Camph., Cic., Ign., Ip., Op., Sec.

COPPERY COLOR: Carb-an., Lach., Merc., Mez., Nit-ac., **Rhus-t.**

COVERS, wants: Tub.

averse to: Acon., Camph., Iod., Puls., Sec., Sulph.

CRACKING IN JOINTS: Benz-ac., Cann-s., Caps., Caust., Kali-bi., Kalm., Led., **Nit-ac.**, PETR., **Rhus-t.**, Sulph., Thuj.

CRACKLING, like tinsel: Acon., Calc., Coff., Hep., Rheum, Sep.

CRACKS, fissures, chaps, etc.: Ant-c., Arum-t., **Calc.**, Caust., Cist., **Ferr.**, Fl-ac., GRAPH., Ign., Lyc., **Merc.**, Merc-c., Mez., Mur-ac., Nat-m., NIT-AC., PETR., Phos., Rat., Rhus-t., **Sep.**, Sil., **Sulph.**

CRAFTY: Tarent.

CRAMP, colic, etc.: **Bell.**, Cact., CALC., Caust., **Cham.**, Cocc., COLOC., CUPR., **Dios.**, Dulc., **Graph.**, Ign., Lach., **Lyc.**, Mag-m., Mag-p., Nit-ac., NUX-V., **Plat.**, Plb., Rheum, Scop., Sil., Stann., Staph., SULPH., **Verat.**, Vib.

Comp. **Constriction.**

coition, Agg.: Coloc., Cupr., Graph.

every where: Hydr-ac.

joints, in: Ang., Calc., Ph-ac., Plat., Sulph.

menses, after: Chin., Cupr., Puls.

muscles, in: Anac., Ang., Bell., Calc., Cina, Con., CUPR., Lyc., Merc., NUX-V., Plat., Sep., Tab.

Comp. Compression

nursing, Agg.: Cham.

pains, after: Sec.

paralysis, then: Tab.

radiating over whole body: Dios., Lyc., Nux-v.

stiffness, then: Sec., Sel.

CRAWLING, see Formication.

CREEPING or running, as of a little animal: Bell., Calc., Lyc., Phos., Rhod., Staph., Sulph.

Comp. Formication.

CREPITATION: Acon., Calc., Coff., Rheum.

CRUSHING, see Compression: Bry., Kali-i., Kalm., Nat-s.

CRUSTS, scabs, see Skin.

CUPPED: Thuj., Vario.

CUTTING: Acon, BELL., Bry., Calc., Calc-p., Calc-s., Canth., COLOC., Con., Dios., KALI-C., Kali-m., Lyc., Nat-m., Nit-ac., Nux-v., Plan., Polyg-a., Puls., Rat., Rumx., Sabal, Sulph., Tell.

smarting: Canth.

squeezing: Thuj.

CYSTS: Apis, Ars., BAR-C., CALC., GRAPH., Lyc., Nit-ac., PHOS., Sabin., SIL., Sulph., Thuj.

DARK, dusky, see Black

DAYS, hot, with cold nights: Acon., Dulc., Merc-c.

DAYTIME only: Agar., Euph., Sep., Sulph.

DEAD FEELING., see Numbness.

DEAD look: Thuj.

DEADNESS: Acon., Agar., Bar-c., Rhus-t., Sec.

DEATH, apparent: Acon., Ant-t., Carb-v., Coff., Op., Petr., Plat.

agony: Tarent.

DEBAUCHERY: Ant-c., Carb-v., Lach., Nux-v., Sul-ac.

DECOMPOSITION: Mur-ac., Sec.

DELICATE, tender, sickly, easily enervated: Ars., Calc., Caust., Con., Croc., Cupr., Ign., Lyc., Nat-c., Psor., Sil., Stront-c., Sulph., Teucr., Verat.

Comp. Nerves.

DELIRIUM, see Perception, changed.

DELUSIONS, see Perception, changed.

DENTITION: See **Teeth.**

DESIRES: See **Craving.**

DESQUAMATION, **branny,
scaly, hair falls, etc.:** Am-c.,
Ars., **Bell.,** Calc., Canth.,
Dulc., **Graph.,** Hep., KALI-
C., **Kali-m.,** Manc., **Med.,**
Merc., Mez., Nat-c., Nat-m.,
Nit-ac., PHOS, Puls., Rad-
met., Rhus-t., Sars., Sel., Sep.,
Staph., SULPH., Thyr., Tub.

Comp. **Crusts.**

branny: Rad-met., Tub.

brown: Am-m.

DESTRUCTIVE: Fl-ac.

DEVELOPMENT: See **Growth.**

DIABETES: Arg-met., Ars., **Carb-
v.,** Coloc., Kreos., **Nat-m.,** Ph-
ac., Ran-b., Sep., Squil.,
Sulph., Thuj., **Uran-n.**

DIARRHEA, **of phthisis:** Ars.,
Bry., Carb-v., Chin., Ferr.,
Hep., Nit-ac., Phos., Ph-ac.,
Puls., Sulph.

cold drink, agg.: Chin.

DIAPHRAGM: Cact., Ign.,
Stann., Strych.

DIGESTION: Aeth., **Ant-c.,** Arg-
n., Ars., Bry., **Calc.,** CHIN.,
Ferr., Merc., NUX-V., Olnd.,
Phos., PULS.

DIRECTION: ASCENDING
sensations: Acon., ASAF.,
Bell., Calc., Cimic., Con.,

Croc., Cupr., Dulc., Gels.,
Glon., IGN., Kali-bi., Kalm.,
Kreos., LACH., Led., **Naja,**
Op., PHOS., **Puls.,** Sabad.,
SANG., SEP., SIL., Stroph-h.,
Sulph., Thuj., **Zinc.**

backward: Bar-c., Bell., **Bry.,
Chel.,** Con., Crot-t., Cupr.,
Gels., **Kali-bi.,** Kali-c., Kali-
i., Lil-t., Merc., Nat-m., Par.,
Phos., Phyt., Prun., Puls.,
Sep., Spig., SULPH.

crosswise, across, etc.: Bell.,
Berb., Calc., **Chel., Chin.,**
Ferr., Hell., Kali-bi., Kali-
m., **Lac-c.,** Sep., **Sil., Sulph.,**
Valer., **Verat.,** Zinc.

Comp. **Alternating.**

distant parts, to: Berb., Cupr.,
Dios., Mag-p., Plb., Tell.,
Valer., Xan.

diagonal: Agar., **Alum.,** Ambr.,
Apis, Borx., Kali-i., **Kalm.,**
Lach., Lyc., Mang., Murx.,
Nat-c., Nux-v., **Phos.,**
RHUS-T., Stict., Sul-ac.,
Tarax.

downward: Aloe, Arn., Aur., Bar-
c., **Berb.,** Bry., Caps., **Cic.,**
Coff., **Hyper.,** KALM.,
Lach., Lyc., Puls., **Rhod.,**
Rhus-t., Sel., Zinc.

forward: Berb., Bry., Carb-v.,
Gels., Lac-c., Sabin., Sang.,
Sep., Sil., SPIG.

outward: Asaf., Bell., Berb., Bry.,
Chin., **Kali-bi.**, Kali-m.,
Kalm., Lith-c., Prun., Sep.,
Sil., **Valer.**, Zinc.

radiating: Agar., Arg-n., Ars.,
Bapt., **Berb.**, Caust., Cham.,
Cimic., **Coloc.**, **Cupr.**,
Dios., Kalm., Kali-bi., Kali-
c., **Mag-p.**, **Merc.**, Mez.,
Nux-v., Phyt., Plat., Plb.,
Sec., Sil., Spig., Xan.

up and down, falling and rising,
etc.: Ars., Bapt., Bry., Calc.,
Cimic., Eup-per., **Gels.**,
Glon., Kali-c., Lach., Lil-t.,
Lyc., Osm., **Phos.**, **Plb.**,
Podo., **Sulph.**, Verat.

DISCHARGES, bloody, streated,
etc: Phos., Sang., Sulph., Zinc.

excessive: Ars., Podo., Verat.

hair destroying: Nat-m.

hot: Borx., Kreos.

increased: see **Moisture**.

milky: Kali-p., Nat-s., Sep.

redden parts: Ars., Kreos., Merc.

retained, ceasing, etc.: Camph.,
Hydr., Thlasp.

vicarious: **Bry.**, Con., Dig., Ferr.,
Ham., **Lach.**, Lycps., Mill.,
Nux-v., PHOS., **Puls.**, Sec.,
Senec., **Sep.**, Sulph.

yellow, tenacious: Sumb.

green: Merc., Puls.

DISLOCATED, sprained, as if,
etc.: Asaf., Arn., **Ign.**, **Phos.**,
Nat-m., Petr., **Puls.**, RHUS-T.,
Sulph., Thuj.

Comp. **Sprains**.

DISLOCATION, spontaneous
easily: Ars., **Calc.**, Carb-an.,
Chel., Hyper., Lyc., Prun.,
Rhus-t., Ruta.

DISORDERLY: Stram.

DISTENSION: Mag-c., Ran-b.,
Ruta.

Comp. **Bursting**.

DISTORTIONS: Agar., Caust.,
Guaj., Ruta.

DISTRACTION: Thuj.

DOUBLING UP, see **Lying bent**.

DRAFT, see **Wind**.

DRAGGING, see **Falling**: Lil-t.,
Sil.

DRAWING: Arn., **Bry.**, Carb-v.,
Caust., Cham., Chel., Chin.,
Cimic., Kali-bi., Kali-c., Lach.,
Lyc., Merc., Nux-v., Puls.,
Rhod., RHUS-T., Sep.,
Sulph., Valer.

DRAWN or gathered together, as
if: Carb-v., **Chin.**, Merc., Naja,
Nat-m., Nux-v., Par., Puls.,
Rhus-t., **Sel.**, **Sulph**.

Comp. **Constriction**.

back: Croc.

DRINKS much, eats little: Sulph.

sips in: Kali-n.

DROPSY, edema, etc.: **Acet-ac.,** Agar., Ant-c., **Apis, Ars.,** Aur., Bell., Bry., Canth., **Chin.,** Colch., Dig., Graph., **Hell.,** Just., Kali-c., Lob., Lyc., **Merc.,** Olnd., Op., **Phos.,** Puls., Rhus-t., **Sep.,** Sil., Squil., Stront-c., **Sulph.,** Til., Zinc.

Comp. **Oedema**

in a.m.: Apis, Aur, Just., Kali-chl., Phos., Sep., Sil.

after exanthema: Ars., Hell., Rhus-t., Sulph.

angio-neurotic: Apis, Ars., **Rhus-t.**

saccular: Apis, Ars.

DRUGS, abuse of: Ars., Camph., Cham., Hep., **Hydr.,** Kali-i., Nat-m., Nit-ac., NUX-V., **Puls., Sulph.**

DRYNESS: Acon., **Ars.,** BELL., **Bry.,** Iod., Lach., Lyc., Melia., Nat-m., Nat-s., NUX-M., Phos., Plb., Puls., Rhus-t., Sanic., Sang., Sec., Sulph., Thyr., Tub., Ust., Visc.

cold: Acon., Nux-m., Samb.

internal: Bell., Bry., Graph., Op., Petr., Rumx.

profuse secretion, with: Euph., Lyc., Merc., Nat-m.

DUALITY, in pieces, separated, as if some one else, etc.: **Anac.,** Arg-n., BAPT., Calc-p., Cann-s., GELS., Nux-m., PETR., Phos., **Pyrog.,** Sil., **Stram.,** Ther., Thuj., Tril., Xan.

DUSKY COLOR: Ail., **Ant-t.,** Ars., BAPT., Crot-h., **Gels.,** Hell., Lach., Nit-ac., **Nux-v.,** OP., Sec.

Comp. **Bluish.**

DUST, feathers, etc., as of: **Ars.,** Bell., CALC., Chel., Chin., DROS., Hep., Ign., **Lyc.,** Phac., Puls., Rumx., Sulph.

Comp. **Vapor.**

DWARFISH: Ambr., **Bar-c., Con.,** Med., Op., Syph.

DYSPNEA: See **Respiration.**

EARTHY, see **Yellow.**

EBULLITION, see **Waves.**

EDGE, on an: Ruta, Valer.

EFFUSION, deposits, etc.: Apis, **Bry.,** Canth., Hell., Kali-n., Ran-b., Sulph., Sul-i.

Comp. **Reabsorbant.**

EGG, albumen: Ol-an.

foul: Asclp., Psor., Staph.

ELONGATED, as if: Alum., Hyper., Kali-c., Lac-c., **Phos.,** Stram., Tab.

EMACIATION, atrophy, etc.:
Arg-met., ARS., Bar-c., Bism.,
Calc., CALC-P., Caust., Chin.,
Ferr., Graph., IOD., Led.,
Lyc., Nat-m., Nit-ac., Nux-v.,
Op., Phos., PLB., Sanic., Sars.,
Sil., Sulph., Syph., Thuj.,
Thyr., Tub.

appetite, with: Abrot., Ars.,
Calc., Cina, Iod., Lyc., Nat-
m., Petr., Psor., Sulph.

descending: Sanic.

glands, of: Con., Iod.

infantile, marasmus: Abrot.,
Aur., Calc., Chin., Lyc.,
Sulph., Tub.

partial: Bry., Calc., Graph.,
Mez., Phos., Plb., Puls.,
Sec., Sel., Sulph.

senile: Bar-c., Chin., Fl-ac., Iod.,
Lyc., Op.

sensation of: Naja.

spare habit: Arg-met., Calc-p.,
Kreos., Nux-v., Sec.

upper parts: Calc., Plb.

EMOTIONS: Acon., Ant-c.,
ARS., Aur., Bell., Cham.,
Cina, Coff., Coloc., Croc.,
Gels., Hyos., IGN., Lach.,
Lyc., Nat-m., Nit-ac., NUX-
V., Pall., Phos., Ph-ac., Plat.,
Psor., PULS., Staph., Stram.,
Sulph., Sumb., Verat.

EMPTY, hollow, sinking, etc.:
Chin., Cocc., Dig., Hydr.,
IGN., Kali-c., Murx., Nux-v.,
Olnd., PHOS., Podo., SEP.,
Stann., Sulph., Tab., Tell.,
Verat-v.

ENLARGED, see Swelled.

EPILEPSY: Arg-n., Ars., Art-v.,
Bufo, Calc., Cupr., Hydr-ac.,
Lach., Oena., Op., Plb., Sil.,
Zinc-p.

sexual: Bar-c., Bufo, Calc., Visc.

status epilepticus: Absin., Acon.,
Oena.

EPISTAXIS, heat, with: Thuj.

lying on sides: Sulph. (r).

menses, Agg.: Graph., Lach.,
Sep.

absent: Apis, Bry., Carb-an.,
Cham., Dulc., Ferr., Lach.,
Lyc., Merc., Puls., Sil.

profuse: Acon., Meli-a.

puberty, at: Abrot., Kali-c., Phos.

sweat, with: Bry., Caust., Con.,
Nux-v., Op., Phos., Tarax.,
Thuj.

washing face, Agg.: Bry.

ERETHISM, false: Merc., Mur-
ac., Phos.

ERYSIPELAS: Acon., APIS, Arn.,
Bell., Canth., Crot-h., Euph.,
Graph., Lach., Merc., Puls.,
RHUS-T., Sec., Sulph.

recurrent: Graph., Hydr., **Rhus-t.**

swelling, great: Apis, **Bell.,** Merc., Rhus-t.

wandering, creeping: Graph., Hydr., Rhus-t., Sulph., Syph.

EXCITEMENT, **mental, nervous, etc.:** ACON., **Bell.,** COFF., Gels., **Hyos.,** Lach., NUX-V., Op., Pyrog., **Stram.,** Teucr., Valer., Verat., Zinc-val.

Comp. **Nerves.**

EXCORIATION, see **Rawness.**

EXCRETIONS, **suppressed:** Stram., Verat.

EXPLOSIONS, see **Shattered.**

EXUDATION: see **Effusion.**

EXUDATIVE DIATHESIS: see **Psora.**

FAG, **enervation, etc.:** Colch., Kali-p., Pic-ac., Tab., Zinc.,

Comp. **Exertion.**

FAINT, **faints, etc.:** Acon., ARS., Bry., Camph., **Carb-v.,** Cham., Chin., Crot-h., Dig., Hep., **Ign.,** LACH., Mosch., Nux-m., NUX-V., Op., Puls., SEP., Stroph-h., Sulph., Thyr., Verat.

heated, if: Tab.

looking up, Agg.: Tab.

pain, Agg.: Nux-m., Ran-s., Stront-c.

rising, on: Bry., Merc-i-f., Phyt., **Verat-v.,** Vib.

stool, at: Con., Podo., Sulph.

Comp. **Collapse, Empty, Raising up.**

FALLING, **sinking:** Aloe, Aur., **Bell.,** Borx., Brom., **Calc.,** Caust., Cimic., Coll., Con., Cupr., Frax., Gels., Glon., Helo., Hydr-ac., **Ign.,** Kali-cy., Kreos., Lach., **Laur.,** Lil-t., **Merc.,** Mur-ac., Nat-c., Nat-m., Nux-v., Pall., Ph-ac., Phos., Plat., **Puls.,** Rat., **Rhus-t.,** Senec., Sep., Stann., Verat.

FALLING, **as if:** Bell., Thuj.

backward: Bry., Chin., Led., Rhus-t.

out: Podo., Sep.

FAR OFF: Med.

FASTING: Ars., **Bry.,** Chin., Puls., Verat.

FEATHERS, see **Dust.**

FEET, **higher than head, as if:** Spig.

FIBROUS TISSUE, **tendons:** Bry., **Calc.,** Calc-f., Colch., FL-AC., **Graph.,** GUAJ., **Kali-m., Lyc.,** Phyt., Rhod., RHUS-T., Ruta, Sabin., **Sec., Sil.,** Staph.

injured: Anac.

pains in: Rhus-t., Sabin.

sheath of: Bry., Iod., Rhus-t.

tense, short, etc.: Am-m., Caust., Graph., Guaj., Nat-m., Ol-j.

FIDGETY: Apis, Borx., Cimic., Graph., Sil., Tarent.

Comp. Restlessness

FILM: See Leaf.

FINE PAINS; needle, splinter, thread or hair, like a: Agar., All-c., Alum., Apis, ARG-N., Ars., Caps., HEP., Kali-bi., Kali-c., Nat-m., NIT-AC., Paeon., Rat., Rhus-t., Sabad., SIL., Sulph., Syph., Thuj., Valer., Verat.

FISHY: Calc., Graph., Med., Olan., Sanic., Tell., Thuj.

FISTULAE: Berb., CALC., Calc-f., Calc-p., Caust., Fl-ac., Lyc., Nit-ac., Petr., Phos., Puls., SIL., Sulph.

chest symptoms and: Berb., Calc-p.

FITS AND STARTS, pains in: Bar-m., Cupr., Mez.

FLABBY: Merc-d.

FLOATING, flying, etc., as if: Acon., Arg-n., Asar., Cann-s., Cocc., Hyper., LAC-C., Lach., Nat-m., Nux-m., Op., Phos., Spig., Stict., Thuj., Valer., Zinc-i.

Comp. Vertigo.

FLOWING, see Trickling: Bufo, Lam., Sumb.

FLUSHES, see Waves.

FLYING TO PIECES see Shattered.

FOAMY, frothy: Arn., Apis, Ascl., Chel., Cob., Elat., Form., Grat., Ip., Kali-bi., Kali-c., Kali-i., Kreos., Led., Mag-c., Merc., Nat-s., Oena., Podo., Rheum, Rhus-t., Rumx., Sabad., Sep., Sulph., VERAT.

FOGS: see Cloudy weather.

FONTANELLES, open: Calc., Calc-p., Puls., Sil.

FORCED, through a narrow opening, as if: Asaf., BAR-C., Bell., Bufo, Carb-an., Coc-c., Cocc., Dig., Glon., Lach., Op., Plb., Puls., Sil., Sulph., Tab., Thuj., Valer.

apart: see Separated.

FOREIGN BODIES: Acon., Calc-f., Sil.

FORMICATION, crawling, etc.: Acon., Agar., Arn., Calc., Carb-an., Coca, Colch., Lyc., Merc., Nux-v., Oena., Op., Osm., Phos., Plat., Rhus-t., SEC., Sep., Sulph., Stram., Stront-c., Tell., Vario., Zinc.

sweat, with: Rhod.

Comp. Alive.

FRAGILE: See **Breaking.**

FRAIL: Sars.

FROSTBITE: AGAR., Ars., Carb-v., **Nit-ac., Nux-v., Petr., Puls.,** Sulph.

FULL: **Acon., Chin.,** Lil-t., Melia., Nat-s., **Sulph.,** Vip-t.

FULLNESS, see **Bursting, Congestion.**

FUMES, see **Vapor.**

FUNGOID GROWTH, see **Skin.**

GAIT, stooped, bent, etc.: **Arg-n., Carb-v.,** Cocc., **Coloc.,** Con., Gels., **Mang., Phos., Sulph.,** Verat.

dragging: Rhus-t.

limping: Caust., Dulc., Kali-c., Tab.

reeling: Agar., Alum., Cocc., Lol-t., Phos.

shuffling: Ol-an.

slovenly: Sil.

spastic: Zinc.

staggering: Alum., Calc., Nat-c., Onos., Pic-ac., Puls.

stooped: Am-m., Nat-m., **Sulph.**

stumbling: Agar., Arg-n., Bar-c., Con., Hyos., Nat-c., Nux-v., Phos., Ph-ac., Ruta.

tottering: Phos., Rhod., Verat.

unsteady: Agar., Arg-n., Bar-c.,

Caust., Cocc., Kali-br., Lil-t., Nat-c., Sec., Stann., **Sulph.**

GANGLION, Bursae: Am-c., Apis, Arn., Benz-ac., Phos., **Ruta,** Sil., Stict., Sulph.

Comp. **Cyst.**

GARLICKY: Art-v., Asaf., Lach., Petr., **Tell.**

GATHERED TOGETHER, see **Constriction** and **Drawn together.**

GELATINOUS: **Aloe, Arg-n.,** Berb., COLCH., Coloc., Dig., HELL., **Kali-bi.,** Laur., Podo., **Rhus-t.,** Sabin., Sel., Sep.

Comp. **Albuminous.**

GIRDLE PAINS: Sulph.

GLAIRY, see **Albuminous.**

GLANDS: Apis, Ars., Arum-t., Aur., BAR-C., **Bell.,** Bry., CALC., Carb-an., Chin., **Clem.,** Con., Hep., Iod., **Kali-m., Lach., Lyc.,** MERC., Nit-ac., **Phos., Phyt.,** PULS., Rhod., Rhus-t., SIL., Spong., Staph., Sulph., Tab., Tub.

cervical: Bar-c., Calc., Lyc., Merc., Viol-t.

flaccid: Cham., Con., Iod.

hard: Bar-m., Calc., Calc-f., Carb-an., Con., **Phyt.,** Sil., Spong.

inflamed: Acon., Bell., Bry., Merc.

itching: Con., Sil.

knotted cords or beads, like: Aeth., Bar-m., Berb., Nit-ac., Sul-i.

mesenteric: Calc., Iod.

submental: Glech., Led.

swelled: Bell., Carb-an., Cist., Dulc., Iod., Merc., Phyt., Rhus-t., Sil., Sul-i., Tub.

over body in fever: Bell., Kali-c., Sep.

GLISTENING: Acon., APIS, Aur., Bell., Bry., Calc-f., Carb-ac., Caust., Cist., Euphr., Glon., Kali-bi., LAC-C., Lach., Mang., Nat-m., Phos., Rhus-t., Sabin., Sil., Syph., Ter.

GLUEY: Graph., Mez.

GLUTTONY, gross feeders, etc.: All-s., Ant-c., Chin.

GNAWING, eating, festering, pains: Agn., Am-m., Berb., Bry., Cham., Coloc., Graph., Guaj., Ign., Kreos., Lach., Lyc., Mag-m., Nat-s., Nit-ac., Olnd., Ox-ac., Phos., Plat., PULS., Ran-s., Rhus-t., Sec., Sep., SIL., Staph., Sulph., Sul-ac., Thuj., Verat., Zinc-chr.

burning: Ruta.

grinding: Zinc-chr.

GONORRHEA: Arg-n., Cann-s., Merc., Puls., Sep., Sulph., Thuj.

effects of sycosis: Arg-n., Kali-i., Kalm., Merc., Puls., Sabad., Sep., Staph., Sulph.

suppressed: Nat-m., Puls.

GOUT: Colch., Coloc., Kali-i., Led., Lyc., Nux-m., Rad-met., Ran-s., Sulph., Urt-u.

acute: Colch., Sabin., Urt-u.

diarrhea, after: Ant-c., Benz-ac., Colch., Merc-d., Nat-s.

rheumatic: Rhod.

GRACILE: Phos.

GRANULAR, sandy appearance: Apis, Carb-v., Cub., Graph., Hep., Lac-c., Lyc., Nat-m., Ph-ac., Phos., Plb., Podo., Sars., Zinc.

GRANULATION, poor: Carb-v., Hep., Kreos., Nit-ac., Sil.

warty: Arg-n.

GRAPES, like: Aloe.

GRASPED AND RELAXED alternately, see Opening and Shutting.

GRASPING, see Fingers, Conditions: Cact., Gels., Sep.

GRAYISH, dirty, etc.: Arg-met., Ars., Berb., Calc., Caust., Chel., Cupr., Dig., Diph.,

Ferr-p., KALI-C., Kali-m., Lach., Lyc., Merc., Merc-cy., Ox-ac., Ph-ac., PHOS., Sil., Still., Sulph.

GREASY, oily, fatty: Asc-t., Bry., CAUST., Dulc., Fl-ac., Iod., Iris, Kali-p., MAG-C., Maland., Merc., Nat-m., Nat-s., Ol-an., Phos., Psor., Puls., Sel., Tarent., Thuj., Valer.

sweat: Merc., Thuj.

GREEN: Gels., (tea), Thuj., (grass), Kali-bi., Med., Rhus-t., Sec., Sul-ac.

dark: Ars.

scum: Asc-t., Bry., Grat., Mag-c., Merc., Sanic.

turns: Arg-n., Borx., Calc-f., Nat-s., Psor., Rheum, Sanic.

GREENISH: Acon., ARS., Carb-v., Cham., Con., Ip., Kali-i., Lyc., Mag-c., MERC., Nat-s., Phos., PULS., Sep., Stann., Sulph., Verat.

yellow: Merc., Puls.

GRINDING, see Boring.

GRIPPING, see Cramp.

GRIPPE, see Influenza.

GRISTLY: Nit-ac., Sil.

GRITTY FEELING, in joints: Con.

GROUND, gives way: Arg-n., Con., Kali-br., Visc.

GROWING PAINS: Calc-p., Guaj., Mang., Ph-ac.

GROWTH, affected: Bar-c., Calc., Calc-p., Phos., Ph-ac., Sil.

disorders of: Bar-c., Calc., Calc-p., Phos., Ph-ac., Sil.

GROWTHS, new: Ant-c., Ars., Bell., Calc., Carb-an., Carb-v., Caust., Clem., Graph., Lyc., Nit-ac., Ran-b., Sil., Staph., Sulph., Thuj.

fleshy: Merc., Nit-ac., Staph., Thuj.

grapes, like: Calc.

horny: Ant-c., Ran-b., Sil., Sulph.

rapid: Iod.

GUMMAE: Carb-an.

GUMMY: Viol-t.

GURGLING: Agar., ALOE, Berb., Brach., Cic., Cina, Crot-t., Cupr., Gamb., Hydr-ac., Jatr., Kali-c., Kreos., LAUR., Lil-t., Lyc., Podo., Puls., Squil., Sulph., Thuj.

Comp. Babbling, Rattling.

GUSHING: Ars., Bell., Berb., Bry., CROT-T., Elat., Gamb., Grat., Ip., Jatr., Kali-bi., Mag-m., Nat-c., Nat-m., Nat-s., Phos., Podo., Psor., Sabin., Stann., Thuj., Tril-p., Verat.

Comp. Swashing.

HACKING, like a hatchet: Am-c., Ars., Aur., Clem., Kali-n., Lyc., Ph-ac., Ruta, Staph., Thuj.

HAIR, thread, etc., see Fine.

HANGING DOWN, loose, suspended, etc., as if: Alum., Aur., Bar-c., Ign., Ip., Kali-c., LACH., Lil-t., Med., Merc., PHOS., Sabad., Sep., Sulph., Valer.

Comp. Fine, Loose, etc.

HARD BED, sensation: Arn., Bapt., Brom., Con., Dros., Flac., Gels., Kali-c., Merc-i-r., Nux-v., Phos., Plat., Pyrog., Rhus-t., Sil., Spong.

bed: Til.

pain: see Aching.

stony: Calc-f., Carb-v., Kali-bi., Kali-m., Merc-i-r., Sulph., Tarent-c.

HARDNESS, induration: Alum., Ant-c., Ars., Bar-c., Bell., Bry., Calc., Calc-f., Carb-an., Cist., Clem., Con., Graph., Iod., Kali-m., Lyc., Merc., Petr., Phos., Phyt., Plb., Rhus-t., Sars., Sep., SIL., Sulph., Tarent.

HEATED, being early: Kali-n., Nit-ac.

HEAVINESS, load, etc.: Alet., Aloe, Alum., Apis, Arg-n., Bry., Calc., Con., GELS.,

Helo., Lach., Lil-t., Lith-c., Lyc., Nat-m., NUX-V., Phos., Ph-ac., Pic-ac., PULS., Rhust-t., Scop., Sep., Stann., Sulph.

HEMOPHILLA: Arn., Ars., Carban., Crot-h., Ham., Kreos., Lach., Nat-s., Phos., Sil.

HEMOPTYSIS: Acal., Acon., Amc., Ars., Bell., Bry., Chin., Ferr., Hyos., Ip., Mill., Nit-ac., Phos., Plb., Puls., Rhus-t., Sabin., Sec., Sulph., Sul-ac.

HEMORRHAGE, bloody discharges, etc.: Acon., Alum., ARN., Ars., BELL., Cact., CALC., Canth., Carb-v., CHIN., Croc., Crot-h., Erig., FERR., Ham., Hydr., Ip., Kreos., Lach., Led., Lept., Lyc., Lycps-v., MERC., Mercc., Mill., NIT-AC., Nux-v., PHOS., PULS., Rhus-t., Sabin., Sec., Sep., Solid., Sulph., Sul-ac., Ter., Thlasp., Tril-p., Urt-u., Ust., Vib., Vipt.

acute: Acon., Bell., Croc., Ferr., Hyos., Mill., Puls.

acrid: Kali-c., Sil.

altered blood, of: Crot-h., Puls., Sec.

bright: Acon., Arn., Bell., Carbv., Dulc., Ferr., Hyos., Ip., Led., Mill., Phos., Plb., Sabin., Sulph.

with dark clots: Ferr., Sabin., Sang.

clots, mixed with: Sabin., Ust.

dark: Acon., Canth., Chin., Carb-v., Cham., Croc., Crot-h., Ham., Lach., Nux-m., Nux-v., Puls., Sec., Sep., Sul-ac., Ust.

clotted, see Lumpy Effects

gushing: Acon., **Bell.**, Cham., Ham., Ip., Lac-c., Puls., Sabin., Sec., Tril-p.

heart symptoms, with: Crat., Lycps-v.

hot blood: **Bell.**, Sabin.

lumpy, clots: Arn., **Bell.**, Canth., Chin., Ferr., Hyos., Ip., Nux-v., Puls., Sabin., Sulph.

menses, between: Sabin.

offensive: Bell., Bry., Carb-v., Sabin.

passive, oozing, etc.: Bov., Bufo, Carb-v., **Chin.**, Crot-h., Fer-p., Ham., Ph-ac., Sec., Ter., Ust.

scratching, Agg.: Psor.

slight, causes great aggravation: Bufo, Carb-an., **Chin.**, Ham., Hydr., Sec.

streaked: Ars., Asaf., Bell., Bry., Caust., Chin., Crot-h., **Ferr.**, Hep., Ip., Lach., **Merc.**, Nit-ac., Ox-ac.,

Phos., Pyrog., Sil., **Sulph.**, Zinc.

stringy: Coc-c., Croc., Graph., Kali-bi., Merc., Naja, Phyt., Sul-ac., Ust.

thick: Agar., Bov., Canth., Croc., Cupr., Graph., Kali-m., Merc-cy., Nat-m., **Nux-m.**, Plat., Psor.

thin: Crot-h., Laur., Sec., Sul-ac.

clot, won't: Lach., Phos.

watery, thin: Carb-v., Graph., Iris, Kali-i., Nit-ac., Sabin.

weakness undue: Alum., Bry., Carb-an., Ham., Hydr.

HERE AND THERE: Acon., Agar., **Am-c.**, Aur., Bar-c., Calc., Chel., Chin., Cimic., Cina, COCC., Graph., IGN., Lyc., Mag-c., Mag-p., Op., Ph-ac., Phos., Rat., Rhus-t., Sec., Stann., Staph., **Sulph.**, **Thuj.**, **Valer.**, Verat-v., **Zinc.**

Comp. **Wandering**.

HOLLOW, see **Empty**: Kali-c., Tab.

HORSE-BACK, see **Riding**.

HOT: Euphr., Kreos., Op., Sulph.

irons, wires, needles etc. as of: Alum, Apis, **Ars.**, Bar-c., Mag-c., Naja, Nit-ac., Ol-an., Rhus-t., Spig., Vesp.

HUMMING, buzzing, whizzing, purring: Caust., Kali-m., Kreos., Mosch., Nux-m., Olnd., Puls., Spig., Sulph.

Comp. **Vibrating.**

HYDROAE see **Eruptions.**

HYDROGENOID: Dulc., Nat-m., Nat-s., Thuj.

HYDROPHOBIA: **Bell.**, Canth., Cupr., **Hyos.**, Merc., Phos., Sabad., **Stram.**

prophylactic: **Bell.**, Hyos., Stram.

HYGROMA: see **Ganglion.**

HYPERTROPHY: **Ant-c.**, Ars., Calc., **Clem.**, **Dulc.**, **Graph.**, Ran-b., Rhus-t., Sep., **Sil.**, Sulph.

HYPOSTASIS: Rhus-t.

HYSTERIA: Cham., Cocc., **Ign.**, Mag-m., Mosch., Nux-m., Nux-v., Plat., Tarent.

coition, **Agg.**: Lac-c.

ICY COLD: Agar., Apis, **Carb-v.**, Elaps, Helod., Hydr-ac., Med., Meny., Nit-ac., Ol-an., Phos., Sil., **Verat.**

Comp. **Chill, Collapse.**

ILL OR SICK FEELING: Acon., Ant-t., Ars., Bapt., Chel., Nux-v., **Podo.**, Puls., Stront-c.

sick feeling: Cimic., Lach., Lob., Petr., Psor., Sang., Serp., Tab., Tarax.

sick, says, is not: **Arn.**, Iod., Op.

Comp. **Nothing.**

IMMOBILE: Lycps-v., Mang., Stront-c.

INACTIVE, apathetic, lies down, lethargic: Ail., Ant-t., **Arn.**, Ars., Calc., Carb-v., Caust., Chin., Gels., Hell., **Nux-v.**, Olnd., OP., PHOS., PH-AC., Psor., SEP., **Stram.**, **Sulph.**, Zinc.

Comp. **Reaction, Relaxation.**

INCONTINENCE, stool, urine, sexual, etc.: **Aloe, Arn.**, Ars., **BELL.**, **CAUST.**, Chin., Con., Dios., **Gels.**, **Hyos.**, Mur-ac., Nux-m., **Phos.**, PH-AC., **Podo.**, **Puls.**, Sel., **Sep.**, Staph., **Sulph.**

INCOORDINATION: Gels.

INCREASING AND DECREA-SING gradually, sun-pains, etc.: Arg-n., Ars., Gels., **Glon.**, Kali-bi., Kalm., Lach., Nat-m., Phos., PLAT., Puls., **Sang.**, **Spig.**, STANN., **Stront-c.**, Sulph., Syph.

quickly, see **Shooting.**

INCREASES gradually, ceases suddenly: Ign., Puls., Sul-ac.

suddenly and leaves suddenly: Bell., Kali-bi., Nit-ac.

leaves gradually: Sabin.

INDIFFERENT, see **Placid.**

INDURATION, see **Hardness.**

INFILTRATION: Calc., Carb-an., Graph., Kali-m., Rhus-t., Sulph., Sul-i.

INFLAMMATION: **Acon.,** Apis, Ars., **Bell., Bry.,** Calc., Cann-s., Canth., Cham., Ferr-p., **Gels.,** Hep., Hyos., Iod., Kali-c., **Merc., Nux-v., Phos., Puls., Rhus-t.,** Sep., **Sil.,** Staph., Sulph., **Verat-v.**

INFLUENZA: Ars-i., Bapt., Bry., Camph., Caust., Cupr., Eucal., **Eup-per.,** Ferr-p., **Gels.,** Merc., **Nux-v., Rhus-t.,** Sabad.

INJURIES, shocks, wounds, bruises, etc.: ARN., Bell-p., **Calen.,** Cic., **Con.,** Glon., Ham., Hyper., Kali-i., **Lach.,** Led., Lith-c., Nat-s., Nit-ac., **Puls., Rhus-t., Ruta,** Staph., Stront-c., **Sul-ac.,** Zinc-chr.

Comp. **Sprained.**

bones, to: Arn., Calc., Iod., **Petr.,** Phos., Ph-ac., Puls., **RUTA,** Staph.

bones or cartilage: Ruta, Symph.

crushing: Arn., Con., Ruta, Staph.

cuts: Staph.

gaping wounds: Hyper.

head, to: Arn., Calc., **Cic.,** Glon., Hyper., **Nat-s.,** Sil., Symph.

incisions, stabs, etc.: Arn., Lach., **Phos., Puls., Staph.,** Sul-ac.

lacerations: Hyper.

old: All-c., Symph.

pain in: All-c., Kali-i., Sil.

muscles to: Rhus-t.

pains, returning: Glon., Nat-m., **Nit-ac.,** Nux-v.

punctured, shot-gun, etc.: Arn., **Hyper.,** Led., **Nit-ac.,** Sul-ac.

reopening of old: Carb-v., Crot-h., Fl-ac., Lach., Nat-m., **Phos.,** Sil.

scars: Dros.

burn: Tell.

pimples about: Fl-ac.

twitching: Led.

INSENSIBILITY, see **Numbness.**

INSTEP, ulcer: Lyc.

INTERMITTENCY: ARS., Calc., **Chin.,** Ip., Lach., **NAT-M.,** Nit-ac., **Nux-v.,** Ph-ac., **Puls.,** Sec., Sulph.

Comp. **Paroxysms, Periodicity.**

INTERNAL AFFECTIONS: Calc., Canth., Nux-v., Phos.

itching: Apis, Coc-c., Phos., Rhus-t., Sang., Samb.

INTOXICATION, easy: Bov., Con., Zinc.

INSENSIBLE, unconscious, etc.: Ars., Bapt., BELL., Cupr., HYOS., Nat-m., OP., PH-AC., STRAM.

IRREGULAR, inco-ordinate effects: Agar., Cimic., Con., Echi., Ferr., Gels., Glon., Graph., Ign., Kali-p., Nux-v., Plat.

ISCHIAS ANTICA: Podo.

ISOLATED EFFECTS: Agar., Gels., Verat., Zinc.

Comp. Spots.

JERKING PAIN: Asaf., Bell., Calc., Caust., Chin., Ign., Kali-c., Meny., Nat-m., Nux-v., Puls., Rhus-t., Sil., Tarax.

starts pain, Agg.: Arg-n., Lyc.

JERKS: Bell., Borx., Calc., Cic., Colch., Lyc., Merc., Nux-v., Plat., Puls., Rat., Sep., Spig., Stann., Sulph., Sul-ac., Tab., Zinc-i.

local: Thuj.

pain: Rhod.

sleep, on falling to: Ars., Ign.

together: Ther.

Comp. Spasmodic.

JOINTS: Arn., Bell., Benz-ac., BRY., Calc., Caust., Cham., Cimic., COLCH., Dros., Dulc., Graph., Guaj., Kali-bi., Kalm., Led., Lith-c., Lyc.,

MERC., Nux-v., Phyt., Puls., Rad-met., RHUS-T., Ruta, Sabin., Sil., Staph., SULPH.

colds, Agg.: Calc-p., Rumx.

deep in: Cimic., Rad-met.

digging: Colch.

dryness in: Canth., Lyc., Nux-v., Puls.

loose: Chel., Ph-ac., Psor., Thuj.

quaking: Colch.

red spot on: Bell., Stict.

small: Act-sp., Benz-ac., Caul., Colch., Kali-bi., Led., Lith-c., Nat-p., Ran-s., Rhod., Sabin., Sal-ac., Stict., Thuj.

sores, blisters, ulcers on: Ars., Borx., Lap-a., Mez., Nat-c., Psor., Sep.

sprained, easily: Phos., Rhus-t.

suppurating: Calc-hp., Merc., Phos., Psor., Sil.

swelled: Puls.

swelling, pale, (white swelling), etc.: Ant-c., Ars., Coloc., Iod., Kreos., Merc., Rhus-t., Sil., Sulph.

synovitis: Apis, Bry., Iod., Puls., Sil., Sulph.

tuberculosis of: Apis, Calc., Calc-p., Kali-c., Kali-i., Ph-ac., Puls., Sil.

ulcerated: Coloc., Hep., Ph-ac., Sep., Sil.

water in: Sulph.

weak: Bov., Calc., Sep.

KERATITIS: Merc-c.

KNOT, see **Ball.**

LABOR-LIKE., see **Pressing down.**

LACERATIONS: Staph.

LANCINATING: **darting, lightning:** Cupr., Hydr-ac., Hyos., Kali-m., Mag-m., Rad-met.

LASSITUDE, see **Inactive.**

LETHARGY, see **Inactive.**

LIE DOWN, see **Inactive:** Ferr., Rad-met., Thyr.

LIFTED UP: Phos., Stroph-h.

LIFTING, see **Sprains.**

LIGAMENTS, see **Fibrous Tissue.**

LIGHT, see **Sensitive.**

LIGHTNING, see **Shooting:** Alum., Sec., Verat.

           Comp. **Lancinating.**

LIMPING: Coloc., Rhus-t.

LINEAR PAINS: Syph., Tell.

           Comp. **Streaks.**

LITHEMIA: see **Uric acid.**

LIVID., see **Black:** Ox-ac., Rhus-t.

LOOKING INTENTLY, see **Reading.**

   sidewise: Nerc-c.

LOOSE, as if: **Am-c.,** Bar-c., Bov.,

Carb-an., Caust., Chin., Croc., Hyos., **Kali-c.,** Kali-m., Laur., Med., Nat-s., NUX-M., Nux-v., Psor., RHUS-T., Sul-ac., Thuj.

       Comp. **Rolling, Swashing, Hanging down.**

LUMPY EFFECTS, **discharges,** etc.: Aeth., Aloe, **Ant-c., Cham., Chin.,** Coc-c., Croc., **Graph.,** KALI-B1., **Kreos.,** LYC., **Merc.,** Merc-i-f., PLAT., Rhus-t., Sep., Sil., Stann.

LYING DOWN, see **Inactive.**

MALIGNANCY: Crot-h., Lach., Nit-ac., Tarent.

MAPPED, see **Mottled.**

MARASMUS: Nat-m., Sanic., Syph.

           Comp. **Emaciation.**

MEASLES, **measly:** ACON., Ars., **Bry.,** Camph., Coff., Dros., Euphr., Ferr-p., **Kali-bi.,** Kali-m., Phos., PULS., Stict.

complications or sequelae of: Am-c., **Ant-t.,** Ars., **Bry.,** Camph., Cupr-act., **Kali-c., Puls.,** Sulph., Zinc.

hemorrhagic: Crot-h., Ferr-p.

receding: Bry., Phos., Puls., Rhus-t.

MEAT WATER, **like:** Ars., Kali-i., Nit-ac., Rhus-t., Stront-c.

MEATUS, morning drop, clear: Phos.

green: Merc.

yellow: Fl-ac.

red: Merc., Sulph.

MEDICINE, sensitive to: Nux-v., Puls.

Comp. **Reaction.**

MEDULLA: Verat-v.

MEMBRANE, as of a, see **Coated.**

MEMBRANES, **mucous:** Acon., All-c., Ant-t., Apis, **Arg-n.,** **Ars., Bell.,** Borx., **Bry.,** Caps., **Cham., Dulc.,** Eucal., Euphr., Hep., Hydr., Ip., Kali-bi., Kali-c., **Merc., Nux-v.,** Phos., **Puls.,** Rumx., Sabad., Sang., Seneg., Squil., **Stann., Sulph.,** Syph., Ter., Thuj.

Comp. **Moistness.**

dark: Aesc., Bapt., Carb-v., Cham., Ham., Lach., Merc-i-r., Mez., Nit-ac., Phos., Phyt.

dry: Alum., **Bell.,** Bry., Caust., Kali-c., Nux-m., Stict.

pale: Ars., Chin., Ferr., Kali-c., Mang., Phos.

patches: Arg-n., Lach., Merc-i-c., Merc-p-r., Nit-ac., Phyt., Puls.

raw: Arum-t., Nux-v.

red, bright: Acon., Bell., Canth.

serous: Acon., Apis, **Bry., Canth.,** Hell., Kali-c., Ran-b., Seneg., Squil., Sulph.

spongy: Caps., Phyt.

sulci of: Kali-bi.

ulcerated: Arg-n., Ars., Hydr., Kali-i., Kreos., Merc-c., Nit-ac., Phyt., Sil., Sul-ac.

vesicles: Apis, Borx., Canth., Carb-v.

wrinkled: Ars., Elaps, Merc.

MENSES, gushing, see **Hemorrhage.**

METASTASIS: Abrot., Cupr., Puls.

MOBILITY: Camph., Cros., Stram.

MOIST: Graph., Ip., Jab., **Med., Nat-s.,** Squil., Stroph-h., Sul-ac.

MOISTNESS, **fluidity in general, discharges increased, etc.:** Ant-t., **Ars.,** CALC., Carb-v., Cham., **Chin., Dulc., Ferr.,** Graph., **Hep.,** Iris, Kali-i., Lyc., MERC., Nux-v., Op., Phos., Ph-ac., **Puls., Rhus-t., Samb.,** Sel., SEP., **Sil.,** Stann., SULPH., Thuj., **Verat.**

MOLASSES, **like:** Croc., Ip., Mag-c., Phos.

MOON, new: Nux-v., Rhus-t., Sil.

first quarter: Ars., Bry., Nat-m.

full: Calc., **Phos.**, Sulph.

last quarter: Lyc., Sep.

MOTION, absent: **Bry.**, Cocc., Gels., Hell., Rhus-t.

agility: Apis, Coff., Lach., Nux-v., Stram., Tarent., Valer.

automatic: Bell., Calc., Hell., Hyos., Lyc., Nux-m., Phos., Stram., Zinc.

averse to: Acon., **Bry.**, Calad., Caps., Guaj, Lach., Nat-m., **Nux-v.**, Sulph.

difficult: Bell., **Bry.**, Caust., Lyc., Petr., Rhus-t., **Sep.**

erratic: Verat-v.

exaggerated: Agar.

stepping backwards: Stram.

festination: Alum., Mang., Syph., Tarent.

fetus, lively: Lyc., Op.

high: Agar., Rhus-t.

MOTTLED, **patchy, blotchy, etc.:** AIL., Apis, **Ars.**, Bapt., Bell., **Carb-v.**, Con., CROT-H., Glon., Kali-bi., Kali-m., LACH., Led., Lil-t., Manc., Merc-p-r., **Nat-m.**, **Nux-v.**, Ox-ac., Phos., Rhus-t., Sars., Sec., Sep., Syph., **Thuj.**, Verat-v.

                                    Comp. **Spots.**

MOULDY: Crot-h.

MOVEMENTS: Agar., Elaps, Stram.

MUCUS SECRETIONS, **altered:** Ant-t., Arg-met., Arg-n., **Ars.**, CALC., Calc-s., Caust., **Cham.**, Cist. (increased), Graph., Hep., Hydr., KALI-BI., **Lyc.**, **Merc.**, NAT-M., **Nit-ac.**, Nux-v., **Phos.**, PULS., SEP., Sil., **Stann.**, **Sulph.**

MUSCLES: Agar., Anac., Arn., Ars., BELL., **Bry.**, **Calc.**, CAUST., Cimic., Cocc., Con., **Eup-per.**, Gels., Hell., Hyos., Kali-c., **Mur-ac.**, Nux-v., RHUS-T., Sec., Til., Valer., Verat., Zinc.

atrophy: Ars., Caust., Plb., Thuj.

belly of: Cimic., Thuj.

jumping: Colch., Dios., Hydr., Puls.

knots: Cupr., Phys., Senec., Syph.

lax, flabby: Aeth., Ant-t., Calc., Caps., Carb-ac., **Chin.**, Cocc., **Gels.**, Lyc., Merc-d., Mur-ac., Ph-ac., Spong., Stram., Sulph.

obey feebly: Gels., Hell., Phys.

short, see **Contraction.**

tense: Acon., Kali-n., Lach., Mag-p., Nit-ac., **Nux-v.**, Phos., Senec., **Sep.**, Stront-c., Visc.

undeveloped: Nat-m.

MUSTY, mouldy: Borx., Crot-h., Rhus-t., Sanic., Stann., Staph., Teucr., Thuj, Thyr.

NECROSIS: Calc-i., Rad-met.

NEEDLES, see Fine: Agar. (cold), **Ars.** (hot), Bry.

NERVE PAIN, neuralgia, etc.: ACON., ARS., BELL., Bry., Caust., **Cham.,** Chin., Cimic., Coff., COLOC., Dios., Gels., Hyper., IGN., **Iris, Kali-bi.,** Lach., **Lyc.,** Mag-c., **Mag-p.,** Merc., Nat-m., **Nux-v.,** Phos., **Psor.,** Puls., Ran-b., **RHUS-T., Sang., Spig.,** Stann., **Sulph.,** Thuj., **Verat.,** Verb.

NERVES, nervous patients, etc: Acon., Arg-n., Asaf., Aur., Bell., Borx., Carb-v., Castr., Caul., **Caust.,** Cham., **Chin.,** Cimic., **Cocc., Coff., Con.,** Cupr., IGN., **Hyos.,** Iod., Kali-p., LACH., **Lil-t.,** Mag-c., Mag-m., Mag-p., Merc., **Mosch.,** Nat-m., **Nit-ac.,** Nux-m., NUX-V., **Phos.,** Pic-ac., Prun., PULS., Sabal., Senec., Sep., SIL., Staph., Stict., **Stram., Sulph., Tarent.,** Ther., Thyr., Vib., Visc., Zinc., Zinc-val.

Comp. **Mind.**

alternating with: Sabad.

injured: Hyper.

paralysis: Prun.

prostration: Ol-an., Onos., Kali-p., Pic-ac., Phos., Viol-o.

NETTED CAPILLARIES: see Nevi.

NEURALGIA: Mag-c., Ran-b., Stann., Thuj.

orbital: Cedr., Chinin-s.

shingles, after: Kali-chl., Kalm., Mez., Zinc.

stump, of: All-c., Arn., Hyper.

NIGHT, blindness: Stram.

sweats, of phthisis: Ars., Bry., Calc., Carb-v., Chin., Ferr., Phos., Ph-ac., Samb., Sep., Sil., Stann., Sulph.

first sleep in: Ars.

after: Lach.

all night: Phos.

awaking an: Samb.

watching: see Sleep, **loss of.**

NODES: Ant-c., CALC., Carb-an., Caul., Caust., Cinnb., Dulc., **Graph.,** Iod., Kali-s., Lach., Lyc., Mag-c., Mez., **Puls.,** Rhod, Rhus-t., Ruta, Sars., Sil., Staph., **Sulph.**

Comp. **Growths.**

NOISE, see Sensitive: Tarent., Tub.

penetrating: Asar., Bar-c., Chin., Cocc., Iod., Lil-t., Lyc., Mur-ac., Sabin., Ther.

Comp. **Hearings**

NOMA: Tarent-c.

NOTHING ails him: Arn., Iod., Op.

NUMBNESS, insusceptibility, absence of or benumbing pain, etc.: ACON., Apis, Ars., Carb-v., Caust., Cham., COCC., Con., Crot-h., Gels., Glon., GRAPH., Kali-c., LYC., Nux-m., Nux-v., Olnd., Op., Phos., Ph-ac., Plat., Plb., PULS., RHUS-T., Sec., Stram., Thuj., Zinc.

NUMB, painless, etc.: Anac., Cadm-s., Con., Diph., Lappa, Mag-c., Med., Nat-m., Rad-met., Sul-i., Tarent., Tell., Xan.

diagonal: Thyr.

general: Chel.

one-sided: Ars., Caust., Chel., Nat-m., Phos., Puls.

pain, from: Cham., Coloc., Kalm., Plat., Puls., Rhus-t.

part lain on: Puls., Rhus-t.

partial, spots, etc.: Lyc., Sul-i.

wooden feeling: Kali-n.

NUTRITION: Calc., Calc-p., Sil.

OBESITY: Am-c., Ant-c., Bell., Bufo, CALC., Caps., Ferr., Graph., Kali-bi., Phyt., Puls., Seneg., Sulph.

OESOPHAGUS: see Gullet

OFFENSIVE: Ail., Asaf., Carb-an., Con., Crot-h., Eucal., Graph., Kreos., Meph., Merc., Mur-ac., Osm., Phos., Sabin., Sul-ac., Til., Tub., Ust.

body: Bapt., Guaj., Graph., Hep., Kali-i., Kali-p., Med., Nit-ac., Psor., Pyrog., Sep., Sil., Stann., Sulph., Syph., Thuj.

sweat: Bapt., Bar-c., Merc., Petr., Staph., Sulph., Vario.

OFFENSIVENESS, fetor: Arn., Ars., Bapt., Bry., Calc-f., Carb-ac., CARB-V., Graph., Hep., Kali-p., LACH., Nit-ac., Podo., PSOR., Rhus-t., Sec., Sep., Sil., Sulph., Tel., Thuj.

OLD AGE, senility: Ambr., Ant-c., Ars., Aur., BAR-C., Carb-an., Carb-v., Chin., Con., Fl-ac., Gins., Hydr., LACH., Lyc., Nit-ac., Op., Phos., Sanic., Sars., Sec., Sulph., Sul-ac., Syph., Tub., Verat.

maids: Plat.

ONIONS: Kali-p.

OPENING AND SHUTTING or contracted, then relaxed alternately: Cact., Calc., CANN-S., Cimic., COCC., Glon., Lil-t., Sep., Spong.

Comp. Alternating.

OPISTHOTONOS: Ign., Verat-v.

ORGASMS, see **Waves**: Spong.

sexual: Stann.

ORIFICES, see **Skin**, **Edge**: **Aesc.**, **Aloe**, **Bell.**, **Caust.**, **Graph.**, **Ign.**, **Kali-c.**, **Lach.**, **Lyc.**, **Merc.**, **Mur-ac.**, **Nat-m.**, **NIT-AC.**, **NUX-V.**, **Phos.**, **Podo.**, **Rat.**, **Sep.**, **Sil.**, **SULPH.**

OSTEOMALACIA: **Iod.**, Merc-c.

PAIN, see **Sensitive**: Sul-ac.

absence of: Ant-c., Ant-t. see, **Numbness**.

can't stand: Vip-t.

cold: Arn.

fits and starts, in: Bar-m., Cupr., Mez.

fleeting: Ictod., Nux-m., Pall., Stront-c., Valer.

maddening: Verat.

many: Med.

sudden: see **Shooting**.

symptoms, Agg.: Nat-c.

PAINLESSNESS., see **Numbness**.

PARALYSIS, **paralytic pains, etc.**: Ant-t., Arn., Ars., Bell., Carb-v, CAUST., Chin., Cocc., Colch., Con., Dulc., Gels., Hell., Helod., Hyos., Lach., Lyc., NUX-V., Op., PLB., RHUS-T., Sec., Sil., Sang., Staph., Sulph., Verb.

agitans: Agar., Ant-t., Arg-n., Bar-c., Gels., Lol-t., Merc., Nux-v., Phys., Rhus t., Zinc.

apoplexy, after: Arn., Bell., Cocc., Nux-v., Stann., Zinc.

ascending: Con.

cold bathing, Amel.: Con.

descending: Zinc.

diphtheritic: Cocc., Diph., Gels., Lach., Rhus-t.

emotions, from: Coff., Croc., Gels., Lach., Nat-m., Pall., Stann., Stram.

joints, in: Aur., Caps., Euphr., Puls., Staph., Valer.

limbs: Caust., Cocc., Nux-v., Rhus-t., Ruta, Sec., Sil.

localized: Caust., Plb.

organs (single): Ant-t., Bar-c., Bell., Caust., Dulc., Gels., Hyos., Nux-v., Op., Phos., Puls., Sec., Sil., Sulph.

painless: Cocc., Con., Lyc., Plb., Rhus-t.

side, right: Chel., Crot-h., Merc-i-r., Nat-m., Plb.

left: Gels., Op., Stroph-h., Vip-t.

spasms then: Tarent.

twitching: Stram.

paraplegia: Arg-n., Ars., Bapt., Nat-m., Nux-v., Ruta, Sulph.

rheumatism, after: Bar-c., Chin.,
Ferr., Ruta.

sense of (internal): Lyc.

spasms, after: Cocc., Cupr.,
Elaps, Sec.

suppression, after: Caust., Lach.,
Mez., Merc., Stram., Sulph.,
Thuj., Verat.

unilateral: Caust., Cocc., Lach.

PAROXYSMS, repeated: Agar.,
Ars., Bell., Calc., Caust.,
CHAM., Chin., COCC.,
COLOC., Cupr., Dios., Gels.,
Ign., Lach., MAG-P., NUX-V.,
Plat., Plb., Puls., SEP., Stann.,
Sulph., Tab.

Comp. Spasmodic.

PATCHY, see Mottled.

PECKING, hacking: Chin., Ruta.

PERCEPTION, changed (mental
or visual): Acon., Arg-n., Ars.,
Bar-c., BELL., Calc., Cann-s.,
HYOS., Kali-br., Lac-c.,
Lach., Merc., Nux-m., Op.,
Phos., Ph-ac., Plat., Pyrog.,
STRAM., Sulph., Verat.

PERIODICITY: Aran., ARS.,
Cact., Cedr., CHIN., Eup-
per., Gels., Hep., Ip., Kali-c.,
Lyc., NAT-M., Nux-v., Puls.,
Rhus-t., Spig., Sulph., Tarent.

Comp. Intermittency.

exact: Ars., Cedr., Chinin-s.,
Nat-m., Tarent.

yearly: Psor.

PERIOSTEUM, pain in: Merc.,
Rhus-t.

PERITONITIS: see Abdomen.

PHAGEDENA, slough, etc.:
ARS., Carb-v., Caust., Chel.,
Crot-h., Hep., Lyc., Merc.,
Merc-c., Merc-cy., Merc-p-r.,
Mez., NIT-AC., Petr., SIL.,
Sulph.

Comp. Gnawing.

PHOTOPHOBIA: See Light.

PHTHISIS, relapsing: Ferr., Kali-
n.

PICKING bleeds, until: Arg-n.,
Arum-t., Cina, Con., Phos.

one spot, sore: Arum-t., Ph-ac.,
Zinc.

PIECES, in a see Duality.

PIERCING, : Apis, Nat-s.

PINCHING, see Compression.

PITCHY: see Tarry.

PLETHORA, full-blooded, etc.:
Acon., Bell., Ferr., Nux-v.,
Phos., Puls., Sulph.

Comp. Obesity.

PLUG, nail, wedge, clavus, etc.:
Agar., Anac., Arn., Asaf.,
Coff., Hep., IGN., Lith-c.,
Mosch., Plat., Ran-s., Rat.,
Spong., Sulph., Sul-ac.,
THUJ., Ust.

of pus, etc.: Kali-bi., Nit-ac.,
Comp. **Ball.**

POISONED FEELING: Caj.,
Lac-c., Lach., Naja, Vip-t.

POLYPI, see **Fungoid growth.**

POSITION, rest, can't in any:
Lyc., Rhus-t., Sanic., Sulph.

PTOMAINE: poisoning: **Ars.**

POWER **higher:** Lach., Thuj.

POWERLESS: Anac.

PREGNANCY, childbed, etc.:
Acon., Alet., **Arn., Bell., Bry.,**
Calc., Caul., Cham., Cimic.,
Cocc., Con., **Gels.,** Helo.,
Ign., Ip., **Kali-c., Kreos.,** Nux-
m., NUX-V., Plat, PULS.,
Pyrog., Rhus-t., Sabin., Sec.,
SEP., Sulph., Tab., Verat., Vib.

diarrhea of: Ant-c., Chin., Dulc.,
Lyc., Merc., Petr., Phos.,
Puls., Rheum, Sep., Sulph.,
Thuj.

warts: Cinnb., Sep., **Thuj.**

PRESSING OR BEARING
DOWN, **straining, tenesmus,**
etc.: Agar., Apis, Bell.,
CANTH., Castm., Cimic.,
Con., Erig., LIL-T., MERC-
C., Nat-m., **Nux-v.,** Pall., Plat.,
Puls., SEP., Sil., **Sulph.,** Thyr.

PRICKINGS: Crot-h., **Nit-ac.**

PRICKLING: Acon., Apis, Bry.,
Kali-p., Lyc., Nat-m., **Plat.,**

Ran-s., Rhus-t., Sulph.,
Symph., Tarent., Urt-u., Verat-
v.

PRICKLY HEAT: Ant-c., Urt-u.

PRODROME: Chel., Chin.,
Corn., Eup-per.

PROLAPSE, see **Falling.**

PROPORTION: Agar., Calc.,
Cann-s., Onos., Plat., Stram.

PROTRUSION, **also sense of; of
internal parts, as eyes, hernia,**
etc.: **Acon.,** Aur., **Bell.,** Cocc.,
Ferr., **Glon.,** Hyos., Iod.,
LACH., **Lyc.,** Lycps-v., NUX-
V., Op., Spig., Stram., Sul-ac.

PSORA: Ars., Bar-c., **Calc.,**
Graph., Hep., Iod., Merc.,
Phos., **Psor.,** Sil., **Sulph.,** Tub.

PUBERTY: Caust., Croc., Ferr.,
Guaj., Viol-o.

PUBERTY AND YOUTH: Bell.,
Calc-p., Ferr-p., Hell., Kali-
br., **Kali-c., Lach.,** Nat-m.,
PHOS., Ph-ac., PULS., Senec.

PUFFINESS: APIS, ARS., Bov.,
CALC., Caps., **Ferr., Kali-c.,**
Kreos., Led., Lith-c., Med.,
Nat-c., Nux-v., Op., Phos.,
Phyt., RHUS-T., Rumx.,
Ruta, Ust.

Comp. **Swelling.**

lying **Agg.: Glon.,** Sep.

PULSATION, see **Throbbing.**

PUNCTURED wounds: Led., Plan.

PUSHED down: Lyc., Psor.

PYEMIA: Phos.

QUIVERING: Asaf., Kali-c., Mez., Nat-c.

Comp. Trembling, Vibrating.

RADIATING, see Direction.

RAGING PAIN: Led.

RANCID: Alum., Carb-v., Puls., Tell., Thuj., Valer.

RATTLING: Am-m., ANT-T., Cact., Calc-s., Chin., Cupr., HEP., IP., Kali-s., Lob., Lyc., Op., Squil., Sulph., Verat.

Comp. Gurgling.

RAWNESS, smarting, etc.: ARG-MET., Arum-t., Calc., Canth., Carb-v., CAUST., Cist., Fl-ac., Graph., Hep., Hydr., Ign., Iod., Kreos., Lach., Lyc., Meli-a., Merc., Nit-ac., NUX-V., Ol-an., Phos., Polyg-s., Puls., Ran-s., Sang., Sep., Stann., Staph., Sulph., Sul-ac.

internal: Brom., Carb-v., Nux-m., Nux-v., Phos., Sang.

scratches himself: Arum-t., Psor.

REABSORBENT: Arn., Kali-i., Sulph., Sul-i.

REACTION, poor: Aeth., Am-c., Ambr., Calc., Caps., Carb-v.,

Cupr., Dig., Ferr., Laur., Med., Mosch., Op., PSOR., SULPH., Syph., Tub., Valer., Zinc.

Comp. Inactive.

violent: Bell., Cupr., Nux-v., Zinc.

RECLINING, half: Gels., Sang.

RECOVERY, despairs: Ars., Calc., Psor.

RED: Jab., Sabin.

bluish, dark, etc.: Bapt., Phyt, Rhus-t.

discharges: Ars-i., Kreos., Merc., Rhus-t.

fiery: Med., Stram.

orifices: Aloe, Sulph.

rosy: Apis, Pyrog.

spot: Stict.

streaks: Bry., Bufo.

REDNESS: ACON., Apis, Arg-n., Ars., BELL., Bry., Cham., Chin., Ferr., Lach., Meli-a., Merc., Nux-v., Op., Phos., Rhus-t., Sang., Sep., SULPH.

REELING, tottering, staggering, etc.: Ars., Bell., Bry., Caust., Gels., Ign., Lach., Nux-v., Op., Rhus-t., Stram., Sulph., Verat., Verat-v.

REELING: see Gait.

RELAPSES, recurrences: Bar-c.,
Bar-m., Coloc., Hep., Kali-i.,
Mez., Phos., **Psor.**, Sulph.

Comp. **Reaction.**

RELAXATION: **Aeth.**, **Aloe**, **Ant-
t.**, Ars., **Calc.**, **Caps.**, CAUST.,
Chin., Cocc., **Colch.**, GELS.,
Graph., Hell., **Hyos.**, Lob.,
LYC., Merc-cy., MUR-AC.,
Nat-c., Nat-m., Op., PH-AC.,
Seneg., Sep., Verat.

Comp. **Inactive.**

RELAXED: Graph., Lob., Seneg.,
Sep.

REMITTENCY: **Gels.**

REPEATED: Lyc., Zinc.

RESTLESSNESS: ACON., **Apis**,
ARS., **Bell.**, Cham., Cimic.,
Cina, Cupr., **Ferr.**, **Hyos.**,
Mag-p., **Merc.**, Phos., RHUS-
T., **Sep.**, Stram., Sulph.,
Tarent., Teucr., Vib., Zinc.

in blood: Iod.

RETRACTION, **drawn back, etc.**:
Ast-r., Cic., Clem., Crot-t.,
Cupr., Hydr., Lach., **Merc.**,
Nat-m., Nux-v., Op., Par.,
Phyt., PLB., Sars., Sil., Thuj.,
Zinc.

RHEUMATISM: Acon., Bell.,
Bry., Caust., Colch., Ferr-p.,
Led., Lyc., Merc., Phyt., **Puls.**,
Rhus-t., Sulph.

cold, **Amel.**: Am-c., **Led.**, Sec.

hives, with: Urt-u.

hot weather: Rhod.

paralysis: Colch.

tonsilitis, after: Echi., Guaj.,
Lach., Phyt.

RHUS POISON: Rhus-t.

RHYTHMIC: Lyc., Stram.

RICKETS: **Calc.**, **Calc-p.**, Kali-i.,
Phos., Sil., Sulph.

RIGID, see **Stiff.**

RISING THEN FALLING
SENSATION: Bar-c., Lach.

RISING, efforts at: Aesc., Agar.,
Petr., Ruta, Sulph.

from bed, **Amel.**: Ph-ac., Puls.

RIVET: Lil-t.

ROAMING: Lyss.

ROBUST HABIT: Acon., Asaf.,
Bell., Caps.

ROCKING: Cina, Merc-c., Sec.

ROLLING or **turning over**: Am-
c., Ars., BELL., Cact., Crot-
h., Cupr., Gels., **Graph.**, Kali-
c., LACH., Lyc., Phos., Puls.,
Rhus-t., Sabad., SEP., Tarent.

Comp. **Loose, Ball, etc.**

ROUGH, **scratchy; as of a rough
body, etc.**: Aesc., **Alum.**,
Ambr., Am-m., Arg-n., **Berb.**,
Calc-f., Carb-v., Graph., Kali-

bi., Mang., Naja, Nat-m., Nux-v., Par., Phos., Phyt., Ruta, Sang., Sulph.

Comp. Smarting.

RUNNING, see Creeping.

SALTINESS: Ars., Calc., Carb-v., Kali-i., Lyc., MERC., Merc-c., Nat-c., Nat-m., Phos., Puls., Sel., SEP., Tell.

SALTY: Fl-ac., Graph., Iod., Sanic.

SARCOCELE: Iod.

SAWING, as if: Aesc., Brom., Hypr., Phos., Spig., Spong., Sulph., Syph., Tarent.

SCOOPED OUT: Thuj., Vario.

SCORBUTIC SYMPTOMS: Am-c., Carb-v., Kali-m., Merc., Mur-ac., Nux-v., Staph., Sulph.

SCORCHED: See Burnt.

SCRATCHING: Sang.

SCRAWNY: Calc-p., Nux-m., Sec.

SCREWED together: Coloc., Sars.

Comp. Compression.

SCROFULA: Bar-c., Calc., Calc-p., Cist., Hep., Iod., Lyc., Merc., Sil., Sulph.

Comp. Consumption.

erethistic: Calc-p., Psor., Tub.

torpid: Calc., Sulph.

SEASICKNESS, see Swaying.

SECRETIONS, discharges, expectoration, etc., see Discharges: Tab.

bland: Euphr., Kali-m., Hep., Merc., PULS., Sil., Sulph.

bloody, see Hemorrhage.

briny odor: Bell., Graph., Ol-an., Sanic., Sel., Tell., Thuj.

burning: All-c., Ars., Calc., Kali-i., Kreos., Merc., Merc-c., Puls., Sin-n., Sulph.

curdy: Borx., Helo., Merc.

hair, destroying: Bell-p., Lyc., Merc., Nat-m., Nit-ac., Rhus-t., Sil.

hot: Acon., Bell., Borx., Iod., Kreos., Puls., Sabin.

increased, see Moistness.

itching, causing: Calc., Fl- ac., Led., Mang., Med., Par., Rhod., Rhus-t., Sulph., Tarent.

milky: Calc., Kali-m., Kali-p., Nat-s., PH-AC., Puls., Sep.

musty, mouldy: Borx., Carb-v., Coloc., Crot-h., Merc., Nux-v., Phos., Puls., Rhus-t., Stann.

scanty, bringing great amelioration: Apis, Arg-met., Lach., Squil.

slimy: Borx., Calc., Chin., Kali-bi., Lyc., Mag-c., Merc-d., Nat-m., Par., Ph-ac., Phos., Puls.

stain, indelibly: Merc., Sil., Thlasp.

stains, fast: Carb-ac., Lach., **Mag-c.**, Mag-p., Med., Pulx., Thuj., Vib.

　　yellow: Bell., Carb-an., Graph., Lach., **Merc.**, Sel.

tarry: Lept., Mag-c., Mag-m., Nux-m., Plat.

urinous odor: Benz-ac., Canth., Coloc., Nat-m., Nit-ac., Olan., Sec., Urt-u.

watery, thin: Ars., **Asaf.**, Caust., Cham., Crot-h., Cupr., Flac., Gamb., **Graph.**, Grat., Iris, Kali-i., Mag-m., **Merc.**, Mur-ac., Nat-s., Phos., **Podo.**, Rhus-t., Sabin., Sec., Sil., **Sulph.**, Verat.

　　　　Comp. **Moistness.**

SENILITY: Sumb.

SENSES, SPECIAL, DULLED: Bell., **Calc.**, Caust., Gels., Hyos., Lyc., Merc., **Nat-m.**, Nit-ac, Phos., PULS., Sil., **Sulph.**

　　　　Comp. **Numbness.**

blunted: Hell., Laur.

special: Asar., Cimic.

vanishing, as if: Alum., Calc., Cann-s., Carb-an., **Cupr.**, **Plat.**, Stram.

　　　　Comp. **Faint.**

pains, from: Plb.

SENSITIVE, susceptible, etc.: Coc-c., Croc., Mang., Paeon., Sul-i., Tarent., Tell., Ter., Tub.

SENSITIVE, also to noise, light, odors, pain, touch, trifles, etc.: **Acon.**, **Ambr.**, Arn., Ars., Asaf., Aur., **BELL.**, Carb-ac., **Cham.**, CHIN., **Coff.**, Colch., Cupr., Dros. (sour), Ferr., **Hep.**, **Ign.**, LACH., Mag-c., Merc., **Nit-ac.**, NUX-V., **Phos.**, Sep., Sil., Syph., Tarent., Teucr., Ther., Thuj., Tub., Vario., Zinc.

　　　　Comp. **Jarring.**

SENSORIUM, depressed: Bapt., Hell., Ph-ac., Pyrog., Rhus-t.

SENTIMENTAL: see **Reverie.**

SEPARATED, as if: Agar., Arg-n., Calc-p., Cocc., Daph., Dulc., Hyper., **Psor.**, Sabin., Sep., Tril-p., Verat.

SEPSIS, see **Blood, Heart, Circulation and Pulse.**

SEVERE PAIN, see **Tearing.**

SEXUAL DISTURBANCES: Agn., Bar-c., Calc., CANTH., Chin., **Con.**, Graph., Lil-t., LYC., **Nux-v.**, PHOS., Ph-ac., Pic-ac., Plat., Sel., **Staph.**, Stram., Sulph.

SEWING, see **Fingers.**

SHADE, see **Twilight.**

SHAKING, see **Spasmodic.**

SHARP, **pressure:** Ign.

see **Cutting, Fear.**

SHATTERED or **flying into pieces, explosions, etc., as if:** Aeth., Ars., **Bell.,** Bry., Carban., **Coff.,** Dig., Glon., **Murac., Nit-ac., Nux-v., PULS., RHUS-T.,** Sil., **Stann.,** Staph., Sulph., Verat.

Comp. **Bursting.**

SHIFTING: see **Wandering.**

suddenly: Ambr., Colch., Radmet.

SHINY see **Glistening.**

SHOCKS **as of:** Podo., Thuj., Valer.

SHOCKS **through body:** Ambr., Arg-met., **Ars., Bell.,** Cic., Cocc., Colch., Cupr., Kreos., Lyc., Nux-v., Op., Ran-b., Stront-c., Sulph., Thuj., Verat., Zinc., Zinc-chr.

mental: Acon., **Arn.**

nervous: Acon., Am-c., **Arn.,** Camph., Coff., Gels., Hyos., Ign.

surgical: Acon., Camph., Strontc.

SHOOTING, **darting, like lightning, quick pains, etc.:** Acon., **Agar.,** Alum., Arg-n., Ars., **BELL., Berb., Cimic., Coloc.,**

Cupr., **Dios.,** Ferr., Hydr-ac., Hyos., Hyper., Kali-bi., Kalic., Kali-m., Kalm., **Lyc.,** Magc., Mag-m., **Mag-p.,** Nit-ac., Nux-v., Ox-ac., Paeon., Plb., Prun., Rad-met., Ran-b., Rhus-t., Sabin., Sec., Sep., Spig., **SULPH.,** Verat., Xan., Zinc.

laming pain: Colch., Iris.

SHORT, **as if too:** Alum., **Am-c.,** Am-m., **Caust., Coloc.,** Dig., Dios., Graph., **Guaj.,** Lach., Merc., Nat-m., Nux-v., **Rhust., Sep.,** Syph.

Comp. **Lying bent.**

SHUDDERING, **nervous: Acon.,** Am-m., **ARN., Bell., Cimic.,** Cina, Cocc., Gels., Glon., **Ign.,** Led., Mez., **Nat-m., NUX-V.,** Puls., Rhus-t., Sep., Sil., Spig.

shivers: Ars., Cham., Cimic., Dios., Hell., **Hyper.,** Mosch., Phys., Ran-b., Rheum, Thuj., Zinc.

SIDE, **lain on, pain goes to:** Ars., **Bry.,** Calc., **Kali-c.,** Merc., **Phac., PULS.,** Sep., Sil.

not lain on, pain goes to: Bry., Cupr., Fl-ac., Graph., **Ign.,** Kali-bi., Puls., **Rhus-t.**

right: Apis, BELL., Bry., **CALC.,** Canth., Chel., Coloc., Gels.,

Iris, Kalm., LYC., Naja, Nux-v., Puls., Rumx., Sang., Sil., Tarent.

to left: Acon., Ambr., Am-c., **Apis**, **Bell.**, Calc-p., Caust., Chel., Cupr., Lil-t., LYC., Merc-i-f., Phos., Rumx., **Sabad.**, Sang., Sul-ac., Syph., **Verat.** —

left: ASAF., Calc-f., Cina, Clem., **Euph.**, LACH., Lil-t., Mags., **Mez.**, Phos., **Rhus-t.**, Squil., SEP., Spig., Stann., SULPH., Thuj.

to right: All-c., Ars., Brom., Calc., Ferr., LACH., Merc-i-r., Nux-m., Puls., **Rhus-t.**, Sabad., Stann., Tarax.

one: Mez.

alternating: Rad-met.

uppermost, Agg.: Bry.,Graph., Ign., Rhus-t.

SINGLE PARTS, in: Plb.

SINKING, see **Empty.**

down, see **Falling:** Cupr., Glon., Hydr-ac., Laur., Verat.

sensation: Alum., Bry., Dulc., Glon., Kali-c., **Lach.**, Lyc., Nat-m., **Phos.**, Rhus-t., Tab., Xan.

through floor: Hyos., Phos.

SIT, inclines to: Chin., Con., Graph., Nux-v., Phos., Squil.

desires: Caps., Cocc., Lil-t., Merc., Stann.

hands, support body: Berb., Sulph.

SIZE: See **Proportion.**

SKIN, as of a, see **Valve,** and **Coated.**

SLIDES DOWN IN BED: Ars., Bapt., Colch., Hyos., Mur-ac.

SLIMY: Merc-d., Ph-ac.

SMALLER seems: Agar., Cact., Tab.

SMALLPOX: Ant-t., **Ars.**, Bapt., Merc., **Rhus-t.**, Sulph., Thuj., **Vario.**

SMARTING: Berb., Polyg., Staph.

SMOOTH: Alum., Phos., Ter.

SNOW AIR: Mag-m.

SORE: Ham., Hyper., Kali-m., Lap-a., Ol-an., Onos., Plan., Pyrog., Ter., Til.

bruised: Chion., Kalm., Mill., Pyrog.

pains, after: Acon., **Arn.**, Graph., Onos., **Plat.**, Sel., Tell.

SORENESS, bruised, smarting, etc.: **Apis**, ARN., Aur., **Bapt.**, **Bell.**, Berb., BRY., Canth., **Carb-v.**, **Caust.**, **Chin.**, Cimic., **Con.**, EUP-PER.,

Gels., Hep., **Lach.**, **Nit-ac.**,
NUX-V., Phos., Phyt., Polyg-
s., **Puls.**, Pyrog., Ran-b.,
RHUS-T., RUTA, SIL.,
Staph., **Sulph.**

Comp. **Rawness.**

glands: Con.

internally: Bell-p., Cann-s., Puls.

joints: Arg-met., Aur., Puls.,
Sulph.

pains, after: Chin., Gels., Glon.,
Graph., Plat., Sel.

SOURNESS: CALC., Chin.,
Hep., **Lyc.**, **Mag-c.**, Merc.,
Nat-c., Nat-m., Nat-p., NUX-
V., Phos., Puls., Rheum, Sep.,
Sil., SULPH., Sul-ac.

SOUR: Cob., Iris, Kali-c., Lap-a.,
Lith-c., Nat-s., Ox-ac., Ph-ac.,
Rob., Tarax.

bitter: Iris, Nux-v.

SPARKS: Lyc., Sec.

SPASM: Castm., Med., Mill.,
Stroph-h., Tarent., Verb., Vib.,
Zin-val.

clonic and tonic alternately: Ign.,
Mosch.

degenerative: Aur-m., **Phos.**,
Zinc-p.

dentition, Agg.: **Calc.**, **Cham.**,
Gels., Zinc.

pain, Agg.: **Bell.**, Coloc., Ign.,
Kali-c., Lyc., Nux-v.

uremic: Apis, Ars., **Verat-v.**

worms: Art-v., Cic., **Cina**, Indg.

SPASMODIC OR CONVUL-
SIVE EFFECTS, **twitchings,
jerks, etc.:** Agar., Ambr., Ars.,
BELL., Calc., Camph., Caust.,
Cham., Chin., **Cic.**, Cimic.,
Cina, CUPR., HYOS., **Ign.**,
Ip., KALI-C., LACH., Mez.,
Nux-v., Op., Plat., Plb., Puls.,
Sil., STANN., STRAM.,
Sulph., Thuj., Verat-v., ZINC.

Comp. **Paroxysms**

during sleep: Ars., BELL., Kali-
c., Sep., **Sil.**, **Sulph.**

SPEECH, **affected:** **Bell.**, **Caust.**,
Crot-c., **Gels.**, Glon., **Hyos.**,
Kali-br., LACH., Lyc., **Merc.**,
Nat-c., Nat-m., Nux-m., **Nux-
v.**, Phos., Stann., STRAM.

babbling: Lyc.

jerky: Agar.

lost: Caus., Laur., Onos., Stram.

speaking, etc.: Arg-n., Coll.,
Kali-i., Merc-c.

thick: Agar., Caust., Dulc., Gels.,
Lach.

SPHINCTERS: Sil., Staph.

SPITTING: Ant-t., Bor-c., Lyss.,
Stram., **Tab.**, Zinc-chr.

SPLASHING, see **Swashing.**

SPLINTER, see **Fine.**

SPOTS, pain etc., in: Agar., **Alum.**, Arg-met., Ars., **Berb.**, Bufo, **Calc-p.**, Caust., **Cist.**, Colch., **Con.**, Fl-ac., Glon., Hep., Ign., KALI-BI., LACH., Lil-t., Lyc., **Nat-m.**, Nux-m., Ol-an., Ol-j., **Ox-ac.**, **Phos.**, Ran-b., Rhus-t., Sars., Sel., Sep., Sil., SULPH., Thuj., Zinc.

Comp. **Mottled.**

cold: Calc-p., Petr., Sep., Tarent.

moist: Petr.

painful, sore: Glon., Kali-bi., Merc., Phos., Sulph.

SQUEEZING, see **Constriction.**

SQUIRMS: Valer.

STARTS, see **Spasmodic:** Stann.

STICKING, **fine, splinter-like,** see **Fine.**

STICKY, **stringy, etc.:** Ant-t., Arg-n., Bov., Bry., Caust., Croc., **Graph.**, Hydr., KALI-BI., Kali-c., Kali-m., **Lach.**, Lappa, Lyc., Mez., Myrt-c., Nat-m., Osm., **Phos.**, Plat., **Puls.**, Rumx., Stann., Sul-ac., Thuj., Verat.

Comp. **Adhesive.**

STIFF: Ign., Kalm., Onos., Rat., Stict., Sul-ac., Ter.

cramp from: Verat.

pain, **Agg.:** Nit-ac.

STIFFENING OUT (of body): Ang., Camph., Cham., **Cina,** Cupr., **Ign., Ip.,** Just., Phos., Stram.

STIFFNESS: Apis, Bell., Bry., **Caust.,** Chel., Dulc., Kalm., Lach., Led., Lyc., Nux-v., RHUS-T., **Sep.,** Sil., **Sulph.**

STINGS: Apis, Hyper., Latr., Led., Pulx.

STINGING: Acon., APIS, **Ars.,** Berb., Bry., Kali-c., Lyc., Merc., Nit-ac., **Phos.,** Puls., Sabal., **Sep.,** SIL., **Sulph.,** Ther., Zinc.

smarting: Staph.

Comp. **Burning, stinging.**

STAINS, fast: Carb-ac., Lach., **Mag-c.,** Mag-p., Med., Pulex., Thuj., Vib.

yellow: Bell., Carb-an., Graph., Lach., Merc., Sel.

STEPPING, **high:** Agar., Bell., Carb-v., Merc., Nat-m., Onos., Rhus-t.

STERTOR: Op.

STITCHES: Acon., Ars., Bell., Berb., Borx., BRY., Caust., Colch., KALI-C., Kali-m., **Merc., Nit-ac.,** Puls., Ran-b., **Rhus-t.,** Sep., **Sil., Spig.,** Stroph-h., SULPH., Symph., Zinc-chr.

burning, in muscles: Apis, Asaf., Cocc., Glon., Mez., Nux-v., Rhus-t., Staph., Sul-ac., Thuj.

crawling: Arn.

glands, in: Ign., Merc., Puls.

jerky: Cina, Nux-v.

joints, in: Apis, Colch., **Hell.**, **Kali-c.**, Mang., **Merc.**, **Rhus-t.**, Sil., Tarax., **Thuj.**

needles, splinters, etc., as from, see **Fine.**

pressive, in muscles: Sars.

sides, loins, etc.: Abrot., Acon., Bry., Chel. (r), Kali-c. (r), Nat-s. (r), Puls., Ran-b., Sang., Sulph.

tensive: Spig.

STONE CUTTERS (phthisis): Calc., Lyc., Sil.

STRANGLING, **stifling pain:** Sulph., Valer.

STREAKS: Bell., Caust., Ox-ac., Pyrog.

Comp. **Linear.**

STREPTOCOCCUS INFECTION: Arn.

STRETCH, **impulse to: Alum.**, **Ars.**, Bry., **Carb-v.**, CAUST., Cham., Graph., Lyc., NUX-V., Puls., Rhus-t., Ruta, Squil., Zinc.

STRETCHES, **twists, turns:** Alum., **Bell.**, **Calc.**, Chel., **Cina**, Ign., Nux-v., **Rhus-t.**, Sulph.

with chill: Ferr-p.

Comp. **Stiffening out.**

STRICTURE: see **Fontanelles:** Fl-ac.

STRINGY, see **Sticky:** Coc-c., Graph., Kali-bi., Phyt., Sul-ac., Ust.

STUFFED UP: Coc-c., Spong.

STUMP painful: Hyper.

STUNNING: Fl-ac.

SUBSULTUS: see **Twitchings.**

SUDDEN: Acon., Apis, Ars., **Bell.**, Coloc., Cupr., **Hydr-ac.**, Mag-c., Mag-p., Nat-s., Tab., Tarent-c., Verat.

changing about: Berb., Cimic., Dios.

SUN OR RADIATED HEAT, see **Heat.**

SUNBURN: Camph.

SUNSTROKE: Acon., **Bell.**, **Glon.**, Hyos., Nat-c., Nux-v., Verat-v.

Comp. **Heat exhaustion.**

SUPPURATION: Arn., Ars-i., **Calc.**, **Calc-s.**, Calend., HEP., Kali-s., **Lach.**, Lyc., MERC., Merc-d., Phos., Pyrog., SIL., Sulph., **Tarent.**

abscess: Calend., Echi., Rhus-t.,
Sul-i., Syph.

bones: Puls., Sil.

fibrinous parts of: Mez.

chronic: Sulph.

deep: Caps., Tarent.

glands: Bell., Carb-an., Dulc.,
Hep., Lyc., **Merc.**, Nit-ac.,
Rhus-t., **Sil.**, Sulph.

impending, suppressed, etc.:
Ars., Bell., Calc., **Hep.**,
Kreos., Lach., Lyc., Merc.,
Sil.

pus, acrid: Ail., **Ars.**, Bell-p.,
Brom., Echi., Euphr., Gels.,
Kali-i., **Nit-ac.**, Ran-b.,
Sabad., Sanic., Sars., **Sulph.**

bloody: Merc., Nit-ac.

burrowing: Asaf., Sil.

excessive: Asaf., Hep.,
Merc., Puls., Sep., **Sulph.**

foul: **Ars.**, Asaf., Bapt.,
Carb-v., Hep., **Lach.**,
Led., Nit-ac., **Psor.**,
Pyrog., Sep., Sil., **Sulph.**,
Syph.

green: Sec., Syph., Tub.

hair distroys: Bell-p., Lyc.,
Merc., Rhus-t.

profuse: Ars., **Calc.**, Dulc.,
Kali-i., **Merc.**, Nat-m.,
Nux-v., Puls.

salty: Iod., Kali-i.

scanty: Acon., **Bry.**, **Hep.**, Lach.,
Sil.

slimy: Merc.

slow: **Merc.**

sour: Sulph.

suppressed: Bry., Dulc., Lach.,
Puls., Sil., Stram., **Sulph.**

tenacious: Borx., Coc-c., Con.,
Hydr., Kali-bi.

thick: Arg-n., Euphr., Hep., Kali-
bi., Puls., Sanic.

thin: Ars., **Asaf.**, Caust., **Fl-ac.**,
Merc., Nit-ac., Phos., **Sil.**,
Sulph.

unhealthy: Asaf., Hep., Merc.,
Phos., Sil.

watery: Asaf., Merc., Sil.

yellow: Euphr., Mez., Puls.

green: Ars-i., Kali-bi., Kali-s.,
Merc., Puls.

SURGINGS, see **Waved.**

SUTURES, see Fontanelles.

SWASHING, splashing, etc., as of
water: Ars., **Bell.**, Carb-ac.,
Carb-an., **Chin.**, **Crot-t.**, Dig.,
Glon., **Hep.**, **Hyos.**, Kali-c.,
Nat-m., Ph-ac., **Rhus-t.**, **Spig.**
    Comp. **Gushing**, **Loose.**

SWEETISH: Thuj.

SWELLED, enlarged, as if: Acon.,
Alum., ARAN., ARG-N.,
Bapt., **Bell.**, Cocc., Gels.,

Glon., Ign., Nux-v., Par., Puls.,
Ran-b., **Rhus-t.**, Spig.

SWELLING: Acon., **Apis, Ars.,**
Bar-c., **Bell.,** Bry., Calc.,
Cham., Graph., Hep., **Lach.,**
Led., Lyc., MERC., Nit-ac.,
Phos., **Puls., Rhus-t.,** SIL.,
SULPH.

**absent, in affected or inflamed
parts:** Ars., Camph., Carb-
v., Con., Laur., Op., Ph-ac.,
Sulph.

baggy: Apis, Ars., Kali-c.

cold: Asaf., **Cocc.,** Dulc., Merc.,
Sulph.

cord, like: Dulc., Iod., Ox-ac.,
Rhus-t.

feeling, large, as if: Coll., Op.,
Sanic.

glands: Calc., Merc., Sil., Sulph.

hard: Ars., Bell., Hep., Lach.,
Merc., Puls., Sil., **Tarent.**

pale: Bar-c., **Bry.,** Lach., Lyc.,
Rhus-t., **Sulph.**

receding: Ars., Calc., Hep.,
Kreos., Lach., Lyc., Merc.,
Sep., Sil.

sacular: Kali-c., Rhus-t.

SYCOSIS: Apis, Ars., Calc.,
Graph., **Med.,** Nat-s., Nit-ac.,
Ph-ac., Sabin., Sel., Sep., **Thuj.**

Comp. **Fungus growth.**

suppressed: Merc., Nit-ac.,
Staph., Thuj.

SYMMETRICAL: Arn., Kali-i.

SYMPTOM, **goups, recurring:**
Anac., Caust., Cham., Cocc.,
Cupr., Plb., Sil.

SYNALGIAS: Apis, Tarent.

SYPHILIS: Am-c., Aur., Carb-an.,
Cinnb., Iod., Kali-bi., Kali-i.,
Merc., Nit-ac., Phyt., Thuj.

phagedenic: Ars., Merc-p-r., Nit-
ac.

TALK, **can't:** Dig., Phos., Stann.,
Sulph.

fast: Bell.

must: Frax., Stict.

troubles, of her: Arg-n., Mag-p.

TEARING, **very severe pain:**
Acon., Anac., **Arn.,** Ars., Bell.,
Bry., **Calc.,** Caps., **Carb-v.,**
Caust., Cham., **Chin.,** Colch.,
Con., Kali-c., **Lyc.,** Merc.,
Nat-c., **Nit-ac.,** Nux-v, P'at.,
Puls., Rhod., RHUS-T., Sep.,
Sil., Staph., Stront-c., Xan.,
Zinc.

Comp. **Drawing.**

glands, in: Chin.

joints, in: Arn., **Chin.,** Ferr.,
Guaj., **Hell., Hep.,** Merc.,
Olnd., **Puls.,** RHUS-T.,
Stront-c.

paralytic: Carb-v., Chin., **Kali- c., Staph.**

pressive: Carb-v., Stann.

stitching, prickling: Anac., Bry., Calc., Colch., Guaj., Kali- m., Kali-p., Led., Mang., Merc., Puls., Staph., Stroph- h., Symph., Tarent., Thuj., **Verat-v., Zinc.**

twitching, jerking: Chin., **Puls.**

TEMPERATURE, **high, hyper- pyrexia:** Bapt., Chinin-ar., Iod., Phos., Verat-v.

osocillations of: Chinin-ar., **Pyrog.,** Sal-ac., Verat-v., **Zinc.**

sweat, with: Verat-v.

TEMPESTUOUS **action:** Acon., Glon., Tab.

TENACIOUS: see **Sticky.**

TENDONS, see **Fibrous tissue.**

TENDER: See **Delicate.**

TENESMUS, see **Pressing.**

TENSION, **tightness:** Bry., Caust., Kali-m., Lyc., Mag-p., **Nat-m., Nux-v., PHOS., PULS.,** RHUS-T., Senec., Stront-c., Sulph., Visc., Viol-o.

glands, in: Phos.

joints, in: Bry., **Caust.,** Lyc., Nat- m., Puls., Seneg., Sep., **Sulph.**

TERROR: Acon., Spong., Stram. see **Fear.**

TETNUS: Bell., Cic., Cocc., Cupr., Hydr-ac., Hyos., **Hyper.,** Nux-v., Petr., Stram., Stry., Tab.

TETANY: Calc., Plb., Sol-n.

THICK, **discharges, etc.:** Arg- met., **Ars., Calc.,** Calc-s., Canth., Carb-v., Con., Croc., Dulc., Graph., **Hydr., Kali-bi.,** Kali-m., Merc., Merc-cy., Nat- m., Psor., PULS., Sil., Sulph.

THREAD: See **Fine.**

THROBBING, **pulsating:** Acon., Asaf. (hard), Ast-r., BELL., Bry., **Calc.,** Chin., Ferr., GLON., Jab., Kali-c., Kreos., Lach., Nat-m., **Phos.,** Polyg-v., PULS., **Sep.,** Sil., Stroph-h., Sulph.

blood-vessels, in: Bell., **Glon.**

fever, with: Urt-u.

general: Acon., Graph., Lyc., Sang., Sulph., Verat-v.

glands, in: Con., Merc.

lying, Agg.: Glon., Sel.

painful: Acon., Am-m., **Bell.,** Ferr., Ign., Sep.

universal, all over: Alum., Ant- t., **Bell.,** Calc., **Carb-v.,** Ferr., GLON., **Graph.,** Kali- c., Kreos., Lach., **Nat-m.,** PHOS., PULS., Sang., Sep., Sil., Zinc.

THINNESS, spare habit: Arg-n., Calc-p., Fl-ac., Mag-m., Mur-ac., Nux-v., Phos., Sec., Sulph.

THRUSTS, stings, etc.: Apis, Arn., Cina, Plat., Ruta, Sul-ac., Thuj.

TICKLING, (itching) internal: Ambr., Caust., Cham., Con., Ferr., Hyos., IOD., Ip., Kali-c., Lach, Nat-m., NUX-V., PHOS., Rumx., Sang., Sep., Stann., Sulph.

TIGHTNESS: Cact.

all over: Cact.

TIME, sense: Alum., Cann-s.

TINGLING, see Itching.

TIRED: see Weak.

TO AND FRO: see Alternations.

TOPERS: Caps., Sul-ac.

TORN loose, see Adhesive.

to pieces, see Shattered.

out feeling: Alum., Bry., Calc., Elaps, Ol-an., Prun., Rhus-t.

TORPID: Asaf., Dros., Led., Op., Sil.

TOSSING ABOUT: Acon., Bell.

TOUCH, see Sensitive.

TOUGH., see Sticky.

TOURISTS: Plat.

TOUSY: Borx., Med., Sulph.

TREMBLING: Agar., Arg-n., Ars., Calc., Cic., Cimic., Crot-h., Gels., Graph., Iod., Lil-t., Merc., NUX-V., Op., Puls., Rhus-t., Staph., Stram., Stront-c., Sul-ac., Zinc.

quivering: Con., Jab., Lach., Lycps-v., Merc-v., Naja, Ol-an., Plat., Sang., Tub., Verat-v.

delirium, with: Acon., Apis, Ars., Bell., Bry., Calc., Chin., Hyos., Ign., Nat-m., Op., Phys., Plat., Puls., Rhus-t., Sabad., Samb., Stram., Sulph., Verat., Verat-v.

direction, downward: Iod., Merc.

upward: Sil., Spig.

internal: Hep., Staph., Sul-ac.

nervous: Cimic., Coff., Gels., Mag-p., Phos.

pains, during: Puls., Zinc.

senile: Bar-c., Con.

spasmodic: Ign., Nux-v., Sabad.

sweat, with: Merc.

waking, on: Verat.

weakness from: Chin., Nat-m., Stann.

TRENCH MOUTH: Merc-c.

TRICKLING, dropping or flowing, as of water: Arg-n., Bufo, Cann-s., zCaust., Glon., Graph., Kali-bi., Lam., Nat-

m., Petros., Phos., Rhus-t.,
Sep., Stann., Staph., Sumb.,
Tarent., **Thuj.**, Vario., Verat.

TRICKY: Cupr.

TRIFLES, see **Sensitive**: Thuj.,
Tub.

TRISMUS: see **Lockjaw.**

TUBE, **metallic**: Merc-c.

TUGGING, pulling, etc., see
Drawing.

TUMID: see **Puffy.**

TUMORS, erectile: Lyc.

TURNING OVER, see **Rolling.**
over.

rises to: Bry., **Nux-v.**

rotating: Coloc.

TWINGES, **nips, etc.**: Am-m.,
Laur., Mosch., Plb.

TWISTING: Ars., Bell., Calc.,
Cina, **Coloc.**, DIOS., Ign.,
Nux-v., Puls., Rhus-t., Sil.,
VERAT.

TWITCHING, see **Spasmodic.**

TYPHOID STATES, see **Blood**
and **Sepsis.**

TYPHUS FEVER: Ars.

UGLY: Bufo, **Cham.**, Cina, Nux-
v.

ULCERATION: ARS., Asaf.,
Calc., Carb-v., Caust., **Hep.**,
Kali-bi., **Lach.**, Lyc., MERC.,
Nit-ac., PULS., Rhus-t., Sep.,
SIL., Sulph., Sul-i., Syph.

areola, **edge, etc.**: Ars., Asaf.,
Hep., Lach., Lyc., Merc.,
Puls., Sil.

elevated: Ars., **Merc., Sil.**

eruptions, **pimples, etc., in:**
Carb-v., **Hep.**, Lach.

dark: Aesc., **Lach.**

hard: Brom., Fl-ac., Graph.,
Merc-i-r., Sil., Spong.

smaller ones: Calc., Hep.,
Mez., Phos., rhus-t.

atonic: Ars., Lach., Sil., Sulph.

bedsores: Arn., **Fl-ac.**, Sul-ac.

black: Kali-ar.

bleeding: Arn., Carb-v., Lach.,
Phos., Sul-ac., Thlasp.

bloody water, **from:** Carb-ac.,
Rhus-t.

bluish: Crot-h., **Lach.**, Tarent.,
Thuj., Vip-t.

break and **heal, recur:** Kreos.,
Vip-t.

burning: Ars., Sil.

coitus, **Agg.:** Kreos.

cutting: Merc.

deep, **perforating, etc.**: Calc.,
Kali-bi., Kali-c., Mez., Nit-
ac., Puls., Rad-met., Ran-b.,
Rat., Sil., Tarent.

dotted: Arg-n., Ars., Kali-bi.

dropsical persons, in: Ars.,
Graph., Hell., Lyc., Merc.,
Rhus-t., Squil., Sulph.

edge, over-hanging: Kali-bi.

flowing: Kali-ar., Kali-s., Nat-s., Rhus-t. (followed by Lyc.), Zinc-s.

dirty: Lach., Merc., Nit-ac.

heat, Agg.: Puls.
  Amel.: Ars., Clem., Con., Hep., Lach., Rhus-t., Sil.

honey combed: Cinnb.

irregular: Kali-bi., Merc.

pain, as if, see Gnawing.

painful: Ars., Carb-v., Graph., Hep., Sabin., Sil.

painless, indolent: Carb-v., Op., Ph-ac., Sulph.

rapid, malignant: Arg-n., Ars., Carb-an., Carb-v., Hydr., Merc-c., Nit-ac., Sil., Thuj.

round: Kali-bi., Merc., Phyt.

scooped out: Vario.

septal: Aur., Kali-bi., Sil.

shallow, flat: Ars., Hydr., Lach., Lyc., Merc., Nit-ac., Thuj.

small, etc.: Med.

suppressed: Clem., Lach., Sulph.

swelled: Merc., Rhus-t, Sep., Sil.

syphilitic: Asaf., Iod., Merc., Nit-ac.

varicose: Lach., Lyc., Puls.

UNCONSCIOUSNESS, prolonged: Cic., Gels., Hydr-ac., Laur.

UNDULATIONS: See Waves.

URIC ACID diathesis, lithemia: Berb., Cocc-c., Lyc., Nat-s., Sep., Urt-u.

VALVE, leaf, skin, as of a: Alum., Ant-t., Bar-c., Ferr., Iod., Kali-c., Kali-i., Lach., Mang., Phos., Sabad., Spong., Thuj.
  Comp. Opening and shutting, and Plug.

VAULTS: see Dampness.

VAPOR, smoke, fumes, etc., as of (see Smoke): Apis, ARS., Bar-c., Brom., Chin., Ign., Lyc., Phos., Puls., Verat.
  Comp. Dust.

VEINS, sore: Ham., Puls.

VENOSITY: Carb-v., Puls., Sulph.

VERMIN: Staph.

VIBRATION, fluttering, etc.: Am-c., Bell., Brom., Carb-v., Cimic., Glon., Meli-a., Sang., Sep., Sulph.
  Comp. Hamming, Quivering.

VICARIOUS, see Discharges.

VIGOR, sense of: Coff., Nat-p., Op., Phos., Psor.

VIOLENT EFFECTS: Acon., Alum., Anac., Ars., BELL., Bry., Canth., Carb-v., CHAM., Cupr., Glon., Hep., Hyos., Ign., Iod., Lach., Merc., Merc-c., Mez., NUX-V., Ox-ac., Spig., STRAM., Sulph., Tarent., Verat.

WALK, impulse to: Acon., Arg-n., Ars., Ferr., Fl-ac., Kali-i., Lil-t., Lyc., Mag-c., Merc., Naja, Phos., Sep., **Thlasp.**, Thuj.

Comp. Motion, Amel.

late learning: Calc-p., Sil.

learns to, tardily: Calc., **Sil.**, Sulph.

must: Aur., Calc., Dig., **Dios.**, Iod., Murx., Op., Paeon., Ruta, Stront-c., Tarent.

on hard pavement: Con.

WANDERING, shifting pains: Arn., Berb., **Caul.**, Cimic., Colch., Ferr., KALI-BI., Kali-n., Kali-s., Kalm., **Lac-c., Led.**, Mag-p., Merc-i-r., Nux-m., Plan., Prun., PULS., Rhod., Rhus-t., Sil., Thuj., Zinc-chr.

Comp. Here and there.

suddenly: Ambr., Colch., Rad-met.

WARM WET, see Humid.

WARMTH, sense of: Cann-s., Coff., Sul-ac.

WASH, impulse to: Psor., Syph.

WASHING, averse to: Am-c., Ant-c., **Calc.**, Clem., Nit-ac., Rhus-t., Sep., Spig., **Sulph.**

WATER, see Dampness.

chokes him: Stram.

cold, too: Phys., Ther.

tastes bad: Acon.

bitter: ARS., Calc-p., **Chinin-ars.**

putrid: Aur., Bell., **Nat-m.**

WATERY, see Moistness.

WAVES, flushes, orgasms, fluctuation etc.: **Aml-ns.**, Aur., **Bell.**, Calc., Coll., **Ferr.**, Fl-ac., Gels., **Glon., LACH.**, Mang-met., MELI-A., **Nux-v.**, Phos., Sang., SEP., Stront-c., Sulph., Sul-ac., **Thyr., Tub.**

Comp. Alternations, Ascending and Floating.

WEAK, feeble, etc.: Acon., Alum., Ant-t., Arn., ARS., **Bapt.**, Bar-c., **Bry., Calc., Calc-p.**, CARB-V., Caust., **Chin.**, Cocc., Cupr., Echi., Ferr., GELS., Graph., Hep., Ign., Iod., Ip., **Kali-c.**, Kali-p., **Lyc.**, Merc-cy., **Mur-ac.**, Nat-c., **Nat-m.**, Nit-ac., **Nux-v., PHOS., Ph-ac., Pyrog.**, Rhus-t., Sel., **Sep., Sil.**, Solid., Stann., Staph., **Sul-i.**, Sulph., Tab., **Thyr., Tub.**, VERAT.

A. M in: Carb-v., Lach., Lyc., Sep., Staph.

11 A. M.: Phos., Sep., SULPH., Zinc.

appetite, increases with: Sec.

attacks: see Collapse.

cough, after: Cor-r., Verat.

emissions, Agg.: Cob., Dios.

flushes: Dig., Sep.

internally: see Empty.

joints: Acon., Arn., Calc., Kali-c., Lyc., Merc., Rhus-t., Sep., Sulph.

pains, from: Kali-p., Pic-ac.

paralytic: Chin., Ferr., Sulph.

restless and: Ars., Rhus-t., Zinc.

sensitive and: Ter.

sickness, after, debility, etc.: Chin., Psor., Verat.

single parts: Valer.

stool, after: Ars., Cocc., Con., Merc., Tub.

suddenly, see Collapse.

waking, on: Syph.

acute diseases in: Aeth, Ail., Ant-t., Apis, Ars., Gels., Merc-cy., Mur-ac., Verat.

WEARINESS: Cann-s., Croc., Puls.

WEIGHT, as of a heavy: Acon., Alet., Ars., Bar-c., Bell., BRY., Cact., Dios., Helo., Lach., Lil-t., Lith-c., Nux-m., NUX-V., Petr., PHOS., Puls., Sep., Scop., Stann., Zinc.

hanging to part: Cur., Nit-ac.

WELL, unusually, then Agg.: Bry., Nux-v., Phos., Psor., Sep.

thinks is: Apis, Arn., Ars., Cann-s., Coff., Iod., Op.

WHISPERS: Ol-an.

WHITE , chalky: Ant-c., Mez.

turning: Sul-io

WHITENESS: Ant-t., Ars., CALC., Carb-v., Chel., Chin., Cina, Dig., Ferr., Graph., Kali-m., LAC-C., MERC., Nat-m., Phos., Ph-ac., Puls., Sep., Sulph., Verat.

WIND, DRAFT, AIR BLOWING on part, through a hole, etc., as of: Aur., Camph., Chel., Chin., Cor-r., Croc., Culx., FL-AC., Helo., HEP., Lac-d., Lil-t., Med., Mez., Naja, Nat-m., Petr., Sep., Sulph., Syph., Ther., Thyr., Thuj.

blowing on: see Wind.

WORK, dislikes: Psor., Zinc-chr.

WRAPS UP in summer: Hep., Psor.

WRIGGLES: Valer.

WRITING, mistakes, in: Lach., Lyc., Thuj. (see also Fingers).

WRONG, can't tell what is: Thuj.

X-RAY BURNS: Calc-f.

YELLOW: Acon., Ars., Bry., Calc., Carb-an., Cham., CHEL., Chin., Chion., Con., Crot-h., Eup-per., Ferr., Hydr., Iris, Kali-bi., Kali-c., Kali-s., Lach.,

LYC., MERC., Merc-i-f., Nat-s., Nit-ac., Nux-v., Ol-j., Phos., Plb., Podo., PULS., SEP., Sulph., Tarax.

golden, bright or orange: Aeth., Aloe, Alum., Card-m., CHEL., Cina, Colch., Kali-c., Kali-p., Merc., NUX-M., Phos., Sang., SUL-AC.

green: Ars-i., Mang., Merc., Puls.

sticky: Hydr., Kali-bi., Sumb.

ZIGZAG: Calc., Rhod., Sars., Sul-io.

INTELLECT

ACON., Anac., Aur., Bapt., BAR-C., BELL., Cann-s., Cocc., HELL., HYOS., Ign., LACH., Laur., LYC., Merc., Nat-c., Nux-v., OP., PHOS., PH-AC., Plat., Puls., Rhus-t., SEP., STRAM., Sulph., VERAT.

MIND

MIND: Acon., Ars., Aur., BELL., Bry., Calc., Cham., Chin., HYOS., Ign., LACH., Lil-t., Lyc., Nat-c., Nat-m., NUX-V., Op., Phos., Ph-ac., Plat., PULS., Sep., STRAM., Sulph., Valer., Verat.

ABSENCE OF, (absentminded), abstracted, etc.: Acon., Apis,

Asar., Calc-p., CAUST., CHAM., Laur., Olnd., Plat., PULS., SEP., Sulph.

ABUSIVE, scolding, quarrelsome: Aur., CHAM., Hyos., Ign., LYC., NUX-V., Ran-b.

ACTIVE, acute: COFF., OP., Phys.

ALTERNATIONS: Alum., Aur., Bell., Croc., Con., Ferr., IGN., NUX-M., Plat., Stram., Sul-ac., Valer., Verat., Zinc.

mental with physical: Arn., Cere-b., Cimic., Ign., Lil-t., Murx., Plat.

nervous with physical: Sabad.

Comp. Changing.

AMATIVE, erotic, amorous, etc.: Agn., Canth., HYOS., Lach., Lil-t., Lyc., Murx., Phos., Plat., Senec., Squil., Stann., Staph., Verat.

menses, before: Stram.

ANGER, irritability, fretfulness, bad temper, vexation, etc.: Acon., Ant-c., Apis, Arum-t., Aur., Bry., Calc., Calc-p., CHAM., Cina, Coloc., Hep., Ign., Iod., Kali-i., Kali-m., Kreos., LYC., Lyss., Nat-m., Nit-ac., NUX-V., Phos., Samb., Sel., Senec., Sep., Staph., Sulph., Sul-ac., Syph., Tub., Zinc.

Comp. Emotions.

awaking on: Kali-c., Lyc., Phos., Sanic., Tub.

ANGUISH: Acon., ARS., **Aur.,** Dig., Lach., Stram., Verat.

ANIMATION, vivacity, cheerful-ness, exaltation: Aur., Bell., CANN-S., COFF., **Croc.,** Hyos., Nat-c., **Op., Plat.,** Spong., **Stram.**

ANSWERS, slow: Bapt., Gels., Hyos., Lyc., **Merc., Ph-ac.,** Thuj., Zinc.

sleeps then: Arn., **Bapt., Hyos.,** Ph-ac.

ANTHROPOPHOBIA, bashful, shy, etc: Ambr., Anac., BAR-C., Cocc., **Hyos.,** Kali-p., **Lyc.,** Nat-m., PULS., Sil.

Comp. **Company, Cowardly.**

ANTICIPATIONS: Arg-n., Ars., Carb-v., **Gels.,** Lyc., Med., Plb., Ph-ac., **Sil.**

ANXIETY, see **Fearsome:** Merc-c., Murx., Psor.

waking, on: Spong.

APATHY, see **Inactive.**

APPROACHED, see **Touched.**

AVARICIOUS, greedy, miserly: Lyc., Pal., Sulph.

AVERSION to his own: Crot-h., Fl-ac., Iod., Kali-p., Lyc., Phos., Plat., Senec., Sep.

AWAKES, anxious: Spong.

confusion: Puls.

cough, causes: Samb.

horror, in: Tub.

nervous: Rhus-t.

palpitation: Rad-met.

panting: Rad-met.

stupor, then: Hyos.

BAD PART, takes everything in: Nux-v., Puls.

BESIDE HIMSELF, frantic, mad-ness from pain, etc.: ACON., Ars., Calc., CHAM., **Coff.,** Lyc., Nat-m., **Nux-v.**

Comp. **Sensations.**

BEWILDERED, dazed, things look strange, loss of sense of location, etc.: **Arg-n.,** Bapt., Bry., Calc., Cann-s., Cocc., Crot-h., Fl-ac., GLON., Graph., Hell., Hyos., **Nux-m.,** Op., **Petr., Plat.,** Sep., Sil., Stram., Tub., Valer.

Comp. **Confusion.**

BITE, impulse to: Bell., Phyt., Podo.

BLANK: Cor-r., Stann.

BOLDNESS, daring: Ign., **Op.**

BORROWS trouble: Sang.

CARE AND WORRY: Con., Ph-ac., Puls.

CAUTION: **Ign.**, Nux-v., **PULS.**, Verat.

CHANGING MOODS, erratic, fitful, moody, capricious: Acon., **ALUM.**, Ambr., Asaf. (touch on), Croc., **FERR.**, Graph., **IGN.**, **LACH.**, **Nux-m.**, **PLAT.**, **PULS.**, Rhod., Sep., **Stram.**, **SUL-AC.**, Tab., Tarent., Tub., **Valer.**, Verat-v., Zinc.

Comp. **Alternations.**

CLAIRVOYANCE: Acon., **Nux-m.**, Phos.

COMPLAINING, lamenting: Coff., **Verat.**

COMPREHENSION: Lycps-v.

CONFUSION, dazed, incoherence, muddled, etc.: **BELL.**, **Bry.**, **CALC.**, Caps., Cimic., Coloc., **Gels.**, **HYOS.**, Lyc., **Nux-v.**, **PHOS.**, **PH-AC.**, Plb., **RHUS-T.**, Sep., **Stram.**, Tub., **Verat.**

awaking, on: Bov., Chin Gels.

Comp. **Bewildered.**

CONTRADICTION, **Agg.: Asar.**, Ferr., **Ign.**, **Lyc.**, Nux-v., Sep.

CONTRARINESS: Anac., **Ant-c.**, **Ant-t.**, Ars., Bry., **CHAM.**, Kali-c., Nux-v.

Comp. **Discontent.**

COWARDICE: Ambr., Kreos., Lach., Nux-m., Ol-an.

COWARDLY: Bar-c., Gels., Puls., Sil., **STRAM.**

Comp. **Anthropophobia.**

CRITICAL, **exacting: Ars.**, Lyc., Sil., Sulph.

CROSSNESS: Ant-c., Ant-t., **Cham.**, Cina, Iod.

Comp. **Anger.**

CRUELTY: Kali-i.

DEATH, **fears: ACON.**, **Ars.**, Gels., Plat.

wants: Aur., Lac-c., Lach., Sep.

DECEIT, duplicity, lying, tricky, etc.: Bufo, Cupr., Merc., **Op.**, Plb., Tarent., **Verat.**

DELIRIUM: **Acon.**, Agar., **BELL.**, **Cupr.**, **Dulc.**, **HYOS.**, Lach., Nux-v., Op., **STRAM.**, Syph., VERAT.

anxious: Acon., Apis, **Stram.**

easy: Agar., Dulc.

erotic: Bufo, Canth., **Hyos.**, Lilt., Murx., Phos., Senec., Squil., Stann., Staph., Stram., Zinc.

foolish: Bell., Stram., Sulph.

frightful visions, with: Bell., Calc., Stram.

hemorrhage, after: Arn., Ars., Bell., Ign., Lach., Lyc., Phos., Ph-ac., Sep., Squil., Sulph., Verat.

maniacal, furibund, wild, raving: Acon., Ars., BELL., Bry., HYOS., Stram., VERAT., Vip.

sleeplessness, and: Aur., Bell., Bry., Calc., Chin., Coloc., Dig., Dulc., Hyos., Ign., Lyc., Nat-c., Nux-v., Op., Phos., Ph-ac., Plat., Puls., Rhus-t., Sabad., Samb., Sel., Spong., Sulph., Verat.

tremens: Cimic., Hyos., Op., Stram.

Comp. Perception, changed.

variable: Lach., Stram.

waking, on: Zinc.

DELUSIONS, see Perception, changed.

DEMENTIA: Anac., Bell., Lyc., Nux-v., Phos.

DESPAIR, hopelessness: Acon., Ars., Aur., Calc., Ign., Kali-i., Lept., Lyc., Ph-ac., PSOR., Syph., Tab., Verat.

DETERMINED: see Stubborn.

DIPSOMANIA: Ars., Caps., Lach., Nux-v.

DISEASE, fears: Arn., Calc., Kali-c., Lac-c., Lil-t., Nux-v., Phos., Sel.

DISCOURAGED: Kali-m., Myrt-c.

see Despair.

DISCONTENT: Bism., Cham., PULS., Sulph., Tub.

DISTRACTION, can't collect ideas; scattered thoughts: Acon., Alum., Am-c., Anac., Ang., Cocc., Hell., Lach., Nat-c., Olnd., Ph-ac., Sulph., Thuj., Zinc.

DOMINEERING: Lyc., Plat., Verat.

DULL, dim, dazed, beclouded, stupefied, difficult, comprehension: Ail., Ant-t., Arn., Bapt., Bar-c., BELL., Bry., CALC., GELS., Glon., Hell., HYOS., LAUR., LYC., NAT-C., Nux-m., NUX-V., Olnd., OP., Petr., PH-AC., Puls., RHUS-T., SEP., SIL., STRAM., Sulph., Verat.

Comp. Indifference.

DROPS THINGS: see Awlward.

ECSTATIC, see Reverie.

ERRATIC: Verat-v.

ESCAPE, impulse to: Bell., Bry., Cupr., Hyos., Mez., Nux-v., Op.

EXCITEMENT, see Nerves.

EXPRESS, herself can't: Puls.

EXTREMES, goes to: Valer.

FALTERING: Arg-n.

FASTIDIOUS: Ars., Graph., Nux-v.

FATIGUE, mental: Agar., Bell., Calc., **Lach.**, Nat-c., **Nux-v.**, **Psor.**, **Puls.**, Sulph.

FAULT FINDING: Ars., Sulph.

FEARSOME, anxious, fright, etc.: ACON., Arg-n., ARS., Borx., Bry., **Calc.**, **Carb-v.**, Cist., Gels., Graph., Hyos., **Ign.**, Lyc., Med., Nat-m., Nit-ac., **Nux-v.**, **Op.**, PHOS., Plat., **Puls.**, Rhus-t., Spong., Stram., Sulph., Ther., Tub., **Verat.**

animals, dogs, etc.: Chin., Tub.

approach: **Arn.**, Bar-c., Caust., **Lyc.**, Petr., Phos., Plb., Sep., Tarent.

crowds: Acon., Arg-n., Aur., Gels., Nat-m., Puls.

dark: Camph., **Cann-s.**, Hell., Sec., STRAM., Valer.

death: Acon., Ars.

dogs, of: Tub.

falling: Borx., Gels., Sanic., Sil., Zinc.

frightened or startled easily: Acon., **Arn.**, Cocc., IGN., Lyc., **Nat-m.**, Petr., **Phos.**, Stram.

frightful: Plat.

future, death, misfortune, evil forebodings, presentiments, etc., dread of: ACON., ARS., CALC., Caust.,

Cham., Chinin-s., Cimic., Dig., Graph., Lil-t., Merc., Nat-m., **Nux-v.**, Phos., Plat., PSOR., PULS., Thuj., Verat.

ghosts, of: Carb-v., Phos., **Stram.**

glistening objects, water, fluids, etc.: Lach., Stram.

long lasting: Acon., Hyos., Op.

ordeals, of: Arg-n., Arn., **Gels.**, Kali-br., Stroph-h.

people, yet Agg., if alone: Clem., Con., Lyc., Sep., Stram.

places, buildings, etc.: Arg-n., Kali-p., Visc.

pursuit: Hyos.

robbers: Ars., Nat-m.

sharp or pointed things: Alum., Apis, Ars., Bov., Merc., Plat., Sil., **Spig.**

stool, after: Caust., Kali-c.

thunderstorms, of: Lyc., Nat-c., **Phos.**

waking, on: Ant-t., Cina, Psor., Tub.

FEROCIOUS: see **Mania.**

FOOLISH, childish, silly, imbecile: ANAC., BAR-C., BELL., Bufo, HYOS., NAT-C., PH-AC., Stram.

FORGETS errand: Manc.

word in mouth: Bar-c., Rhod.

FORSAKEN, lonely: Aur., Bar- c., Calc., **Meny.**, Plat.

GENTLE, see **Timid.**

GLOOM: see **Sad.**

GRIEF: **Caust., IGN.,** Lach., Lyc., Nat-m., Petr., **Ph-ac., Puls., Staph.**

prolonged: Nat-m., Ph-ac.

GRUMBLING: Sang.

HARSH: Kali-i.

HATEFUL: Lyc., Nit-ac., Tarent.

HAUTEUR: Plat.

HEADSTRONG: see **Stubborn.**

HESITATES: Arg-n., Kali-br.

HOMESICK: **Bry., CAPS.,** Carban., Hyos., **IGN.,** Op., Merc., **Ph-ac.,** Sil.

HOPEFUL: Sulph.

HORROR: Calc., Plat., Zinc.

HOWLING: Acon., Arn., **Bell.,** Cham., Cic., Verat.

with anger: Arn.

HURRY, impatience: Alum., Apis, **Arg-n., ARS., BELL.,** Cham., **HEP.,** Hyos., **IGN.,** Ip., Lach., **Lil-t.,** Lycps-v., Med., **Merc.,** Nat-m., **NUX-V.,** Rheum, **Stram.,** Sulph., **Sul-ac.,** Tarent., Verat.

Comp. **Motion, rapid, Amel.**

HURT, **fears being: Arn.,** Chin., Hep., Kali-c., Ruta, Spig.

HYPOCHONDRIA: Ars., **AUR.,** Con., Ign., **Nat-c.,** Nat-m., **NUX-V.,** Plat., **PULS., Sep.,** Stann., **Sulph.,** Valer.

HYSTERIA: **Asaf., Aur., Cocc., Con., IGN.,** Mag-m., Mosch., **Nux-m., Nux-v.,** Plat., Puls., Sulph., **Tarent., Valer.**

coition, **Agg.:** Lac-c.

IDEAS, compelling: Nit-ac.

erroneous: Sabad.

vanish: Anac., **Nux-m.,** Verat.

wander: Dulc., Phos., Thuj.

IMAGINATIONS, illusions, fancies, etc.: Acon., Anac., **BELL.,** Calc., **Cann-s., COCC., Hyos., Ign.,** Lac-c., Op., Mosch., **PH-AC.,** Plat., **SABAD., STRAM., SULPH.,** Thuj.

snakes: Lac-c., Tub.

sensory: Rhus-t., Thuj.

voices, of: Acon., Chlol., Stram.

IMAGINARY disease: Mosch., Sabad.

IMPULSES, **horrid:** Alum., Argn., Ars., Caust., Iod., Lach., Merc.

fears his: Alum.

IMPULSIVE, emotional: Croc., Cupr., **IGN., PULS.**

INDIFFERENCE: Apis, Arn., Ars., **Bapt., CALC., Carb-v.,**

Chin., Clem., **Con.**, Gels., **HELL., Ign., Nat-c., Nat-m.,** Op., PHOS., PH-AC., **Plat.,** PULS., SEP., Sulph., Tab.

to his own: Phos., **Sep.**

Comp. **Dull and inactive, Placid.**

INDOLENT, **sluggish, slovenly, dirty:** Borx., **Caps., Chel.,** Coca, **Graph.,** Kali-bi., Kalim., Lach., **Merc.,** Nux-v., Olnd., Onos., Phos., Plb., Psor., Sep., Sil., SULPH.

Comp. **Slowness and Motion.**

INDIGNATION: Staph.

INFERIORITY: see **Cowardly, Anthropophobia** and **Company.**

INQUISITIVE: Agar., Aur., Laur.

INSANITY, **craziness:** Ambr., BELL., **Cupr.,** HYOS., Med., Op., STRAM., Syph., Tarent., VERAT.

dreads: Alum., **Calc., Cann-s., Cimic.,** Kali-br., Lil-t.

females, of: Acon., **Bell., Plat., Puls.,** Stram., Verat.

unconsciousness, prolonged: Cic., Gels., Hydr-ac., Laur.

uncouth: Bar-c., Caps.

INTOXICATION: **Caps., Gels.,** Lach., NUX-V., **Op.,** Ran-b.

INTROSPECTIVE: Puls.

INTROVERTED: Ol-an.

IRRESOLUTE: Onos.

JEALOUSY: Apis, HYOS., **Lach.**

JESTS, **jokes:** Caps, Hyos.

JOYOUS: Acon., **Coff.,** Croc., Op.

KLEPTOMANIA: Tarent.

LAUGHTER: **Bell.,** Croc., **Hyos., Stram.**

and cries by turns: Asaf., Croc., Ign., Mosch., Nux-m.,

screams then: Tarent.

LAZINESS: Ars., **Caps.,** Chin, Lach., Nat-c., Nat-m., **Nux-v.,** Sep., **Sulph.**

LEARNS, **with difficulty:** Agn., **Anac., Ars., Bar-c.,** Calc., Calc-p., Caust., Con., Nat-m., Olnd., **Phos., Ph-ac.**

easily: Camph., Coff., **Lach.,** Phos., Plat.

LECHEROUS, **lewd:** Fl-ac., Picac.

LIFE, SATIETY of: Ant-c.

LOOKED AT, **Agg.:** ANT-C., Ant-t., **Ars., Cham., Cina, Nat-m.,** Puls.

LOQUACITY: Agar., Cimic., **Hyos.,** LACH., Podo., Pyrog., **Stram.,** Verat., Verat-v.

chill and heat, with: Podo., Zinc.

rambling: Ambr., Arg-n., Cimic., Hyos., **Lach.,** Onos., Podo., Sel., Teucr., Tub.

sweat with: Sel.

LOVE pangs: Am-c., **Hyos.**, **Ign.**, **Ph-ac.**

unhappy: Aur., Ign.

MALICE, **hatred:** ANAC., **Cham.**, Cupr., Lyc., Nat-m., Nit-ac., NUX-V., Tarent.

MALIGERING: Sabad., Tarent.

MANIA, see **Delirium.**

MASTURBATION: Con., Sep.

MEAN: Sulph.

MELANCHOLY: Ars., Graph., **Puls.**, **Lach.**, Plb., Sulph., Verat-v.

MEMORIES, **disagreeable, recur:** Ambr., Am-c., Calc., Cham., Hep., **Hyos.**, **Lyc.**, **Nat-m.**, Nit-ac., Phos., Psor., Sep., Sulph., Thuj.

MEMORY: ANAC., Arn., Aur., **Bar-c.**, Bell., Calc., Cann-s., Con., Hell., HYOS., **Lach.**, LYC., **Merc.**, NAT-M., NUX-M., Op., **Ph-ac.**, Rhod., Staph., **Sulph.**, **Syph.**

active: BELL.

bad: Acon., **Agn.**, ANAC., Arg-met., **Arg-n.**, Ars., **Bar-c.**, BELL., CALC., **Con.**, Guaj., Hyos., Kali-br., Kali-p., Lach., Laur., **Lyc.**, **Merc.**, Nux-m., Petr., Phos., Sep., Staph., VERAT., **Zinc.**

bad suddenly from pain etc.: Am-c., Arg-n., Bell., Hep., Laur., Nux-m., Pall., Prun., Puls.

lost: BELL., HYOS., VERAT.

MENSES, **Agg.:** Nat-m., Stann., Stram.

before, Agg.: Stann.

MISERABLE: Kreos., Sabad.

MISTAKES, **of speech, etc.:** Alum., **Calc.**, **Chin.**, Graph., Hep., Lac-c., LYC., Nat-c., **Nat-m.**, Nux-v., Sep., Thuj.

MOANING, **groaning:** Acon., **Bry.**, Cham., Graph.

MOCKERY: Nux-m.

MORAL PERVERSIONS: **Anac.**, BELL., Bufo, HYOS., Nux-v., Op., Ph-ac., **Plat.**, STRAM., Tarent., VERAT.

MORBID: Staph.

MOROSE AND SULLEN: NUX-V., Puls., **Sang.**, Sil., Sul-ac., Tab.

MUTTERING: **Hyos.**, **Mur-ac.**, STRAM.

NAGGING: Lyc., Nux-v., Plat.

NOISY: BELL.

OBTUSE, see **Dull.**

OFFENSE, **takes:** Ars., Calc., Cocc., Ign., Lyc., Nux-v., Pall., Plat., **Puls.**, Staph.

OVERPOWERED, as if: Thuj.

PEEVISH, petulant: Acon., Ant-c., **Calc.**, **Cham.**, **CINA**, Cocc., Kali-c., Lyc., Staph., Sulph.

PERSECUTED, as if: Chin., Dros.

PERSECUTION, ideas of: Con., Thyr.

PERSEVERE, can't.: Alum., Lac-c., Lach., Nux-v., **Sil.**, Sulph.

PHILOSOPHIC: Sulph.

PLACID, tranquil: Apis, Arn., Chin., **Hell.**, **Op.**, **Phos.**, PH-AC., SEP., Staph., Sulph.

PLAINTIVE: Crot-h.

POISON, fears: **Hyos.**, Kali-br., Lach., Rhus-t.

POMPOUS, **important**: Bell., Cupr., **Lyc.**, Phos., PLAT., **Verat.**

PRAYING: Stram., Verat.

PRIDE, **arrogance**: Lil-t., Lyc., PLAT., Sulph., **Verat.**

PRIM: Plat.

PROFANITY: ANAC., Lil-t., Lyc., Nit-ac., Stram., Tarent., Verat.

PRYING: Sulph.

PURSUED, as if: Hyos., Lach., Rhus-t.

QUARRELSOME: Nux-v.

Comp. **Anger.**

RECKLESS: Tub.

RECOVERY, despairs: Ars., Calc., Psor.

RELIGIOUS IDEAS: Hyos., **Lach.**, Lyc., Puls., **Stram.**, **Sulph.**, VERAT.

REMORSE, **sense of guilt**: Ars., Chel., **Cocc.**, Croc., Dig., Hyos., Kalm., **Med.**, VERAT.

REPROACHES: **Acon.**, ARS., NUX-V.

REPUGNANCE **to everything**: Ant-c., Merc., Puls.

RESERVE: Lyc., Nat-m.

RESTLESSNESS, **anxious**: ARS., **Calc.**, Cimic., Iod., Merc., Phos., **Tarent.**

Comp. **Generalities.**

REVENGEFUL, **spiteful**: Calc., Lach., Nit-ac., **Nux-v.**

REVERIE, (sentimental) **ecstasy, dreaminess**: ACON., Agar., Ambr., **Anac.**, Ant-c., Cann-s., **Lach.**, Nux-m., Olnd., OP., PHOS., Sep., Sulph., Verat.

SADNESS, **low spirits, depressed melancholy, etc.**: Acon., **Ars.**, AUR., **Carb-an.**, Chin., Cimic., **Graph.**, IGN., Kali-br., Kali-p., Lach., Lyc., **Nat-c.**, NAT-M., **Nat-s.**, **Nit-ac.**, Psor., PULS., Rhus-t., Sel., **Stann.**, **Sulph.**, Syph., Tarax., Zinc.

eating Agg.: Graph.

walking on: Coc-c.

SARCASM, satire: Ars., Lach.

SCOLDING: Cham., Dulc., Lyc., Merc., Mosch., Nit-ac., Nux-v., Sep., Sil., Staph.

SELF, selfish, etc.: Senec.

reproaches: Kali-br., Stram.

torture: Acon., Ars., Bell., Lil-t., Plb., Tarent., Tub.

SENSITIVE, see Generalities.

SHRIEKS, cries, screams: APIS, BELL., Borx., Calc., Cham., Cic., Cina, Cupr., Glon., Hydr-ac., Ign., Jal., Lyc., Mag-p., Phos., Plat., Puls., Rheum, Stram., Syph., Verat., Verat-v., Zinc.

anger, from: Nux-v.

cephalic: Apis, Bell., Hell.

cough, Agg.: Arn., Bell., Cina.

night, at: Kreos.

pains, with: Acon., Bell., Cact., Cham., Coff., Mag-p., Sep.

sleep, during: Apis, Hell., Zinc.

touch, on: Kali-c., Ruta.

u⁻nating: Lyc., Sars.

urinating, before: Borx., Lyc.

Comp. Shrieks.

SIGHS, groans, takes deep breaths, etc.: Acon., Apoc., Arg-n., Cimic., Coca, IGN.

SIGHT of knives, Agg.: Alum., Plat.

SINGING: Ferr-p., Hyos., Sang., Spong., STRAM.

SLOWNESS, sluggish: BAR-C., Bry., Carb-v., Con., HELL., Kali-bi., Kali-m., Olnd., Onos., Ph-ac., Plb., Puls., SULPH.

Comp. Indolent.

SLY: Tarent.

SNAPPISH: Lil-t.

SORROW: Acon., IGN., Nat-m., Ph-ac., Puls., Staph.

SPEECH, see Generalities.

STARTLED EASILY, see Sensitive.

STRANGE, see Bewildered.

STUBBORN, obstinate: Alum., Ant-c., Bell., BRY., Calc., Cham., Chin., Cina, Kreos., NUX-V., Sil.

SUICIDAL IMPULSES, weary of life, etc.: ARS., AUR., Chin., Dros., Lach., Merc., Nat-s., Nit-ac., Nux-v., Psor., Puls., Thuj., Tub.

SUSPICIOUS, distrustful: Acon., Anac., Ars., BAR-C., CAUST., CIC., Cimic., Hyos., Lach., LYC., Merc., Nat-s., Nux-v., PULS., Stram., Sulph.

Comp. Fearsome.

TACITURN, silent, reticent: Ars.,
Bell., Bry., Cocc., Hell., Ign.,
Kali-m., MUR-AC., PH-AC.,
Puls., Stann., Thuj., Verat.,
ZINC.

THINKING, difficult: Anac.,
Bapt., Con., Gels., Lyc., Nat-
c., NUX-M., NUX-V., Olnd.,
Op., Phos., PH-AC., Pic-ac.,
Sep., Zinc.

fixed ideas: Anac., Chin., Nat-
m., Sabad., Sulph., Thuj.

strange ideas: Arg-n.

THROWS THINGS: Coloc.,
Dulc., Staph., Tub.

TIMID, shy, wild: Bar-c., Cocc.,
Graph., Ign., Kali-n., Kali-p.,
Lyc., Nat-c., Petr., PULS., Sil.,
Sulph.

TOUCHED, or approached,
averse to or fears being: Acon.,
ANT-C., Ant-t., Arn.,
CHAM., Cimic., Cina, Con.,
Cupr., Ign., Lyc., Sanic.

TRIFLES, seem important: Ars.,
Calc., Caust., Graph., Hep.,
Ign., Nat-m., Nux-v., Sil.,
Thuj., Tub.

Agg.: Ars., CHAM., Cina, Hep.,
Ign., Nit-ac., NUX-V., SIL.

UNCOUTH: Bar-c., Caps.

UNEASY: Verat-v.

UNHAPPY: see, Sad.

UNREAL: Med.

VACILLATING, wavering: Ars.,
Bar-c., Ign., Lyc., Nux-m.,
PULS.

VANITY: see, Pride.

WEAK, exhausted, relaxed, brain-
fag: Anac., Bar-c., Echi.,
Graph., Kali-p., Lob., Lyc.,
Merc-cy., Mur-ac., PH-AC.,
Phos., Pic-ac., Plb., Pyrog.,
Seneg., Sep., Sil., Solid.,
Staph., Sulph., Sul-i., Tab.,
Thyr., Tub.

after spasm: Sec.

WEEPING: Aeth., Apis, Aur.,
Bell., CACT., Calc., Caust.,
Cham., Graph., Ign., Lyc.,
Nat-m., NUX-M., Plat.,
PULS., Rhus-t., Sep., Sulph.,
VERAT.

anger with: Ant-t., Ars., Sulph.,
Zinc.

WHINING, whimpering: Ant-t.,
Carb-an., Cham., Cic., Cina.

WILD FEELING: Ambr., Cimic.,
Lil-t.

WILFUL: see Stubborn.

WORD HUNTING: Arg-n.,
Lach., Ph-ac., Plb., Thuj.

WORK, dread or dislike for: Arg-
n., Carb-v., Chin., CON.,
GRAPH., Lach., NAT-M.,
Nux-v., Phos., Psor., Puls.,
Rhus-t., Sulph., Zinc-chr.

Comp. Indolent.

WORRY: see **Grief.**

ZEALOUS: Nux-v.

VERTIGO

Acon., **BELL., BRY., Calc.,**
Chel., Cocc., Con., Cupr.,
Ferr., **Gels., Nat-m.,** NUX-
V., Petr., PHOS., PULS.,
Rhus-t., Sil., Sulph., **Tab.,**
Zinc.

ASCENDING, **Agg.:** Borx., Gels.

BENDING BACK, **Amel.:** Ol-an.

BLOOD, **rushes, with:** Bell., Dig.,
Glon., Hell., Merc., Verat-v.

DESCENDING, **Agg.:** Borx.,
Gels.

EATING, **Amel.:** Nux-v.

EYES, CLOSING, **Agg.:** Lach.,
Nat-m.

FAINT **like:** Bry., Cocc., Ther.

FALLS **backward:** Spig.

left, to: Sil.

FELT IN, **forehead:** Arn., Croc.,
Euon., Gels., Phos., Sulph.

occiput: Bry., Carb-v., Con.,
Gels., Petr., Sil., Verat., Zinc.

vertex: Calc., Chel., Lyss.,
Med., Stroph-h.

FEMALE **symptoms, with:** Cycl.

FEVERS, **with:** Eucal.

HEADACHE, **with:** Calc-act.,
Croc., Iod., Lac-c.

HEART **symptoms, with:** Kali-c.,
Lach., Phos., Verat.

INTOXICATED, **as if:** Gels.,
NUX-V., Puls.

LIE DOWN, **must:** Cocc., Nat-s.,
Phos., Puls., Spig.

LYING, **Agg.:** Apis, Con., Kali-m.,
Puls.

side left, Agg.: Lac-d., Onos.,
Zinc-i.

right Agg.: Gels., Rhus-t.

MOTION, **Agg.:** Bry., **Con.,** Dig.,
Kali-br., Lil-t.

NOSE, **blowing, Agg.:** Cod.,
Culx., **Sep.**

PAIN, **Agg.:** Cimic.

PREGNANCY, **Agg.:** Alet.

RAISING UP, **Agg.:** Acon., BRY.,
Merc-i-f., Phyt., Verat-v., Vib.

REELING: Arg-n., Bell., Lol-t.,
Nux-v., **Rhus-t.**

SENILE: Ambr., Arn., Bar-c., Bell-
p., Bry., Con.

SITTING, **Agg.:** Apis, Phos., **Puls.,**
Sulph.

SPASM: Tarent., Visc.

STOOL, **Amel.:** Cupr., Phos.,
Zinc.

STUPOR, **with:** Zinc.

SUN, facing, Agg.: Glon., Kali-p.

SWEAT, Amel.: Nat-s.

with: Tab.

TALKING, Agg.: Alum.

TINNITUS, with: Chinin-s.

TREMULOUS: Gels., Zinc.

TURNING, Agg.: Con., Hydr., Lach. (r).

VISION affected: Cycl., Gels., Stroph-h.

WEAKNESS, with: Colch., Sel.

WHIRLING: Nux-v., Con., Puls.

HEAD

BELL., Bry., Calc., Carb-v., Chin., Gels., Glon., Lach., Lyc., Nat-m., Nux-v., Par., Phos., Puls., Sang., Sep., Sil., Spig., Sulph., Tub.

BRAIN: Bell., Hyos., Pic-ac., Stram., Zinc.

CEREBRO-SPINAL AXIS: Agar., Arg-n., Chin., Cocc., Gels., Ign., Nux-v., Phos.

DEEP IN: Acon., Arg-n., Bov., Calc., Dulc., Lach., Nux-v., Phos., Sulph., Syph., Tub.

FONTANELLES OPEN: Calc., Calc-p., Sil.

FOREHEAD: Acon., Am-c., Arn., Ars., BELL., Bry., Chin., Ign.,

Lach., Lyc., Merc., Nat-m., NUX-V., Phos., Phyt., Prun., Puls., Sep., Sil., Spig., Sulph., Thuj.

alternating: Sabad.

arch, orbital: Asaf., Aur., Bar-c., Bar-c., Cinnb., Kali-bi., Merc., Zinc., Mez., Zinc-s.

eyes, over: Arn., Ars., Bar-c., Bell., Bism., Bry. (l), Carb-v., Cedr., Chel., Chinin-s., Gels., Iris, Kali-bi., Lach., Lil-t., Lyc., Naja, Nat-m., Nux-v., Phos., Puls., Sang., Senec.(r), Sil., Spig. (l), Syph.(r), Thyr., Zinc.

right: Bell., Cedr., Chel., Lyc., Nat-m., Puls., Sang., Sep., Syph.

left: Ars., Bry., Ferr., Kali-c., Nux-m., Sep., Spig.

nose to: Lach., Phys.

occiput to: Caust., Senec. (l), Tub.

root of nose: Acon., Arum-t., Cupr., Hyos., Ign., Kali-bi., Kali-i., Lach., Puls., Sang., Staph., Stict., Sulph., Zinc.

upper: Coloc.

MENINGES: Bell., Bry., Canth., Lyc., Zinc.

OCCIPUT, nape and neck: Bell., Bry., Calc., Carb-v., Chin.,

CIMIC., Cocc., GELS., Ign., Nux-v., Onos., **Petr.**, **Phyt.**, Sanic., Sep., SIL., Sulph., Vario., **Verat-v.**, Zinc., Zinc-ar.

right: Bell., Chel., Sang.

left: Kali-bi., Nat-m., **Onos.**

alternating sides: Sep.

ascending through: Arg-n., **Bell.**, **Calc.**, Carb-v., **Cimic.**, GELS., **Glon.**, **Kali-bi.**, Lac-c., Lach., Lil-t., Onos., **Par.**, Petr., Phos., Sabad., SANG., **Sars.**, Sep., SIL., **Spig.**, Sulph., **Verat-v.**

base: Cimic., Gels., Syph., Verat-v.

downward: Phos., Zinc.

eyes, to: Med.

forward from: Sang., Sil.

    left: Arg-n., Cimic., Lach., Lil-t., **Spig.**, Thuj.

    right: Bell., Gels., Sang., Sil.

nose, root of: Sars.

shoulder to: Kali-bi., Onos., Stict.

side, left: Lyc., Nux-v., Sep., Spig., **Sulph.**

up and down, from: **Onos.**, Sep.

ONE SIDED SYMPTOMS: Alum., Anac., Arg-n., **Ars.**, Asaf., Calc., **Chin.**, Chinin-s., Coff., **Coloc.**, Con., IRIS,

Kali-c., Kali-i., NUX-V., **Ph-ac.**, Plat., PSOR., **Puls.**, SANG., Sars., **Sep.**, Spig., Sul-ac., Verb., Zinc.

begins on one, goes to and is Agg. on other: Arg-n., Ferr., Iris, Lac-c., LYC., Mang., Nat-m., Tub.

right: BELL., Cact., Calc., Carb-v., Chel., IGN., Iris, Kalm., Lyc., Nat-c., Plat., Plb., Prun., Puls., Rhus-t., **Sabad.**, SANG., Sars., **Sil.**

left: Arn., Ars., Asaf., Brom., Chinin-s., **Coloc.**, Ip., Kali-c., **Lach.**, **Lil-t.**, **Merc.**, Mur-ac., Naja, Nit-ac., Nux-m., **Nux-v.**, Onos., Rhod., Sel., Sep., SPIG., **Sulph.**

alternating: Agar. (O), Arg-n. (S), Aloe, Alum., Ars., Bism., Cina, Gels., Glon., Hell., Hyper. (T), Ign., **Iris**, (F), Kali-c. (O), Lil-t. (F), Lyc. (T), **Nit-ac.**, Phos. (F), PSOR., Sep. (O), Sil., Stroph-h., Sulph., (T).

ears, over: Merc., Puls.

PAINS, EXTENDING, **backward:** Arn., BELL., BISM., BRY., **Cimic.**, **Glon.**, Kali-bi., Lac-d., Lach., Lyc., Med., Mur-ac., Nat-m., **Nit-ac.**, Par., Prun., Ruta, Sep., Syph., **Thuj.**, Tub., Verat-v., Verb., Zinc.

downward to nose, face, neck, etc.: **Agar.**, Ant-t., Bism., Calc., Calc-p., Cham., **Chin.**, Dulc., Guaj., Hyper., Ign., IP., **Lach.**, **Led.**, **Med.**, Meny., **Mez.**, NUX-V., **Phos.**, Pic-ac., Plat., **Puls.**, Rhus-t., Sep., **Staph.**, Stront-c., VERB., **Zinc.**

arms, over: Ars., Lac-c., **Puls.**

into eyes: Carb-v., **Chin.**, Cimic., Ign., LACH., Lith-c., Mang., Nat-c., NIT-AC., PHOS., Ph-ac., Puls., **Sil.**, SPIG., **Sulph.**, Valer., **Zinc.**

jaw, into: Phos., Stront-c.

neck, to: Bry., Cimic., Cocc., Kali-c., Lach., Nux-m., **Nux-v.**

forward: Acon., Alum., Arg-n., **Bell.**, Canth., **Carb-v.**, Chel. (l), **Chin.**, Cimic., **Con.**, GELS., Kali-c. (r), Laur., Lyc., Mur-ac., Ph-ac., **Rhus-t.**, Sabad., Sabin. (l), SANG. (r), **Sil.** (r), SPIG. (l), Thuj. (l), Verb.

inward: Agar., Anac., Arn., Ars., Calc., Canth., Hep., **Ign.**, Nit-ac., **Stann.**, Thuj.

outward: Acon., Arn., **Asaf.**, BELL., Bism., **Bry.**, Canth., Cham., Chin., Con., Dulc.,

Ign., Lach., Lyc., **Mez.**, Nat-c., Rhus-t., Sep., Sil., Spig., Sulph., Valer.

Comp. **Bursting.**

upward, ascending: Acon., BELL., Bry., **Calc.**, Canth., Chel., Chin., Cimic., Gamb., **Gels.**, **Glon.**, Kalm., Lach. (F), Mang., MENY, Merc., Nat-m., Phos., Plb., SANG., Sep., SIL., SPIG., Zinc. (F).

right: Aloe, **Bell.**, Gels., Ign., Meny., Nat-m., Nux-v., Phos., SANG.

left: Arg-n., Chel., Cimic., Colch., Lac-c., Lil-t., Par., Petr., Sabin., **Sil.**, SPIG.

left, to face and neck: Tarent.

TEMPLES: **Anac.**, **Arg-met.**, BELL., CHIN., Cycl., Glon., Kali-c., Kreos., Nux-m., Par., Ph-ac., Plat., **Puls.**, Rhus-t., Sabin., Thuj., Verb., **Zinc.**

VERTEX: **Cact.**, Calc., **Calc-p.**, Carb-an., Caust., Cimic., Cupr., Glon., Hyper., **Lach.**, Lyc., Meny., **Nit-ac.**, Phos., Ph-ac., RAN-S., **Sil.**, SULPH., VERAT., Verat-v.

across (ear to ear): Chel., Kali-m., Naja, **Nit-ac.**, Pall., Phys., Sabal, Sil.

AWAKEN by pain: Acon., Chin., Sil., Sulph.

BALD: Syph.

BAND, constriction, etc.: Anac., Ant-t., Carb-v., Carb-ac., Caust., Coca, Cocc., Gels., Glon., Graph., Merc., Nit-ac., Rad-met., Rat., Sulph.

BEATS, the: Acon., Hyos., Syph., Tub.

BIG, with big belly: Calc.

BINDING UP, Amel.: Arg-n., Puls., Sil.

BLOW, shock, thrust, etc., as of a: Apis, Cann-s., Croc., Glon., Ign., Naja, Nat-m., Nux-v., Spig., Stront-c., Sul-ac., Tarent., Zinc-chr.

BORING, digging: Arg-n., Caust., Coloc., Hep., Ign., Spig., Sep.

BORES into pillow, drawn backward, etc.: Apis, Bell., Cic., Hell., Med., Op., Podo., Syph., Tub., Verat-v., Zinc.

BRAIN, bruised: Bapt., Chin., Gels.

burning: Acon., Bell., Phos.

coldness: Mosch., Phos.

degeneration, softening: Arg-n., Sil., Stry-p., Zinc-p.

humming, roaring, etc., in: Kreos., Lach., Phos.

loose, brain feels: Acon., Bar-c., Bell., Chin., Glon., Kali-c., Nux-v., Rhus-t., Spig., Sulph., Tub.

needles: Tarent.

numb: Apis, Calc., Hell., Kali-br.

rolling over: Plan.

wrapped: Cycl., Op.

BRUISED, crushed, etc.: Chin., Ign., Ip., Nux-v.

BURNING: Oena.

BURSTING, distended, etc.: Acon., Arn., Bell., BRY., Chin., Ferr., Glon., Mag-c., Meli-a., Merc., Nat-m., Nux-v., Ran-b., Ruta, Sep., Spig.

CATARRHAL: Kali-bi., Merc., NUX-V.

CAP, on: Eup-p.

CHRONIC: Arg-n., Ars., Calc., Nat-c., Nat-m., Psor., Sep., Sil., Zinc.

COLD APPLICATIONS, Amel.: Ars., Glon.

COLDNESS: Agar., Bell., Calc., Calc-p., Cann-s., Chel., Cupr., Dulc., Hyper., Laur., Nat-m., Phos., Sep., Sil., Tarent., VERAT., Verat-v.

COMPRESSION, squeezing, cap, etc.: Agn., Arg-n., Berb., Bry., Cact., Crot-c., Glon., Ign.,

Lach., **Meny.**, Merc., Onos.,
Ph-ac., Plat., **Puls.**, **Staph.**

vise-like: Nit-ac., Puls.

CONGESTION: **Acon.**, Aml-ns.,
Apis, Arn., **BELL.**, **Bry.**, Calc.,
FERR., **Gels.**, GLON., Hyos.,
Lach., **Meli-a.**, NUX-V., **Op.**,
Phos., **Puls.**, **Psor.**, Rhus-t.,
Sang., STRAM., **Sulph.**,
VERAT-V.

COVER, **must:** Brom., **Rumx.**

COUGH, **Agg.**: BRY., Caps.,
Carb-v., Iris, **Nat-m.**, Nux-v.,
Phos., Sulph., Viol-o.

CRAMP: Acon., Ign., Plat.

CRASH or explosion in: Aloe,
Dig., Glon., Phos., Zinc.

CRAWLING, formication, etc.:
Acon., **Arg-met.**, Colch.,
Cupr., Hyos., Phos., **Plat.**,
Puls., **Rhus-t.**, Sulph.

CRUSHING into: Bry., Kali-i.,
Kalm., Nat-s., Nit-ac., Syph.

CUTTING or **sharp shooting
pains**, etc.: Arn., **Bell.**, Calc.,
Lach., Sep. (l), Spig. (r), Tub.

DIARRHEA, **alternating with:**
Aloe, Podo.

DIURESIS, **with:** Acon., Glon.,
Lac-d., Phys., Vib.

DRAFTS, **Agg.**: Borx., Mag-m.,
Naja, Psor., **Sil.**

DRAWING: Carb-v., Cham.,
Chin.

DRAWN **to a point:** Graph.,
Hyper., Lachn., Stront-c.,
Ther.

DULL or **heavy aching:** Acon.,
Agar., Alet., Aloe, Am-c., Ars.,
Bell., Bism., Bry., Cact., Calc.,
Carb-v., **Chel.**, Chin., Echi.,
Erig., Eucal., **Gels.**, Glon.,
Helo., Kalm., Lept., Lil-t.,
Lith-c., **Meny.**, NAT-M., **Nux-
v.**, **Petr.**, Phos., Ph-ac., **Puls.**,
Pyrog., Rad-met., Rhus-t.,
Ruta, Scop., Sep., Sil., **Stann.**,
Sulph., Ter., Thuj., Vario.,
Zinc.

EATING, **Amel.**: Cist., Elaps,
Lyc., Mag-c., Phos.

EMPTY: **Cocc.**, Kali-c., Murx.,
Nux-v., Olnd., Phos., Puls.,
Tab., Verat.

ENLARGED, **as if:** Arg-n., Bell.,
Gels., Glon., **Nux-v.**

EXPANDING and **contracting:**
Calc., Glon., Lac-c.

EYE or **visual symptoms, with:**
Bar-c., Bell., Bry., Cocc., **Gels.**,
Hyos., Lach., Puls., Sep., Sil,
Stram.

EYE STRAIN, **Agg.**: Gels., Nat-m.,
Onos., Ruta.

FEAR, **with:** Acon., Cimic., Glon.

FLYING **to pieces:** Xan.

FOREHEAD, ball, lump: Ant-t., Carb-ac., Caust., Con., Kali-c., Staph.

band: Cact., Gels., Merc., **Sulph.**

brown: Kali-p., Sep.

brown-yellow at edge of hair: Caul., Kali-p., Med., Nat-m.

nasal discharge, Amel.: All-c., Kali-bi., **Lach.,** Zinc.

sweat, cold: Ant-t., **Carb-v.,** Chion., Cina, Dros., Ip., Merc-c., Op., Staph., VERAT.

  Agg. drinking: Cupr., Ip.

  Amel. drinking: Verat.

swelled: Apis, Hell., **Nux-v.,** Rhus-t.

tongue, protruding, Agg.: Syph.

veins: Abrot., Calad., Camph., Chin., Cub., Sulph.

vertigo, in: Cocc., Euon., Phos., Sulph.

wrinkled: Hell., **Lyc.,** Sep., Stram.

FULLNESS: **Acon.,** Bry., **Glon.,** Merc., Sulph.

HAIRCUT, **Agg.: Bell.,** Glon., Phos., Sep.

HAIR DOWN, **Amel.: Bell.,** Cina., Ferr., Kali-p., Phos.

HAMMERING: Calc., **Ferr.,** Ham., Lach., Nat-m., Psor., Sulph.

HEAT, **burning: Acon., Bell.,** Borx., Bry., **Frax., Graph.,** Lach., Merc., **Merc-i-r.,** Nat-c., Phos., **Pic-ac.,** SULPH.

HEATED, if, **Agg.: Acon.,** Bell., **Bry.,** Carb-v., **Glon.,** Nit-ac., **Verat-v.,** Zinc.

HEAVY on pillow: Bufo, Glon., Sang.

HOT, **air about:** Ast-r., Fl-ac., Plan., Puls., Verat.

HOT, **with cold limbs:** Acon., **Arn.,** BELL., Bry., Calc., **Chin.,** Ferr., Gels., Lach., Mur-ac.

HOT SPOTS, **on:** Con.

HYDROCEPHALUS: Apis, Calc., Calc-p., Sil., Zinc.

INJURIES, **to: Arn.,** Cic., Con., Hep., Lach., Puls., Rhus-t., Sul-ac.

  stupefaction after: Arn., Cic., Con., Puls., Rhus-t.

  delirium after: Bell., Hyos., Op., Stram., Verat.

JERKS: **Bell.,** Bry., Caust., Chin., **Puls.,** Sep.

          Comp. **Spasmodic.**

LOW, **Agg.:** Puls., Sang.

  Amel.: Bry., Phys., Verat-v.

LYING, **Amel.:** Con., **Nat-m.,** Nux-v., Sang., Sel.

LYING on side: Phos. (r).

MADDENING PAIN (shrieks with):Acon.,Apis,Ars.,Bell., Calc., **Cham.**, Coloc., Cupr., **Meli-a.**, Sep., **Stram.**

MENTAL EXERTION, **Agg.**: Anac., Iris, Kali-br., **Nat-c.**, Pic-ac., Sep., Sil., Zinc.

MENINGITIS: Acon., **Apis**, Arn., **Bell.**, Bry., Cupr., **Gels.**, Hell., Merc-d., Nat-s., Stram., Sulph., **Zinc.**

with clear, pale urine: Bell., Hyos., Lach., Phos.

nose, into: Cimic., **Lach.**, Mez.

MILK, **Amel.**: Bry., Verat.

MOTION, **Agg.**: Tub.

NAIL, clavus, plug: Coff., **Ign.**, Nux-v., Thuj., Ust.

NERVOUS: Sel.

NODDING, to and fro, etc.: Chin., Hyper., Ign., Nat-m., Sep., Stram.

NOISES in, clang, in: Ars., Chin., Cop., Kali-c., Lyc., **Phel.**, Plat., Puls., Sars., Sil., Sul-ac., Sulph.

NUMB: Graph., **Kali-br.**, Petr., Plat., Tarent.

OCCIPUT, air on, **Agg.**: Sanic.

band: Arg-n.

blow on: Apis, Bell., Cimic., Kali-m., Lach., Naja, Tab., Tarent., Zinc.

bursting: Gels.

cold: Cuel.

cough, **Agg.**: Puls.

enlarging, swelled, as if: Bry., Cocc.

hair falls from: Merc.

heat: Aur.

heaviness: Bell., Calc., Carb-v., **Chel.**, Kali-m., Mur-ac., Merc-i-r., **Nat-m.**, Petr.

legs, weak, with: Zinc.

lying on, **Agg.**: Bry., Cact., Carb-v., COCC., Kali-p., Nux-v., PETR., Phos., Sep., Spig.

pillow, **Agg.**: Bufo, Glon.

pressure, outward: Aesc.

sore, bruised: Prun., Staph.

tension: Lyc.

throbbing: Cann-s., Phos., Sep.

OPENING AND SHUTTING, as if: Calc., Cann-s., Cimic., **Cocc.**, Glon., Sep., Sulph.

PAIN, eyes and: Bell., Gels., Kali-c., Nat-c., Sang., Zinc.

motion of, **Agg.**: Bry.

out thro': Nat-c., Sil.

strain, **Agg.**: Gels., Nat-m., **Onos.**, Ph-ac.

feet and: Mag-m.

heart and: Cact., Dig., Glon., Kalm., Naja, Spig.

POLYURIA, with: Gels., Ign. (>), Lac-d., Ol-an., Sel., Sil.

PRESSURE: **Bry.**, Chin., Ign., Nux-v., Sabad., Stann., **Sulph.**

Amel.: **Arg-n.**, Bry., Cact., Meny., Nat-m., Nux-m., Puls., Stann., **Verat.**

REVERBERATION, **buzzing, roaring, clang, etc.:** Ars., Aur., Cop., Iod., Lyc., **Phel.**, Phos., PULS., Sars., Sil., **Staph.**, **Sulph.**, Zinc.

SCHOOL GIRLS, **Agg.:** Calc-p., Nat-m.

SEPARATED **from body, as if:** Agar., Aloe, Alum., Ant-t., Cann-s., Cocc., **Daph.**, Hyper., Nat-c., Nat-m., **Nux-m.**, Psor., Sabin., Ther., Verat.

SHAKING, **Agg.:** Bell., Glon., Nux-v.

Amel.: Lach., Phos.

SHATTERED, **as if:** Aeth., Arg-met., Bar-c., **Bell.**, Bry., Calc., **Chin.**, Cimic., Ign., **Iris**, Merc., **Nux-v.**, Phos., Rhus-t., Sil., Sulph.

SHOOTING: Tub.

SLEEP, **during:** Ther.

SORE, **bruised: Chin.**, Gels., Ip., Nux-v., Prun., Staph.

SPOT, **in a:** Cann-s., Colch., **Ign.**, Kali-bi.

STANDING **on, as if:** Ars., Dios., Elaps, Glon., Lach., Phos., Ph-ac., Thuj.

STITCHES, **stinging, etc.: Arn.**, **Bry.**, Caust., **Kali-c.**, Merc. Nat-m., **Puls.**, Sabal, Sulph., Ther., Zinc.

STOMACH, **alternating with:** Ars., Bism., Ox-ac., Plb., Verat.

STOOL, **Agg.:** Manc.

STOOPING, **Amel.:** Ign., Mez.

STUPEFYING PAIN: **Bell.**, Calc., Cocc., Gels., Hyos., **Nux-v.**, Ph-ac., Spig., Verb.

SUNDOWN, **Amel:** Gels., Sul-i.

SUNSHINE, **Agg.:** Bell., Glon., Lach., Nat-c., Valer.

SUPPRESSIONS, **from:** Ant-t.

SWEAT, **on:** Am-m., CALC., **Cham.**, Chin., Kali-m., **Merc.**, Puls., Rheum, Sanic., **Sil.**

TALKING, **Agg.:** Acon., Chin., **Nat-m.**, Sil., **Sulph.**

TEARING, **rending: Chin.**, Lyc., **Merc.**, Nux-v., Puls., Sulph.

Comp. **Shattering**

TEMPLES, **biting, Agg.:** Zinc.

burning: Coloc., Lyc., Mez., **Phos.**

heavy: Zinc.

throb: Bell., Glon., Zinc-chr.

twitch: Psor.

veins: Ars., Cupr., Fl-ac., Glon., Ham., Puls., Sang., Vip-t., Zinc.

THROBBING: Acon., BELL.,
Bry., Cact., Calc., Chin.,
Cocc., Ferr., GLON., LACH.,
Laur., Lyc., Meli-a., Nat-m.,
Sep., Sil., Staph., Sulph.

TIGHTNESS: Nit-ac., Nux-v.

TOUCH, Agg.: Aur., Chin., Hep.,
Lyc., Mez., Nit-ac., Nux-v.

TWINGING: Bell., Bry., Chin
Puls., Sulph.

TWISTING in: Kali-c., Mur-ac.,
Til.

UNCOVERING, Agg.: Ars., Aur
Bell., Calc-p., Colch., Con.,
Hep., Hyos., Kali-bi., Lach.,
Mag-c., Mag-p., Nux-m.,
Nux-v., Psor., Rhus-t., Samb.,
SIL., Stront-c.

URINATION, Amel.: Gels., Ign.,
Meli-a., Sang., Sil.

UTERINE reflexes, with: Helon.,
Plat., Puls., Sep.

VARIABLE: Zinc.

VERTEX, ache: Ign.

buring heat, etc.: Frax., Graph.,
Sulph.

burst: Cimic., Sil.

cold: Calc-p., Naja, Verat.

dry: Ars., Frax.

fly off, as if to: Bapt., Cann-s.,
Cimic., Iris, Syph., Thlasp.,
Xan.

hair, falls: Bar-c.

lying, Agg.: Manc.

menses, Agg.: Ferr-p.

numb: Glon.

pressure, heavy, crushing, etc.,
on: Aloe, Apis, Cact., Ferr-
p., Hyper., Lach., Lyc.,
Meny., Nat-m., Pall., Ph-
ac., Plb., Zinc-chr.

Agg.: Chin., Lach.,
Phys., Ther.

sides, down: Ferr-p., Hyper.

sore, painful: Chin., Nit-ac.,
Sulph.

tension: Lob.

throbs: Bry., Caust., Cocc.,
Lach., Phos., Sil., Sulph.,
Syph., Visc.

VERTIGO, after: Rhus-t.

VIOLENT: Tub.

VOMITING, with: Dig., Eup-per.,
Ip., Sang.

WASHER-WOMAN'S headache:
Bry., Phos.

WEAKENED by pain: Ars., Nux-
v.

WEEKLY: Calc., Epiph.

WIND thru: Aur.

WOBBLING about: Abrot., Aeth.,
Bell., Calc-p., Cham., Dig.,
Hyos.

WRAPPING, Agg.: Led., Lyc.

Amel.: Cor-r., Hep.,.Led., Nux-
v., Phos., Rhus-t., Rumx.,
Sil.

EXTERNAL HEAD; BONES AND SCALP

Acon., Apis, **Arn.**, **Ars.**, **Aur.**, **Bar-c.**, **Bell.**, CALC., CALC-P., Caps., Chin., Clem., Hep., **Lyc.**, **Merc.**, Mez., **Nit-ac.**, **Nux-v.**, **Olnd.**, **Phos.**, **Ph-ac.**, RHUS-T., Rhod., **Ruta, Sil.**, **Staph.**, Sulph., **Viol-t.**

right: **Calc.**, Canth., Con., Mez., Sil.

left: Clem., Ruta, Thuj.

FRONT: Hep., Led., Ph-ac., Sulph.

bregma: Ars., Merc.

SIDES: Zinc.

TEMPLES: Nat-m.

EARS, behind: Bar-c., Caust., **Graph.**, Petr., Sil., Staph.

OCCIPUT: Carb-an., **Carb-v.**, Petr., Sil.

VERTEX: Carb-v., Graph.

BURNING in vertex: Graph., Lach., **Sulph.**

DAMP, **Agg.**: Led.

DANDRUFF: Ars., Graph., Kali-m., **Phos.**, Staph., Thuj.

white: Ars., Kali-m.

yellow: Calc., Kali-s.

ERUPTION: ARS., Bar-c, Calc., Graph., HEP., **Lyc.**, Merc., Mez., OLND., **Petr.**, RHUS-T., **Sulph.**, Viol-t.

FISSURE: Kali-i.

GATHERED, as if: Chin., Sel.

GLABELLA, puffy: Fl-ac.

HAIR, affected: Bell., Borx., Calc., Carb-an., Carb-v., Con., **Graph.**, **Hep.**, **Kali-c.**, **Lyc.**, Merc., **Nat-m.**, Nit-ac., **Sulph.**, Ust.

blond: Brom., **Calc.**, Caps., Cocc., Hyos., Puls., Sel., Seneg., Sil.

body, over: Thyr.

bristling erect: Acon., **Bar-c.**, Canth., Cham., Chel., Glon., **Laur.**, Meny., Mur-ac., Sul-i., **Verat.**, **Zinc.**

cold: Sulph.

combing: Carb-ac.

dark: Acon., Cina, Iod., Nit-ac., **Nux-v.**, Phos., Ph-ac., Plat., Sep.

dry: Kali-c., Psor., Sulph., Thuj.

falling: **Ars.**, Ars-s-f., **Aur.**, **Calc.**, GRAPH., **Hep.**, **Kali-c.**, Lach., Lyc., NAT-M., PHOS., Sep., SULPH., Thuj., Thyr.

bregma: Ars., Nat-m., Phos.

eyebrows: Kali-c.

headaches, after: Hep., Nit-ac.

occiput: Carb-v., Phos.

sides: Graph., Phos.

spots in: Alumn., Graph., Hep., Lyc., **Nat-m.**, **Phos.**

temples: Kali-c., **Nat-m.**

vertex: Bar-c., Graph., Lyc., Sep., Zinc.

foul: Vinc.

gray, early: Ars., **Lyc.**, Nat-m., Ph-ac.

letting down, Amel.: Bell., Ferr., Kali-m.

margins, of: Kali-p., Med., Mez., Nat-m., Petr., Sep.

matted: Ant-c., Graph., Lyc., Ust., Vinc., Viol-t.

painful, touch to, etc.: Ars., Chin., Nux-v., Sel., **Verat.**

pulls hair: Ars., **Bell.**, Cina, Cupr., Med., Tarent., Tub., Xan.

sensation of: see **Formication.**

split: Thuj., ZINC.

stiff: Sel.

tangled, tousy: Borx., Fl-ac., Lyc., Med., Mez., Nat-m., Ph-ac., Sulph.

ITCHING: Graph., Lyc., Nat-m., Olnd., Phos., Sep., **Sulph.**

LUMPS, nodes: Graph., Sil.

MILK CRUSTS: Calc., Graph., Lyc., Ol-j., Psor., Sep., **Sulph.**, Tub., Ust.

eroding: Staph.

foul: Staph.

MOTION of: Alum., **Bell.**, Camph., Cic., Cina, **Cupr.**, Hyos., Ign., Sep., Spong., Stram.

NUMB, one side: Mez.

PLICA POLONICA: Graph., Vinc., Viol-o.

ROLLING OF: Agar., Am-c., Apis, Ars., **Bell.**, Cina, **Hell.**, Lyc., **Nux-m.**, Phos., PODO., Tarent., Verat-v., **Zinc.**

SENSITIVE, painful: Ars., Bell., Chin., Kali-i., Merc., Nit-ac., Nux-v., Sil., Spig., Tub.

SKULL, painful: Mez.

STIFF: Rhus-t.

SWEATS: Calc., Cham., **Puls.**, Rheum.

TENSION: Merc.

EYES

Acon., **Agar.**, Apis, **Arg-n.**, **Ars.**, BELL., CALC., Caust., Euphr., **Gels.**, Graph., **Lyc.**, MERC., NAT-M., Nux-v., Phos., PULS., **Rhus-t.**, **Ruta**, Sep., SULPH., Verat., Zinc.

RIGHT: Am-c., **Bell.**, Calc., Cann-s., **Coloc.**, Euphr., **Lyc.**, Nat-m., Nit-ac., Petr., Phos., Plat., Rhus-t., Seneg., Sil.

LEFT: Apis, Ars., Asar., Bry., Chel., Chin., Hep., Laur., Mez.,

Nux-v., Plb., **Spig.**, **Spong.**, Squil., Stann., Sulph., Tarx., Thuj.

ALTERNATING BETWEEN: Acon., Agar., Ang., **Ars.**, Bell., **Chin.**, Cupr., **Lyc.**, Puls., **Ran-b.**, Seneg., Sil.

ASCENDING, into: Sang. (r), Spig. (l).

BACKWARD (drawing, etc.): Astr., Bry., **Crot-t.**, Graph., Grin., Hep., **Lach.**, Nicc-s., Olnd., Par., Phos., Prun., **Puls.**, Rad-met., **Rhus-t.**, Seneg., Sil., Spig.

BROWS: Bell., Caust., Kali-c., Par., Sel.

outward, along: Cinnb., Echi., Kali-bi., Mez., Viol-o.

hair falling: Kali-c., Med., Plb., Sel.

CANTHI: Agar., Calc., Carb-v., Kali-n., Nat-m., Nux-v., Phos., **Puls.**, Sil., **SULPH.**

inner: **Agar.**, Bell., **Staph.**, Zinc.

outer: Calc., Ran-b., Sulph.

gum in: **Agar.**, **Ant-c.**, Calc., Graph., Lyc., Staph.

inflamed: Ant-c., Arg-n., Euphr., **Graph.**

red: Apis, (pale), Rhus-t. (dark).

COROID: Phos.

CONJUNCTIVA: **Acon.**, Apis, **ARG-N.**, **Ars.**, **Bell.**, **All-c.**, **EUPHR.**, Merc., **PULS.**, Rhus-t., **Sulph.**

chemosis: Apis, Arg-n., Kali-i., Lyc., Rhus-t.

granular: Apis, Arg-n., Ars., Kali-bi.

inflamed: Acon., **Arg-n.**, **Ars.**, **Bell.**, Euphr., Puls., Rhus-t., Sulph.

phlyctaenae: Ars., Graph.

pouting: Nit-ac.

raw: Kali-i., Lyc.

saccular: Apis, Ars.

CORNEA: **CALC.**, **Cann-s.**, Con., **Euphr.**, Hep., Merc., Merc-i-f., **Puls.**, Sulph.

inflamed: Syph.

opacity: Arg-n., Calc., **Cann.**, Lach., Puls., Sil., **Sulph.**, **Zinc-s.**

spots on: Nit-ac.

ulcer: Arg-n., **Ars.**, Calc., Euphr., Hep., **Kali-bi.**, **Merc-c.**, Sil., Sulph.

EYEBALL: **Acon.**, Bell., Calc., Cimic., Euphr., Hep., Lyc., Phyt., Prun., Spig., **Sulph.**

behind: Bad., **Bry.**, Chel., **Cimic.**, Gels., Lac-f., **Lach.**, Lith-c., Manc., Merc.,

Podo., Puls., RHUS-T., Sep., Ther.

big, feel: Arg-n., Chel., Glon., Guaj., Meli-a.

bursting: Phos., Prun., Sulph.

falling out, as if: Brom., Carban., Coloc., Guaj., Hell., **Ign.,** Lyc., Puls., **Sep.,** Tril-p.

motions of: Agar., **Bell.,** Cham., Cupr., Hyos., Stram.

oscillation: Agar., Cocc., **Cupr.,** Gels., **Zinc.**

sore, aching, bruised, as if: Arn., Bapt., **Bry.,** Chion., **Cimic.,** Com., EUP-PER., **Gels.,** Merc., Onos., Phos., **Phyt.,** Rhus-t., Sang., Spig.

IRIS: Bell., Merc., **Merc-c.,** Nit-ac., Sulph.

jagged: Sil., Staph., Thuj.

LENS: Euphr., **Puls., Sil., Sulph.**

cataract: Calc., Calc-p., **Caust.,** Euphr., Phos., Sec., **Sil., Sulph.**

LIDS: Acon., Agar., Apis, Bell., Calc., **Caust.,** Hep., Merc., Rhus-t., **Sep.,** Spig., **Sulph.**

upper: Caust., GELS., Kalm., Sep., Spig.

lower: Calc., Ph-ac., Ruta, Seneg.

adhere: Asaf., Glon., Guaj.

agglutinated, suppuration: Caust., Euphr., Lyc., **Nux-v.,** Phos., **Puls., Rhus-t.,** Sep., Sulph.

closed, drawn, shut: Coloc.

closed tightly, spasm: Ars., Bell., Cham., Croc., Euphr., **Hyos.,** Ip., Kali-c., Merc., Nat-m., Sil., Stram.

Agg., by: Bry., Lach., Sep., Ther.

dry: Rhus-t., Verat.

edges, tarsi: Borx., Merc., PULS., Staph., **Sulph.,** Valer.

eczema: Tub.

inflamed: Graph., Mag-m., Petr., Puls., Sulph.

itching: Calc., Sabad.

pustules: Ant-c.

red: Ars., Euphr., Graph., Merc., Puls., Sep., Sulph.

scaly: Ars., Graph., Mag-m., Med., **Merc.,** Sep.

thick, swelled: Calc., **Euphr.,** Graph., Hep., Merc., Puls., Tell.

everted: Psor.

gummy: Psor.

heavy, falling, drooping, paralysis, etc.: **Caust.,** Cham., Cocc., Con., GELS., KALI-P., Manc., Nux-v., Rhus-t., Sep., Spig., Verat.

droop, left: Bar-c., Coloc., Kali-p., Thuj.

right: Caust.

inflamed: Acon., Ars., Bell., **Lyc.**, **Puls.**, **Staph.**, Sulph.

gonorrheal: Acon., **Puls.**, Sulph., **Thuj.**

inner surfaces: **Arg-n.**, Ars., Rhus-t.

inverted: Borx., Psor., Puls., Sil.

nodes: Graph., Staph.

open, half open, etc.: Bapt., Bell., Cupr., Hell., **Lyc.**, Op., Phos., **Podo.**, Samb., Stram., Thuj.

one: Ant-t., Chin., Ign., Verat.

red: Acon., Lyc.

stiff: Apis, Kalm., Nat-m., Onos., Rat., **Rhus-t.**

styes: Calc-f., Graph., Kreos., Puls., Sil., Staph., Sulph., Zinc.

swelled, upper: Kali-c., Sep.

lower: Apis, Ars., Phos.

swelling, inner angles, over: Com., Kali-c., Puls.

thickened: Alumn.

twitch: Agar., Cic., Phys., Sulph.

thick, swelled: Alumn., Calc., **Euphr.**, Graph., Hep., Merc., Puls.

warts, on: Caust., Thuj.

ORBITS: Ang., **Apis**, Aur., Bar-c.,

Cinnb., Merc-i-f., Rhus-t., Spig., Syph., Valer., Zinc.

neuralgia: Ars., Cedr., Chinin-s., Kali-bi., Nat-m., Spig., Stann.

PUPILS, adherent: Nit-ac.

contracted: Acon., **Chel.**, Cocc., **Op.**, Sep., Sil., Sulph., Thuj., **Verat.**

dilated: BELL., CALC., Hep., **Hyos.**, Op., Spig., **Stram.**

dilate and contract alternately: Arn., Stroph-h.

fixed: Bell., Cupr., **Op.**

irregular: Merc., Sulph.

mobile: Stroph-h.

unequal: Colch., Hyos.

SCLERA: **Acon.**, Ruta, Sulph.

sclerotitis: Thuj.

ARCUS SENILIS: Calc., Kali-c., Merc., Phos., Vario.

BLOODSHOT: Acon., Arn., Ham., **Nux-v.**

BURNING: ARS., BELL., Brom., Bry., Cimic., Graph., Merc-c., Phos., Rumx., Sulph., Zinc.

CLOSING, **Agg.**: Bry., Carb-an., Lach., Stront-c., Ther.

sees visions: Bell.

COITION, **Agg.**: Kali-c., Nat-m.

COLDS: Dulc., Merc., Puls., Rhus-t.

COLDNESS: Calc., Croc., Fl- ac.

COVERED: Puls.

CRAMP: Viol-o.

CROSSED, as if: Bell., Calc., Con., Kali-bi., Nat-m., Op., Podo., Puls., Zinc.

DRAWN TOGETHER, as if: Lach., Lyc., Merc., Naja, Nat-m., Op., Par., Puls., Zinc.

DRY: Acon., Alum., Bell., Ign., Lyc., NUX-M., Puls., SULPH.

burning: Arum-t., Croc.

DULL: Op.

EARS, and: Viol-o.

EYEGUM, sticky: Euphr., Kali-bi.

FORWARD, PRESSURE: Bry., Kali-m., Merc-c., Nux-v., Prun., Sang., Spig.

GLAUCOMA: Phos.

HEAT of fire, Agg.: Phos.

INJECTED: Acon., All-c., Apis, Arg-n., Arn., BELL., Glon., Led., Merc., Nat-m., Nux-v.

INJURIES: Symph.

INTO, PAINS: Staph.

ITCHING: Calc., Puls., Sulph.

KERATITIS: Merc-c.

KIDNEYS, and: Viol-o.

LACHRYMAL DUCT: Apis, Fago., Hep., Merc-d., Petr., Puls., Sil., Staph.

LACHRYMATION: All-c., Ars., Bell., Calc., Euphr., Kreos., Merc., Nat-m., Puls., Rhus-t., Ruta, Sabad., Sil., Staph., Stram., Sulph.

affected side, Agg.: Lach., Nat-m., Nux-v., Puls.

biting: Com.

eating, Agg.: Ol-an., Zinc.

pain, Agg.: Chel., Nat-m., Ran-b.

LASHES, falling: Med.

ingrown: Graph., Tell.

LIGHT, Agg.: Bell., Calc., Nat-s., Rhus-t.

LIPPITUDE: Acon., Euphr., Merc., Puls., Rhus-t., Stram.

LOOKS down, before him: Stann., Verat.

MENSES, before: Naja.

OPHTHALMIA, gonorrheal: Arg-n., Kali-bi., Puls.

OUTWARD, pulled: Glon., Lach.

OVARIES, with: Onos.

PRESSED, apart: Asar., Prun.

out: Cedr., Gymn., Nat-m.

PINK EYE: Euphr.

PROTRUDING: Acon., Bell., Chlor., Guaj., Hyos., Iod., Lycps-v., Nat-m.

PUCKERED, as if: Ars.

RADIATING PAIN: Mez., Spig.

RAW: Arg-n., Kali-i., Lyc.

RED: Asar., Bell., Merc., Merc-i., Myrt-c., Rad-met., Rhus-t, Spig.

Agg.: vomiting or hiccough: Apis, Arn., Asar., Bry., Chin., Lyc., Nux-v., Puls., Sep., Sil., Verat.

RETINITIS: Kali-p.

RUBS: Gamb., Sanic., Seneg.

RUBBING, **Amel.:** Cina, Croc., **Puls.**

SMALL, as if: Lach.

SMART: Manc., Rad-met., Ran-b.

SPARKLING: Bell., Stram.

SQUINT: **Alum.,** BELL., Calc., Cic., Con., Cupr., **Cycl.,** HYOS., Nat-m.

divergent: Hyos., Nat-m.

STARING: Bell., Cic., Hell., **Hyos.,** Ign., Op., Stram.

STRAIN, sprained, etc.: Croc., Lilt., Naja, **Nat-m.,** Onos., Phys., Rad-met.

SUNKEN: **Abrot.,** Ant-c., Ant-t., **Ars.,** Camph., **Chin.,** Cina, Ferr., **Ph-ac.,** Sec., Spig., Staph., Sulph., Verat.

SWEAT on: Mag-c. (r).

SWELLED, as if: Coll., Com., **Guaj.,** Mez., **Nat-m.,** Op.,

Par., Prun., Rhus-t., Rumx., Sanic., Seneg., **Spig.,** Spong.

TEARS: Colch., Ip., Kali-p.

hot: Phyt., Rhus-t.

itching, causing: Ars., Senec.

music, Agg.: Graph.

pains: Ran-b.

thick: Tarent.

varnish mark, leave: Euphr., Graph., Nat-m., Petr., **Rhust.,** Thuj.

TINEA CILIARIS: Mag-m.

TOUCH, **Agg.:** Aur.

TWISTING **or revolving,** as if: Phos., Phys., Pop-c.

UPWARD, from: Berb., Graph., Lach.

VERTEX, to: Lach., Thlasp., Violo.

WIND, **blowing on:** Cham., Flac., Lach., Mez., Puls., Sep., Syph., Thuj.

WINKING: Merc-d.

WIPE, **must:** Euphr.

YELLOW: Nux-v., Spig.

night: Stram.

VISION

Arg-n., Aur., BELL., **Con., Cycl., Gels., Hyos.,** Jab., Lyc., NAT-M., Nux-v., Op., **Phos.,**

Puls., Ruta, Sep., **Sil.**, **Stram.**, SULPH.

ACCINMMODATION: Phys.

ASTHENOPIA: Jab.

ACUTE: Hyos.

AFFECTED, glittering, motes, dim, etc., **then headache**: Gels., Glon., Graph., Iris, KALI-BI., Lach., **Nat-m.**, Phos., Podo., PSOR., Sep., Sulph., Ther., **Tub.**

BLACK, suddenly, blind spells, etc.: BELL., Caps., Cic., **Con.**, Cycl., Glon., Graph., Hyos., Merc., **Nat-m.**, Olnd., Phos., Puls., Sep., Sil., Stram., Sulph.

BLINDNESS: Con., **Hyos.**, Op., Puls., Sil., **Stram.**

COUGHING, **Agg.**: Ign., Kali-m.

CROSSED: Con., Kali-bi.

DAZZLED: Kali-c., Sil.,

DIM, blurred, etc.: Calc., Cann-s., **Caust.**, Con., Cycl., **Euphr.**, Gels., Hep., Nat-m., Phos., **Puls., Sil.**

EYES, **closing, Agg.**: Bell., Bry., Calc., Thuj., Verat-v.

FARSIGHT: Calc., Nat-m., SEP., SIL.

FIELD, of: Phos., Thuj.

sees, objects besides: Calc., Camph., Cann-s., Coloc., Graph., Ign., Lac-c., Nux-m., Nux-v., Stram., Thuj.

FLICKERING, flames, red, etc.: BELL., **Cycl., Graph.**, Hyos., Kali-c., **Phos.**, Sep., **Spig.**

GLIMMERINGS, glitterings: **Graph.**, Iod., Lach., **Nux-v.**, Ol-an., Phos., Stroph-h., Syph.

HEADACHE, during: Bell., Iris, Ph-ac., Podo., **Puls.**, Zinc.

follows: Sil.

after, **Agg.**: Caust., Con., Lach., Phos., Sil., Sulph.

ILLUSIONS of: Bry., **Hyos.**, Op., Spig., **Stram.**, Verat.

animals, bugs, etc.: Cimic., **Hyos., Stram.**

bright objects: Hyos., Nat-c., Valer.

colors: Bell., Osm., Phos.

black: Caps., Cycl., Graph., Phos., Sep., Sil., **Stram.**, Sulph.

blue: Crot-c., Lyc., **Zinc-ar.**

dark, rich, etc.: Stram.

green: Phos., Phyt., Vario.

purple: Verat-v.

rainbow: Ph-ac.

red: BELL., Hyos., Merc-i-f., Myrt., **Phos.**, Rad-met., Ruta, Sulph., **Verat-v.**

rings, of: Calc., Elaps.

striped: Sep.

streaks: Bell., Caust., Ox-ac., Pyrog.

yellow: Dig., Sep.

diplopia: Aur., Bell., Cic., GELS., **Hyos.,** Nat-m., Nit-ac., Phos., Puls., Sulph., Verat., Verat-v.

vertical: Atrop., Kali-bi., Rhus-t., Seneg., Stram., Syph.

distances, of: Cann-s., Carb-an., Onos., Stram.

fantastic, apparitions, etc.: Bell., Stram., Verat.

fiery, bright, etc.: Ars., Bell., Cinnb., Hyos., **Kali-c.,** Kreos., Nat-c., **Phos.,** Spig.

Comp., **Red.**

flies, musca volitantes, etc.: Agar., Sil., **Stram.**

right: Chinin-s., Cimic., Sel., **Sil.**

left: Agar., Calc., **Caust.,** Merc., **Sulph.**

hair, as of a: Lach., Plan.

halos: Lach., PHOS., Puls., **Sulph.**

hemiopia: Chion., Lach., **Lyc.,** NAT-M.

imaginary, on closing eyes: Bell., Bry., **Calc.,** Thuj.

large, as if too objects seem: Hyos., Nux-m., Phos.

letters running together: Nat-m., Sil., Thlasp.

lightnings: Spig.

mist: Calc., Caust., Croc., **Phos.**

near, too: Bov.

small, objects appear: Berb., Carb-v., Cycl., Nat-s., Plat.

spotted (like drops before): Amm., Kali-c., **Phos.,** Sil.

veil, as of a: Phos.

wavering: Morph., Zinc-chr.

zig-zags: Con., Nat-m., Sul-i.

IMAGES, **retina retains, too long:** Gels., **Jab., Lac-c.,** Nat-m., **Tab.,** Tub.

LIGHT, **artificial, Agg.:** Nat-m.

LIGHT, **aversion to:** Hyos.

desires: Gels., Stram.

LOOKING **down:** Stann., Verat.

LUMINOUS: Valer.

MENSES, **before, Agg.:** Dict.

during, Agg.: Cycl., Graph., Puls., Sep.

ONE **eye, using, Amel.:** Kali-bi., Phos., Phys.

NEARSIGHT: Con., **Nit-ac., Phos.,** Ph-ac., **Puls.**

PALE: **Sil.**

PARALYSIS OF OPTIC NERVE: Bell., **Caust.,** Con., **Gels.,** Hyos., **Phos.,** Puls., Sec., Sil., Stram., Sulph.

PHOTOPSIES: Sec., Sep.

RETINA, retains images too long: Gels., Lac-c., Nat-m., Phos., Tab., Tub.

SCINTILLATIONS: Kali-m.

SHADE, Amel.: Con., Phos.

STOOPING, Agg.: Ther.

WEAK: Anac., Bell., Chin., Nat-m.

EARS

Aur., Bell., Calc., Cham., FERR-P., Graph., Hep., Lyc., Mang., MERC., Petr., Phos., Pic-ac., Plan., Psor., PULS., SIL., SULPH., Tell., Zinc-chr.

RIGHT: Bell., Fl-ac., Iod., Kali-c., Kali-n., Nit-ac., Nux-v., Plat., Sil., Spong.

LEFT: Anac., Asaf., Borx., Graph., Guaj., Ign., Olnd., Viol-o.

LEFT TO RIGHT: Graph., Mur-ac.

ALTERNATING SIDES: Bell., Bry., Caps., Caust., Chel., Cocc., Ferr-p., Glon., Kali-c., Mag-m., Med., Mosch., Nit-ac., Sulph.

and teeth alternate: Plan.

EXTERNAL: Alum., Kali-c., Kreos., Merc., Ph-ac., Sep., Spig.

red: Acon., Puls., Sulph.

left: Ant-c., Carb-v., Kreos.

INTERNAL: Calc., Caust., Graph., Kali-c., Mang., Nux-v., Phos., Psor., Puls., Sep., Spig.

BEHIND, (also mastoids): Aur., Bar-c., Calc., Canth., Caps., Caust., Graph., Lach., Lyc., Merc., Olnd., Petr., Phos., Psor., Sanic., Sil., Staph., Zinc-chr.

mastoiditis: Calc-p., Caps., Ferr-p., Lach., Phos., Sil.

moisture: Graph., Lyc.

nape to: Mur-ac.

BELOW: Bell.

BETWEEN: Plan.

LOBULES: Bar-c., Caust., Chin., Kreos.

GLANDS: Bell., Cham., Con., Lach., Merc., Rhus-t., Sil.

ABSCESS: Calc-pic., Merc., Syph.

ACHING: Cham., Ferr-p., Nux-v., Puls.

BURNING, drum (tympanum): Ang.

COLD, Agg.: Caps.

Amel.: Bell.

COLDS, Agg.: Ferr-p., Merc-d.

CRASHING: Acon., Glon., Phos., Rhus-t., Sil.

CRACKED, behind: Caust., Cist., Fl-ac., **Graph.**, Merc-c., Mez., Mur-ac.

CRACKING in: Ars., Dig., Glon., **Phel.**

CRACKLING: Coff.

DISCHARGE: Calc., Con., **Lyc.**, Merc., Psor., Puls., Sil., Viol-o.

briny: Graph., Sel., **Tell.**

suppressed: PULS.

DRUM, perforated: Sil.

DRYNESS: Graph., Lach.

EUSTACHIAN TUBE: Bar-m., **Kali-m.**, Merc-d., Nux-v., Petr.

itching: Nux-v., Petr., Senec., Sil.

EXCORIATED, raw: All-c., **Ars.**, **Kali-bi.**, Merc., PSOR., Sulph., Tell.

FETOR: **Calc.**, Carb-v., **Caust.**, Hep., Kali-p., Nat-c., PSOR., **Sil.**, **Sulph.**, Thuj.

INFLAMED: FERR-P., Phos., Sulph., Tell.

KIDNEYS and: Thuj., Viol-o.

LYING ON FACE, **Amel.**: Rad-met.

MENSES, before: Acon.

MOISTURE, behind: Graph., Psor.

NOISES, tinnitus, Meniere's disease: Arn., Benz-ac., Chinin-s., Eucal., Kali-m., Rad-met., Thyr.

OUTWARD in: Agar., Calc., Canth., Chel., Merc., Psor.

PUS, from: **Calc.**, Con., Hep., Merc., Phos., Puls., Sil.

SCABBY: Rad-met.

SCARLATINA, after: Mur-ac., Sulph.

STITCHES in: **Bell.**, Cham., Con., **Kali-c.**, Merc., Nux-v., **Puls.**, **Sulph.**

STOPPED, as if: Con., Kali-m., Lyc., Merc., **Puls.**, Sil.

SWASHING in: Sulph.

TICKING: Zinc-val.

URINARY SYMPTOMS, with: **Viol-o.**

WAX, foul: Caust.

WIND, **Agg.**: **Cham.**, Lach.

HEARING

ACUTE: Caust., Op., Sabal.

and dull alternately: Cic.

BAD: Aur., **Bell.**, Calc., Caust., Chinin-s., **Cic.**, **Con.**, Hyos., Kali-n., Led., **Lyc.**, MERC-D., **Nit-ac.**, Op., Petr., Phos., **Ph-ac.**, Puls., Sec., Sep., SIL., **Sulph.**

for the human voice: Chen., Phos.

DEAFNESS: Kali-m., Mag-c. (sudden), Verat-v.

spinal fever, after: Sil., Sulph.

COLDS, **Agg.**: Ferr-p., Kali-m., Merc-d., Phos.

ILLUSORY SOUNDS, **tinnitus**: Bell., Calc., Caust., **Chin.**, Chim-s., Graph., Kali-i., Kali-m., Puls., Spong., Sulph.

crashings, cracking, explosions: Aloe, Bar-c., **Dig.**, Kali-bi., Kalm., Mosch., **Rhus-t.**, Sabad., Zinc.

echoing, reverberations: Caust., Coloc., Phos.

fluttering: Spig.

humming, buzzing: Calc., Caust., **Chin., Puls.**, Sulph.

pulsating: Bell., **Calc.**, Cann-s., **Ferr-p.**, Nit-ac., **Phos.**, Puls.

ringing: Calc., Cann-s., **Chin.**, Nux-v., Puls.

roaring, rumbling, etc.: Aur., Bell., Caust., Graph., Nux-v., Puls., Staph., Sulph.

rushing: Petr., Phos.

MOTION, **Agg.**: Verat-v.

NOISE, **Agg.**: Acon., BELL., Coff., Nux-v., Op., Spig., **Ther.**

Amel.: Calen., **Graph.**, Jab., Nit-ac.

PARALYSIS, **auditory**: Bell., Hyos., Puls., Sil.

SENSITIVE: **Acon.**, Aur., **Bell.**, Cham., Chin., COFF., Lyc., Nux-v., Sep., Sil., Spig., **Ther.**

SNAP, **Amel.**: Sil.

SOUNDS, **location of:** Arg-n., Carb-an., Kali-bi.

TICKING **sounds:** Zinc-val.

VARIABLE: Chen.

VOICES, **hears:** Acon., Cham., Chlol., Nit-ac.

NOSE AND ACCESSORY CAVITIES

Acon., Aesc., Alum., **Ars., Aur.**, Calc., Graph., **Hep.**, Hydr., Ign., Iod., KALI-BI., **Kali-i.**, Lyc., **Merc.**, Merc-i-f., **Nat-m.**, Nit-ac., Nux-v., Phos., PULS., Sabad., **Sep.**, SIL., Spig., **Sulph.**, Zinc-chr.

ONE SIDE OF: Am-m., Hep., Ign., Nux-v., Phos., Phyt., **Sabad.**, Sin-n., Sil.

right: Con., Spig., Teucr.

left: Carb-v., Nat-m., Rhod., Sep.

alternating between: Kali-i., Lacc., Lach., Mez., Nux-v., **Phos.**, Phyt., Rad-met., Rhod., **Sin-n.**, Sulph.

EXTERNAL: **Aur.**, Carb-v., Caust., Kali-c., **Merc.**, Nat-c., Ph-ac., Puls., **Rhus-t., Sep.**, Spig., Sulph.

INTERNAL: All-c., Ars., Ars-i., Aur., Bell., **Calc.**, Euphr,

Graph., **Kali-bi.**, Kali-i.,
Sabad., Sil., Spig., Stict.,
Teucr.,

posterior: Cinnb., Elaps, Hydr.,
Lyc., **Merc.**, Merc-c., Merc-
i-r., **Nat-c.**, **Nat-m.**, Phos.,
Rumx., Sep., **Spig.**, **Staph.**,
Sulph., Ther.

ROOT **and above:** Acon., Ars.,
Calc., Cimic., **Cupr.**, Gels.,
Hep., **Hyos.**, **Ign.**, Iod., Kali-
bi., Kali-i., Merc., Par., Phos.,
Puls., Sang., Sars., Stict.,
Sulph., Verat-v., **Zinc.**

BONES: Aur., **Merc.**, Phos.

BRIDGE: Ph-ac., **Sep.**, Thuj.

bones: Kali-bi., Rhus-t.

SINUSES: Cinnb., Kali-bi., Lach.,
Phos., Syph.

TIP: Carb-an., Carb-v., Caust.,
Sep.

WINGS: Lyc., Thuj.

ABSCESS, **septal:** Anthraci.

tip: Acon., Anan.

AIR, **inspired, agg.,** see Conditions.

open, Amel.: All-c., Acon.,
Hydr., Iod., Nux-v., Puls.,
Tab., Tarent., Tell.

ALAE, **fanning:** Diph.

motions: Ant-t., Ars., Bapt.,
Bell., Brom., **Chel.**, Cupr.,
LYC., PHOS., Pyrog.,

Rhus-t., Spong., Sul-ac.,
Zinc.

BLOWING: Mang., Stict.

but no relief: Kali-bi., Psor.,
Stict., Teucr.

BORING into, with fingers, pick-
ing at, **itching:** Anac., **Arum-
t.**, **Aur.**, Carb-v., Caust.,
C1NA, Hep., Lyc., Merc.,
Nat-m., Nat-p., Phos., **Ph-ac.**,
Sabad., **Sil.**, Spig., Sulph.,
Teucr., Thuj., Zinc.

BURNING, **external:** Agar.

internal: Ars., Merc., Sang.

CARIES: Aur., Nit-ac.

COLD: Apis, **Verat.**

Agg.: Sulph.

CORYZA (fluent discharges):
Acon., **All-c.**, ARS., Camph.,
Cham., Euphr., Ferr-p.,
GELS., Hep., Kali-i., Lach.,
Merc., Merc-c., NUX-V.,
Puls., Rhus-t., Sel., Sulph.

aged, of: Am-c., Ant-c., Camph.

annual (hay fever): Ars, Am-br.,
Chen., Gels., **Kali-i.**, Kali-p.,
Nux-v., Phos., Psor., Sabad.,
Senec., Sep., **Sil.**, **Sulph.**

asthma: Ars., Chlor., Naja,
Sep.

autumn: Merc.

chronic: Hep., Kali-bi., Sil.,
Sulph.

coughing, Agg.: Agar., **Lach.**, Nit-ac., **Squil.**, Sulph., Thuj.

day, by: Nux-v.

diarrhea, then: Alum., Calc., Sang., Sel., Tub.

dries up: Stict.

eating, Agg.: Sanic.

epistaxis, with: Sil.

fluent, indoors: All-c., Calc-p., Nux-v.

hoarseness, with: Ars-i.

menses, at; menstrual colds: Am-c., **Graph.**, Kali-c., **Lach.**, Mag-c., Phos., Zinc.

stopped: Ars., **Arum-t.**, Brom., Calc., LACH., **Lyc.**, **Nit-ac.**, NUX-V., Teucr.

stuffy with: Calc.

CRAWLING, formication: Merc., Nat-m., Ran-b., Teucr.

CRUSTS, scabs: Alum., Aur., **Graph.**, Kali-bi., Merc., Nit-ac., Psor., **Sep.**, Stict., Sulph., Thuj.

CUTTING: Nit-ac.

DARK, sooty nostrils: Ant-t., Crot-h., Hell., Hyos.

DILATED alae: Cupr.

DISCHARGES, acrid: **Ars.**, **Ars-i.**, Arum-t., Merc., Nit-ac.

burning, hot, etc.: Acon., Nat-m.

changing: Staph.

cold: Ambr., Ichth., Lach.

cough, Agg.: Agar., **Lach.**, Nat-m., Nit-ac.

crusts, scabs, from: **Kali-bi.**, Sep., Thuj., Zinc-chr., Zinc-i.

dark: Cinnb., Merc-d.

eating on: Carb-an., Clem., Nux-v., Plb., Sanic., Sulph., Trom.

frothy: Merc., Sil.

glutinous: Hep., KALI-BI., Merc-c.

green: Kali-bi., Kali-i., Merc., Nit-ac., PULS., Sep.

lumpy: Alumn., Cinnb., KALI-BI., Merc-d., Phos., Sel., Sep., Sil., Solid., Zinc-i.

musty: Nat-c.

night: Nat-s.

salty: Aral., Cimic., Nat-m.

stopped, and: Bry., **Kali-bi.**, **Lach.**, Merc., Nux-v., Puls., Sil.

yellow-green: Kali-bi., Merc.

DRIPPING: All-c., Am-c., **Ars.**, Ars-i., Arum-t., Calc., Euph., Euphr., Graph., Kali-i., Nit-ac., Nux-v., Phos., Rhus-t., Sabad., Sulph., Tab.

DRY: Bell., Bry., Calc., GRAPH., Kali-bi., Lyc., Nat-m., Nux-m., Phos., Samb., **Sep.**, **Sil.**, Sin-n., Stict., Sulph., Thyr., Zinc-i.

DYSPNEA in: **Ars.**, Kreos., Lach., Puls., Sabad., Sulph.

EPISTAXIS: **Ferr-p.** (recurrent), HAM., Phos., Vip-t.

from coughing: Bell., Dros., Lach., Nux-v., **Phos.**

Comp. **Hemorrhage.**

EXCORIATED: **All-c.**, ARS., Ars-i., Arum-t., Gels., Iod., Kali-i., **Merc.**, Merc-c., Nit-ac., Nux-v., Phos., Sin-n.

FETOR: **Aur.**, **Calc.**, Graph., Hep., Kali-bi., Merc., Nit-ac., Nux-v., **Puls.**, Sulph.

FLOWS, but is stopped: **Ars.**, Calc., Osm.

FOREIGN **body**, plug, etc., in: Psor., Ruta, Sep.

FOUL, **ozena**: Aur., Cadm-s., Calc., Kali-bi., Kali-i., Merc-c., Sep., **Thuj.**

GUSHES, **fluid**: Agar., Dulc., Euphr., Fl-ac., Hydr., Kali-bi., Lach., **Nat-c.**, NAT-M., Phos., Sel., **Thuj.**

HEAVY: Kali-bi., Merc., Phyt.

HOT: Sabad.

ITCHES: Caust., **Cina**, Sabad.

LYING, **Agg.**: Puls.

NOSTRILS, **dark**: Ant-t., Colch., Hell.

dirty: Merc.

drawn in: Cina.

sore: Nux-v.

NUMB: Acon., Bell.

OBSTRUCTED, **at night**: Am-c., Lyc., Zinc-i.

fresh air, by: Dulc.

ODORS in: Puls., Zinc-chr.

PAINFUL: Hep., Merc.

PEELING: Nit-ac., Phos.

POLYPI: CALC., Merc-i-r., Phos., Sang., **Teucr.**, Thuj., Zinc-chr.

PRESSURE **(of glasses)**, **Agg.**: Argn., Chin., Cinnb., Con., Cupr-ar., Fl-ac., Kali-bi., **Merc.**, Phos.

root: Cimic., Sep., Stict., Zinc.

PUS, from: Aur., **Calc.**, Con., Hep., LACH., **Merc.**, **Puls.**, Zinc-chr.

QUINSY: **Hep.**, Lach., Lyc., Nat-m., Psor., **Sil.**

RAW, **sore posteriorly**: Acon., Aral., Arum-t., CARB-V., Caust., Kali-n., Nat-m., Sep.

RED: Agar., ALUM., Apis, **Aur.**, Bell., Calc., Cann-s., Chel., Merc., Nit-ac., Phos., Rhus-t., SULPH.

ROSACEAE: Carb-an., Kali-bi., Rhus-t.

SADDLE across, brown: Carb-an., Lyc., Op., Sanic., SEP., Sulph.

pain: Cinnb., Thuj.

SENSITIVE to inspired air: Acon., Aur., Brom., Camph., Cimic., Cist., Cor-r., Ign., Med., Nux-v.

SEPTUM, perforated: Kali-bi., Merc., Merc-c.

SMELL: Aur., BELL., Calc., Colch., Graph., Hep., Lyc., Nat-m., NUX-V., PHOS., Puls., Sep., Sil., SULPH.

acute: Ars., Aur., Bell., Carb-ac., Chin., Coff., Colch., Graph., Lyc., Nux-v., Phos., Sabad., Sep., Sulph.

Comp. Odors, Agg.

illusory: Bell., Calc., Par., Sulph.

catarrh, as of: Puls., Sulph.

earth, as of: Verat.

foul: Bell., Par., Puls.

sulphur, as of: Nux-v.

and taste, lost: Anac., Crot-t., Just., Mag-m., Nat-m., Puls., Sil.

weak: Bell., Calc., Hyos., Nat-m., Plb., Puls., Sep., Sil.

SNEEZING: All-c., Ars., Ars-i., Carb-v., Cina, Gels., Ign., Kali-i., Nat-m., NUX-V., Puls., Rhus-t., Sabad., Seneg., Sil., Squil., Sulph.

abortive: Carb-v., Nux-v.

odors, Agg.: Phos.

cough, with: Agar., Bell., Psor., Squil.

persistent: Cycl., Sabad., Sang.

violent: Agar., Nux-v., Sabad.

SNEEZING, Agg. least uncovering: Nux-v., Pyrog., Rhus-t., Sil.

SNUFFLES: Kali-bi., Med., Phos., Osm., Sabad., Samb., Vib.

SWELLED: Bell., Caust., Kali-c., Merc., Nat-c., Ph-ac., Puls., Rhus-t., Sep.

thick: Bar-c., Calc., Nat-c., Phos., Sars., Sulph.

SYPHILIS: Aur.

TENSION: Eucal., Ham., Kali-i.

TWITCHING: Ambr., Am-c., Aur., Calc., Chel., Con., Hyos., Kali-bi., Nat-m., Plat.

ULCERS: Ars., Merc., Puls., Nat-m.

WEATHER, changing, Agg.: Ars.

WINTER, Agg.: Amm-c., Am-c., Ars.

FACE

Acon., Ant-c., Apis, Ars., **Bell.**, Bry., Caust., Cham., Chin., Ferr., Hyos., Lyc., Mag-p., **Merc.**, **Nux-v.**, Op., **Rhus-t.**, Stram., **Sulph.**, Verat.

RIGHT: Apis, **Bell.**, Cact., Calc., Canth., Chel., **Kalm.**, Lyc., Nat-c., Nux-v., **Sang.**, Zinc.

to left: Graph.

LEFT: Acon., **Coloc.**, Con., **Lach.**, Rhus-t., Sep., **Spig.**, Staph.

ALTERNATING SIDES: Chin., Lyc., Phos.

TEMPLES (see **Head**): Ang., **Bell.**, Lyc.

ZYGOMA: **Aur.**, **Kali-bi.**, Olnd., Stann., Staph., Verb.

CHEEKS: Bell., Caust., Ign., Merc., **Rhus-t.**, Staph.

hang down: Apis.

heat, one: Tab., Tub. (affected side).

red: Sep. (one).

EYEBROWS: Nat-m.

hair, falling: Kali-c., Med., Plb., Sel.

EYES, around: Asaf., **Cinnb.**, Hep., Ign., Kali-bi., Merc.

Comp., **Orbits.**

JAW-BONES: Phos., Sil.

ache: Merc., Phyt.

angles, of: Ign., Merc., Phyt., Sang.

boring: Plat.

cracking: Nit-ac., Rhus-t.

cramp: Tab., Verat.

dislocation, easy: Ign., Petr., **Rhus-t.**

drop: see **Mouth open.**

lower jaw: Bell., Caust., Cham., Cocc., Lach., Laur., Nat-c., Plb., Staph., **Zinc.**

painful: Caust.

snap shut: Bell., Cic., **Ign.**, Lyss., Merc., Nux-v., Plat., Rhus-t.

spasms: Tab.

thickened: Hecla (lower).

throbbing, lower: Nat-m.

upper: Phos.

upper jaw: Am-c., Carb-v., Chin., Kreos., **Phos.**, Zinc.

wagging: Bry.

MALAR BONES: **Ars-i.**, Coloc., Glon., Kali-bi., Kali-i., Mag-c., Mez., Ol-an., Sep., Stront-c., Thuj., Tub.

MAXILLARY JOINT: Bell., Ign., Merc., **Rhus-t.**, Thuj.

MAXILLAE, cracks: Rhus-t.

MASSETERS: Hydr-ac., Ign.

cramp: Cocc., Cupr., Stram., Strych.

ABOUT MOUTH: Ars., Bry., Cina, Kali-m., **Kreos.**, Nat-m., Rhus-t., Sep., Staph., **Sulph.**

LIPS: Ars., Arum-t., **Bell.**, Bry., **Nat-m.**, **Rhus-t.**, Sep., Sil., **Sulph.**

upper: Bar-c., Carb-v., Kali-c., Sulph., Zinc.

lower: Bry., Ign., Puls., Sep.

corners: Ant-c., Bell., Merc., Phos.

black: ARS., **Chin.**, Merc., Ph-ac., Verat.

bleeding: Arum-t., Lach.

blue: Camph., **Cupr.**, **Dig.**, Lyc., Nux-v., Spong., Verat.

changing color: Sulph.

cracked, chapped: Ars., Arum-t., **Bry.**, Calc., Graph., Ign., Meny., Merc., Mur-ac., **Nat-m.**, Puls., Sep.

corners: Arum-t., Cund., Graph., Mag-p., Merc., Mez., Nit-ac.

middle: Calc., **Cham.**, Hep., **Nat-m.**, Phos., **Puls.**, Sep.

crusty, scabby, at angles: Ars., Graph., Merc., Mur-ac., Nat-m., Ph-ac., **Rhus-t.**, Sep., **Sil.**, Staph., Thuj.

drawn up, retracted: Ang., Ant-t. (up), **Camph.**, Nux-m., Nux-v., Tab.

droop: Bar-c., Merc., Nux-v.

dry: Caust., Nux-m., Puls., Rhus-t., Thyr.

egg, albumen on: Ol-an., Ph-ac.

herpes, on: Ars., **Nat-m.**, Rhus-t.

jerked up: Tell.

licks: Agar., Aloe, Ars., Lyc., Nat-m., **Puls.**, Stram.

numb: Acon., Nat-m.

peeling: **Arum-t.**, Cham., Con., Kali-c., **Lac-c.**, Nat-c., **Nat-m.**, Nit-ac., Nux-v., Puls.

picking at: Ars., Arum-t., Kali-br., Tarent.

pouting, thick: Bar-c., Calc., Graph., Merc., Nat-m., Psor., Syph.

raw, angles: Ant-c., Arum-t., Graph.

red: Aloe, **Ars.**, Bell., Calc. (up), Merc-c., Nat-m. (up), Sep. (low), SULPH., Thyr.

upper: Ars-i.

salty: Merc., Nat-m., Sulph.

shrivelled: Ant-t.

sore: Mur-ac.

sticky: Merc-i-r., Nux-m., Zinc.

sweat, upper: Med.

swelled: **Ars.**, Bell., Merc-c.

upper: **Calc.**, Hep., **Nat-m.**, Nit-ac., Psor.

lower: Asaf., Lach., **Merc.**, Sep., **Sulph.**

twitching, trembling, spasm: Carb-v. (up), Cham., Olan., Senec., Vip-t.

ulcerated: Borx.

vesicles, cold sores, etc.: **Ars.**, NAT-M., Phos., **Rhus-t.**, Sep.

CHIN: Caust., Plat., Sil.

ACHE: Rhus-t., Stann., Staph.

pregnancy, in: Mag-c.

BESOTTED, stupefied: Arn., Bapt., Bry., Crot-h., Gels., Hyos., **Op.**, Stram.

BLUISH: Acon., **Ars.**, Bell., CUPR., Ip., Kali-m., **Lach.**, Op., **Verat.**, **Verat-v.**

about eyes: Ant-t., Ars., **Chin.**, Ip., Merc-i-f., Olnd., Rhus-t., Sec., Staph., Thuj., Verat.

about mouth: Cina, Cupr., Verat.

Comp. **Color in General.**

BORING: **Aur.**, Hep., Mag-c., Mez., Plat.

BROWN: Anthraci.

CHANGING COLOR: Acon., Bell., Ferr., **Ign.**, Phos., Plat., Sep., Stram.

CHEWING MOTIONS: Acon., Bell., BRY., Calc., **Cham.**, Cina, **Hell.**, **Lach.**, **Lyc.**, Verat-v.

swallows, and, in sleep: Cina, Ign.

CHLOASMA: Caul., Kali-p., Sep.

Cobweb, on: Graph.

COLD: Abrot., Arn., **Ars.**, Camph., **Carb-v.**, Cina, Colch., Lyc., VERAT.

wind on, Agg.: Arg-n.

CONGESTED: Acon., **Bell.**, Hyos., Nux-v., Op., **Stram.**

COUGH, Agg.: Samb.

CRAMP: Coloc., Mez., **Plat.**, Verb., Tab., Verat.

DEAD, look: Thuj.

DEATHLY, pinched, collapsed, etc.: Ars., **Verat.**

Comp. **Collapse.**

DISTORTED: Ars., **Bell.**, Cocc., Hyos., Ip., Lyc., Op., **Stram.**

DUSKY, **dark, sooty**: Ant-t., **Bapt.**, Colch., Gels., Hell., Iod., Murac., Op., **Phos.**, Psor., Sec., Stram., Tub

EARTHY, **dirty brown**, etc.: Ars., Calc-p., **Chin.**, **Ferr.**, Ferr-pic., Iod., Lyc., Merc., Nat-m., Nux-v., Op., Petr., **Psor.**, Sulph.

EATING, **Amel.**: Rhod.

EMACIATED, thin: Alum., Ars., Calc., Carb-v., Ferr., Iod., Nat-m., Sel., Staph., Tarent.

ERUPTIONS: Ant-c., Kreos., Led., Rhus-t., Sep.

about lips: Ars., **Nat-m.**, Rhus-t.

eczematous: Ars., Borx., Calc., Cic., Graph., Kreos., Merc., Mez., Rad-met., **Rhus-t.**, Sars., Solid., Vio-t.

eyebrows, eyes about, etc.: Ant-c., Apis, Ars., Bar-c., Caust., Hep., Merc., Sil., Sulph.

menses at: Graph.

pimples: Carb-v.

EXPRESSION, changed: **Acon.**, Apis, Arg-n., ARS., Bell., Camph., **Gels.**, Hyos., Lyc., Mang., **Op.**, Phos., Ph-ac., Sec., STRAM., Verat.

FORMICATION, starts in: Nux-v., **Sec.**

FRECKLES: **Ant-c.**, Calc., Lyc., Nat-c., **Puls.**, Sulph.

FRIGHTENED LOOK: Acon., Cupr., Stram.

FROWNING: Cham., Hell., Hyos., LYC., Sep., Stram., Sulph., Verat.

FUZZY: Psor.

GLISTENS, **waxy**: Ars., Thuj.

GRIMACES: Agar., **Hyos.**, Plat., Stram.

HEAT, of, affected side: Tub.

rises into: Kali-bi., Sang.

HECTIC SPOTS: Acon., Ars., Calc., **Chin.**, Ferr., Iod., Kali-c., Kreos., Lyc., Ol-j., **Phos.**, Ph-ac., Puls., **Sang.**, Sil., Stann., **Sulph.**, Tub.

HOT: **Bell.**, Calc., Cham., Ferr., Nux-v.

IMMOBILE: Lycps-v., Mang.

INJURIES: Symph.

ITCHING: Calc.

LOCKJAW, mouth clenched, etc.: Ang., **Bell.**, Camph., Cann-s., Cic., Cham., Hyper., Ign., Merc., Merc-i-f., **Nux-v.**, Op., Sec., Verat.

MOTTLED, **spotted**: Ferr-p., **Lach.**, Lachn., Led., Manc., Oena., Stroph-h.

NUMB: Acon., Asaf., Cham., Gels., Kalm., Mez., PLAT., Sep., **Verb.**

OLD LOOK: **Arg-n.**, Bar-c., **Calc.**, Lyc., OP., Sanic., Sars., Sul-ac., Sulph., Syph., Tub.

PAIN, **neuralgia, migraine, proso-palgia**, etc.: Ars., Bry., Caust., Chin., Chion., **Coloc.**, Gels., Kali-bi., Kalm., **Mag-c.**, Mag-p., Mez., Nat-m., Nat-s., **Nux-v.**, Onos., Phos., Prun., Psor., Ran-b., Rob., **Sang.**, Sep., Sil., Spig., Stann., Ther., Thuj., Verb.

orbital: Cedr., Chinin-s.

radiating: Sang., Spig.

sleepy before: Sulph.

PALE: Stroph-h.

hot and: Cimic., Cina, Croc., Hyos., Op.

around mouth: Arum-t., Bell., Cic., Merc-c.

and nose: Carb-ac., Cina, **Phos.**

linea nasalis: Aeth., Ant-t., Carb-ac., **Cina,** Ip., Merc-cy., **Phos., Stram.,** Tarent.

rising, on: Acon., Verat.

PARALYSIS: Caust.

PEAKED: Staph.

POINT, **drawn to:** Bism., Brom., Kali-n.

PUFFY, **bloated:** Acet-ac., **Acon.,** APIS, Apoc., **Ars., Bry., Calc.,** Crot-h., **Lach.,** Laur., Lyc., Merc., Merc-d., Phos., Psor., Verat-v.

pale: Apis, Ars., **Calc.,** Graph., Lyc.

red: Acon., Chin., Lach., Op., Stram.

RED cheeks: Acon., Arn., Bell., CHAM., Chin., **Ferr., Ign.,** Lyc., Mosch., Nux-v., Phos., **Puls.,** Sulph., Tarent.

circumscribed: Chin., Ferr, Lyc., Phos., Sulph.

cold, but: Caps., Mosch.

cough, **Agg.:** Tub.

eating, after: Caps., Nux-v., Sulph.

eyes around: Apis, Borx., Chinin-ar., **Elaps,** Lappa, MALAND., Merc-i-f., Myrt., Puls., Rad-met., **Rumx.,** Sil.

flushes: Amyl-ns.

hot, and: Bell.

one side: Acon., Arn., Bar-c., Bell., CHAM., Chel., **Ign.,** Lac-c., Merc., Mosch., Nux-v., **Phos.,** Puls., Ran-b., Spig., Sulph.

right: Ars., **Calc.,** Lachn., Merc., Mosch., Nat-c., Sang., Sul-ac., Tab.

left: Acet-ac., Agar., Am-c., Apis, Borx., Cham., **Lyc.,** Nat-m., PHOS., **Rhus-t.,** Stram., **Sulph.,** Thuj., Verat.

alternating: Chel., Lach., Nat-p., **Phos., Rad-met.**

and pale, alternately: Aloe, Ferr-p., Glon., Op., Stram.

pimples: Led.

stool, during: Caust.

reddish-yellow: Chel., Gels.,
Lach., NUX-V.

RUDDY, florid: Arn., Ferr.

SICKLY: Chin., Nux-v., Psor., Sul-
ac., Teucr.

SPOTTED, blotched: Acon., Ars.,
Carb-an., Kali-bi., Kreos.,
Lach., Rhus-t., Sil., Sulph.

STUPID look: Bar-c., Hell.

SUNKEN: Ars., Camph., Chin.,
Hydr., Kali-m., Op., Par.,
Rhus-t., Sec., Verat.

SWEAT on: Lyc.

cold: Ant-t., Ars., Carb-v., Cina,
Merc-c., Tab., VERAT.

eating, Agg.: Cham., Nat-m.

hot: Cham.

SWOLLEN, turgid: Am-m., Apis,
Arn. (r), ARS., BELL., Bry.,
Cham., Kali-c., Kali-chl.
[A.M.], Lac-d., Lycps-v., Lyc.,
Merc., Merc-i-f., Nux-v., Op.,
Phos., Polyg. (r), Rhus-t.,
Sang. (r.), Stram., Tarent.

cheeks: Arn., Cham., Merc.

eyes, under: Apis, Ars., Phos.

between and brows: Kali-c.

one side: Arn., Bell., Bry.,
Cham., Merc., Merc-c., Sep.,
Spig.

veins of temples: Ars., Glon.

TENSION: Puls., Verb., Viol-o.

TERRIFIED, look: Acon., Spong.,
Verat.

TONGUE, protruding, Agg.:
Syph.

TWITCHING, trembling, etc.:
Agar., Ars., BELL., Cham.,
Gels., Ign., Lyc., Mygal., Op.,
Rheum, Senec., STRAM.,
Tell., Thuj.

about mouth: Op., Thuj.

lower jaw: Ant-t., Carb-v., Gels.,
Phos.

WHITE about nose and mouth:
Carb-ac., Phos.

WRINKLED: Abrot., Alum.,
Calc., Lyc.

YELLOW: Ars., Bry., Chel., Chin.,
Coll., Ferr., Lyc., Mag-c.,
Merc., NUX-V., Plb., Podo.,
SEP.

about eyes: Coll., Mag-c., Nit-
ac., Nux-v., Spig.

across, nose: SEP.

hair, at edge of: Caul., Kali-p.,
Med.

nose and mouth, about: Nux-v.

red spots: Kreos.

TEETH

ACON., Ant-c., Bell., Bry.,
Calc., Calc-p., Caust.,
CHAM., Chin., Coff., Kreos.,

Lach., MERC., Mez., Nux-v.,
Plan., Podo., PULS., **Rhus-t.**,
SEP., Sil., Spig., STAPH.,
Sulph.

RIGHT: Bell., Fl-ac., Staph.

LEFT: Caust., Cham., Clem.,
Euph., Mez., Sep., Sulph.,
Thuj.

ALTERNATING SIDES: Ambr.,
Am-m., Caps., Chel., Iod.,
Kali-n., Lyc., Psor., **Puls.**,
Stram., Sulph., **Zinc.**

between upper and lower:
Acon., Laur., Nat-m., Puls.,
Rat., Rhod.

CHANGING ABOUT: Bry.,
Cycl., Graph., Hyos., Hyper.,
Kali-bi., Kali-c., Mag-c.,
Mang., Nat-m., Nux-m.,
Prun., Puls., Rhod., Sil., Thuj.

RADIATING: MERC.

ROW, in a whole: Ars., Aur., Carb-
v., Glon., Lach., Mag-c., Mag-
p., **Merc.**, Nat-m., **Nux-v.**,
Psor., Sep., Spig., **Staph.**, Zinc.

UPPER: Am-c., Bell., Carb-v.,
Chin., Kreos.

LOWER: Bell., Canth., **Cham.**,
Nat-c., Plb., Staph.

CANINE: Calc., Nux-v., Sep., Sul-
ac.

INCISORS: **Colch.**, Phos., Sulph.

behind: **Phos.**

MOLARS: Bry., **Kreos.**, Staph.,
Zinc.

ROOTS: Mag-c.

ABSCESSED roots: Calc., Hep.,
Kreos., Phos., **Sil.**, Staph.

ACIDS, **Agg.**: Mur-ac.

AIR, **Agg.**: Rat., Tub.

BITES, cheek or tongue: Cic., **Ign.**,
Nit-ac.

BITING, **Amel.**: Caust., Mur-ac.,
Ol-an., **Phyt.**, **Podo.**

BLACK: Merc., **Staph.**

BLUNT: Mez., Ran-s., Rob., Sul-
ac.

CHATTER: Nux-v.

CLENCHING: Merc-i-f., **Phyt.**

COATED, as if: Colch., Dios.,
Phos.

COLD, **Agg.**: Rhod.
    Amel.: Coff., Ferr., Puls.

COLDS, **Agg.**: Mag-c.

CRUMBLING: Plan.

DECAY at roots: Fl-ac.
    on sides: Thuj.

DENTITION: Calc., Calc-p.,
Cham., Rheum, Sulph., Tub.

EARS, head, etc., to: Merc.

EATING, **Amel.**: Ign., Rhod.

EDGE, on: Calc., Chion., Dig.,
Iris, Lyc., Merc-i-f., Rob.

of gums, at: Am-c., Calc., Fl-ac.,
Mez., Syph., Thuj.

ENAMEL, thin: Fl-ac.

EXTENDING to ears, head or
face pain: Ant-c., Cham.,
Lach., Merc., Mez., Plan.,
Puls., Rhod.

GRINDING, clenching: Ars.,
BELL., Cina, Hyos., Lyc.,
Mag-p., Med., Phyt., Podo.,
Xan., Zinc-chr.

in sleep: Ars., Calc., Cann-s.,
CINA, Ign.

HEAVY: Fl-ac., Verat.

HOLLOW, early decay, soft,
brittle, broken, etc.: Ant-c.,
Bell., Borx., Calc., Cham.,
Cupr., Euph., Fl-ac., Kreos.,
Lach., Med., Merc., Mez.,
Nat-c., Par., Plb., Sep., Staph.

ICE water, Amel.: Clem., Coff.,
Ferr.

INTO, pains go: Chin., Ferr., Kali-
bi., Merc., Mez., Staph., Thuj.

JAMMED: Lach., Merc-i-f., Tub.

JERKING: Merc., Puls., Rhod.

LOOSE: Bry., Caust., Hyos.,
Merc., Merc-c., Nit-ac., Nux-
v.

LYING, Agg.: Rat.

MENSES, Agg.: Bar-c., Calc.,
Carb-v., Cham., Lach., Sep.,
Staph.

NIGHT: Cham., Lyc., Merc., Rat.,
Sulph.

NOISE, Agg.: Plan.

NUMB: Chin., Dulc., Phos., Plat.,
Rhus-t.

PREGNANCY, Agg.: Chin., Kali-
bi., Kreos., Sep.

PULLED: Calc.

QUIVERING: Phys.

RADIATING PAIN: Kali-bi.,
MERC., Mez., Nux-v., Staph.

ROUGH: Phys.

SENSITIVE fangs: Gels., Sulph.

SMOOTH, as if: Aesc., Colch.,
Dios., Phos., Sul-i.

SOFT: Med.

SORDES, slimy: Bry., Phos., Ph-
ac., Rhus-t.

STICKY: Arg-met., Crot-h., Eupi.,
Psor., Sang., Syph.

SWEETS, Agg.: Mur-ac.

TARTAR: Ars., Asc-t., Calen.,
Carbn-s., Chin., Epiph.,
Merc., Plb., Thuj.

TEMPLES to: Merc.

TOOTHACHE, see Teeth.

WORM in: Syph.

GUMS

Borx., Carb-v., Kali-c., Kreos.,
Merc., Nux-v., Staph.

UPPER: Calc., Ruta.

LOWER: Sars.

INNER: Phos., **Staph.**

ALTERNATING SIDES: Aeth.

ABSCESS: Echi., Merc., Sil.

BLEEDING: Ph-ac., Staph.

BORING: Merc.

CLENCHES: Lyc., **Phyt.**, Podo.

EXCORIATED: Carb-v., Sep.

INCISORS, behind: Merc-cy., **Phos.**

PALE: Staph.

RECEDING: Carb-v., Merc.

SORE: Carb-v., Merc.

SPONGY: Kali-p., Kreos., Merc., Mez., Sep., Thuj.

SUPPURATING, pyorrhea: Calc., Carb-v., Cist., Hep., **Merc.**, **Phos.**, **PULS.**, **Sil.**, Staph.

SWELLED: Merc., Nux-v., Sep., Staph., Sulph.

PALATE

Aur., Bell., Crot-h., **Merc.**, **Nux-v.**, Phos.

ABSCESS: Phos.

APHTHAE: Borx., **Kali-bi.**, Sars.

CRAWLING: Ars., Carb-v., Phos., Polyg-s., Ran-b., Sil.

DRY: Ph-ac.

EDEMA: Apis, Kali-i.

GREASY: Asaf., Card-m., Kali-p., Ol-an.

HARD: Bell., **Nit-ac.**, Nux-v., **Phos.**

ITCHING: Arum-t., Kali-p., Nux-v., Polyg-s., Sabad., Stry., Teucr.

RAW: Caust.

SCALDED: Sang., Sanic.

SOFT: Apis (uvula), Merc., Merc-c. (uvula), Merc-i-f. (rim).

SORE: Arum-t., Bell., Caust., Iris, Lach., Merc., NIT-AC., Nux-v., **Phos.**, Phyt.

STIFF: Crot-h., Grat., Nat-m.

SWELLED: Apis (uvula), Arg-met., Lach.

TONGUE

Bell., Hyos., **Merc.**, Mur-ac., **Nux-v.**, **Phos.**, **Plb.**, **Puls.**

ACROSS: Acet-ac., Asar., Cob., Kali-p., LACH., Merc.

DIAGONALLY: Rhus-t.

DOWN CENTER (stripe): Ant-t., **Arn.**, Ars., **Bapt.**, Caust., Lach., **Phos.**, Pyrog., **Rhus-t.**, VERAT-V.

EDGES: Apis, Nat-m., Phyt.

SIDE, one: Bell., **Calc.**, Lob., Mez., **Nat-m.**, RHUS-T., Sang., Sil., Thuj.

TIP: **Rhus-t.**, Sulph.

ROOT: Bapt., Kali-bi., Kali-i., Lach., Nat-s., Phyt.

STITCHING: Merc.

TEARING: Merc.

APHTHAE: **Borx.**, Carb-v., Kali-chl., Merc., Mur-ac., Sulph., Thuj.

BITES the: **Cic.**, **Ign.**, **Nit-c.**, Vip-t.

BLACK, blue, etc.: Ars., Carb-v., **Chin.**, Crot-h., Dios., Gymno., Lept., **Merc.**, **Phos.**, Rad-met.

BLUISH: Ars., Dig., Gymno.

BROAD: Mag-m., Merc.

BURNING, **tip**: Caps.

BURNT, scalded, as if: Acon., Ars., Bell., Calc-p., Hydr., Ign., **Iris**, Kali-i., Mur-ac., Nat-s., Plat., Ptel., **Puls.**, Sabad., Sang., **Verat-v.**

tip: Coloc.

CATCHES on teeth: Lach.

CENTER, down: Iris, Maland., Merc-c.

CLEAN: Cina, Dig., **Hyos.**, Ip., Mag-p., Sec.

COATED: Bell., **Bry.**, Chin., Merc., **Nux-v.**, Phos., Puls.

on one side: Daph.

white: Ant-c., Ars., Bell., Chin., Kali-m., Puls., Sulph.

yellow: Bry., Chin., **Merc-i-f.**, (base).

COLD: Camph., Iris.

CRACKS, fissures: Arum-t., **Bell.**, Hyos., **Kali-bi.**, Kali-i., Nit-ac., Phos., RHUS-T., Sulph.

center: Nit-ac., Syph.

CRAWLING: Plat., Sec.

DIRTY: Cean., Chin., Nat-s.

DOTTED : Ant-t., Bell., Graph., Stram.

DRY: **Ars.**, **BELL.**, **Bry.**, Calc., Nux-m., Phos., RHUS-T., Sulph.

half of: Bell., Sang.

ERUPTION on: Sars.

FILMY: Merc-i-f.

FLABBY: Merc.

FURRY: Merc.

FOAM, beads (edge): Aeth., Am-c., Apis, Iod., **Nat-m.**, Phos.

glands: Bar-c.

GLISTENING: Apis, Ars., Cist., **Kali-bi.**, Lach., Phos., Ter.

GRAY: Kali-m.

GREEN **at base**: Caps., Chion.

yellow: Nat-s.

HAIR on: Kali-bi., Nat-m., Nat-p., Sil.

HEAVY: Bell., **Gels.**, Glon., Kali-bi., Lach., Mur-ac., Nat-m., Nux-m., Nux-v.

INDENTED: Ars., Chel., Hydr., Kali-i., Mag-m., MERC., **Podo.**, Puls., Rhus-t., Stram.

INDURATED: Hydr., Merc-d.

INFLAMED: Acon., Apis, Bell., Crot-h., **Merc.**, Merc-c.

NEURALGIA: Crot-t., Mang.

NUMB, painless: Acon., **Anac.**, Cadm-s., **Con.**, Diph., **Gels.**, Lappa, Mag-c., Med., Nat-m., Nux-m., Puls., Rad-met., Sul-i., Tarent., Tell., Xan.

OILY: Phys.

PAINFUL: Agar., Caps., Thuj. (tip).

PALATE, sticks to: Kali-p., Nux-m.

PAPILLAE, **showing**: Arg-n., Ars., Bell., Caust., Kali-bi.

PARALYSIS: Bar-c., CAUST., Gels., Hyos., Lach., **Op.**, Plb.

PATCHY, mapped, spots, etc.: **Ars.**, Dulc., Hydr., Kali-bi., Lach., Merc., **Merc-c.**, NAT-M., **Nit-ac.**, Ran-s., **Rhus-t.**, Sep., Syph., **Tarax.**, Tub.

POINTED: Ip.

PROTRUDING, **Agg.**: Cocc., Cist., Cupr., **Kali-bi.**, **Phyt.**, Syph., Vario.

RANULA: Merc., **Thuj.**

RAW: Carb-v., **Nux-v.**, Sil.

RED: APIS, **Ars.**, Bell., Hyos., **Kali-bi.**, Lach., Merc., **Phos.**, Rhus-t.

along centre: Verat-v.

edges: Ars., Bell., Chel., **Merc.**

edges and tip: Apis, Sulph.

fiery: Apis, Pyrog., Sang.

tip, at: Ars., Merc-i-r., Phyt., **Rhus-t.**

triangle at tip: Arg-n., **Rhus-t.**, Sep.

ROUGH: Arum-t.

SANDY: Apis, Cist.

SHRIVELLED: Chion.

SLIMY: Eucal., **Puls.**

SMOOTH, glazed: Apis, Lach., Pyrog., Sul-i., Ter., Tub.

SORE, **painful**: Agar., Calc., Carb-v., Ign., **Nit-ac.**, Puls., Sabad., Sep.

edge: Apis, Zinc.

tip: Calc-p., **Kali-c.**, Lyc., RHUS-T., Sep., **Thuj.**

spot: Agar., Ant-c., **Sil.**, Tarax.

STIFF: Apis, Bell., Lyc., Merc-i-r., Mur-ac., Nat-m., **Rhus-t.**

STRAWBERRY: Bell., Ter.

STRIPE, widens toward tip: Calad.

SWELLED: **Acon.**, **Apis**, Ars.,
Bell., Caust., Crot-h., **Merc.**,
Polyg-s., Zinc.

THICK: **Gels.**

TICKLING: Stann.

TIP: Thyr., Zinc.

TREMULOUS: Agar., Apis,
Camph., Gels., **Lach.**, **Merc.**,
Phos., Sulph.

TWITCHINGS: Castm.

ULCER, **edge on:** Apis (1), Sil. (r),
Thuj. (r).

ULCERATED: A..g-n., Bapt.,
Carb-v., Mer..

VESICLES: Manc., Urt-u.

    edge: Am-c., Con., Lach., Nat-
m., Phos.

    tip: Apis, Caust., Kali-c., Lyc.,
Nat-c.

WEAK: Bar-c., Caust., Con.

WHITE at base: Kali-m., Nat-m.,
Sep.

WHITEWASH: Ant-c.

WRINKLED: Merc-i-r.

YELLOW: Hydr., Kali-p.

    at base: Merc-i-f., Nat-p., Nat-
s., Phyt.

MOUTH AND THROAT

Apis, Arg-n., Arum-t., **Bar-c.**,
BELL., **Caust.**, Gels., **Hep.**,
Kali-bi., Lac-c., **LACH.**, **Lyc.**,
MERC., **Merc-c.**, Merc-cy.,
Merc-i-f., Merc-i-r., **Nit-ac.**,
Nux-v., **Phos.**, Phyt., Puls.,
Rhus-t., Sulph.

RIGHT: **Agar.**, Am-c., **Apis**, **Bell.**,
Bry., Carb-ac., **Ign.**, Kali-m.,
Kreos., **LYC.**, **Merc.**, Merc-d.,
Merc-i-f., Phyt., Sang., Stann.,
Sulph., Syph., Tarent.

    to left: Apis, **BELL.**, Calc.,
Caust., LYC., MERC-I-F.,
Phos., Sabad., Sang., Sul-ac.

    cold drinks, Amel.: Apis, Calc.,
Merc-d., Merc-i-f., Phos.,
Phyt.

    hot, Amel.: Alum., **Lyc.**, Nux-v.

LEFT: Calc., Caust., Crot-h.,
Diph., Ferr., Hep., Kali-c.,
Lac-c., LACH., Merc-c.,
Merc-i-r., Naja, Petr., Ph-ac.,
Rhus-t., **Sabad.**, **Sep.**, **Sil.**,
Teucr., Til.

    to right: Calc., LACH., **Merc-i-
r.**, RHUS-T., Sabad., Stann.

    cold, Agg.: Lac-c., Manc., Merc-
i-r., Rhus-t., Sabad., Sil.

    Amel.: Daph., **Lach.**

    in A.M.: Cimic., Rhus-t.

ALTERNATING SIDES: **Alum.,**
Arn., Cocc., Coloc., **LAC-C.,**
Podo., Puls., Sulph.

THROAT PIT: Apis, Arg-n.,
Cham., Chlor., Hep., Kali-bi.,
Phos., **Rumx.,** Sang., **Sep.,**
Zinc-chr.

pressure: Calc.

BACK OF: Acon., Cocc., Kali-c.,
Merc., Nit-ac., Rhus-t.

TONSILS: Bar-c., **Bell.,** Guaj.,
Lach., Merc., **Merc-i-f., Merc-**
i-r., Nit-ac., Phyt.

chamois, skin, wash leather, etc.:
Phyt., **Rhus-t.**

chronicity: Bar-c., Bar-m.,
Brom., Hep., Kali-i., Lyc.,
Mez., Nat-m., Sul-i., Thuj.

enlarged: Bar-c., Calc-f., Calc-i.,
Calc-p., Lyc., Merc., Merc-
i-f., Merc-i-r., Nit-ac.,
Staph., **Tub.**

foul: Ail., Bapt., **Lach.,** Lyc.,
Merc., Nit-ac.

glisten: Apis, **Lac-c.**

gray: Kali-m., Merc-cy.

indurated: Alum., Bar-c., Phyt.

menses, at, Agg.: Lac-c.

red, bright: Acon., **Bell.,** Phyt.

dark: Aesc., Bapt., Carb-ac.,
Lach.

throb: Am-m., Phyt.

suppurating: Bell., Hep., Lach.,
Lyc., Merc., SIL., Tarent.

ADENOIDS: Agra., Calc., **Calc-**
p., Merc., Tub.

EUSTACHIAN TUBE: Fag.,
Hydr. (r), **Kali-m., Merc-d.,**
Sang. (l).

GULLET, **burning, in typhoid:**
Ars., Bell., Bry., Nux-v., Phos.,
Rhus-t., Sulph.

constriction, acute: Nux-v., Ran-
b.

chronic: Phos., Zinc.

cutting: Vinc.

inflamed: Verat-v.

lump in: Chel., Podo.

GLOTTIS, **spasm:** Bell., Calc.,
Calc-p., Gels., **Ign.,** Mosch.

UVULA: Apis, Kali-bi., Merc.,
Merc-c., Phyt.

dripping: All-c., Hydr., Merc-c.,
Spig.

edema: Apis, Kali-bi., Merc-c.,
Phyt., Rhus-t.

elongated, flaccid: Hyos., Sulph.

one side, hangs to: Apis (r),
Lach., Nat-m. (r).

swelled: Caps.

ulcerated: Kali-bi., Merc-s-cy.

ANGINA, **simple sore throat:**
Acon., Bell., Merc., Merc-i-f.,
Phos., Sep.

APHTHAE: Ars., Bapt., Borx., Kali-chl., Kali-m., **Merc.**, Rhus-t., Sulph., Sul-ac., **Thuj.**

APPLE core, choke pear, etc.: Merc., Nit-ac., Phyt., Plan., **Verat.**

BITTER: Chin., Con., Kreos., Menis., Phos., Sil., Verat., Zinc.

BROWN-RED: Lyc.

BURNING: Acon., ARS., **Arum-t.**, **Bell.**, Borx., Canth., Caps., Iris, Lach., MERC-C., Mez., Petr., **Phos.**, Phyt., Sang., Sulph., **Verat.**

heat in throat: Oena, Phyt., Ran-b.

burnt mouth: Iris, Puls., Sep.

CHEESY LUMPS FROM: **Agar.**, **Hep.**, **Kali-bi.**, KALI-M., Kali-p., **Mag-c.**, Merc-i-f., Phos., PSOR., Sanic., Sep., Sil.

old: Bry., Hep., Sanic.

CHOKING, constriction, spasms, narrow, as if: Arg-met., Bapt., **Bell.**, Canth., Caust., Cham., Con., Graph., Hyos., **Ign.**, **Lach.**, Laur., Lyc., Lycps-v., **Meph.**, Merc-c., Merc-i-r., NAJA, Nux-v., Phos., Plb., Rad-met., Rat., Spong., Stram., Stroph-h., Sulph., Ter., Thyr., **Verat.**

bending head back, Amel.: Hep., Lach.

goitre, in: Meph.

sleep, Agg.: **Lach.**, Spong.

from water: Bapt., Bell., Canth., Hyos., Stram., Sumb.

water, Agg.: Stram.

CLAMMY: Bell.

CLOTHES, Agg.: **Kali-c.**, **Lach.**

COATED FEELING: Carb-v., **Puls.**

COLD, Agg.: **Ars.**, Hep., Kali-n., Lob., LYC., Manc., Merc-i-r., Rhus-t., Sabad., Sil., Syph., Tell., Verat.

Amel. (heat Agg.): Apis, Ign., Kali-m., **Lach.**, Merc-d., Merc-i-f., Phyt., Sang.

taking, Agg.: Bell., Calc., **Dulc.**, Lach., **Merc.**, Nat-s., Nux-m., **Nux-v.**, Phos., Rhus-t.

COVERS IT: Am-c., Arg-n., Cor-r., Cupr., Ip., Kali-bi., **Lach.**, Rumx., Thuj.

CRAWLING: Kali-c., Kali-m.

CUTTING: Merc-cy., Nit-ac.

DARK: Aesc., Ail., Arg-n., Bapt., Crot-h., **Lach.**, Phyt.

DIPHTHERIA, TONSILITIS, etc.: APIS, Ars., Kali-i., Lac-c., LACH., Lyc., MERC-CY.,

Merc-i-f., Merc-i-r., Mur-ac.,
Phos., Phyt., Rhus-t, Spong.,
Sul-ac.

laryngeal: Brom., Iod., Kali-bi.,
Lac-c., **Lach.**, Merc-cy.

nasal: Kali-bi., Manc.

painless: Apis, Carb-ac.

DRIPPING from uvula: All-c.,
Aral., Cupr., Kali-bi., Merc-c.

DRY, in general: Acon., Aesc.,
BELL., Bry., Lyc., Merc.,
Phos., Ph-ac., Sep., Stram.,
Sul-i., Thyr., Tub., Sulph,
Verat.

anterior: Ars., Bry., Nux-v.

posterior: Mez., Thuj.

with chill: Petr.

with increased saliva: Alum.,
Aral., Kali-c., Lyc., Mag-m.,
Merc., Nat-m., Plb.

but no thirst: Apis, Bry., Cocc.,
Kali-c., Lyc., NUX-M.,
Nux-v., **Puls.**, Spig.

EAR, extending to: Hep., Kali-bi.,
Kali-m., Lach., MERC., Merc-
d., Phyt.

EXERTION, Agg.: Caust., Lac-c.,

FAUCES, itching: Phyt., Rhus-t.

sensitive: Coc-c.

FULL: Arn.

speaking, Agg.: Iod.

FISSURES, cracks: Arum-t., Bell.,
Caust., Cist., Fl-ac., Kali-bi.,
Merc-c., Mez., Mur-ac.

FOAM, from: Bell., Hyos., Ign.,
Stram.

GLISTENING: Apis, Kali-bi.,
Lac-c., Petr., Phos., Stram.

GRASPS the: See **Larynx.**

GRAY: Phyt.

HAIR in: See **Fine.**

GREASY mouth: Iris.

HANGING loose, as if, in: Alum.,
Berb., Iod., **Lach.**, Merc.,
Phos., Plat., Sabad., Sulph.,
Valer.

Comp. **Fine.**

HAWKING (mucus): Arg-n.,
Caust., Con., **Kali-bi.**, Kali-c.,
Lach., Lyc., Nat-c., Nat-m.,
Phos., Puls., Rhus-t., Sep.

lump from throat: Merc., Sep.

posterior nares, from: Cinnb.,
Elaps, **Hep.**, Hydr., Kali-bi.,
Mag-c., Nat-m., Nit-ac.,
Nux-v., Rumx., Sel., Spig.,
Sulph., Ther.

Agg: Nux-v.

discharge: Syph.

hot: Zinc-i.

itch: Ail., Kali-p.

lumps, foul: Kali-m., Med.

solid: Calc., Merc-i-f.,
Teucr.

lumps in: Cist., Hydr.,
Kali-bi., **Lach.**, Nat-m.,
Phos., Sep., Spig., Stict.,
Sulph., Teucr., Zinc.

mucus: Merc., Nat-m., Rumb., Sel.

bitter: Arn., Ars., Cist., Menis., Nat-s.

cold: Sin-n.

eating, Agg.: Sil., Tub.

salty: Nat-m.

tough: Aesc., Ol-an., Par.

sticky: Arg-n., Coc-c., KALI-BI., Lach., Mag-m., Phyt.

HEAT, mouth: Cham., Med.

HOLLOW, empty (throat): Calc-p., Fl-ac., Iris, Lach., Lob., Phyt., Rumx., Sanic., Xan.

INFLAMED: Acon., Alum., Am-m., Apis, Bapt., Bar-c., Bell., Brom., Bry., Caps., Cham., Chin., Cocc., Coff., Dulc., Hep., Hydr., Ign., Lach., Mang., Merc., Merc-c., Nit-ac., Nux-v., Phos., Puls., Rhus-t., Sulph., Sul-ac., Verat.

ITCHING: Apis, Arum-t., Caps., Con., Nux-v., Phyt., Rhus-t.

LEFT: Merc-c., Til.

in A. M.: Cimic., Rhus-t.

LIFTING, Agg.: Caust., Sil.

LOOSE skin, in mouth: Phys.

LUMP, plug, globus, stick, etc.: Asaf., Hep., IGN., Lach., Lyc., Naja, Nat-m., Phys., Puls., Sep.

descends and rises, as she swallows: Aloe, Asaf., Bar-c., Calc., Chel., Kali-c., Lac-c., Lach., Lil-t., Plb., Rumx.

hot: Lach., Phyt.

left: Lach., Sil.

rises and is swallowed again: Asaf., Bar-c., Camph., Chel., Con., Lach., Spong.

and sticks: Calc., Lyc.

MENSES, at: Bar-c., Lac-c., Mag-c.

NASO-PHARYNX: Elaps, Merc-c., Spig., Thuj, Zinc-i.

discharges, from: Mag-c., Nat-c., Phyt.

dripping: All-c., Hydr., Merc-c., Spig.

hot, dry: Acon., Aesc., Lyc., Sep., Zinc-i.

itching: Ail., Kali-p., Nux-v.

lump, in: Aesc., Cist., Lappa.

lumps, from: Cimic., Merc-i-f., Sep., Syph., Teucr.

mucus, drops into: Cinnb., Lith-c.

NOSE, ascending into: Brom., Lac-c., Merc., Sep.

NUMB: Bapt., Mag-m., Stront-c.

ODOR from, bad breath: Ail., Arn., Ars., Arum-t., Aur., Bapt., Carb-v., Cham., Crot-

h., Hell., Kali-chl., **Lach.,**
Merc., Merc-cy., Nit-ac., **Nux-**
v., Petr., Puls., Pyrog., Rheum,
Sulph., Verat-v.

OFFENSIVE **pellets from throat:**
Lach.

OPEN MOUTH, **hangs: Ail.,** Ars.,
Bapt., Bar-c., Carb-v., Colch.,
Hell., Hyos., **Lach.,** LYC.,
Merc-c., Mur-ac., Nat-c., **Op.,**
Rhus-t., Zinc.

PAINFUL: Lach., Merc-c.

PARALYSIS **throat noisy swallow-**
ing, etc.: **Caust.,** Cocc., Cupr.,
Gels. (palate), Hydr-ac., Lach.,
Laur., Phos., Thuj.

PHARYNX, **burning:** Bell., Carb-
v.

  chronic conditions: Aesc.,
  Cinnb., Rumx., Sep.

  dry: Bell., Nux-m.

  fissured: Elaps, Kali-bi.

  glistening: Apis.

  inflamed: Bell., Merc.

  scraping: Mez., Sang.

  tickling: Stict.

PRESSURE **towards throat:** Asaf.

PUFFY **throat:** Arg-n., Phyt.

RAW: ARUM-T., Carb-v., Nit-ac.,
NUX-V., **Phos.,** Rad-met.,
Sulph. (nursing), Sul-i.

  sleep, after: Rheum.

REGURGITATION: Ant-c., Asaf.,
Bry., Carb-v., Ferr., Ferr-p.,
Hydr., Lach., Merc., NUX-V.,
PHOS., **Puls., Sulph.,** Sul-ac.,
Vario.

SCRAPING, **rough: Nux-v.**

SKIN **in: see Hanging.**

SLEEP, **after:** Rheum.

SLIMY, **sticky:** Bell., Caps., Chel.,
Kali-bi., **Lach.,** Merc., Petr.,
PULS., Tub.

SMOKING, **Agg.:** Caps.

SOPPY: Sul-ac.

SPLINTER, **stick,** etc. **as of a:**
Agar., Alum., **Arg-n., Hep.,**
Ign., Kali-c., Nat-m., **Nit-ac.,**
Paeon., **Phyt.,** Rat., Thuj.,
Thyr.

                              Comp. **Fine.**

SPEAKING, **Agg.:** Acon., Alum.,
Bar-c., Bry., Dulc., Ign.,
Mang., Merc., Phos., Rhus-t.,
Sulph.

  Amel.: Hep.

SPOT, **dry, sore,** etc.: **Apis,** Caust.,
Cimic., **Cist.,** Con., Crot-h.,
Hep., Hyos., Lac-c., **Lach.,**
Lith-c., Merc-cy., **Nat-m.,** Nit-
ac., **Phos.,** Phyt., **Sil.**

  left, cough, from: **Caust., Hep.,**
  Lach., Rhus-t.

  right, cough, from.: Dros.,
  Stann., Stict.

STICKY, clammy, pasty: Aesc.,
Ant-t., Bapt., Chel., Ferr.,
KALI-BI., **Lach.**, Lappa, Mez.,
Myrt-c., Osm., Ph-ac., Plat.,
Puls., Sec., Sul-ac.

STIFF: Merc-i-r.

SWALLOWING, **food lodges:**
Arg-n., Ars., Bar-c., Caust.,
Chin., Cina, Graph., Hydr-
ac., Ign., Kali-c., Laur., **Lyc.**,
Meph., **Nat-m.**, PULS.,
Sulph., Sul-i.

drink, must: Bar-c., Bell., Calad.,
Nat-c.

noisy: Arn., **Ars.**, Cupr., Hell.,
Hydr-ac., Laur., Phos.,
Thuj.

painful: Ars., Bell., Canth., Lac-
c., **Lach.**, Merc-c., **Phyt.**,
Sul-i.

painless: Apis, Carb-ac.

returns through nose: Arum-t.,
Cocc., Gels., Kali-per.,
Lach., **Lyc.**, Merc., **Phos.**,
Sul-ac.

sleep, in: Calc., Cina.

solids, Amel.: Ign.

urging to: Bell., Caust., Lach.,
Merc.

won't go down: Bar-c., Calc.,
Graph., Lyc., Sep.

SWEETS, **Agg.:** Bad., Lach.,
Spong.

SWELLED: **Apis**, Lach., **Merc.**,
Nux-v., Puls. (as if).

TASTE, in: Nux-v., Sil.

ULCERS, aphthae, etc.: Ail., **Ars.**,
Borx., Kali-bi., Kali-chl., Kali-
m., Lach., Merc., **Merc-c.**,
Mur-ac., **Nit-ac.**, Nux-v.,
Rhus-t., Sul-ac., THUJ.

behind: Ars., Merc.

UPWARD **through or from:**
Acon., Ars., BROM., Calc.,
Carb-v., Ferr., Kali-bi., **Kali-c.**,
Lac-c., **Lyc.**, Merc., Nat-m.,
Nux-v., Phos., **Sep.**

VALVE, see **Generalities.**

VAPOR, in: Apis, Ferr., Ol-an.,
Sulph.

WASH LEATHER, throat: Phyt.

WEAK: Lac-c., Stann.

WINTER, **Agg.**: Mez.

WIPE, **must mouth:** Kali-bi., Sec.

YELLOW **mouth:** Plb.

SALIVA

Merc., Sulph.

ACRID: Arum-t., Kreos., Merc-c.,
Nit-ac.

BLOODY: Merc., **Nit-ac.**, Phos.,
Rhus-t.

FLOWS, **pain, headache, etc.**

during: Epiph., Gran., Helo.,
Merc., Phos., Plan.

DIMINISHED: **Bell.**, Kali-bi., Nux-v., Phos., Stram., Sulph., **Verat.**

FOUL: Lach., **MERC.**, **Nit-ac.**, Petr.

FROTHY, snowy, cottony, etc.: Apis, **Bell.**, **Berb.**, Dulc., Caul., **Ign.**, Kali-bi., Lach., **Nux-m.**, Ol-an., Onos., Phos., Ph-ac., Pic-ac., **Puls.**, Sabin., Spig.

GUSHES of: Carb-v., Nat-m.

IN SLEEP: Cupr., **Merc.**, Phos., Rhus-t., Syph.

INCREASED: Dig., Dulc., **Merc.**, Nit-ac., Nux-v., Phos., Puls., **Rhus-t.**, Stram., **Verat.**

cough, with: Am-m., Lach., Verat.

dryness, with: Lyc., **Merc.**, Nat-m.

headache, with: Epiph., Merc.

pregnancy in: Kreos., Lob., Zinc-s.

sleep, Agg.: **Bar-c.**, Ign., Ip., Lac-c., Lach., Nit-ac., **MERC.**, **Phos.**, **Rhus-t.**, Syph.

MENSES, **Agg.**: Phyt.

MUMPS: Merc., Phyt.

septic: Anthraci., Lach., Syph.

ROPY: Coc-c., Sabad., Sulph.

SALIVARY GLANDS: Calc-f., Cham., Iod., Lach., Merc., Phyt., Puls., Sil.

SALTY: Sanic.

SOAPY: Ign., Iod., Kali-bi., Ph-ac.

SOUR: Con.

STICKY: Bell., **Kali-bi.**, **Lach.**, Plb.

SWALLOW, **must:** Ip., Merc.

SWEET: Cham., Iris, Phos., Plb., **PULS.**

THICK: **Cimic.**, Glon., Lach., Lyc.

TASTE

ACUTE: Chin., Coff.

AFTERTASTE, of food eaten: Ant-c., Caust., Dios., Nat-m., **Phos.**, **Ph-ac.**, Puls., Sil.

ALTERED, in general: Chin., **Puls.**, Rhus-t.

ASTRINGENT: Alum., Arg-n., Ars., Chion., Graph., Hydr-ac., **Merc-c.**, **Phos.**

BAD, foul, nauseous, repulsive, etc.: Arn., Merc., **Nux-v.**, **Puls.**, Rhus-t., Staph.

in the morning: Bry., Nat-s., **Nux-v.**, **Puls.**

to water: Acon., Apis, Ars., Ferr., **Kali-bi.**, **Nat-m.**, **Puls.**, Sil., Thlasp.

BITTER: Acon., Ant-c., Ars., **Bry.**, Cham., **Chin.**, Lyc., Merc., Nat-s., **Nux-v.**, Podo., **Puls.**, Sep., Solid., Sulph., Verat.

sour: Arg-n., Asar., Cupr., Lyc.,
Merc., **Nux-v.**, Phos., Stann.

to food: Chin., Puls.

BLOODY: Ip.

CHEESY: Sep.

COUGHING, **Agg.**: Lach., Nux-
v., Sang.

DULLED, flat, watery, etc.: **Bry.**,
Chin., Ign., **Puls.**, Staph.

EARTHY: Puls.

FISHY: Sep.

GREASY, fatty: **Alum.**, Asaf.,
Caus., Iris, Kali-p., Petr.,
Puls., Tril-p.

HERBY: Nux-v.

LOST: Anac., Bell., Cycl., Hyos.,
Nat-m., Puls., Sil.

METALLIC, coppery, etc.: Cocc.,
Cupr., Iod., Kali-bi., **Merc.**,
Nux-v., Rhus-t., Seneg., Thyr.,
Vario., Zinc-chr.

MUSTY: Staph., Teucr.

PEPPERY: Hydr., **Lach.**, Mez.,
Rad-met., Sulph., Xan.

PUTRID, filthy: Psor., Syph.,
Vario.

RANCID, also of eructation:
Alum., Carb-v., Thuj., **Valer.**

SALTY: **Ars.**, Con., Kali-i., Lyc.,
Merc., Phos., Puls., **Sep.**

SLIMY: Kali-bi., Puls.

SOUR: Arg-n., Asar., Bell., **Calc.**,
Chin., **Lyc.**, Mag-c., **Nux-v.**,
Phos., Puls., Sulph., Zin-val.

salty: Cupr.

SWEET: Calad., Iris, Lil-t., Phos.,
Plb., Puls., Sabad., Squil., Stan.

WOODY: Ruta.

APPETITE

Merc-cy., Stroph-h.

AFFECTED, changed, in general:
Ant-c., Ars., **Calc.**, CHIN.,
Cina, Graph., Iod., **Lyc.**, Nat-
m., NUX-V., Petr., Phos.,
PULS., Sil., SULPH., Verat.

CRAVES, coarse, raw food, chalk
etc.: Abies-c., Alum., Ant-c.,
Calc., Cic., Ign., **Nit-ac Nux-
v.**, Psor., SIL., Sulph., **Tarent.**

condiments, spices, pickles, etc.:
Ars., Caps., Chel., **Chin.**, Fl-
ac., **Hep.**, Nux-v., **Phos.**,
Puls., Sang., Staph., **Sulph.**,
Tarent.

HUNGER: Calc., Chin., **Cina**,
Graph., Phos., Puls., Sabad,
Sep., Stann., Sulph.

11 a. m.: Hydr., Phos., SULPH.,
Zinc.

attacks of sickness, before: Bry.,
Nux-v., **Phos.**, **Psor.**, Sep.

eating, after: **Cina**, Kali-p., Lyc.,
Murx., **Phos.**, Sars., Sil.

headache, with: Bry., Phos., Psor., Sel.

loathing after first bite: Caust., Lyc., Prun.

lost: Chin., Gins., Nux-v., Puls.

by day only: Arn.

nausea, with: Valer.

navel, from: Valer.

nightly: Phos., Psor.

ravenous: Calc., **Chin.**, **Cina**, **Iod.**, Lyc., Nux-v., **Phos.**, Psor., Rumx., Sabad., Sil., **Sulph.**, Verat.

relish, without: Nat-m., Op., Rhus-t.

spine, from: Lil-t.

stools, after: Kali-p.

sudden: Sulph.

weak and: Phos., Sulph., Zinc.

NIBBLING: **Aeth.**, Calc., Mag-c., Mag- m., Nat-c., Petr., Rhus-t.

VARIABLE, capricious: Calc., **Cina**, **Coc-c.**, Ferr., Gran., **Iod.**, Lach., Merc., Nat-m., Petr., **Phos.**, Syph.

AVERSIONS

TO FOOD, etc.: **Ars.**, **Nux-v.**, Puls.

eating: Zinc-chr.

in chronic diarrhea: Ant-c., Ars., Chin., Nux-m., Phos., Puls.

loathing, disgust, etc., with: **Ant-c.**, Arn., **Ars.**, Cham., **Colch.**, Ip., **Kali-c.**, Nux-v., Op., Phos., Puls., Sep.

ACIDS: Sulph.

BEER: Chin.

BREAD: Kali-c., **Nat-m.**, Puls., Sulph.

COFFEE: Nux-v.

EGGS: Ferr.

FATS: Nat-m., **Petr.**, **Puls.**

MEAT: Graph., Mur-ac., **Petr.**, **Puls.**, Sep., Sil., **Sulph.**

MILK: **Ign.**, Sep., **Sil.**

MOTHER'S MILK: Sil.

SWEETS: **Caust.**, Rad-met., Senec., Sulph.

TOBACCO: Calc., **Ign.**, Nux-v.

WINE: **Lach.**, Merc.

THIRST

Acon., Arn., Ars., Bell., Bry., Calc., Caps., Cham., Chin., Cina, Croc., Dig., Lyc., **Merc.**, Nat-m., Phos., Rhus-t., Sep., Sil., **Stram.**, Sulph., Verat.

with aversion to drinks: Hell., Stram.

with the chill: Bry., Caps., **Ign.**,
Nat-m.

ABSENT, aversion to water, flu-
ids, etc.: Aeth., **Apis**, Bell.,
Canth., Chin., Ferr., **Gels.**,
Hell., Hyos., Ign., Ip., **Nux-
m.**, PULS., Sabad., Sep.,
Stram.

during the heat: **Apis**, Carb-v.,
Gels., Hell., Ign., Ip., Nux-
m., **Puls.**, Sabad., Sep.

CHILL, before: Carb-v., Chin.,
Eup-per.

COLD DRINKS, for: Acon.,
ARS., Bism., Bry., Chin.,
Merc-c., PHOS., Rhus-t.,
VERAT.
Amel.: Manc.

LITTLE AND OFTEN, for:
Acon., Ant-t., Apis, ARS.,
Bell., Chin., Hyos., Kali-n.,
Lil-t., **Lyc.**, Nat-m., Rhus-t.

MUCH AT A TIME, **large drinks
for:** Bry., Lil-t., Nat-m.

eats little: Sep., Sulph

NIGHTLY: Calc., **Cham.**

THIRSTLESS: Ant-t., **Nux-m.**,
Puls., Sel.

VIOLENT, **burning:** Acon., Ars.,
Bry., Coloc., Cupr., Merc.,
Nux-v., Sabad., VERAT.

CRAVINGS AND DESIRES

APPLES: Ant-t.

BACON: Calc., Calc-p., Rad-met.

BEER: Stront-c., **Sulph.**

BITTERS: Dig., Nat-m.

BUTTERMILK: Chinin-s., Elaps,
Sabal, Thlasp.

CABBAGE: Cic.

COARSE or **raw food:** Abies-c.,
Alum., Ant-c., Calc., Ign., Sil.,
Sulph., Tarent.

COFFEE: Ang., Bry., Nux-v.,
Stroph-h.

COLD THINGS: **Ars.**, Lept.,
Verat.

CONDIMENTS, **spices, pickles,
etc.:** Caps., Nux-v., Staph.,
Tarent.

FATS, etc.: Calc-p., Nit-ac., Nux-
v.

FINERY: Lil-t., Sulph.

HOT THINGS: Ars., Bry., Chel.,
Ferr., Lac-c.

ICE **water:** Acon., Ars., Phos.,
Verat.

INDEFINITE THINGS: Bry.,
Chin., Ign., Puls., Zinc-chr.

JUICY FOODS, **fruit:** Ph-ac.,
Staph., **Verat.**

LEMONADE: Bell.

LIQUIDS: Staph., Sulph.

MEAT: Viol-o.

MILK: Rhus-t., Sabad., Sanic.

PREGNANCY, during: Sep.

REFRESHING THINGS: **Puls.**

REFUSED, **what is:** Bry., Cham., Kreos., Phys., Staph.

RELISH, **what can't:** Bry., Ign., Mag-m., Puls.

SALTY THINGS: **Carb-v.**, Caust., **NAT-M., Phos.**, Verat.

SOUR THINGS: **Acon., Arn.,** Ars., Bell., Cham., **Hep.**, Puls., **Sulph.**, Verat.

SPIRITS, **alcoholic:** Arn., **Ars., Calc., Lach.**, Led., Nux-v., **Op.**, Staph., Stroph-h., Sulph., Syph.

STIMULANTS: Crot-h.

SWEETS AND DAINTIES: Arg-n., **Chin., Kali-c., Lyc.**, Sabad., Sulph.

THINGS **that are refused, when offered:** Bry., Cham., Phos., Staph.

WINE: Calc.

WATERBRASH

(Also raising mucus)

Ars., **Bry., Calc., Carb-v.**, Mez., Nat-m., **Nux-v.**, Par., **Phos.**, Sabad., Sep., **Sil.**, Staph., Sulph.

COLD: Caust., Verat.

TOBACCO, **Amel.:** Ol-an.

HEARTBURN

Calc., Carb-v., Con., Croc., **Nux-v., Puls.**, Sumb.

QUALMISHNESS

Ars., Caust., Nat-s., Sulph.

HICCOUGH

Am-m., Cic., Cina, **Cycl.**, Gins., **Hyos., IGN.**, Mag-p., **NUX-V., Puls.**, Ran-b., Ruta, Tab., Teucr., Zinc-val.

BREATH, **short** with: Phys.

ERUCTATIONS, with: Dios., Ign.

FEVERS, **after:** Ars., Lach.

VOMITING, **before:** Cupr.

with: Bell., Bry., Lach., Ruta.

NAUSEA

Aeth., Ant-c., Ant-t., Ars., Bry., Carb-v., Cham., **Cocc.**, Colch., Cupr., Dig., Hep., Ign., Ip., Lyc., Nit-ac., Nux-v., Phos., Puls., Rhus-t., Sep., Sil., Sulph., Tab., **Verat.**

IN A. M.: Med.

ABDOMEN, **in:** Polyg.

CHEST, **in:** Ant-t.

CHILL, **with:** Echi.

CONTINUOUS: **Ip.**, Iris, Nux-v., Sil.

DEATHLY, **anxious:** Ant-c., Ant-t., Cocc., Crot-h., Ip., **Lob.**, Puls., Tab.

EATING, **Amel.**: Sang.

EYES, **closing:** Ther.

using, Agg.: Jab., Puls.

HEAD, **felt in:** Colch.

HUNGER, **Agg.**: Petr.

LYING **on right side, Agg.**: Cann-s., Crot-h., Iris, Sang., Sul-ac.

MORNING: Cimic., Nux-v., **Puls.**, Sep.

NOSE, blowing, sneezing, etc., **Agg.**: Hell., Lach., Sang., Sulph.

ODORS (cooking, etc.), **Agg.**: Ars., Cocc., COLCH., Dig., Ip., Merc-i-f., Sep., Stann., Vario.

SPINE, **pressure on, Agg.**: Cimic.

STOMACH, **felt in: Verat.**

THROAT, **in:** Cycl., Ph-ac., Stann., Valer.

REGURGITATION

Aeth., Ant-t., Arn., **Bry.**, Nux-v., PHOS., **Puls.**, Sars., Sulph., Sul-ac.

INGESTA, **of:** Bry., **Phos.**, Puls.

RETCHING AND GAGGING., Bell., Bry., Cham., Colch., Dros., Eup-per., IP., **Nux-v.**, **Podo.**, Puls., Rhus-t., Sulph., Tab., Verat.

empty: Sec.

hawking, Agg.: Arg-n., Nux-v.

yawns then: Tell.

VOMITING

Ant-t., Apoc., Arn., **Ars.**, Bry., Cham., Cina, Cupr., Ferr., IP., Kreos., Lob., **Nux-v.**, Op., Puls., Sil., Sulph., Stroph-h., Tab., **Verat.**, Verat-v.

ACRID, **scalding,** etc.: Chion., Kali-c., Kali-m., **Kreos.**, Lyc., Med., Rob., **Sang.**, Sil.

ALBUMINOUS: Kali-bi.

ANXIOUS: Ars., Tab.

AT ONCE: Apoc., ARS., Cadm-s., Zinc.

BILIOUS, **Amel.**: Card-m., Sang.

BITTER: Eup-per., Kali-bi., **Nux-v.**

BLACK: **Ars.**, Cadm-s., Kreos., Mez., **Nux-v.**

BLOOD: Cadm-s., Carb-v., Chin., Crot-h., Ham., Ip., Phos.

at close of vomiting: Verat.

bluish: Kali-c.

brown: Bry., Carb-v., Mez., Rhus-t.

BURNING, hot: Med.

CHILL, after: Eup-per., Nat-m.

CONTINUOUS: Ars., Hell., Ip., Merc.

CURDS: Aeth., Calc., Nat-p., Sanic., Sil., Valer.

DELAYED, after a while: Bism., PHOS.

DRINKING, Agg.: Ant-c., Ars., Bry., Kali-bi.

after a while: Phos., Pyrog.

EARLY: Stann.

EASY: Ars., Cham., Ip.

EXHAUSTING: Aeth., Ant-t., Podo., Verat., Verat-v.

FECAL: Op., Rhus-t.

FLUIDS only: Ars.

after they become warm: PHOS.

FORCIBLE: Ant-t., Apoc., Verat.

FROTHY: Aeth., Arg-n., Ars., Kreos., Led., Mag-c., Nat-c., Phos., Sil., Verat.

GREEN: Ars., Bell., Cham., Chel., Eup-per., Ip., Merc-d., Nat-s., Verat.

HEADACHE, with: Bry., Cocc., Ip., Iris, Nux-v., Puls., Sang., Sep., Verat.

INGESTA: Ars., Bry., Cina, Ferr., Ign., Nux-v., Puls., Sil., Sulph.

LONG after meals: Aeth., Ferr., Kreos., Plat., Puls., Sabin., Sang.

LYING on left side, Agg.: Sul-ac., right side, Amel.: Ant-t.

MILK: Aeth., Calc., Mag-c.

mother's, anger, after: Valer.

MUCUS: Dros., Ip., Puls.

NAUSEA, without: Apoc., Arn., Ars., Chel., Kali-bi., Lyc., Verat-v., Zinc.

at once: Ars.

OFFENSIVE: Ars., Nux-v., Sep.

PAINFUL: Verat.

PERITONITIS, Agg.: Op.

PREGNANCY, Agg.: Anac., Cocc., Goss., Ign., Ip., Kreos., LOB., MED., Nux-v., Sep., Sulph.

PURGING, with: Aeth., Apis, Ant-t., Arg-met., ARS., Asar., Borx., Camph., Cham., Colch., Cupr., Ip., Iris, Merc., Phos., Podo., Sec., Seneg., Sulph., Sul-ac., VERAT., Verat-v.

bilious: Eup-per.

blood: Ars. (black), Erig.

SEPTIC: Bapt., Crot-h., Lach., Vip-t.

SLEEP, then: **Aeth.**, Ant-t., Cupr., Nat-m.

SOLIDS: Arn., Ferr., Sep.

SOUR: Calc., Iris, Lyc., Mag-c., Med., Nat-p., Rob., Sulph., Sul-ac.

STOMACH, from full: **Bism.**, Grat.

STRINGY: Croc., Cupr., Kali-bi.

SUDDEN, **projectile:** Ant-t., Kali-bi., Kali-chl.

SWEAT, **cold, with:** Ars., Cup-ar., Tab., **Verat.**

TEETH, sets, on edge: Chion.

THIRST, with: Ars., Canth.

UREMIC: Apoc., Ars., Samb., Scopar., Senec.

UTERINE: Caul., Senec.

VIOLENT: Ant-t., Ars., Canth., Cupr., Kali-bi., **Nux-v.**, Phyt., Stann., **Verat.**

WATERY: Ars., **Bry.**, Caust., Dros., Tab., **Verat.**

WORMS: Cina.

YELLOW, **bright:** Kali-bi.

ERUCTATIONS

Arg-n., Asar., Bell., **Bry.**, Carb-v., Cocc., Con., **Lyc.**, Merc., Nat-m., **Nux-v.**, Sabad., Sep., Sulph., Verat.

ABORTIVE: Ars., Con., Graph.

ACRID, **hot:** Fago., Merc.

COUGHING, **when:** Ambr., Kali-bi., **Sang.**, Sul-ac., Verat.

COUGH, with: Ambr., Arn., Carb-v., Chin., Lob., Sang.

DIFFICULT: Calc-p., Cocc.

EGGS, **like bad:** Arn., Cham., Plan.

EMPTY: Bry., Calc., Carb-v., Con., Graph., Phos., Sep., Sulph.

FECAL: Plb.

FOAMY: Sep.

FROTHY: Kreos.

GALL-STONES, with: Dios., Lyc.

GREASY: Alum., Asaf., Caust., Iris., Mag-c., Thuj., Valer.

INCOMPLETE: Lyc.

INGESTA, tasting of: **Ant-c.**, Bry., Puls.

LOUD, **noisy:** Arg-n., **Asaf.**, Kali-bi., Petr., Phos., Thuj., Vip-t.

NAUSEOUS, **foul:** Asaf., Carb-v., Puls., Sulph.

PUTRID: Kreos.

RANCID: **Asaf.**, Carb-v., Tell.

RELIEF, **without:** Carb-v., **Chin.**, Lyc.

SOUR: **Calc.**, Caps., Carb-v., Chin., Lyc., Mag-c., Nat-m., **Nat-p.**, Nux-v., Puls., Rob., Sep., Sulph., Sul-ac.

hot: Fago., Gymno.

STALE: Fl-ac.

TOUGH: Sep.

URINOUS: Agn-c., Ol-an.

EPIGASTRIUM

ARS., **Calc.**, Chel., Cocc., Coloc., **Ign.**, Ip., KALI-C., **Lach.**, Lob., **Lyc.**, **Nat-m.**, NUX-V., Phos., **Puls.**, Sep., Sulph., Tab.

ABOVE: Nat-m., PHOS., Puls.

ACHING: Sil.

ANXIETY **at:** Ars., Lyc., Nux-v., Puls.

BURNING: Ars., Nux-v., Sep., Sil., Ter.

CHILL, **from:** Arn.

COLD: Kreos.

COUGH, **from:** Bry., Nit-ac., Phos., Ph-ac.

CRAMP, pinching, etc.: Lach., Laur., Merc-c., Sil., **Verat.**, Vip-t.

CUTTING: Puls.

EMOTIONS: see **Stomach.**

LUMP **above, as of:** Agar., Arn., Chel., Con., Cupr., **Lach.**, Nat-c., Nat-m., Phos., Puls., **Sep.**

PAIN **in:** Ars., Nux-v., Verat., Vip-t.

PRESSURE: Cupr., Lyc., Nat-m., **Nux-v.**, **Phos.**, **Puls.**, Verat.

PULSATION: Ars., Bry., Chin., Lach., **Nat-m.**, Nux-v., Olnd.

SENSITIVE: Bry., Calc., Carb-v., Chin., Hyos., Kali-c., **Lach.**, Lyc., Nux-v., **Verat.**

SINKING, **faint, etc.:** Ant-t., Apoc., Dig., Glon., Ign., Kali-c., Lob., **Sep.**, Stroph-h., **Sulph.**, Tab.

SORE: Lach., Phos.

STICKING: Arn., Bry., **Nit-ac.**, Rhus-t., **Sep.**, Sulph.

STOPPAGE in: Guaj.

SWEAT: Kali-n.

SWELLED: **Calc.**, Manc., Nux-v.

TENSE: Sang.

THROBBING: Asaf., Kali-c., Puls., Rhus-t., Sep.

TICKLING in: Puls.

TREMOR: Sul-i.

UPWARD (up throat, etc.): **Acon.**, Ars., Calc., Carb-v., Ferr., Kali-bi., **Kali-c.**, Lyc., Nat-m., Nux-v., Phos.

STOMACH AND ABDOMEN

Aeth., Arg-n., ARS., Bry., **Calc.**, Carb-v., **Chin.**, Coloc., Ip., Lach., LYC., NUX-V., PHOS., PULS., Sep., Sil., **Sulph.**, Verat.

BEHIND STOMACH: Arn., Cact., Ham., Kali-c., Stram.

DUODENUM: Podo., Uran-n.

UPPER ABDOMEN: Caust., Cham., Chin., Cocc., Nux-v., Puls.

NAVEL (about): Bry., Coloc., Dios., Ip., Kreos., Nux-v., Ph-ac., Rhus-t., Spig., Verat., Verb.

breasts, to: Pall.

bubbling: Hyper.

burning, in: ACON., Bov., Kali-i., Lach., Lyc., Phyt., Plb., Sep.

cramp, colic, etc.: Coloc., Dios., Ip., Nat-s., Rhod.

cutting: Colch., Coloc., Nux-v., Verat-v.

empty: Cob.

festers: Abrot., Calc-p., Nux-m.

hard: Puls.

hernia: Plb.

inflated: Calc.

lump, at: Kreos., Nux-v., Rhus-t., Sep., Verb., Zinc.

moisture, at: Calc-p.

pelvis, uterus, etc., to: Pall., Rumx., Sep.

pouting: Dulc.

rectum, to: Aloe, Ars., Crot-t., Dios., Lach. (reverse), Lyc.

retracted: Plb., Puls., Stann., Verat., Zinc.

rumbling: Tarax.

sore: Nux-m.

suppurating: Phos.

ILEO-CAECAL REGION: Ars., Bapt., Bell., BRY., Carb-v., Chin., COLOC., LACH., Lyc., Merc-c., Mur-ac., Nux-v., Phos., Ph-ac., Plb., Puls., RHUS-T., Sep., Sulph., Thuj.

SIDES: Asaf., Carb-v., Chin., Ign.

right: Ars., Lach., Lyc., Rhus-t.

to left: Sep.

left: Alum., Arg-met., Asaf., Brom., Dulc., Fl-ac., Hep., Plb., Rheum, Sil., Sulph., Tarax.

to right: Nux-v.

alternating: Arn., Puls., Sulph.

LOINS (flanks): Canth., Plb., Rheum, Thuj., Zinc.

burning: Bar-c.

hollow: Pall.

sticking: Berb., Plb.

LOWER: Bell., Bry., Carb-v., Lyc., Merc., Ran-b., Squil., Sep.

backward, right: Caust., Phos., Sep., Ust.

left: Acon., Carb-v.

UPWARD, right: Acon., Kali-c., Mag-m., Murx., Seneg., Sep.

left: Alum., Ign., **Naja**, **Nat-s.**, Spong., Zinc.

diagonally: Lach.

ACHES, **sick in:** Lept., Podo., Puls., Rhus-t., Verat-v.

ALTERNATING, **with:** Bry., Coloc., Nux-v., Rad-met., Ran-b.

ANXIETY, emotions felt in, etc.: **Ars.**, Aur., Carb-v., Cham., Coloc., Cupr., **Ign.**, **Kali-c.**, Mez., Nat-m., Nux-v., Phos., Tarent., Verat.

BACKWARD, **pain goes:** Arn, **ARS.**, **BELL.**, Berb., Bism., Borx., Carb-v., Chel., Con., Cupr., Ferr., Kali-p., **Lyc.**, **Nux-v.**, **PHOS.**, Plb., Puls., Sep., Sulph., **Tab.**

BALL, **lump, as of a, etc.:** Anac., Kreos., Verb.

BAND **about:** Caust., **Chel.**, Chion., Plb., **Puls.**, **Sulph.**

BORING **in, grinding:** Fl-ac., Plb., Polyg-s., Sars., Stann.

BOWELS: Psor.

cancer: Ruta.

inactive: Phys.

knotted: Sabad.

obstructed, paralysis: Bry., Con., Lyc., Mag-m., **Op.**, Plb., **Rhus-t.**

BURNING **in:** **Ars.**, Canth., Caps., Carb-v., **Caust.**, Cic., Manc., Merc-c., **Phos.**, Ran-b., Sec., Sep., **Sulph.**, **Verat.**

CANCER: **Ars.**, Aur., Calc., Carban., Con., Cund., Hydr., Lyc., Phos., Phyt., **Sec.**, Sil., Symph., Thuj.

CHANGING, **about in:** Dios., Mur-ac., Nux-v.

CHEST, **to:** Aeth., **Cham.**, Nux-v.

CLAWING: Bell., Lyc.

COLDNESS: Ambr., **Ars.**, Cadms., Calc., Colch., Kali-c., Meny., Phos., Sec., Sul-ac., **Verat.**, Zinc.

CONTRACTED: Mag-p.

COUGHING, **Agg.:** Ant-t., Bry., Dros., **Nux-v.**, Phos.

COVERS, **lifts:** Bell., Lac-c., **Lach.**, Lil-t., Phos., Sec., Staph., Tab.

CRAMP, **colic, griping, squeezing:** Bell., Cham., **COLOC.**, Cupr., Dios., Dulc., Ign., Kreos., Magm., Mag-p., Nux-v., Op., Plb., Polyg-s., Rad-met., Rheum, Tob., Scopar., Stann., Staph., Stroph-h., Sulph., Verat., Zinc-val.

nightly: Cham., Chin., Cycl.

CUTTING: Bell., **Bry.**, Chin., **Coloc.**, Dios., Ip., Merc., Nit-ac., Nux-v., **Puls.**, Rat., Rheum, **Sulph.**, Verat.

DIARRHEA, sense of: Dulc., **Nux-v.**, Puls.

DIGESTION DISORDERED: **Ant-c.**, Arg-n., Carb-v., **Ip.**, Nat-c., **Nux-v.**, **Puls.**

DISTENDED, tympanitic, inflated, swelled. etc.: Acon., **Arg-n.**, Ars., CALC., CARB-V., **Chin.**, Colch., Graph., **Kali-c.**, **Lyc.**, Merc., Nat-c., Nat-m. (side), Nux-m., NUX-V., **Phos.**, Rhus-t., Stram., Sulph., **Ter.**, Vario., Verat.

DRAWING: Puls.

DRINKS, **Agg.**: Rhod.

DRINKING (water), **Agg.**: Ars., Phos., Zing. (bad).

DRYNESS, in: Calad.

EATING, **Amel.**: Anac., **Chel.**, **Graph.**, Ign., Lach., Petr., **Zinc.**

averse to: Zinc-chr.

fatigue, **Agg.**: Kali-c., Lyc., **Nat-m.**, Ph-ac.

no relief: Carb-an.

satiety, quick: Chin., Lyc.

tired too: Bar-c., Stann.

too much, **Agg.**: Ant-c., Ant-t., Coff., Ip., Nat-p., **Puls.**

EMPTY, hollow, weak, sinking, etc.: Carb-an., Cupr., **Dig.**, Glon., Hydr., Hydr-ac., Ign., Ip., Kali-c., Laur., Nux-v., **Phos.**, Podo., Sec., **Sep.**, Stann., Staph., Sul-ac., **Sulph.**, Tab., Verat., Zinc.

at 11 A.M.: Ign., Petr., Phos., Sep., **Sulph.**

not Amel. by eating: Cina, Lach., Lyc., Mur-ac., Phos., Sep, Verat.

Comp. **Generalities.**

ENLARGED: Bar-c., Sil.

EXTENDING to: Bism., Colch., Dulc., Kali-bi., Lappa.

FEVER, **Agg.**: Ip., Verat-v.

FATS, **Agg.**: Carb-v., **Puls.**

FERMENTATION in: Chin.

FOOD SPOILED, **Agg.**: Ars.

FORWARD into: Thuj.

FULLNESS: Carb-v., Chin., Kali-c., Kali-m., **Lyc.**, **Nux-v.**, **Sulph.**

GASTRITIS: Acon., Bry., Nux-v., Phos.

GNAWING, eating, ulcerative pain: **Carb-v.**, Coloc., Guaj., Nat-s., Nit-ac., Ox-ac., Phos., Sep., Sul-ac., Zinc-chr.

burning: Ruta.

eating, **Amel.**: Anac., Kali-p.

GRIPING: Rat.

GUMMY: Viol-t.

GURGLING in: **Aloe**, Berb., Brach., Crot-t., Gamb., Kali-c., Kreos., Lil-t., Podo., Squil., **Sulph.**

then gushing stools: Aloe, Berb., **Crot- t.**, GAMB., Ip., Iris, Jatr., Kali-bi., Mag-m., **Nat-s.**, Phos., Podo., Sabin., Sec., Stann., **Sulph.**, Thuj., Tril-p., Verat.

GROINS, to: (Kali-c.), Puls.

HANDS, on, **Agg.**: Zinc-chr.

HANGING **or fallen down or weak:** Acet-ac., Ign., Laur., Merc., Phos., Podo., **Sep.**

HARD: Bar-c., Calc., Graph., Merc., Sil.

HEAD, alternating with: Aloe, Bry., Calc-p., Podo., Thuj.

HEAVY, weight as if, oppression: **Aloe**, Am-m., Bry., Cupr., **Graph.**, Kali-c., Lyc., **Nux-v.**, **Puls.**, Sep., Spig., Tab. (r).

HOLDS the: Agn., Diph., Lil-t., Merc., Sep., Staph., Sul-ac.

HYPOGASTRIUM, **bearing down:** Dict., Lil-t., Sep., Sulph.

heavy: Med., Sulph.

weak: Am-c., Apoc., Calc., Chion., Phos., Plb., Sulph., Verat.

ICE: Acon., Caust., Tab.

ILEUS: Nux-v., **Op.**, Plb., Rhus-t., Tab., Thuj.

INFLAMED: Acon., Ant-t., **Ars.**, Bry., Ip., Merc-c., Nux-v., **Phos.**, Puls.

INGUINAL GLANDS, **swelled:** Clem., Hep., **Merc.**, Nit-ac., Sulph.

LYING side, **Amel.:** Squil. (l).

LUMPS, knots, ball, **stone**, etc.: Abies-n., Ant-t., Arn., Ars., Bov., Bufo, **Calc.**, Cocc., Coloc., Hydr. (sharp), Ign., Manc., Naja, Nux-m., **Nux-v.**, Osm., Plb., **Puls.**, **Rhus-t.**, Sabad., Scopar., Sep., Sulph.

MESENTERY: Calc., Sul-i.

MILK, **Amel.:** Graph., Merc., Mez.

OVERLOADING, **Agg.**: **Nux-v.**, Staph.

PAIN, dull, aching, indefinite, etc.: Ars., Coloc., Cupr., Echi., Erig., Eucal., Kalm., Lept., **Nux-v.**, Plb., Puls., Pyrog., Rad-met., Ruta, Sep., Ter., Vario., Verat.

radiating: Plb.

spasmodic: Caust.

PERISTALSIS: Asaf., Nux-v., Rhus-t.

PLUG: Chel.

PRESSURE, **load**, etc.: Agar., Arn., Ars., **Bry.**, Calc., Cham.,

Chin., Hyos., Lyc., **Nux-v.**, Ph-ac. (lower), **Puls.**, Sep., Sil., **Sulph.**

Agg.: Ars., Bry., Calc., Chin., Merc-c.

Amel.: Arg-n., Castr., COLOC., Stann.

PUSHINGS: Thuj.

QUIVERING: Sabin.

RAWNESS: **Ars.**, Bell., Canth., Carb-v., **Nux-v.**, Ran-b.

RAW: Carb-v., **Nux-v.**

REFLEXES: Ol-an.

RETRACTED: Hydr., **Plb.**

RUBS: Aran., Kali-c., Mag-c., Nat-s., **Phos.**, Plb.

RUBBING, **Amel.**: Podo.

SHOULDER to: Sang. (r).

SORE SPOT in: Arg-n., Bar-c., Bism., **Kali-bi.**, Phos., **Rhus-t.**

SPINE to: Arn., Verat-v.

SPOT in: Arg-n., Bar-c., Bism., Kali-bi., Lyc.

SQUEEZING in: Ant-t., Cocc., **Coloc.**, Scopar., Staph.

STANDING, **Agg.**: Nat-p.

STIFF: Lil-t., **Rhus-t.**

STITCHES: Bry., **Sulph.**

worse from motion: Bry., Spig.

STOOL, **Amel.**: Colch., **Coloc.**, **Gamb.**, Mag-c., NUX-V., Verat.

Agg.: Sul-ac.

SUNKEN: Apis, **Calc-p.**, Cupr., **Hydr.**, Kali-br., PLB., Verat., Zinc.

SWASHING: see **Gurgling.**

SWEAT on: Bell., Borx.

TEARING, **shooting**: Cham.

TENSION: Apis, Arn., Caps., **Carb-v.**, Chin., **Coloc.**, Lil-t., **Rhus-t.**, Scopar., Sil.

THIGHS, into: Lil-t., Mag-p., Sabal, **Staph.**, Thyr.

THROBBING: Nat-m., Nux-v., Ol-an., **Puls.**, Sel., Sep.

TREMBLING: Sang.

ULCER and ulcerative feeling: Kali-bi., Phos., Ran-b.

UNCOVERING, **Amel.**: Camph., Med., Sec., Tab., Vip-t.

UPWARD, extending: Acon., Ars., Calc., **Carb-v.**, Kali-bi., Kali-c., Lact-ac., Sabad.

from: Kali-m., Phos.

WARM (foods), **Amel.**, Lyc., Mag-p., **Nux-v.**, Sul-ac.

WEAK, sinking, hanging, etc.: Ign., Kali-c., Lil-t., Med., Merc., Phos., Sep.

EXTERNAL ABDOMEN

Apis, Bry., Merc., Nux-v., Plb., Puls., Sel.

BRUISED, sore: Acon., **Apis, Ars.,**
Bell., Bry., Chin., **Lach.,** Lyc.,
Merc-c., NUX-V., Stann.,
Sulph., Ter.

NUMB: Acon., **Bry., Plat., Puls.,**
Sars.

PENDULOUS, enlarged, pot-
bellied: Alum., **Calc.,** Carb-v.,
Caust., Colch., **Sep.,** Sulph.,
Syph., Tub., Vario.

HYPOCHONDRIA

Acon., Chin., Ran-b., Staph.

RIGHT, **liver, gall-ducts,** etc.:
Acon., Aloe, Am-c., Am-m.,
Ars., **Aur.,** Bar-c., **Bell.,** Berb.,
Bry., **Chel., Chin.,** Cocc.,
Colch., Dios., Gels., Hydr.,
Iris, **Kali-c., Lach.,** Lept., **Lyc.,**
Mag-m., Merc., **Nat-s.,** Nux-
v., **Phos.,** Podo., Rheum,
Sang., Sep.

  posterior: Calc., Kali-bi., Lept.,
  Rhus-t.

LEFT, **spleen and pancreas:**
Alum., Arn., Ars., **Asaf., Carb-**
v., Cean., **Chin.,** Con., Fl-ac.,
Helia., Ign., Iris, Kali-bi., Naja,
Nat-m., Nat-s., Nit-ac.,
Polym., Ran-b., Ruta, Squil.,
Sulph., Ther.

ABSCESS: Bell., Bry., Lach., Nux-
v., Puls., Ruta, Sep., Sil.

ACHE: Squil.

AROUND: **Ran-b.**

BACKWARD (to scapula); (r):
Acon., Aesc., Berb., **Borx.,**
Calc., CHEL., Dios., Dulc.,
Graph., **Hydr.,** Kali-bi., Lept.,
Lyc., Mag-m., Merc., **Myrt-c.,**
Nat-m., Sep.

BAND **about:** Acon., Card-m.,
Dros., Ign., Nux-v.

BURNING, **heat,** etc., l.: Aloe,
Aur., **Lach., Lept.,** Merc.,
Myrt-c.

BRUISED, sore: Bry., **Chin., Eup-**
per., Ran-b., Visc.

COUGHING, **Agg.:** Dros., **Eup-**
per., Kali-c., Nat-s.

CRAMP: Merc. (r).

GALL BLADDER, **gall-stones,**
etc.: Bell., Berb., **Bry., Calc.,**
Card-m., **Chel.,** Chion.,
CHIN., Euon., **Lach., Lept.,**
Lyc., Mag-p., MERC., Merc-
d., Myrt-c., **Nat-s.,** Nux-v.,
Phos., Podo., Sang., Sulph.

  bile ducts: Chel., Gels., Merc-d.,
  Rheum.

  burning: Lept., Myrt-c.

  bursting: Bapt., Lept., Myrth.

  clawing: Lyc., Med., Nat-s.

  griping: Sep.

  septic: Bry., Bufo, **Lach., Phos.,**
  Quas.

sore: Bapt., Lept., Myrt-c.

stooping, Agg.: Sep.

HOLDS: Dros.

INDURATION: Graph. (liver).

INFLAMMATION (liver): Lach.
(gall-bladder), Mag-m., **Phos.**
(gall-bladder).

JAUNDICE, infants of: Myrt-c.

urinary symptoms, with:
Carb-v., Cham., Chin., Ign.,
Lyc., Nux-v., Plb.

LIVER AND RIGHT ARM: Bry.,
Iris.

with lung symptoms: Card-m.,
Chel., Hydr.

lying on left side, Agg.: Arn.,
Bry., Card-m., Mag-m.,
Nat-s., Ptel., Sep.

pressure, Agg.: Bell., Bry., Carb-
v., Card-m., Lach., Lyc.,
Mag-m., **Merc.**, Phos.

scapula, left, to: Dios., Dulc.,
Lept., Myrt-c.

urticaria, with: Astac., Myrt-c.,
Polyg-s., Urt-u.

LIVER, burning: Aur-m.

bursting: Bry., Lept., Nat-s.

cramp: Astac., Mag-m.

cutting: Hydr., Thyr.

deep in: Lach.

breath, Agg.: Ptel., Thyr.

epigastrium to: Mag-m.

symptoms, with: Con.

griping: Phys.

heart, with: Myrt-c.

heavy: Bry., Nat-s.

lump: Aesc.

below: Arn., Borx., Echi.,
Gels., Lach., **Nat-s.**,
Thuj., Verat., Zinc.

navel to: Dulc., Lept., Myrt-c.,
Sep.

pain: Bry.

posterior: Arn., Borx., Echi.,
Thuj.

rash over: Sel.

shoulder to: Kali-c., Nux-v., Sep.

sore, sensitive: Aur-m., **Bell.**,
Bry., Iod., Iris, Kali-i., Lach.,
Lyc., **Nat-s.**, Nux-v.

spine to: Lept., Sil.

sticking: Nux-v.

swelled: Acon., **Chin.**, **Lyc.**,
Mag-m., **Merc.**, **Nat-s.**,
Nux-v., Podo., Sep., Vip-t.

tension: Chel.

throbs in: Crot-h., Lappa.

STICKING: Ign. (spleen), Sil.

TENSION: Acon., Lyc.

FLATULENCE

Arg-n., Arn., Asaf., CARB-V., **Cham.**, **CHIN.**, Cocc., **Graph.**, **Ign.**, Kali-c., LYC., Nit-ac., NUX-V., Phos., Puls., Scopar., Sil., **Sulph.**, Ter., Valer., Vib.

right: Bism., CALC., Graph., Lil-t., **Nat-s.**, Ox-ac., **Phos.**, Thuj.

left: Am-m., **Aur.**, **Carb-v.**, CON., Crot-t., Dios., Euph., Lyc., Nat-m., Ph-ac., Seneg., Staph., SULPH.

ABDOMEN, **upper, in:** Carb-v., Puls.

lower: Acon., Lyc., Nat-m., Nux-m., Sil., Sulph., Zinc., Zinc-val.

CROAKING: Coloc.

DISCHARGE of: **Carb-v.**, Chin., Graph., Kali-c., **Olnd.**

FERMENTING, **as if:** Rhus-t.

FLATUS, **coughing,** on: Sang.

hot: Teucr.

FOOD, **all turns to gas:** Carb-v., Kali-c., Nux-m., Nux-v.

FOUL, **putrid:** Ars., Asaf., **Carb-v.**, Cocc., Puls., Squil., Sulph.

GENERATION OF: Carb-v., Kali-c., Teucr.

HYSTERICAL: Asaf., Ign., Puls.

MENSES, with: Kali-p., Nux-m., Vib.

NOISY, rumbling, growling, etc.: Ant-c., **Carb-v.**, Caust., Chin., Hell., **Lyc.**, Nat-m., **Nat-s.**, **Nux-v.**, Phos., Ph-ac., Puls., Sep., Sil., Sulph., Verat.

OBSTRUCTED, retained: Ant-t., Aur. (l), Carb-v., Cham., Chin., **Cocc.**, Graph., **Ign.**, **Lyc.**, Nat-c, Nit-ac., Nux-v., Plb., Puls., **Raph.**, **Staph.**

PAINFUL, **wind colic:** Carb-v., **Cham.**, Chin., Coll., Lyc., Mag-p., Nat-s., **Nux-v.**, Ox-ac., Puls., Rhod., Staph., Verat., Zinc-val.

PRESSING, **on bladder: Carb-v.**, Ign., Kali-c.

on rectum: Calc., Ign., Nat-s.

upward: Arg-n., Asaf., Carb-v., Graph., Thuj.

PUSHING: Nat-s.

RECTUM, in: Hep., Nux-v., Sep.

ROLLING: Thyr.

SOUR: Calc., Mag-c., Nat-c., Rheum.

UP AND DOWN, passing, **Amel.:** Arg-n., Goss., Graph., Kali-c., SANG., Verat.

WANDERING: Carb-v., Chin., **Lyc.**, Nat-m., Puls., Sil.

GROINS

Aloe, Am-m., Cocc., Gran., Guaj.

RIGHT: Calc., Cham., Kali-c., Lach., **Lyc.**, Nux-v., Puls., Rhod., Rhus-t., Sul-ac., Thuj.

LEFT: Euph., Mag-c., **Zinc.**

ALTERNATING between: Coloc.

BODY, as of a: Plan.

EXTERNAL ring: Ars., Merc.

GLANDS: Calc., **Hep.**, **Merc.**, Nit-ac., Oci., Thuj.

HERNIA: Am-m., Aur., Cham., Lyc., **Nux-v.**, Sulph., Sul-ac., Verat.

    incarcerated or protruding: Nux-v., Verat.

    infantile: Calc., Cham., Lyc., Nit-ac., **Nux-v.**, Sul-ac.

    strangulated: Acon., Alum., Aur., Bell., Calc., Caps., Cham., Coloc., Lach., Lyc., Nit-ac., Nux-v., Op., Plb., Sil., Sulph., Sul-ac., **Verat.**

INTERNAL ring: Am-m., Aur., Lyc., **Nux-v.**, Sul-ac.

MONS VENERIS: Rhus-t.

SORE, **before menses:** Bry.

TENSE, sprained, etc.: Am-m., Nat-m.

ANUS AND RECTUM

ANUS: Aesc., Carb-v., Graph., Kali-c., Lach., Mur-ac., Nit-ac., **Nux-v.**, Paeon., Phos., Sabad., Sep., **Sulph.**

RECTUM: Aesc., **Aloe,** Calc., **Ign.**, Lyc., **Merc-c.**, Nat-m., **Nux-v.**, Phos., **Podo.**, Rat., Sep., **Sulph.**

ACHING: Rat.

BORING: Bry.

BUBBLES (anus): Coloc., Nat-m.

BURNING: **Ars.**, Caps., Carb-v., Iris, Kali-c., Lyc., Merc., Scopar., **Sulph.**

COITION, **Agg.:** Merc-c., Sil.

CONSTRICTION, **spasm, etc.:** **Ign.**, **Lach.**, Lyc., Merc-c., **Nit-ac.**, Nux-v.

COUGH, **Agg.:** Ign., Nit-ac., Tub.

CRAWLING in, **rectum:** Sulph.

CRUSTS, **anus in:** Paeon., **Petr.**

CUTTING, **rectum in:** Sil.

DRAWING: Lach.

DRY (anus): Aesc., Rat.

ERUPTION, **anus around:** Merc-c., **Nat-m.**, Nit-ac., **Petr.**, Polyg-s.

EXCORIATION: Sulph.

FIERY (anus): Med.

FISSURE: Alum., Caust., **Graph.**, Ign., Nat-m., **Nit-ac.**, Paeon., Rat., Syph., Thuj.

FISTULA: Calc-p., Nit-ac., **Sil.**, Sulph.

FULLNESS in rectum, with frequent urination: Ferr-pic.

GENITALS to: Chin., Lil-t., Rhod., Sil., Zinc.

HEMORRHOIDS: Aesc., **Aloe**, Caust., Coll., Graph., Ham., Kali-c., Lach., **Mur-ac.**, Nit-ac., NUX-V., SULPH.

blind: Nux-v.

painful: Mur-ac., Nit-ac., Paeon., Staph.

protruding: Aloe, Calc., Mur-ac., Sulph.

INACTIVE, powerless, open, etc.: Ail., **Aloe**, Alum., Apis, Ign., Kali-c., Op., **Phos.**, Sec.

ITCHING: Caust., Lyc., Nit-ac., **Sulph.**, Viol-o.

LABOR, after: Ruta.

LIVER, to: Dios., Lach.

LUMP, **plug**, etc.: Anac., Cann-s., Crot-t., Kali-bi., **Lach.**, Lil-t Nat-m., **Plat.**, SEP., Sul-ac.

MOISTURE at: **Ant-c.**, Caps., Carb-an., Caust., Hep., **Nit-ac.**, Op., **Phos.**, Sep., Sil., Sulph., Sul-i.

foul: **Ant-c.**, Sul-i.

NAVEL, to: Coloc., Lach.

PAIN, **continuous**: Kali-chl., Phyt.

PAINFUL, **long after stool**: Aesc., Agar., Aloe, Am-c., Calc., Graph., **Ign.**, Mur-ac., Nit-ac., **Paeon.**, Rat., Sil., Sulph.

PILES, **alternating with**: Abrot., Coll., Sabin.

bathing, cool, Amel.: **Aloe**, Nux-v.

bleeding: Am-c., Caps., Ferr., Kali-c., **Phos.**, Ph-ac., **Puls.**, Sabin., Sep., Sulph.

bluish: Aesc., **Carb-v.**, **Lach.**, Mur-ac.

bursting: Ham.

cough, Agg.: Lach.

foul: Podo.

heat, Amel.: Ars., Lyc., Mur-ac., Petr., Phos., Zin.

lifting, Agg.: Rhus-t.

reflex from: Coll.

sitting, Amel.: Calc.

sore: Ham.

sticking: Sep.

ulcerate: Carb-v., Zinc.

urinating, Agg.: Bar-c.

walking, Agg.: Zinc.

PRESSURE, **down on**: Sulph.

PRESSURE, fullness, etc.: Aesc., **Nit-ac.**, Sulph.

PRESSING, down on: Sulph.

PROLAPSE: **Aloe, Ign.**, Lyc., Merc., **Mur-ac.**, Phos., **Podo.**, Rad-met., Ruta, Sep.

RETRACTED, anus: Nat-p.

SHOOTING: Ign.

SORE, sensitive, smarting, painful: Bell., Carb-v., Graph., Kali-m., **Mur-ac.**, Nit-ac., Onos., Puls., Rad-met., Sulph.

STICKS, burr, splinter etc.: Aesc., Hell., Iris, Sanic.

STOOPING: Ruta.

STRICTURE (rectum): Syph.

SWEAT: Sep.

ULCER: **Carb-v.**, Kali-bi., Nit-ac., **Sulph.**

UPWARD, pain goes: Graph., Ign., Lach., Phos., **Sep.**, Sulph.

URGING: Caust., **Merc.**, Sulph.

abortive: Nux-v.

absence of: Bry., Op.

ineffectual (tenesmus): Caps., Erig., Merc., MERC-C., Rheum, Rhus-t., **Sulph.**

irresistible: Aloe.

passes flatus only: Aloe, Carb-v., Mag-m., Nat-c., Phos., Ruta, Sep.

URINATION, **Agg.**: Mur-ac.

WRIST, alternates with: Sulph.

PERINEUM

Agn., Alum., Carb-an., Carb-v., Cycl., Sulph.

ABSCESS: Crot-h.

BALL: Cann-s., Chim., Kali-m.

LACERATION: Staph.

MOIST: Paeon., Thuj.

PROSTATE GLAND: Bar-c., Chin., CON., Crot-h., Dig., Lyc., Med., Pareir., Phos., Polyg., Pop-t., PULS., **Sabal, Sel.**, Sep., Solid., **Staph.**, Sulph., THUJ.

enlarged: Cann-i., Chim., Sabal., Sil.

inflamed: Aur., Ferr-pic., **Sabal, Thuj.**

PROSTATORRHEA: Con., **Lyc.**, Sel., Sep.

STOOL

ACRID: Arn., **Ars.**, Carb-v., Chin., Colch., Gamb., Ign., Iris, Merc., Puls., Scopar., **Sulph.**

destroys hair: Coll.

AGGRAVATION from: Dios., Merc., **Merc-c.**

AMELIORATION from: Coloc., Gamb., **Nux-v.**

BAD ODOR: **Ars.**, Asaf., Bapt., **Carb-v.**, Nux-v., **Podo.**, **Psor.**, Puls., Sulph.

BILIOUS: Cham., Merc., Puls., Verat.

BLACK: **Ars.**, Lept., Op., Stram., Thuj., **Verat.**

foul, and: Chion., Crot-h., Lept.

tarry: Chion., Lept., Mag-m.

BLADDER, symptoms with: Merc-c.

BLOODY: Canth., Colch., Ferr-p. (water), Ham., **Ip.**, Merc., **Merc-c.** (water), **Nux-v.**, Phos., Puls., Rhus-t. (water), Sep., Sulph. (streaked).

BLUE: Bapt., Phos.

BREAKFAST, **Agg.**: Nat-s., Thuj.

BROWN, gushes: Aster., Kali-bi.

CHANGEABLE: Cham., Dulc., Puls.

CHILL, **with:** Ars., Coloc., Lacc., Merc., **Puls.**, Sulph., Verat.

COLD: Cub.

COLD, **Agg.**: Calc., Rumx., Tub.

COLORS, **several:** Aesc., Colch., Euon., Kali-p., Menis., Sulph., Zinc-cy.

CONSTIPATED: **Bry.**, Calc., Cocc., Graph., Lach., Lyc., **Nux-v.**, **Op.**, Plb., Psor., Sanic., Sil., Staph., Sulph.

alternate days, on: Calc., Cocc., Con., Kali-c., Lyc., Nat-m.

chronic: Bry., Graph., **Nux-v.**, Op., Plb., Sulph., Verat.

hard feces, from: Bry., Mag-m., Nux-v., Op., Plb., Verb.

inactivity, from: Alum., Hep., Kali-c., Nat-m., **Nux-v.**

scaly stools, with profuse nightly urination: Alum., Bry., Caust., Graph., Hep., Kali-c., Kreos., Lyc., Nat-c., Nux-v., Rhus-t., Sabin., Samb., Sep., Spig., Squil., Sulph.

CONSTIPATION, of intants: Plb.

CRUMBLING: Am-m., Mag-m., Nat-m., Sanic.

CURDLED, cheesy: Iod., Tab.

DARK, brown, etc.: Ars., **Bry.**, Graph., Kali-n., Nux-v., **Psor.**, Stram.

DIARRHEA: Aloe, Ars., Cham., Chin., Cina, Coloc., Con., Crot-t., Gamb., Iris, Merc., Nat-s., Phos., Ph-ac., **Podo.**, Psor., Puls., Rheum, Rhus-t., Sulph., **Verat.**

chronic: Ars., Calc., Phos., **Sulph.**

cold drinks, Agg.: Chin.

constipation, alternating with: Abrot., Ant-c., Arn., Berb., Calc., Chel,, Croc., Cupr., Lyc., Nat-s., Nux-v., Phos., Podo., Psor., Puls., Stront-c., Sul-ac., Valer.

debility; none: Calc., Ph-ac.

diarrhea and asthma: Kali-c.

diarrhea, then rheumatism: Dulc.

drinking, Agg.: Arg-n., Ars., Crot-t., Phos., Rhus-t.

debility none: Calc., Ph-ac.

diarrhea, then rheumatism: Dulc.

drinking, Agg.: Arg-n., Aral., Crot-t., Phos., Rhus-t.

early morning: Rumx., Sulph., Tub.

rising, after: Lil-t., Nat-s.

eating, Agg.: Aloe, Ars., Chin., Coloc., Crot-t., Ferr., Nux-v., Podo.

to Amel.: see Generalities.

fluent coryza, with: Calc., Canth., Cham., Chin., Coloc., Iod., Kali-i., Lach., Mag-c., Merc., Op., Phos., Rhus-t., Ruta, Sulph., Sul-ac.

gushes: Chin., Crot-t., Elat.

gurgles out: Aloe, Gamb., Thuj.

menses, Agg.: Bov., Caust., Coloc., Lach., Nat-s., Phos., Ph-ac., Puls., Sec., Sulph., Verat., Vib.

milk, Agg.: Nat-c., Sep.

milky: Tab.

morning: Aloe, Bry., Kali-bi., Lil-t., Nat-s., Podo., Rumx., SULPH.

muddy, dirty water, etc.: Ars., Brom., Ferr-p., Jal., Ox-ac., Ph-ac., Podo.

nervous; emotions, Agg.: Acon., ARG-N., Cham., Coff., Croc., GELS., Hyos., Ign., Op., Pall., Phos., Podo., Puls., Verat.

nightly: Ferr., Rhus-t., Stront-c.

odorless: Verat.

orange, tomato sauce, etc., like: Apis, Nat-c.

painful: Ars., Bry., Cham., Coloc., Merc., Merc-c., Rheum, Rhus-t., Sulph.

pain, long after: Aesc., Nit-ac., Paeon., Rat.

painless: Ars., Bapt., Chin., Ferr., Hyos., Lyc., Phos., Ph-ac., Podo., Puls., Stram., Sulph., Verat.

periodical: Stront-c.

phthisis of: Ars., Bry., Carb-v., Chin., Ferr., Hep., Kali-i., Nit-ac., Phos., Ph-ac., Puls., Sulph.

rice water: Ars., Camph., Jatr., Verat.

rising, after: Bry., Nat-s.

rumbling, with: Coloc., Stroph-h.

running thro' diaper: Benz-ac., Podo.

sago, like: Colch., Phos.

sand in: Lyc., Sars.

starch, like: Arg-n., Borx.

summer, Agg.: Bry., Podo.

watery: Tub.

weather, hot, Agg.: Bry., Podo.

DIFFICULT: Bry., Chin., Mag-m., Nat-m., Nux-v.

although soft: Alum., Chin., Hep., Ign., Nux-m., Plat., Psor., Puls., Sep., Sil., Staph.

DIURESIS, with: Mag-s.

DROPSY, with: Apoc.

DRY: Bry., Nat-m.

DYSENTERIC: Acon., Canth., Caps., Coloc., Ip., MERC-C., Nux-v., Phos., Rhus-t., Sulph.

EGGS, like bad: Cham.

FLATULENT, gassy, noisy, spluttering: Agar., Aloe, Arg-n., Coloc., Crot-t., Ferr., Gamb., Ign., Nat-s., Nux-m., Stroph-h., Thuj., Thyr., Tub.

FLATUS, passing, Agg.: Ars-i., Caust., Mur-ac.

FLOATS: Colch., Mag-c., Sabad.

FLOCCULENT: Kali-m.

FREQUENT: Acon., Calc., Cham., Merc-c., Nux-v., Podo., Verat.

GELATINOUS: Aloe, Colch., Kali-bi.

see also Generalities.

GLISTENS: Aloe, Alum., Calc., Caust., Mez.

particles: Cina, Mez., Phos.

GRANULAR, sandy, etc.: Apis, Arg-met, Ars., Bell., Berb., Bov., Cist., Coll., Cub., Hydr., Lac-c., Lyc., Mang., Mez., Phos., Plb., Podo., Sars., Thuj., Zinc.

GRASS GREEN: Acon., Ant-t., ARG-N., Cham., Gels. (tea), Ip., Iris, Merc., Merc-d., Thuj.

dark: Ars.

scum: Asc-t., Bry., Grat., Mag-c., Merc., Sanic.

turns: Arg-n., Borx., Calc-f., Nat-s., Psor., Rheum, Sanic.

GUSHING, pouring: Aloe, Bry., Crot-t., Gamb., Jatr., Podo., Psor., Sang., Sec., Verat.

see also Generalities

HACKED, chopped: Acon., Cham., Nat-p., Sul-ac.

HARD: Alum., Bry., Graph., Mag-m., Nat-m., Nit-ac., Plb., Sil., Sulph.

HEAVY: Sanic.

HOLD back: Nit-ac., Sil., Sulph., Thuj.

HOT, burning: Aloe, ARS., Asc-t., Bell., Caps., **Cham.**, Gamb., IRIS, **Merc-c.**, Pic-ac., Podo., Scopar., Stroph-h., Sulph.

IMPACTED: Calc., Nat-m., Sanic., Sel., Sep., Sil.

INSUFFICIENT: Arn., Caps., Cham., **Lyc.**, Mag-m., Merc-c., Nat-c., **Nux-v.**, Sulph.

INVOLUNTARY, hurried, etc.: **Aloe**, Apis, **Arn.**, Bar-c., Gels., Hyos., Lycps-v., **Phos.**, Ph-ac., Podo., **Sulph.**, Thuj., Verat.

although solid: Aloe, Ars., Caust., Coloc., **Hyos.**

urinating on: Apis, Mur-ac.

KNOTTY, lumpy, like sheep dung, of little balls: Alum., Bell. (chalky), Calc. (chalky), Chel., Chin., Cob., Graph., Hydr., Kali-m., Lil-t., Lyc., Mag-c. (tallow), **Mag-m.**, Merc., Merc-d., Merc-i-r., Mosch., Nat-m., **Op.**, Plan., Plb., Pyrog., Sanic., Sel., Senec., Sep., Sil., Sulph., Syph., Teucr., Thuj., Ust., Verat., Verb.

LARGE CALIBER: **Bry.**, Graph., Kali-c., Lyc., **Sanic.**, **Verat.**

MEALY: Podo., Stront-c.

MEAT WATER, like: Calc., Canth., Ferr-p., Kali-i., Kreos., Mang., Merc-c., Nit-ac., Phos., Podo., Rhus-t.

MISSHAPEN, angular, square, etc.: Plb., Sanic., Sel.

MUCUS: Arg-n., **Ars.**, Asar., Borx., **Caps.**, **Cham.**, Colch., **Graph.**, Hell., Ip., Kali-m., Merc., Merc-c., Nux-v., Phos., **Puls.**, Rhus-t., Solid., Spig., Sulph.

after: Bry., Sep., Thuj.

bloody: Merc., **Merc-c.**

coated: Am-m., Cham., **Graph.**, Hydr., Nat-m., Puls.

colitis: Asar., Colch., Kali-p., Rhus-t., Zinc-val.

green: Acon., Arg-n., Cham., Gamb., Iris, **Merc.**

lumps, of: Aloe, Ip., Mag-c., Spig.

MUSTY: Coloc.

NOISY: Arg-n., **Nat-s.**, Thuj.

PASTY, sticky: Bry., Chel., Kali-bi., Lach., Merc., **Plat.**, Rheum, Rhus-t., Sulph.

PENETRATING odor: Podo., **Psor.**, Stram.

PERISTALSIS, inactive: **Bry.**, Nux-v., **Op.**, Thuj.

POP'S out: Thuj.

PROSTRATING: Ars., Verat.

not: Apis, Calc., Ph-ac.

PUTTY like: Dig., Plat.

RECEDING: Mag-m., Op., Sanic., Sil., Thuj.

RED: Chel., Lyc., Merc., **Rhus-t.**, Sulph.

RETAINED: **Cocc.**, Sil., **Stram.**

REMOVED, must be: Lyc., Nat-m., Plat., Sanic., Sel., Sep., Sil.

SCANTY, but frequent: Ars., Merc-c., Nux-v.

SCUM, floating on: Asclp., **Bry.**, Cocc., Grat., MAG-C., Sal-ac., Sanic., Zinc-i.

SHREDDY: Arg-n., Canth., Carb-ac., Colch., Coloc., Merc., **Merc-c.**, Phyt.

SLENDER: Caust., **Phos.**

SOFT, mushy, etc.: Bry. (yellow), Chin., Nit-ac., Onos., Phos., Puls., **Sulph.**

SOUR: **Calc.**, Hep., Mag-c., Merc., Nat-p., Rheum, Sulph.

STANDING, **Amel.**: Alum., Caust.

STRAIN, must: Alum., Chin., Nat-m., **Nux-v.**, Rat., Sil.

STRINGY, tough: Colch., Lept., **Phos.**

SUDS, like: Benz-ac., Colch., Elat., Glon., Iod., Sulph.

TARRY: Chion., Lept., Phys., Ptel.

TEARING anus: Mez., Nat-m.

TRIANGULAR: Nat-m., Plb., Sanic., Sep.

UNDIGESTED: Ars., **Calc.**, Calc-p., **Chin.**, Ferr., Graph., Olnd., Phos., Ph-ac.

brown: Kreos., Psor.

UNSATISFACTORY: Alum., Graph., Lyc., Mag-m., **Merc-c.**, Sep., Sulph.

URGING, cramp: Plob.

flatus only, passes: Aloe.

fruitless: Nux-v.

in sleep: Phyt.

URINATING, when: Aloe, Apis, Mur-ac.

WAXY: Kali-bi., Lept., Sin-n.

WHEYEY: Cupr., Iod.

WHITE, gray, ashy, etc.: Ars., Calc., Chel., Dig., Kali-c., Lach., **Merc.**, Op., Phos., Ph-ac., **Podo.**, Tarax. (ashy).

WORMS: **Acon.**, Art-v., **Calc.**, Chin., **Cina,** Cupr-ox., Ign., Merc., Nat-p., **Sabad.**, **Sil.**, Spig., Stann., **Sulph.**

feverish and: Cina.

pinworms: Calc., Chin., Ferr., Ign., Naphtin., Rat., Sabad., Sin-n., Sulph., Teucr., Urt-u.

tapeworm: Calc., Graph., Plat., Puls., Sabad., Sil., Sulph.

YELLOW: Ars., Crot-t., Merc., Nuph., **Podo.**

bright: Aeth., Aloe, Chel., Colch., Gamb., Gels., Kalip., Nux-m., Phos., Podo., Sul-ac., Sul-i.

water: Gamb., Podo.

CONCOMITANTS

BEFORE STOOL: Calc., Merc., **Nux-v., Verat.**

DURING STOOL: Ars., Cham., Merc., Puls., **Sulph.**, Verat.

AFTER STOOL: **Caust., Merc-c.**, Nux-v., **Phos.**, Podo., Sel.

MICTURITION

BEFORE, **Agg., cries,** etc.: Acon., Borx., **Lyc.,** Nux-v., Sanic., Sars.

BURNING: see **Generalities.**

CONTINENCE, **Agg.:** Calc., Con., Lyc., Pic-ac., **Plat.**

COUGHING on: **Caust.,** Nat-m., Puls., Squil., Verb.

CUTTING: Canth., Sep.

DESIRE, **urging,** etc.: Ant-t., Bry., **Canth.,** Caust., Lil-t., **Merc-c., Nux-v.,** Ph-ac., Puls., Sabin., Sars., Squil., Staph., **Sulph.**

SITTING, **Agg.:** Sas.

Amel.: Zinc.

SPURTS, in: Clem., Con., Tub.

diarrhea, during: Apis, Arn., Canth., **Merc-c.**

fruitless: Ars., Canth., Dig., Merc-c., **Nux-v.,** Sars.

DIFFICULT, **dysuria,** painful, drop by drop, strangury, etc.: Cann-s., **Canth.,** Cham., Erig., Lil-t., **Merc-c., Nux-v.,** Pop-t., Prun., Puls., Sabad., Sars., Staph., Sulph., Ter.

in presence of others: **Ambr.,** Hep., Mur-ac., **Nat-m.,** Tarent.

DOUBLING-UP, **Amel.:** Canth., Prun.

DRIBBLING: **Canth.,** Clem., Kali-m., Merc-c., Puls., Sel., Sulph.

senile: Bar-c., Con., Rhus-a.

DRINKING, after: Apis, Arg-n., **Ferr-p., Samb.**

FEEBLE, slow, weak, etc.: Alum., Arn., **Caust.,** Echi., **Hep.,** Lyc., Merc-cy., Mur-ac., Pyrog., Sars., Sep., Solid., Stil-i., Tab., Thyr., Tub.

drops vertically: Arg-n., Caust., Gels., **Hep.**

FREQUENT: Arg-met., Bar-c., Caust., Guaj., Kali-n., Lyc.,

Mang., **Merc.**, **Merc-c.**, **Nux-v.**, Rhus-t., Squil., Staph., Sulph.

HEADACHED, with: Vib.

HURRIED, irresistible: Bry., Kreos., Phos., Puls., Sulph.

sudden: Petros., Sulph.

INFREQUENT: Apis, Canth.

INTERRUPTED, intermittent, stops and starts, etc.: Agar., Ant-c., Apis, Carb-an., Caust., **Clem.**, **Con.**, Gels., Kali-c., Led., Lyc., Op., Sars., Sulph., Thuj.

INVOLUNTARY: **Caust.**, Ferr., Puls., Rhus-t.

bed in, bed-wetting: **Bell.**, Calc., Caust., Cina, Merc., **Puls.**, Rhus-t., Sabal., Sec., Sil., **Sulph.**, Syph., Tub.

during first sleep: Caust., Sep.

coughing, on: Caust., Phos.

lying, Agg.: Bell-p., **Kreos.**, Lach., Lyc., Pic-ac., **Puls.**, Uva.

by day, only: **Ferr.**

rising: Petr.

NERVOUS: Cimic., **Ign.**, Vib.

NIGHTLY: Lyc., Rhus-t.

ODD POSITIONS, in: Zinc.

PAINS, **Agg.:** Ter., Thuj.

PROFUSE, polyuria, etc.: Gels., Kreos., Lac-d., (pain), Ph-ac.

RETENTION, **suppression**, tardy, etc.: **Acon.**, Apis, Arn., Ars., Camph., **Canth.**, Hep., Kali-bi., **Lyc.**, Mez., Op., Puls., **Stram.**, Ter., Thuj., Verat.

Comp. **Discharges** and **Feeble.**

RIDING, **Amel.:** Lyc.

SCANTY: **Apis, Canth.**, Colch., Dig., Graph., **Hell.**, Op., Ruta, Staph.

SENSATION, **without:** Alum., Caust., **Mag-m.**

SITTING, **Agg.:** Sars.

Amel.: Zinc.

SPURTS, in: Clem., Con., Tub.

STANDING, **Amel.:** Caust., Con., Hyper., Sars.

STOOL, strains, **Amel.:** Aloe, Alum., Lil-t., Mur-ac., Tub.

STRANGURY: Canth., Ter.

STREAM, **slender:** Staph.

UNEASY: Verat-v.

WEAKNESS, then: **Ars.**, Caust., Ferr., **Gels.**, Nux-v., **Phos.**

WHITE, **at close:** Ph-ac., Sars.

URINE

ALTERED IN GENERAL: Puls., Sep., Sulph.

ACRID: Hep., Merc., Med., Puls., Urt-u.

ALBUMINOUS: APIS, **Ars.**, **Canth.**, Calc-p., **Ferr.**, MERC-C., **Phos.**, **Plb.**, Phyt., Rhus-t., **Sulph.**, Ter., Tarent.

ALBUMINURIA: Ant-c., Aur., Bry., Kali-c., Lach., Puls., Thuj., Valer.

periodical: Phos.

AMMONIACAL: Med., Pic-ac.

AROMATIC: Eup-per., Onos.

BLACK: Apis, Ars., Colch., Kali-c., Lach., Merc-c., Ter.

BLOODY: **Arn.**, Ars., Merc-c., **Phos.**, Sec., Squil., **Ter.**

CLOUDY: **Cina**, Con., **Merc.**, Phos., Sabad.

turning: Bry., Cham., **Ph-ac.**

DARK: **Acon.**, Ant-t., Bell., **Bry.**, Colch., **Merc.**, Sep., Solid., **Verat.**

flecks, in: Hell.

ENURESIS: Sabal., Sec.

first sleep, in: Caust., Sep.

FLOCCULENT: **Canth.**, Mez.

FILAMENTOUS: Canth.

FROTHY: Aur., Chel., Lach., Scopar., Spong., Syph.

GRASSY: Sars.

GREEN: Merc-c.

GREENISH: Camph., Verat.

HOT, **burning:** Acon., Ars., **Bell.**, Cann-s., Canth., Hep., Merc., Merc-c.

HORSE's, like: Benz-ac., Nit-ac.

ITCHING, causing: Uut-u.

LITHEMIA: see **Acid Diathesis.**

LITHEMIA: see Generalities, Uric **Acid, Diathesis.**

MILKY: Cina, Kali-p., **Ph-ac.**, Viol-o., Visc.

MORE **than drinks:** Apis, Merc., Ph-ac.

ODOR, **ammoniacal, strong:** Asaf., Benz-ac., Nit-ac., Phos.

foul, repulsive: Benz-ac., **Dulc.**, Puls., **Sep.**, Solid., Thuj.

OXALURIA: Berb., Kali-s., Nit-m-ac.

PALE: Con., Kali-c., **Ph-ac.**, Stront-c.

PELLICLE on: Coloc., **Par.**, Phos., Psor., Puls., Sep.

PROFUSE: Arg-met., Lyc., Mur-ac., Phos., **Ph-ac.**, Rhus-t., Squil., Spig., Verb., Vib.

Amel.: Gels., Ign., Sang.

dropsy, in: Squil.

hemorrhage, with: Calc., Gels., Ign., Lach., Mosch., Sars., Stram., Sulph., Vib.

headache, Agg.: Mosch.

menses, with: Med., Vib.

and scanty, alternately: Bell.,
    Berb., Dig., Gels., Nit-
    ac., Senec.

PURULENT: Bapt., Polyg-s., Sul-
    i., Uva.

RECEDES: Prun.

RETAINED, at birth: Acon., Apis,

SACCHARINE: See Diabetes.

SCANTY: Ars., Bry., Chin., Dulc.,
    Led., Lyc., Phos., Puls., Rhus-
    t., Sep., Soli., Stront-c., Til.,
    Verat.

then headache: Iod., Ol-an.

SHREDDY: Seneg.

SMOKY: Ter., Verb.

STRAIN, must, at stool to pass:
    Alum.

STREAM, small: Eup-per.

SUPPRESSED: Canth., Lyc.,
    Solid.

TURBID, sedimentitious : Chim.

UREMIA: Apis, Ars., Bapt., Bell.,
    Canth., Hyos., Op., Stram.,
    Verat.

VALERIAN: Murx.

VISCID: Coloc.

WATERY: Squil.

SEDIMENT

Canth., Coloc., Lyc., Ph-ac.,
    Puls., Sep., Valer., Zinc.

ADHERENT: Apis, Bov., Coloc.,
    Ferr., Ign., Merc-c., Ol-an.,
    Osm., Phos., Polyg-s., Puls.,
    Rumx., SEP., Ust.

BLACK: Colch., Lach., Ter.

BLOODY: Canth., Ph-ac., Puls.,
    Sep.

BRANNY: Ant-t., Merc., Phos.,
    Valer.

CLAYEY, earthy: Zinc.

CLOUDY: Ph-ac.

COARSE: Sel.

COFFEE grounds: Apis, Hell.

FLAKY: Canth., Mez., Zinc.

GRAVEL: Polyg-s., Sars.

LIMY: Sabal.

MEALY: Ant-t., Apis, Berb., Calc.,
    Chin., Graph., Merc., Nat-m.,
    Phos., Ph-ac., Sulph.

MUCUS: Berb., Puls., Ter.

MUDDY: Ter.

RED, brickdust, etc.: Bry., Canth.,
    Chin., Lyc., Nat-m., Puls.,
    Sep., Valer.

ROSY-RED: Apis, Ars., Berb.,
    Bov., Cist., Coll., Led., Lyc.,
    Sars., Sel., Sep., Sul-i. (Brown),
    Tarent., Thuj.

STICKY: Pyrog., Tub.

WHITE: Phos., **Rhus-t.**

YELLOW: Zinc.

CONCOMITANTS

Cann-s., Merc., Puls.

BEFORE URINATION: Borx., Coloc., **Nux-v., Puls.**

AT START OF URINATION: Merc.

DURING URINATION: Cann-s., Canth., Hep., Lyc., **Merc.,** Ph-ac., **Puls.,** Sep., Thuj.

AFTER URINATION: Canth., Coloc., Hep., **Merc-c.,** Nat-m., **Thuj.**

URINARY ORGANS

Acon., APIS, **Ars.,** Arn., Bell., **Berb.,** Calc., Camph., Cann-s., CANTH., **Caust.,** Dulc., Ferr., Hell., Hep., Hyos., Lyc., **Merc.,** Merc-c., Nat-m., Nit-ac., **Nux-v.,** Op., Pareir., Phos., Ph-ac., Polyg-s., PULS., Rhus-t., Sars., Sil., Squil., Sulph., Ter., Thuj., Til., Valer., Verat.

ALTERNATING **with rheumatic symptoms:** Benz-ac.

KIDNEYS: Apis, Ars., Berb., **Canth.,** Merc-c., Polyg-s., Rhus-t., Samb., Scopar., Solid., Squil., Stront-c., Ter.

right: Berb., Coc-c., **Lyc.,** Nux-v., Oci., **Sars.**

left: Chin., Coloc., Merc., Pareir., Zinc.

abscess: Ars., **Canth.,** Chin., Hep., Lyc., Puls., Sil.

ache: Helon., Phyt., Sep., Solid.

boring: Kreos.

bubbling: Berb., Med.

burning: Phyt., Sep., Ter.

colic: Berb., Coloc., Oci-c., Pareir., Polyg-s., Sars., Tab., Ter.

congestion: Acon., Ars., Canth., Kali-bi., Scopar., Solid., Ter.

distended: Helon., Solid.

epigastrium to: Thuj. (l).

fluttering: Brach., Chim.

heavy: Kali-bi.

inactive: Helon., Solid.

nephritis: Acon., Apis, Cann-s., Canth., Ferr., Hep., Kali-chl., Med., Merc-c., Nit-ac., Puls., Rhus-t., Solid., Stront-c., Sulph., Ter., Thuj.

bronchitis with: Ter.

frequency of: Gels., Kali-p.

scarlatinal: Ars., Canth., Hell., Hep., Ter.

suppurative: **Canth.,** Lyc., Puls., Sul-i.

pyelitis: Kali-s., Rhus-t., Sul-i.

coma, with: Bapt.

sore: Cadm-s., Senec., Solid., Vis-a.

thigh, to: Ip.

URETERS: Apis, Bell., Berb., Canth., Lyc., Oci-c., Polyg-s., Sars., Sep., Ter.

cramp: Nit-ac., Polyg-s.

cutting: Verat-v.

sore:Apis, Berb., Hedeo., Oci-c.

BLADDER: Canth., Caust., Dulc., Hyos., Lyc., Merc-c., Nux-v., Puls., Ruta, Sabal, Staph., Sulph.

aching: Ter.

atony: Stann.

back, to: Sars.

burning, heat, etc.: Berb., CANTH., Caps., Merc-c., Senec. (neck), Ter., Zinc-ar.

bursting: Pareir., Zinc.

chill: Sars.

colds, Agg.: Dulc.

cramp: Mez., Puls.

crawling in: Sep.

cutting: Pall.

griping: Canth.

inflamed: Polyg-s., Solid., Ter.

injuries to: Staph.

irritable: Bell., Nux-v., Sabal, Staph.

lump in: Kreos.

neck of: Canth., Merc-c.

painful, sore: Apis, Canth., Equis., Ter.

paralysis of: Ars., Gels., Hyos., Nux-v.

tenesmus: Bell., Cann-s., Canth., Dig., Dulc., Erig., Equis., Merc-c., Pareir., Sulph., Ter.

throbbing in neck: Epig.

ulceration, suppuration: Petr., Puls., Sep., Sulph.

URETHRA: Arg-n., Cann-s., Canth., Caps., Clem., Lyc., Merc., Phos., Puls., Sulph., Thuj.

abscess: Canth., Puls., Rhus-t.

bleeds after urinating: Hep., Merc-c., Sars.

burning: Canth., Merc-c., Sulph.

before urination: Caps.

caruncle: Arg-n., Ars., Cann-s., Hep., Nit-ac., Sulph., Sul-i.

cramp: Clem.

cutting: Canth., Thuj.

discharge, fetid: Carb-v., Sil.

painless : Ferr., Nat-s., Thuj.

persists: Alum., Arg-met., Kali-bi., Sulph.

urinating after: Sars.

thin: Lyc., Nat-m., Nit-ac., Phos., Psor., Sulph.

drawing: Fl-ac., Merc.

heavy: Eup-per., Sabad., Til.

itching: Merc-c., Nux-v., Rhus-t., Sil., **Sulph.**

riding, Agg.: Staph.

stricture: Clem., Fl-ac., Nat-s., Petr., Puls.

trickling: see Generalities.

urinating, Amel., while: Staph.

walking, Agg.: Staph.

GENITALS

Agn., Arn., Berb., Calad., Coff., Erig., Gels., Hyos., Merc., Nit-ac., **Puls.**, Rhus-t., Sabal, Sel., **Sep.**, Sulph.

RIGHT: Apis, Calc., Caust., Clem., Hep., Lyc, Merc., Nux-v., Pall., Spong., Sul-ac., Verat.

LEFT: **Lach.**, Naja, **Puls.**, Rhod., Thuj.

alternating between: Cimic., Coloc., Lac-c., Lil-t., Lycps-v., Ol-an., Onos., Rhod., Ust.

___

DRY: Tarent.

HEAT: Tarent., Tub.

IRRITATION, of: Senec.

ITCHING: Rad-met., Sabin., Tarax.

burning: Nat-m., Urt-u.

MOTION, **Agg.**: Sabin.

OFFENSIVE: Psor., Sars., Sulph., **Thuj.**

PROLAPSE: Bur-p., Podo., Sep.

RAW: Tarent.

RELAXED, coitus, **Agg.**: Nux-v., Ph-ac., Sulph.

SENSITIVE: Coff., Plat., **Staph.**, Tarent., Zinc.

SITTING, **Agg.**: Sulph.

SWEAT, moisture on: Dios., Sars., Sel., **Sep.**, Thuj.

SWELLED: **Rhus-t.**, Tarent.

THIGHS, down: Cham., Chel., Cimic., Kali-c., Ox-ac., Rhus-t., Sep., Ust.

TICKLING: Plat.

UPWARD: Murx.

VARICOSE: Zin.

MALE ORGANS

Agn., Arg-n., **Aur.**, Cann-s., Canth., Cinnb., CLEM., Con., **Graph.**, Lyc., MERC., NIT-AC., **Nux-v.**, Plat., PULS., **Rhod.**, **Rhus-t.**, Spong., Staph., **Sulph.**, Thuj.

PENIS: Arn., **Cann-s.**, Canth., Clem., Cop., Dulc., **Merc.**, Thuj.

constriction: Kali-bi.

priapism: Caps., Oena., Phos., Pic-ac., Staph.

pulsation: Cocc-c., Con.

warts: Ant-t., Med., Thuj.

GLANS: Merc., Nit-ac., Rhus-t., Thuj.

  into: Par-b.

  urinating, Agg.: Prun.

PREPUCE: Apis, Calad., Jac-c., Merc., Rhus-t.

  cracked: Hep., Sul-i.

  edema: Nit-ac., Rhus-t.

  slough: Thuj.

  warts: Cinnb., Sep., Thuj.

SPERMATIC CORD: Berb., Ham., Puls., Spong.

  abdomen to: Rhod.

  burns: Pus.

  sore: Ham., Kali-c., Ox-ac., Phyt.

  thigh, to: Rhod.

TESTES: Arn., Aur., Clem., Merc., Nux-v., Puls., Rhus-t., Sep., Spong.

  alternately: Rhod.

  crushed, as if: Rhod.

  gripe: Phos.

  hanging low: Calc., Clem., Puls.

  indurated: Aur., Clem., Con., Iod., Rhod., Spong.

inflamed: Clem., Ham., Puls.

  mumps, from: Plb., Puls.

orchitis: Acon., PULS.

retracted: Sabal.

soft: Sul-i.

swelled: Clem., Dulc., Puls., Spong.

throb: Ox-ac., Spong.

SCROTUM: Arn., Crot-t., Petr., Rhus-t., Sulph.

bluish: Puls.

edema: Fl-ac.

excoriated: Polyg-s., Sil.

hydrocele: Rhod., Sil.

moist: Cinnb.

scaly: Calc.

spots: Sil.

COLDNESS: Agn., Caust., Gels., Lyc., Sabal, Sulph.

EJACULATION, premature: Carb-an., Chin., Erig., Graph., Lyc., Nux-v., Phos., Zinc.

EMISSION: Calad., Chin., Con., Ferr., Gels., Phos., Ph-ac., Sel., Squil.

bloody: Merc., Puls.

voluptuous: Viol-t.

ERUPTION: Crot-t., Graph., Petr., Rhus-t., Rad-met.

FLACCID, suddenly: Graph., Lyc., Nux-v.

glans: Mag-m., Nat-c.

FUMBLING, grasping: Acon., Bell., Bufo, Canth., HYOS., Merc., Sep., Stram., Zinc.

IMPOTENCY: Tab.

SEMEN, bloody: Fl-ac., Lyc.

hot: Calc., Tarent.

painful: Cann-s., Canth., Sabal.

watery: Sel., Sulph.

FEMALE ORGANS

Ambr., Apis, BELL., Calc., Cham., Cimic., Con., Graph., Kali-c., Kreos., Lach., Lil-t., Lyc., Nat-m., Nux-v., Onos., Phos., Plat., PULS., Sabin., Sec., Senec., SEP., Sulph., Thuj., Til., Tril-p., Ust., Vib., Visc.

external: Sep., Thuj.

OVARIES: Apis, Bell., Canth., Coloc., Guaj., Lach., Lil-t., Lyc., Mag-p., Puls., Sabal, Staph., Thuj., Zinc-val.

back to: Rumx. (r).

breasts to: Murx., Senec.

congested: Apis.

cystic: Apis, Apoc., Aur., Form.

left to heart: Brom., Cimic., Lac-c., Lach., Lil-t., **Naja**, Sulph., Vib.

legs, stretching, **Agg.**: Podo.

mammae to: Murx., Senec.

pains in: Naja.

swelled: Lyc.

tearing: Thuj.

thighs to: Coloc., Graph., Podo., Staph., Ust., Xan., Zinc-val.

VAGINA: Calc., Ferr., Kali-c., Lyc., Merc., Puls., Sep., Sulph.

bloody water: Nit-ac.

cutting: Sil.

dry: Nat-m., Tarent., Zinc-chr.

flatus: Brom., Lyc., Ph-ac.

heat: Tarent.

itches: Carb-ac., Coff., Kreos., Plat., Sep., Thuj.

prolapse: Bur-p., Plat., Podo.

raw: Tarent.

scratching, **Agg.**: Tarent.

sensitive, painful: Kreos., Plb.

shooting up: Rhus-t., Sabin., Sep.

spasm: Bell., Mag-p., Plat., Sep.

VULVA holds: Sanic.

open: Bov., Sabal, Sec., Sep.

sensitive, sore: Plat., Staph., Sulph.

sitting, **Agg.**: Berb., Kreos., Staph., Sulph.

swelled: Hep., Puls., Sep.

UTERUS: Arn., **Bell.**, Castm., Caul., Cham., Cimic., Kali-c., Plat., Pall., **Puls.**, Sabin., Sec., Sep., Vib.

burning: Tarent., Ter.

cancer: **Ars.**, Aur., Bell., Carban., Chin., Clem., Con., Ferr., Iod., Kreos., Lach., Mag-m., Merc., Plat., Puls., Sabin., Sars., Sec., Sep., Thuj.

cutting: Ip., Sulph.

enlarged: Aur., Con., Helon., Mag-m., Plb., Sep.

fullness: Aloe, Helon.

gnawing: Thyr.

hemorrhage: see Generalities.

heavy: Helon., Pall., Puls., Sep.

omert: Alet., Goss., Helon., Kali-c., Plb., Sabin., Sec., Sep.

inflamed: Bell., Rhus-t., Sec., Sulph., Ter.

in a.m.: Bell., Nat-m.

numb.: Phys.

nursing, Agg.: Arn., **Cham.**, Sil.

os rigid: Bell., Caul., Gels., Verat-v.

pain, in: Coloc., Helon., Ign.

reflexes: Bell., Cimic., Goss., Helon., Kali-c., Lil-t., Plat.

septic: **Arn.**, Ars., Pyrog., Rhus-t., Sec.

sore: Gels., Lappa, Murx., Ust.

spongy: Ust. (cervix).

stitching: Sep.

subinvolution: Arn., Frax., Helon., **Sep.**

smelled: Aur., Calc-i., Con., Lappa, Lyc., Plat., Sec., Sep.

tilted, to left: Sep.

to right: Murx., Puls.

ulcer: Carb-an., Hydr., Kreos., Ust.

———

ABORTUS: Apis, Bell., Cham., Croc., Ip., **Sabin.** (3rd month), Sec., Sep., Vib.

habitual: Apis, Ferr., Lyc., Plb., Sil., Syph., Thuj.

tenesmus recti, Agg.: Bell., Calc., Cocc., Con., Ip., Lyc., Merc., Nux-v., Rhus-t., Sep., Sulph.

third month: Bell., Plb., Sabin., Sep.

ABSCESS, labial, pus tubes, etc.: Lach., Merc., **Puls.**, Sep.

ADHERENT PLACENTA: **Puls.**, Sec.

septic: Sec.

AFTER-PAINS: Arn., Cham., **Cimic.**, **Puls.**, Rhus-t., Sabin., Vib.

intolerable: Cham., Cimic.

BACKWARD pains: Bell., Lil-t., Sep.

BURNING: Ars., Berb., **Canth** Carb-an., **Kreos.**, Sec., Sulph., Tarent., Ter.

COITION, **Agg.**: Apis, **Arg-n.**, Kreos., Nat-m., Puls., Sep., Sulph.

DRYNESS: Berb., Lyc., Nat-m., Sep.

ECLAMPSIA: Cic., Cupr., **Hyos.**, Ign., **Strych.**, **Verat-v.**

FIBROID: Calc., Graph., Tril-p.

bleeding: Calc., Nit-ac., Phos., Sul-ac., Tril-p.

GANGRENE: Sec.

HEART, to: Naja, Xan.

ITCHING: **Calad.**, Calc., Carb-v., Con., Lat-m., **Nat-m.**, Sep., Sulph., **Tarent.**

of pregnancy: Sabin.

LABIAE, abscess, swelled: Sep.

eruption: Sep.

LABOUR-LIKE, or bearing down pains: **Bell.**, Castm., **Cham.**, Frax., **Gels.**, Lil-t., **Nux-v.**, Pall., Plat., PULS., Sabin., Sec., **Sep.**, Sil., Thyr., Vib.

LABOR PAINS, ceasing, weak, etc.: Bell., Caul., Gels., Kali-c., Kali-p., Op., **Puls.**, Sec.

easing: Caul., Cimic., Vib.

false: Puls.

inefficient: Caul., Coff., Nux-v.

pains, upward: Calc., Cham., Gels., Lach.

too painful, laborious or violent, etc.: Cham., Puls., Sec., Sep.

spasms, with: Cham., **Hyos.**, Ign., Puls.

weak: Kali-c., Kali-p., Op.

LOCHIA, foul: Echi., Kreos., Sec.

green: Lac-c., Sec.

nursing, **Agg.**: Sil.

suppressed: **Bry.**, Hep., Puls., Sulph.

LYING, **Agg.**: Ferr., Kreos., Murx., **Puls.**

MOTION, **Agg.**, bleeding: Croc., Sec., Tarent.

NURSING, **Agg.**: Arn., **Cham.**, Puls., Sil.

PUERPERAL INFECTION, septic uterus: Ars., Bell., Lyc., Op., **Pyrog.**, **Rhus-t.**, Sec., **Sulph.**

PUERPERAL SEPSIS: Lyc., Phos., Puls., Pyrog., **Rhus-t.**, Sulph.

PUBES backward, lumbar, region, etc., to: Calc., Phos., Sabin.

PUDENDUM, **urine burns:** Scopar.

pulsates: Prun.

SALPINGITIS: **Puls.**, Staph.

SORE, **sensitive, painful:** Apis, Canth., Coff., **Con.**, Gels., **Kreos.**, **Lach.**, Lappa, Lil-t., Murx., **Plat.**, Staph., Sulph., Thuj., Ust.

STOOLING, **Agg.:** Ambr., Podo., Stann.

SWELLED: Apis, Aur., Bell., Calc-i., Canth., Con., **Kreos.**, Lappa, Lyc., Nit-ac., Nux-v., Plat., **Puls.**, Sec., Sep.

THIGHS, **to:** Cham., Staph., Xan.

UPWARD GOING: Alum., Cact., Calc-p., Coc-c., Elaps, Lach., Lil-t., Nit-ac., Puls., Sabin., Sep.

  right: Alum., **Apis**, Croc., Lach., Lyss., Murx.

  left: **Brom.**, Caul., Cimic., Kali-c., Lac-c., **LACH.**, **LIL-T.**, **NAJA**, Sulph.

SEXUAL IMPULSE

DECREASED: Bar-c., **Caust.**, Graph. (F), Lyc., Nat-m. (F), **Onos.**, Ph-ac., Sabal, Sulph.

EXCITEMENT: Manc., Orig., Sumb., Thlasp., Zinc.

  menses, before: Calc-p., Phos., Verat.

  during: Canth., Hyos., Lach., Plat., Puls.

  after: Kali-p.

ERECTIONS (see **Genitals** also): **Canth.**, Graph., Merc., Nat-c., Nat-m., **Nux-v.**, **Phos.**, Pic-ac., Plat., Puls., Thuj.

  deficient, falling: Arg-n., Bar-c., **Con.**, Lyc., Sulph.

  painful: Canth., Merc., Nux-v.

  poor: Sul-i.

IMPOTENCY, **sexual weakness:** Agn., Calad., Con., **Lyc.**, Sel., Tab.

  after onanism: Arg-n.

  imaginary: Stry.

INCREASED: **Canth.**, Carb-v., Chin., Murx., Nux-v., Orig., **Phos.**, **Plat.**, Puls., Sil., Stram., Verat.

  with physical weakness: Calc., Kali-c., Phos.

MINDED: Sep., Staph.

NYMPHOMANIA: **Agn.**, Hyos., Orig., Plat., Stann., Stram., Sumb.

ORGASMS: Stann.

STERILITY: Aur., **Borx.**, Merc., **Nat-m.**, Phos.

TOUCH, **mere, Agg.:** Con., Grat., Nat-c., Plat.

URGE, **futile:** Staph.

MENSTRUATION

Acon., Bell., **Nux-m.**, Plat.,
Puls., Sep., Sulph.

ABSENT: Gins., Lac-d., Nat-s.,
Puls., Senec., Sep.

cold, from: Hell., Senec.

emigrants, in: Plat.

puberty, at: Apis, Kali-c., Mang.,
Puls., Senec., Sep., Sulph.

tuberculosis, in: Solid., Ust.

ACRID: Kali-c., Nit-c., Stram.

ALTERNATE months: Syph.,
Thlasp.

BETWEEN periods, flow: Ambr.,
Bov., Hydr., Lyc.

BLADDER, Agg.: Canth., Sabal.

BROWN: Bapt., Bry., Thuj.

BURNING: Kreos., Sulph.

CHILDBIRTH, after: Tub.

CHOLERAIC symptoms, with:
Am-c.

CLOTS and serum: Lyc., Ust.

COLD BATHS, Agg.: Ant-c.

COLLAPSE at: Merc.

DAY only: Caust., Coff., Ham.,
Puls.

DIARRHEA, Agg.: Bov., Castm.,
Kreos., Mag-c.

EARLY: Ambr., **Bell.**, Borx., Bov.,
Calc., Carb-v., Caul., **Cham.**,
Cocc., Ferr., Ip., Mang., **Nux-
v.**, Phos., **Plat.**, Rhus-t., Sabin.

EVENING only: Coff., Phel.

FAINTS at: Sep.

FEARSOME: Nat-m.

FEEL like coming: Carb-an., Lil-
t., Mosch., Phos., Puls., Senec.,
Vib., Zinc-chr.

FEVERISH during: Pyrog. (see
also **Conditions of Agg. and
Amel., Menses, during, Agg.**)

FOUL: Syph.

GUSHING: see **Hemorrhage.**

GREEN: Graph., Lac-c., Med.,
Puls., Sep.

HOT: Bell.

HYSTERICAL twitchings, before
menses: Cupr., Kali-c., Nat-
m., Phos., Ph-ac., Plat., Puls.,
Sep., Sulph.

during menses: Acon., Bry.,
Calc., Caust., Cham.,
Chin., Cocc., Coff., Cupr.,
Form., Hyos., Ign., Ip., Lyc.,
Mag-m., Merc., Nat-m.,
Nux-v., Puls., Sulph.

after menses: Chin., Cupr., Puls.

INDELIBLE: Mag-c.

INTERMITTENT: Ambr., Bov.,
Ferr., Kreos.

INTERRUPTED, reappearing,
etc.: Kreos., Lach., Nux-v.,
Phos., Puls.

IRREGULAR in time and amount: Cimic., Cocc., Cocc., Ign., Iod., **Nux-m.**, Plat., Sec., Senec.

ITCHING: Sulph., Tarent.

LATE: Caust., Con., Cupr., Dulc., Graph., Kali-c., **Lach.**, Lyc., Mag-c., Nat-m., **Puls.**, Sep., Sil., **Sulph.**, Vib.

LEUCORRHEA, with: Kreos., Sep.

LUMBAR pain: Nux-m.

LYING, ceases on: Cact.

> more on: Kreos., Mag-c.

MAMMAE, **Agg.**: Bry., Calc., Lac-c.

MENSTRUAL BLOOD, see Hemorrhage.

MORNING, more: Carb-an., Sep.

MOTION, less in: Bov., Cycl., Mag-c., **Sabin.**

> only during: Cact., Caust., Lil-t., Manc.

NIGHT only: Bov., Mag-c.

NURSING, **Agg.**: Pall.

PAINFUL: Calc., **Cham.**, Cimic., Cocc., Con., Cupr., **Graph.**, Lyc., Med., Nux-m., Plat., **Puls.**, Sep., **Sulph.**, Tub., Verat., Verat-v., **Vib.**, Zinc-val.

> bending back, **Amel.**: Lac-c.

> fainting, with: Nux-m.

over body: Nux-v.

more flow, more pain: Cann-s., Cimic., Phos., Tarent., Tub.

PALE: **Ferr.**, Graph., Nat-m.

PREGNANCY, during: Asar., Cham., Cocc., Croc., Ip., Kali-c., Lyc., Phos., Rhus-t., Sabin., Sec.

PROFUSE, excessive: Ars., Bell., Calc., **Chin.**, Croc., Ferr., **Ip.**, Mill., Nat-m., Nux-m., **Nux-v.**, Phos., Plat., **Sabin.**, Sec., Stram.

PUBERTY, before: Calc., Sabin., Sil.

PUTRID MEAT, like: Lachn., Syph.

SCANTY: Am-c., Con., Dulc., Graph., Kali-c., Lach., Mag-c., **Puls.**, **Sulph.**

> Comp. **Discharges.**

SHORT: Am-c., **Puls.**, Sulph.

SUPPRESSED: Hell., Lyc., Mez., Phos., Sil., Stram., Sulph., Thuj., Verat.

> Comp. **Discharges.**

TARDY at puberty: Puls., **Senec.**, Sulph.

TARRY: Kali-m.

THROAT, **Agg.**: Gels.

TOO LONG: Calc., Cupr., Lyc., Nat-m., **Nux-v.**, Plat., Sec.

VICARIOUS: Bry., **Ferr.**, Graph., **LACH.**, **Phos.**, **Puls.**, Sec., Senec., **Sulph.**

WATERY: Dulc., Goss.

WEEKS, **every two:** Bov., Brom., Calc-p., Lyc., Mag-c., Phos., Tril-p.

MENSTRUAL BLOOD, see **Hemorrhage.**

LEUCORRHEA

Alum., Calc., Kreos., **Merc.**, Natm., Puls., **Sep.**

ACRID, **eroding:** Alum., Kreos., Phos., Puls., Sec., Syph.

BLISTERING: Phos.

BLOODY **water:** Calc., Mang., **Nit-ac.**

BROWN: Ust.

BURNS, **hot,** etc.: Borx., Kreos., Lept., Lil-t.

CHILDREN, **of:** Calc., Caul., Merc., Senec.

COLIC, **after:** Am-m., Con., Lyc., Mag-m., Sil., **Sulph.**, Zinc.

DIRTY: Sec.

EXHAUSTING: Cocc., Frax., Senec., Visc.

FLOWING **down thighs:** Alum., Lept., Lyc., Onos., **Senec.**, Syph.

GONORRHEAL: Sabin., Sep.

GUSHING: Calc., Graph., Kreos., Lyc., Mag-m., Sil., Stann.

ITCHING, **with:** Helon., Kreos., Staph., Syph.

LUMPY, **curdy:** Borx., Helon., Rad-met., Sil., Tarent. (clear).

MENSES, **after:** Graph., Kreos.

before: Graph., Sep.

instead of: Graph., Nat-m., Xan.

MENSES, **before and after:** Graph.

MILKY: Puls.

PURULENT: Hep., Kali-p., Prun.

STICKY: Kali-bi., Tarent.

THICK: Merc., Senec.

acrid: Bov., Hydr.

URINATING, **when:** Sil.

CONCOMITANTS

Kreos., Merc., Nat-m., Sep.

RESPIRATION

Acon., **Ant-t.**, **Apis**, **ARS.**, **Bell.**, **Bry.**, Carb-v., Cupr., Dig., Dros., Grin., Hep., IP., **Kali-c.**, **LACH.**, Lob., **Lyc.**, Nat-s., OP., **PHOS.**, **PULS.**, **Samb.**, SPONG., Stann., SULPH., Tarent., Vib.

AIR, open, Agg.: Psor.

Amel: Ant-t.

ANXIOUS: Acon., Ip., Phos., Puls., Ran-b., Squil., Stann.

ARMS apart, Amel.: Lach., Laur., Nux-v., Psor., Spig., Sulph.

motion, Agg.: Spig.

ASPHYXIA NEONATORUM: Ant-t., Camph.

ASTHMATIC, wheezing: Acon., ARS., Eucal., Hep., Ip., Kali-c., Lach., Lob., Nux-v., Puls., Samb., Seneg., Sil., Spong., Stann., Stram., Tab., Tub., Visc.

bronchial: Ter.

cardiac: Laur., Naja, Spong., Sumb.

catarrhal: Calad., Caps.

constitutionally: Calc., Iod., Sulph.

consumptives, of: Meph.

coryza, with: Just.

drunkards, of: Meph.

dry weather, Agg.: Cham.

expectoration, Amel.: Ant-t., Zinc.

goitre, in: Spong.

hay fever, of: Arum-t., Chlor.

hives, from: Apis.

humid: Cann-s., Dulc.

hysterical: Cocc.

itchings, with: Calad., Cist., Sabad.

nervous: Cham., Kali-p., Mag-p., Stram.

sycotic: Nat-s., Sil.

BACK, touching, Agg.: Adon.

BREATHE again, can't: Apis, Bell., Coca, Helon., Rumx.

CARDIAC: Crat., Stroph-h.

CHOKING: Naja.

CLOSING EYES, Agg.: Carb-an.

COITION, Agg.: Ambr., Staph.

COLD BREATH, exhalation: Carb-v., Verat.

hot: Bell., Cham., Coff., Kali-bi., Med., Zinc.

COLIC, Agg.: Berb.

COUGH, Agg.: Ars., Cupr., Dros., Ip., Just., Merc-cy., Naja, Phos., Tarent., Tub.

DEEP: Bry., Calc., Caps., Carb-v., Coca, Ign., Ip., Lach., Lil-t., Op., Plat., Sel., Sil., Sulph.

Comp., Sighing.

breath, wants: Cupr., Hydr-ac., Ign., Lach., Mosch., Op.

DEEP ENOUGH, can't get: Lach.

DIFFICULT, short: Kali-m., Nat-s., Spong., Stann., Sumb., Tarent., Verat., Vib.

coryza, with: **Ars.**, Calc., Ip., Nit-ac., Phos., Sulph.

exhalation: see Conditions of **Agg.**, and **Amel.**

inhalation: Brom.

motion, **Amel.**: Bell., Brom., Ferr., Lob., **Puls.**, **Rhus-t.**, **Samb.**

nervous: Arg-n., Ars.

nausea, with: Ip., Kali-n.

sneezing, **Agg.**: Naja.

DIFFICULT, suffocating, choking, etc.: Acon., Ant-t., **Ars.**, Brom., Bry., Chlor., Con., Cupr., Graph., Hep., Ign., Iod., **Ip.**, Kali-bi., Kali-c., Kali-i., **Lach.**, Lycps-v., **Meph.**, Op., Phos., **Puls.**, Samb., **Spong.**, **Sulph.**, Ter., Thyr.

on falling to sleep: Bapt., Dig., Graph., Grind., **Lach.**, **Op.**

bending head back, **Amel.**: Hep., Lach.

goitre, in: Meph.

sleep, **Agg.**: **Lach.**, Spong.

water, **Agg.**: Stram.

DUST, **Agg.**: Ars-i., Brom., Dulc., Ictod., Nat-ar., **Sil.**

EATING, **Agg.**: Lach., Nat-s., **Phos.**, Zinc-val.

EMPHYSEMA, **Agg.**: Sars.

EPIGASTRIUM, from: Guaj., Lach., Nat-m., Sulph.

EXERTION, least, **Agg.**: Calc., Nat-s.

EXPECTORATION, **Amel.**: Ant-t., Aral., Lach.

GASPING: Carb-v., Cor-r., Kali-n., Lob., Mep.

HEART symptoms with: Carb-v., **Kalm.**, Stroph-h., Sumb.

HEAVY: Glon., Verat-v.

HOLDS something to, **Amel.**: Graph.

HUMID AIR, **Agg.**: Aur., Bar-c., **Nat-s.**

INSPIRATION, double: Led.

IRREGULAR: Ang., **Bell.**, Cupr., Op., Sulph.

ITCHING, with: Sabad.

JERKY: **Bell.**, **Ign.**, Laur., Ox-ac., Tab.

KYPHOSIS in: Acon., Ant-c., Asaf., Aur., Bar-c., Bell., Bry., Calc., Camph., Cic., Clem., Coloc., Dulc., Hep., Ip., Lach., Lyc., Merc., Mez., Phos., Ph-ac., Plb., Puls., Rhus-t., Ruta, Sabin., Sep., Sil., Staph., Sulph., Thuj.

LAST BREATH, cease as if: Apis, Bell., Dros., Helon., Laur., Rumx.

LIGHT, shallow: Bell., Phos.

LONG: Lil-t.

LOUD, noisy: **Cham.**, Chin., Samb., **Spong.**

LYING, **Amel.**: Chel., Dig., Kali-bi., Psor., Ter.

on **left side, Agg.**: Merc.

on **right side, Amel.**: Naja.

MOTION, **Agg.**: Calc.

Amel.: Arg-n., Aur., Bell., Brom., Ferr., Lob., Phos., **Puls.**, **Rhus-t.**, **Samb.**

NIGHT, **Agg.**: Ox-ac., Vib.

midnight: Ars., Ferr., Graph., Samb.

OPPRESSED: **Acon.**, **Ars.**, Bell., Bry., **Carb-v.**, Cupr., Ign., **Ip.**, Kali-m., Nux-v., Op., **Phos.**, **Puls.**, Sep., **Sulph.**, Verat.

PAINS, **during the**: Ars., Carb-v., Cocc., Nat-m., Prun., **Puls.**, Ran-s., Sep., Sil., Sulph.

Agg.: Ign., **Onos.**, Verat.

PALPITATION, **with**: Aur., Kalm., Merc-i-f., Puls., Spig., Verat.

PANTING: Bry., Calad., **Ip.**, Stram.

PARALYSIS: Ant-t., Grind., **Lach.**

PUFFING: Naja, Op.

QUICK: **Acon.**, Bell., Carb-v., Cupr., Ip., Lyc., Phos., Sep., **Sulph.**

RATTLING: Am-c., **Ant-t.**, Carb-v., Cupr., **Hep.**, **Ip.**, Kali-s.,

Lyc., Seneg., Squil., Stann.

Comp., **Cough, loose.**

SHALLOW: Laur.

SHORT: **Acon.**, **Ars.**, **Bry.**, Carb-v, Con., Cupr., **Ip.**, Kali-bi., Merc., Nat-m., Rhus-t., Sep., Sil., Sulph.

SIGHING, takes deep breaths: Acon., Apoc., **Ign.**, Lach., Sil.

SLEEP, falling to, on: Am-c., **Ars.**, Cadm-s., Carb-v., Gels., **Grind.**, Kali-c., **Lach.**, Phos., Sulph., Jab.

SLOW: **Bell.**, Hydr-ac., Op.

SMOKE, vapor, fumes, etc., as if: Ars., Bar-c., Brom., Chin., **Ign.**, Lach., Lyc., Phos., **Puls.**

SNEEZING, **with**: Ambro., Ars-i., Phos.

see, **Sneezing, Nose.**

SNORING: Hyos., Merc-c., Op.

TIGHT: see **Chest.**

STOMACH, from: Ars., Chin., Cocc., **Phos.**, Rhus-t.

STOOL, **Amel.**: Poth.

SWEAT, with: Samb.

UNEQUAL: Ant-t., Op.

URINATING, **Agg.**: Chel.

WET WEATHER, **Agg.**: Aran., Nat-s.

WHISTLING, **hissing, etc.**: Ant-s-aur., Aur., Caust., Chin., Hep., **Ip.**, Kali-i., **Samb.**, Spong., Stram.

CONCOMITANTS

Ars., Bell., Cupr., Ip., Phos., Puls., Sep.

COUGH

Acon., **Ars.**, **Bell.**, Bry., Carb-v., Caust., Cham., Chin., Cina, Coc-c., **Con.**, DROS., HEP., **Hyos.**, **Ign.**, Ip., **Kali-c.**, Lach., Lyc., Merc., Nat-m., NUX-V., PHOS., PULS., Rumx., Sang., SEP., **Spong.**, Stann., **Sulph.**

AIR, cool, Amel.: Mag-p.

inhaling, Agg.: **Rumx.**, Sang.

foul, raises: Calc., Caps., Dros., Guaj., Lach., Mez., Sang., Sep., Sulph.

open, Agg.: Kali-n., **Phos.**, Rumx.

ANGER, Agg.: **Cham.**, Sabad.

ARM, raising, Agg.: Tub.

AUDITORY CANAL, touching, Agg.: Kali-c., Lach., Sil.

BARKING: Bell., Dros., Spong.

BELLOWING, **trumpeting:** Verb.

BOUTS, **2-3:** **Merc.**, Phos., Plb., Puls., Stann., **Sulph.**, Thuj.

3 or 4: Bell.

COLD DRINKS, Agg.: Calc., Coc-c., Hep., Sil., Sulph., Verat.

Amel.: **Caust.**, Coc-c., Cupr., Tab.

CONVULSIONS, with: Cina, **Cupr.**, Lach., Meph., Stram.

COUGHING, **Agg.:** Ign., Stict., Teucr., Thyr.

CRIES before: Bell., Bry., Hep., **Phos.**

CROUP: **Acon.**, **Hep.**, Kali-bi., Kali-i., Kali-s., Merc-cy., Phos., **Spong.**

diphtheritic: Iod., **Lach.**, Spong.

CROUPY, crowing: see **Voice.**

DAY: Calc-i., Dulc.

DEEP: Dros., **Hep.**, Spong., Stann., Verat., Verb.

DRY and **loose, alternately:** Ars.

dry at night, but loose by day: Ars., Hep., Puls., Sil.

expectoration, without: Acon., Ip., Nux-v., Phos., Spong., Sulph.

tickling, with burning fever but no thirst: Ars., Con., Phos., Puls., Sabad., Squil.

DUST, feathers, etc., as from: Rumx.

EATING and **drinking Agg.:** Spong.

ERUPTION, receding, **Agg.:** Dulc., Led., Puls.

EVENING, **Agg.:** Tub.

EXERTION, **Amel.**: Rad-met., Stront-c.

EXHAUSTING: Carb-v., Phos., Verat.

EXPECTORATION, **Amel.**: Antt., **Apis**, Aral., **Coc-c.**, Grind., Kali-bi., Sep., **Stann.**, **Zinc.**

Agg.: Coc-c.

astringent: Chion.

bluish: Phos

casts: Iod., Kali-bi.

cheesy: Kali-c., Thuj.

easy: Squil., Stann.

by day: Euphr., Mang., Phos.

foamy: Ip.

foul taste: Asaf., Lach., Puls.,

hard: Nat-c.

heavy: Squil.

little, a **Amel.**: Bell.

loose: Zin-chr.

lying, **Amel.**: Thuj.

morning and evening: Squil.

plugs, balls: Sang., Stann.

profuse: Mag-c.

purulent: Brom., Bry., Carb-v., Chin., Con., Dros., Ferr., Kali-c., Led., Nat-c., Nit-ac., Ph-ac., Plb., Puls., **Rhus-t.**, Samb., Sep., Stann., Sulph.

see also **Suppuration.**

sago, like: Sil., Spong., Stann.

slips back again: Caust., Con., Sang., Zinc-chr.

smeary: Nit-ac., Phel., Thuj.

sweet: Zin-chr.

thick: Kali-s.

tough, sticky: **Kali-bi.**, Zinc-chr.

EYE **symptoms, with:** Nat-m.

FALLS **down:** Nux-v., Phos.

FLATUS passing, **Amel.**: **Sang.**

FOUL AIR, **coughs up:** Calc., **Caps.**, Culx., **Lach.**, Mez., Sang., Sep., Sulph.

HAWKING, **Agg.**: Am-m., Cocc.

HEART, from: Adon., Lycps-v., Nux-v., Spong.

HEAT of bed, **Amel.**: Arg-n., Nuxm.

HOLLOW: **Spong.**

INCESSANT: **Acon.**, **ALUM.**, **Caust.**, Cham., Chin., **Coff.**, Crot-h., Cupr., **DROS.**, **HYOS.**, Ip., Kali-c., Lach., **Nux-v.**, Ph-ac., Puls., **Rhus-t.**, **RUMX.**, Sep., **SPONG.**, Squil., Verat.

JERKING: Ther.

LARYNX, **dry spot in:** Con., Hyos., Nat-m.

LARYNX, **pressure on, Agg.**: Cina.

LOOSE; expectoration, with: Ars., **Calc.**, **Led.**, Lyc., Phos., **Puls.**, **Sep.**, Stann.

in morning: Carb-v., Hep., Par., Phos., Puls., Sep., Squil., Sul-ac.

by day: Ars., Calc., Cham., Hep., Merc., Puls., Sil.

difficult: Ant-t., Caust., Kali-bi.

easy: Arg-met., Stann.

flies from mouth: Arg-n., **Bad.**, **Chel.**, Kali-c., **Kali-m.**, Mang., Mez.

excessive: Coc-c.

night, at: Sep.

swallowed, must be: Caust., Lach.

taste of: see Taste in General.

LYING, **Agg.**: Ars., Hyos., Puls.

Amel.: Calc-p., Euphr., Mang., Psor.

bending backward, Amel.: Med.

on face, Amel.: Eup-per., Med.

side, right, **Agg.**: **Merc.**, Seneg., Staph.

MEASLES, **Agg.**: Dros., Ip., Puls.

MENSTRUATION, **Amel.**: Senec.

MIDNIGHT, after: Aral., Lach.

MORNING and evening: Caust., Ferr-p., Phos., Sep.

MOUTH, **covers**: Rumx.

MUFFLED: Sabad.

NECK, **touch**, **Agg.**: Bell., Brom., **Lach.**

NERVOUS: Ambr., Cimic., Ign., Verb.

NIGHT: Laur.

NOISE, **Agg.**: Tarent.

PAINFUL: **Acon.**, Arn., **Bell.**, BRY., **Caps.**, Caust., Dros., Eup-per., Kali-c., **Nat-m.**, NUX-V., **Phos.**, Rhus-t., Seneg., Spong., **Squil.**, Stann., Stict., Sulph.

PREGNANCY, in: Cham., Puls.

PRODROME, in: Bry., Rhus-t., Sabad., Samb.

RETCHING, **gagging**: Phos.

Amel.: Lach.

REVERBERATING: Cor-r.

ROOM, **entering or leaving, Agg.**: **Phos.**

SALIVA runs: Am-m., Thuj.

SAWING: Spong.

SHAKING, shattering: Mang., Phac., Rumx.

SHORT: Acon., Caust., Merc., Rhus-t.

SIDES, **holds**: **Bry.**, Dros., Eupper., **Ign.**, Nat-s., Phos., Sep.

SINGING, **Agg.**: Kali-bi.

SITS UP: Hyos., Phos., Puls.

SMOKING **Agg.**: Rad-met.

Amel.: Arg-n., Euph., Hep., Ign., Merc., Tarent., Sep.

SPASMODIC, VIOLENT, WHOOPING, etc.: **Bell.**, **Carb-v.**, Cina, Coc-c., Cor-r., Cupr., Dros., Ip., Just., Meph., **Nux-v.**, Puls., Stram., Tub., Verat., Verat-v.

catarrhal phase: Acon., Dulc., Ip., Kali-bi., Merc-d., Nux-v., Phel., Puls., Senec., Verb.

spasmodic phase: Carb-v., Cina, Coc-c., Dros., Kali-c., **Nux-v.**, Puls., **Verat.**

defervescent stage: Ant-t., Phos., Puls.

SPINE, from: **Agar.**, Nux-m, Tell.

STOMACH, epigastrium or abdomen, from: Ant-c., Arg-n., Bell., BRY., Dros., Ign., Kali-bi., **Kali-m.**, Lach., Nat-m. (epigastrium), **Nit-ac.**, Ph-ac., **Phos.**, Puls., **Rumx.**, Sang., SEP.

SUFFOCATING, choking: Ant-t., Brom., Carb-v., Con., Cupr., Dros., Graph., Ip., Lach., Lycpr-v., Meph., Op., Samb., Sang., Seneg., Spong., Stram., **Sulph.**, Ter., Thyr.

SWEETS, **Agg.**: Bad.

TEARING: Rhus-t.

TEETH, cleaning, **Agg.**: Carb-v., Coc-c., Dig., Euphr., Sep., Staph.

TEMPERATURE, change of, **Agg.**: Kali-c., **Phos.**, Rumx., Sep., Verb.

THROAT OR LARYNX, from: **Acon.**, Ambr., Calc., CHAM., **Con.**, Hep., IP., Kali-c., **Lach.**, Nat-m., Nux-v., Phos., **Rumx.**, **Sang.**, **Sep.**

left, from: Caust., Hep., Lach., Lith., **Rhus-t.**, Tell.

right, from: Agar., Dros., Stann., Stict.

back of, from: Dulc.

dry, with: Thuj.

TICKLING: **Acon.**, **Arn.**, Cham., DROS., Hyos., Iod., Ip., **Lach.**, **Nux-v.**, PHOS., Ph-ac., Phyt., **Rhus-t.**, RUMX., Sang, Sep., **Stann.**, Sulph.

TIGHT: Phos., Spong.

UNCOVERING, **Agg.**: Hep., Nux-v., Rhus-t., Rumx.

VAPOR, as from: Brom., Lyc.

VIOLENT: Verat-v.

VOMITING, with: Alum., **Ant-t.**, Bry., Carb-v., Coc-c., Cor-r., Dros., Ferr., **Ip.**, Nux-v., Puls.

WAKES: Spong.

WALKING fast, **Agg.**: Sep.

WARMTH, **Amel.**: Hep., Lyss., Phos., Rumx.

WINTER: Ant-t., Nat-m.

TIME, morning: Lyc.

and evening: Acon., Borx., **Calc.**, Carb-v., **Caust.**, Cina, Ferr., Ign., **Lyc.**, Merc., Nat-m., Phos., **Rhus-t.**, Sep., Sil., **Stram.**, Verat.

evening: Bry., Calc., Nux-v., Rhus-t., Sep.

night: Bar-c., Bell., Calc., Con., Hyos. (dry), Nux-v., Phos., Puls.

at same hour: Lyc., Sabad.

LARYNX AND TRACHEA

Acon., All-c., **Bell.**, Brom., **Caust.**, Dros., Hep., **Iod.**, Kali-bi., LACH., Mang., Nux-v., PHOS., **Puls.**, Rumx., **Sel.**, Spong., Stann., Sulph.

RIGHT: Agar., Kali-n., Puls., Stann., Stict.

LEFT: Caust., **Crot-h.**, **Hep.**, Lach., Rhus-t., **Sul-ac.**, Thuj., Til.

BACKWARD BENDING, **Amel.**: Hep., Med.

CONSTRICTION, **spasm, etc.**: Bell., Cupr., Ign., Lach., Mang., Meph., Mosch., Samb., Verat.

COUGHING, **Agg.**: Acon., All-c., Arum-t., Bell., Phos.

CUTTING: Manc., Merc-c., **Merc-cy.**, Nit-ac., Vinc.

DOWNWARDS: Cham., Glon., Ip., Verat.

DRY: Thyr.

DRY SPOT: see **Throat.**

EAR, to: Zinc-chr. (l).

GRASPS the, clutches: **Acon.**, All-c., Ant-t., Arum-t., Asaf., Dros., Iod., Naja, Phos., Spong.

HANGING in: Lach., Phos., Sang.

LIFTING, **Agg.**: Sil.

MUCUS in: Lyc., Phos., Seneg.

PLUG, **wedge, valve, etc.**: Lach., Phos., Spong.

RATTLING in: Ant-t., Hep., Ip.

ROUGH, **raw, etc.**: Caust., Mang., Nux-v., **Phos.**, Puls., Stann., Sulph.

SPASM: see **Glottis.**

SPEAKING, **singing, etc., Agg.**: Phos., Spong.

STREAK: Caust., Ol-an.

TALKING, **Amel.**: Rhus-t., **Sel.**

TEARING: Cap.

TICKLING **in: Acon., Apis,** Brom., Caps., Cham., **Con.**, **Ign.**, Kali-bi., Lach., Lyc., Nat-m., Nux-v., Op., Phos., Psor., **Puls.**, Rhus-t., RUMX., **Sang.**, Sep., Sil., Stann.

TOUCH, **Agg.**: **Lach.**, Phos., Spong.

TUBERCULOSIS of: Carb-v., Dros., Spong.

UPWARDS: Stann.

WEAK: Alum., Bar-c., **Caust.**, Gels Plb., Lyc.

VOICE AND SPEECH

Acon., Arg-n., **Bell.**, Brom., Canth., **Carb-v., Caust.**, Coll., DROS., Hep., **Iod.**, Kali-i., Mang., **Merc.**, Merc-c., PHOS., Puls., SPONG., Stann., **Stram.**, Verat.

BABBLING: Lyc.

BARKING: **Bell., Canth.**, Lyc., Spong., Stram.

BREAKS, **cracks, fails, changes key**: Ant-c., Arum-t., Bell., Con., Graph., Sep., Spong., Stram.

CHANGEABLE: Ferr.

COLDS, **Agg.**: Sole.

CREAKY: Sec.

CROAKING: Acon.

CROWING: **Spong.**, Stram.

DEEP: Dros.

DIFFICULT: Stram.

EXERTION, **Agg.**: Arn.

HASTY: **Bell.**, Lach.

HOARSENESS: Acon., Arg-n., Bell., Brom., Calc., CARB-V. (P.M.), **Caust.** (A.M.), **Dros.**, Hep., Iod., Kali-bi., Kali-m., Lach., **Mang.** (A.M.), PHOS., Spong., Sulph. (A.M.).

HOARSE, **croupy**: All-c., **Bell.**, Dros., Merc-c., **Sel.**

evening, **in**: Carb-v., Phos.

menses, **Agg.**: Lac-c.

morning and evening: Caust.

HOLLOW: Bell., Spong., Verat.

HUSKY: Merc.

INDISTINCT: **Caust.**, Lyc.

JERKY: Agar.

LOST, **aphonia**: Am-caust., Ant-c., **Carb-v.**, Caust., Kali-bi., Laur., Mang., Onos., Phos., Stram.

aphonia: Kali-bi., Mang.

LOUD: Hyos., Nux-m.

LOW: Ang., Canth., Hep, Verat.

NASAL: Bell., Lyc., Ph-ac., **Staph.**

OVERUSE, **Agg.**: Arum-t., Ferr-p., Graph., **Rhus-t.**, Sel.

ROUGH: Phos.

SHRILL: Acon., Samb., Spong., Stram.

SINGING, **Agg.**: Arg-n., Sel.

SLOW: Ars., Phos., Thuj.

STAMMERING: Agar., Bell., Caust., Cocc., Merc., Stram.

THICK: Agar., Caust., Dulc., **Gels.**, Lach.

TONELESS, **loss of timbre:** Dros.

TREMULOUS: Merc.

UNSTEADY: Seneg.

WEAK: Alum., Carb-an., Cocc., Spong., Stann., Verat.

EXTERNAL THROAT

Bell., Lyc.

RIGHT: Caust., Fl-ac., Lyc., Merc., Nat-c., Nat-m., Nit-ac., Sil.

LEFT: Asaf., Calc., Con., Sulph.

ALTERNATING SIDES: Am-m., Calc-p., Rad-met.

GLANDS of (**Goitre, etc.**): Am-m., Ars. (r), **Bar-c.**, Bell., Brom., Calc., Calc-f., Calc-i., Calc-p., Cham., Graph., Hep., **Ign., Iod.**, Kali-c. (r), Lach., Lyc., **Merc.** (r)., Nat-m., Nit-ac. (r), Rhus-t., Sil. (r), **Spong.**, Staph., Sulph., Vip-t., Zinc-i.

exophthalmic: Bell., Ferr-p., **Iod.**, Lycps-v., **Nat-m.**

hard: Bufo, Iod., Spong.

menses, before, Agg.: Cimic., Lach., Sil.

nodulated: Graph., Phyt.

small, Agg.: Bar-c., Brom., Caust., Crot-h., Graph., Lach., Phos.

toxic: Crot-h.

PAROTITIS: Merc., Phyt., Rhus-t.

PAROTIDS: Lach., Sil.

(see also **Glands, ears.**)

RED, external: Bell., Graph., Sulph., Verat.

SENSITIVE to touch, pressure, clothes, etc.: Ant-t., Apis, Lac-c., LACH., Merc-c., Nux-v.

NECK (Nape)

Acon., Bar-c., **Calc.**, Cimic., Gels., **Nux-v.**, Phyt., Puls., Rhus-t., Sanic., Sep., Sil., Staph., Tub.

ACHING (neckache): **Bry.**, Chin., **Cimic., Gels.**, Hydr., Kali-p., Kalm., **Lach.**, Lil-t., Lyc., Onos., Par., **Phyt.**, Sil., Verat-v.

AIR on, **Agg.: Calc-p.**, Lach., Psor., Sanic., **Sil.**, Stront-c.

ASCENDING, from nape: Meny., Sulph.

BOILS (nape): Pic-ac., Sulph.

BURNS, heat, etc.: Lach.

CHLOASMA: Caul., Sanic.

CONSTRICTION, as of a band, cord: Glon., **Lach.**, Sep., Spong.

CRACKING: Cocc., Nat-c., Petr., Sulph.

CRAMP: Calc-p., Cic., Cimic., Hydr-ac. (nape), Nux-v. (nape), Phyt., Plat., Verat-v.

DRAFT, on Amel.: Sil.

EMACIATION, shrivelled: Mag-c., Nat-m., Sars.

ERUPTION: Arn., Sil., Sul-i.

EXERTION, Agg.: Arg-n., Calc., Lil-t., Sep.

mental, Agg.: Zinc.

FORMICATION starts: Nux-v., Sec.

FULL: Glon.

LEFT HEAD or shoulder to: Spig.

RED: Graph., Phos., Verat.

HEAVY (nape): Meny., Nux-v., Par., Rhus-t.

LAME (nape): Zinc.

PAIN in nape: Stront-c.

SHOOTING: Nat-m.

SHORT: Syph.

SHOULDERS and: Guaj., Lachn., Nux-v. (r), Stict., Sulph., Verat-v., Zinc. (r).

SIDES, alternating: Calc-p., Puls.

SORE: Stict.

STIFF: Bar-c., Bell., Bry., Calc., Caust., Chel., Cimic., Ign., Kali-c., Lach., Lyc., Mag-c., Merc-i-r., Nit-ac., Nux-v., Phos., Rhus-t., Sep., Sil., Stict., Sulph.

left: Bell., Carb-an., Chel., Coloc., Glon., Guaj., Kreos., Lyc.

right: Agar., Caust., Nat-m.

side, on one: Coloc., Stict.

STUPOR, with (nape): Zinc.

SWEAT: Calc., Lach., Mang., Ph-ac., Sanic., Stann., Sulph.

TENSE, nape: Tub.

THROBBING in: Bell., Pyrog., Spig.

TIRED nape: Zinc.

TOUCH, Agg.: Lach.

VERTEBRAE crack: Chel.

WEAK: Abrot., Aeth., Ant-t., Caul., Nat-m., Sep., Sulph., Verat-v.

then stupor: Hyos., Zinc.

WEAKNESS: Calc-p., Cocc., Plat., Verat., Zinc.

WRY neck: Bell., Dulc., Glon., Hyos., Lyc., Nux-v., Rhus-t.

CHEST AND LUNGS

Acon., ANT-T., Arn., ARS., BRY., Calc., Chel., Chin., Dulc., Ferr-p., Guaj., Iod., Ip., Kali-c., Lyc., Op., Phel., PHOS., PULS., Ran-b., Ran-s., Rhus-t., Sang., Senec., Seneg., Spig., Squil., Stann., Sulph., Tub., Verat-v., Verb.

RIGHT: Arn., Ars., **Bell.**, **Bry.**, Carb-an., Chel., Colch., Coloc., Iod., **Kali-c.**, Lach., **Lyc.**, Mur-ac., Psor., Puls., Sil.

into **right arm:** Hydr., Kreos., Lob., Phos., Phyt., Plb., Sang.

to **left:** Acon., Lach., Petr.

LEFT: Am-m., Arg-met., Arg-n. (last rib), Calc., Con., Euph., Fl-ac., Kali-c., Kali-n., Laur., Lyc., Nat-s., Nit-ac., **Nux-v.**, **Phos.**, Rhus-t., Seneg., Stann., Sulph.

to **right:** Apis, Calc., Graph., Kreos., Phos., Plb., Zinc.

CHANGING ABOUT in: **Acon.**, Alum., Arg-n., Bell., Cact., Caust., Colch., Ferr., **Lyc.**, Mag-m., Merc., Nat-c., Phos., **Puls.**, Seneg.

ALTERNATING SIDES: **Agar.**, Apis, Ars., **Calc.**, **Cimic.**, Dulc., Graph., Hyper., Lyc., Mang., Mosch., PHOS., Plb., Rad-met., Ran-b., Rumx., Thuj.

UPPER: Calc., Iod., Mang., Puls., Stann.

MIDDLE: Calc., Dulc., Kali-bi., Phel., Sep.

BACKWARD, EXTENDING: Ars., Bry., **Calc.**, Caps., Carb-v., Chel., Con., Cupr., Kali-bi.,

Lil-t., **Merc.**, Nat-m., Phos., Sep., Spig., **Sulph.**, Ther.

right: Ars, Carb-v., Chel., Merc., Sep.

left: Lil-t., **Lyc.**, Nat-m., Spig., Ther.

INTERCOSTAL: Asc-t., Aml-ns., Bry., Cimic., Mez., Ran-b., Sil., Verb.

RIBS, **along:** Apis.

below: Chin., Sulph., Ter.

right: Am-c., Am-m., Bar-c., Bell., Berb., Bry., Hydr., Kali-c., Lyc., Nux-v.

left: Apis, Ars., Asaf., Chin., Ign., Nit-ac.

to **right:** Graph.

right, lower: Chel., Merc., Merc-i-r., Sang.

left, lower: Phos., Sulph.

DEEP, in: All-c., Arn., Bry., Dros., Eup-per., Kali-c., Kreos.

DOWNWARD: Agn., Kali-bi

right: Dulc., Nit-ac., Sang., Sep.

left: Kali-c., Laur., Phos., Puls., Squil., Zinc.

FORWARD: Berb., Borx., BRY., Castm., **Kali-c.**, Kali-n., Psor., Rat., **Sep.**, Sulph.

right: Acon., Coloc., Merc.

lelt: Agar., Bar-c., **Bry.**, Lac-c., Naja, Phos., **Sulph.**, Thuj., Zinc.

UPWARD: Ars., Calc., Caust., Lach., Mang., Mur-ac., Thuj.

right: Arn., Plat., Thuj.

to left: Petr.

left: Am-m., Bov., **Coc-c.**, Kali-c., Laur., Med., Spig., **Squil.**, Stann., Zinc.

to right: Calc., Carb-v., Graph., Ign., Lil-t.

TRANSVERSELY: Caust., Thuj.

arms, to: Alum.

AIR, in: Chlor., Ther.

ANXIETY in: Bry.

APICES, pains in: Guaj., Myrt. (l), Puls., Ther. (l).

sunken: Thuj.

ARMS, into: Bry., Dig., Dios., Lat-m., Phos. (r).

raising: Tell.

BACKWARD thro' right: Acon., **Chel.**, Dulc., Guaj., Kali-bi., Merc., Nit-ac., Phel., Phyt., Sep., **Sulph.**

left: Bry., Kali-n., Mur-ac., Phys., Rhus-t., Sul-ac.

BAR across: Kali-bi.

BRONCHORRHEA: All-c., Cop., Eucal., Grin., Phel., Puls., Stann., Tub.

BURNING, heat: **Acon.**, Apis, ARS., Canth., CARB-V.,

Euph., Kali-m., Lyc., Naja, **Phos.**, Sang., Spong., **Sulph.**, Tub., Verat-v.

BURSTING, as if: Brom.

CHLOASMA: Card-m., Sep., Sulph.

COLD AIR, draft, etc., Agg.: Act-sp., **Calc-p.**, Petr., Ph-ac., Ran-b.

drinks, Agg.: Phos.

COLDNESS in: **Ars.**, Bry., Carb-an., Kali-c., Lil-t., Nat-c., Olnd., Sulph.

CONGESTION: Acon., Bell., Cact., Ferr., Ferr-p., Phos., Seneg., **Sulph.**, Verat-v.

CONSTRICTION, band, cramp, in etc.: Aeth., Cact., Coloc., Dulc., Ferr., Helon., Ign., Lob., Mag-p., Mosch., Nux-v., Phos., Rheum, Scopar., Stann., Staph., Sulph., Vip.

lower: Cocc., Cupr., **Plat.**

COUGHING, Agg.: **Bry.**, Phos.

CREPITATION: Acon., Calc., Coff., Rheum.

DIRECTIONS of pains, various: Thuj.

DRY: Naja (l), Phos.

EMACIATION: Petr., Senec.

EPIGASTRIUM, to: Ox-ac. (l).

ERUCTATIONS, Amel.: Aml-ns., Canth., Sep.

FIXED: Ox-ac., Stry.

FULNESS: Glon., **Phos.**, Sulph.

HOLD, **must: Bry., Dros.**, Eupper., Nat-s.

HOLLOW, **empty, as if:** Carb-an., Cocc., Kali-c., Med., Murx., Naja, Nux-v., Naja (l), Nux-v., Olnd., Phos., Stann., Tab., Verat.

LOAD, **heavy, on:** Am-c., Cact., Nux-m., **Phos., Puls.**, Seneg., Stront-c., **Sulph.**, Verat-v.

LUMP, **plug, etc., as of:** Ambr., Am-m., **Anac.**, Cupr., **Kali-c., Lach.**, Lil-t., Nat-c., Nux-m., PHOS., **Ran-s.**, Stict., Sulph., Tarax., Thlasp., Zinc.

MORNING, **Agg.:** Calc., **Carb-v.**

NUMB: Stict.

PARALYSIS (of lungs): **Ant-t.**, Ars., Bar-c., Carb-v., Ip., Kali-i., Op., Phos.

PLEURISY: Acon., Arn., Bry., Guaj., Kali-c., Merc-d., Phos., Sulph.

PLEURODYNIA: Acon., Arn., Bry., Chin., Lach., Nux-v., Puls., Sabad., Sulph.

PNEUMONIA & BRONCHITIS: **Acon.**, Ant-t., Bry., Calc., Ferr-p., Hydr., Iod., Kali-bi., Lyc., Merc., **Phos.**, Puls., Rhus-t., Seneg., Sep., Stict., Sulph., Tub., Verat-v.

capillary: ANT-T., **Ferr-p., Ip.**

catarrhal: Ant-t.

cerebral type: Acon., Arn., Bell., Bry., Cann-s., Canth., Hyos., Lach., Merc., Nux-v., Phos., Puls., Rhus-t., Stram., Sulph.

secondary: Ferr-p., Phos.

senile: Am-c., Ant-c., Ant-t., Ars., Kreos.

unresolved: Lyc., Phos., Sulph., Sul-i.

PRESSURE (heavy): Aur., Ferr., Lach., **Nux-v.**, Phos.

Amel.: Bry.

PURRING in: Caust., Spig.

PULSATION: Asaf., Cact., **Sulph.**

right: Asar., Crot-t., **Dig.**, Ign., Ind., Paeon., Phos.

left: Am-m., Cann., Glon., **Meny.**

RATTLING: Hep., Phos.

coarse: Ant-t., Cupr., Kali-s.

fine: Ip.

without expectoration: Am-c., **Ant-t.**, Carb-v., Caust., Con., Hep., Ip., Kali-s., Lob., Phos., Sep., Sulph., Tub., Verat.

RIBS, **dislocated, broken as if:** Agar., Caps., Kali-bi., Naja, Petr., Psor., Stram.

fifth and sternum: Mag-c. (r), Ox-ac. (l), Thuj. (r).

floating: Benz-ac., Berb. (r), Ther. (l).

plug between: Anac., Aur., Caust., Cocc., **Lyc., Ran-s.,** Verat.

RUSHES of **blood:** Kali-n., Phos., Sulph.

SCRAPING: Seneg.

SHUDDERING in: Agar., Aur.

SORENESS: Phos., Stann.

SPINE, **pressure, Agg.:** Sec., Tarent.

SPOTS in: Agar., Anac., Bufo, Nat-m., Ol-j., Seneg., Thuj., Tub.

SPRAINS: Lyc., Rhod., Tell.

STABBINGS: Kali-c.

STERNUM, back to: Kali-bi., Kali-i., Merc-sul.

twisting: Ph-ac.

under: Am-c., Aur., Calc., **Caust.,** Cham., Gels., Iod., Phos., Rhus-t., **Rumx.,** Sang.

heaviness: Aur.

bump: Abies-n., Aur., Chin., Echi., Gels., **Phos.,** Puls., Sil., Thlasp.

STICKING: **Acon., Bry.,** Kali-c., **Phos.,** Rhus-t., Squil., Sulph.

STITCHES: Myrt., Ol-j., Phos. (l),

Pix, **Ran-b.,** Squil.

STRINGY: Kali-bi.

SWEAT: see **Sweat, Partial.**

THROAT, into: Apis, Bell., Calc., Laur., Phos., Sulph., Thuj., Zinc.

TIGHTNESS: Ars., Asaf., **Aur.,** Caust., Ign., Ip., Nat-m., **Nux-v., PHOS.,** Puls., Sulph., Sumb. (l).

right: Am-m., Cocc., Sulph.

left: Graph., Lyc., Sul-ac.

ULCERATIVE **pain:** Ran-b.

UNCOVERING, **Amel.:** Ferr.

WANDERING **pains:** Seneg.

WEAKNESS: Calc., Carb-v., Kali-c., **Laur.,** Nit-ac., Seneg., **Stann., Sulph.**

EXTERNAL CHEST

Arn., Bry., Calc-p., Phos., Ran-b., Ran-s., Sil., Spig., Sulph.

AXILLAE

Carb-an., Carb-v., **Hep.,** Phos., **Sep.,** Sil., Sulph.

ABSCESS: Lyc., Phos.

ACHE in: Latr.

ALTERNATELY: Colch.

ERUPTION in: Lyc., Sep.

EXCORIATION: Carb-v., Mez.

GLANDS, engorged: Sulph.

GLANDS SWELLED: Bar-c., Lach., **Lyc.**, Nit-ac., Phos., Sil.

ITCHING: Phos., Sang.

MENSES, before: Sang.

STITCHES: Dros.

SWEAT: Calc., Lappa (cold), Nat-m., Petr., **Sep.**, **Sil.**, Sulph.

MAMMAE

Bell., Bry., Carb-an., Cham., **Con.**, Hydr., Iod., Lac-c., Oci., Phel., **Phos.**, **Phyt.**, Sil., Urt-u.

RIGHT: Kali-bi., **Sil.**

LEFT: Borx., Bov., **Lil-t.**, **Lyc.**, **Phel.**

ABDOMEN, to: Phel.

ABSCESS: Phos.

ACHING: Puls.

ALTERNATING SIDES: Puls., Rad-met.

ARMS, to: Lith-c.

BACKWARD: CROT-T., Form. (l), Laur., Lil-t., Til.

BELOW, L.: Apis, Bry., Cimic., Phos., Sulph., Thlasp., Ust.

BELOW, R.: Carb-an., Caust.,

CIMIC., Chel., **Graph.**, Laur., Lil-t., **Phos.**, **Sulph.**, Ust.

BURNING: Sulph.

under: Aeth. (r), Laur. (l), Mur-ac. (l), Phos. (r), Rumx. (l).

COLD, **Agg.**: Sabal.

CONGESTED: Acon., Apis, Ferr., Phos.

with milk, in insanity: Bell., Stram.

DWINDLING: Cham., Chin., Con., Ferr., Iod., Nit-ac., Sec., Sil.

FLOWING in: Dict., Kreos.

HARD: Bry., Carb-an., Grap Phyt., Sil.

HEAVY: Bry., Chin., Iod., Lac-c., Phyt.

INFLAMED: Bell., Phyt.

LACTATION: Bell., Cham., Merc., **Puls.**, Sep., Sil.

MENSES, before, **Agg.**: Bry., Calc., **Con.**, KALI-M., LAC-C., Lyc., Ol-an., **Phyt.**, Puls.

MILK in breasts (of non-pregnant): Asaf., Cycl., Merc., Puls., Thlasp.

altered: Bell., Merc.

escaping: Calc.

eroding: Staph.

flowing, as if: Dict., Kreos., Nux-v., Puls.

increased: **Bell., Bry.,** Phyt., **Puls.**

milk, present with absent menses, etc.: Bell., Bry., Calc., Lyc., Phos., Puls., Rhus-t., Sabin., Stram.

increased: Calc., **Sabin.**

in virgins: Cycl., Merc., Puls.

scant, absent, etc.: Agn., **Bry.,** Calc., **Dulc., Lac-c., Lact., Puls.,** Urt-u., Zinc.

spoiled: Aeth., Calc., **Cham.,** Sil.

NODES in: Bel-p., Carb-an., Con., Phyt., **Sil.**

OUTWARD dartings: Arg-met., Clem., Ol-an.

RADIATING: Phyt.

SMALL: Onos., Sabal.

SORE, painful: Arn., Bry., Calc., Con., Kali-m., **Lac-c.,** Phyt., Sabal.

STITCHES in: Con., Nit-ac.

SUCKLING, **Agg.:** Ant-t., Borx., Bry., Crot-t., Lac-c., Lil-t., Phel., Phyt., **Puls.,** Sil.

SWELLED: Bell., **Bry.,** Con., Phos., **Phyt., Puls.,** Sil., Urt-u.

NIPPLES

Arn., Cham., Graph., Lyc., Nat-s. (l), Puls., Rat., Rumx. (l), Sulph.

AIR, from: Cycl.

BACKWARD, from: Crot-t., Phel., Sulph. (l).

BURNING: Senec. (l).

BLEEDING: **Sep., Sil.,** Sulph.

CRACKED: Aesc., Carb-an., Caust., **Graph., Petr.,** Phyt., Rat., **Sars.,** Sulph.

CRAWLING: Sabin.

EXCORIATED: Arn., Fl-ac., Phyt., Sulph.

INVERTED: Graph., Nat-s., Phyt., Sars.

OOZING: Med.

OUTWARD going pains, darts: Berb., **Bry.,** Gels., Kali-bi., Lappa, Lyc., **Mez., Ol-an.,** Spig., Stann.

RETRACTED: Con., Hydr., Lach., **Nat-s., Sars.,** Sil., **Thuj.**

SORE, tender: Arn.

UNDER: Rumx. (l).

HEART, CIRCULATION AND PULSE

ACON., Ars., **Aur., Bell.,** Bry., Bufo, CACT., **Calc.,** Carb-v., Chin., DIG., **Ferr-p.,** Glon., Iod., **Kali-c., Kalm.,** Lach., LIL-T., LYCPS-V., Naja, **Nat-m.,** PHOS., Prun., PULS., Scopar., Sep., SPIG., Spong.,

Squil., Stroph-h., SULPH.,
Tab., Tarent., Thyr., Verat.,
Verat-v., Zinc-i.

BLOOD, sepsis, etc.: Ail., Am-c.,
Arn., ARS., Bapt., Bell., Bry.,
Calc., Carb-ac., Carb-v.,
Chin., Crot-h., Echi., Elaps,
Ferr., Kali-c., Kreos., LACH.,
Merc., Merc-cy., Mur-ac.,
Naja, Nat-m., Nit-ac., Nux-
v., Phos., Puls., Pyrog., Rhus-
t., Sec., Solid., Sulph., Sul-ac.,
Tarent., Ter., Vario., Verat.,
Verat-v., Zinc.

boils: Crot-h.

rushes of: Bell., Ferr., Glon.,
Lach., Sang., Spong., Sulph.

downward: Aur., Meph.,
Thyr.

upward: Acon., Arn., Bell.,
Bry., Ferr., Glon., Kali-
i., Mell., Phos., Sang.,
Stront-c.

stasis: Carb-v., Ham., Puls., Sep.,
Sulph.

streaked: Rhus-t., Sang., Senec.,
Seneg., Sulph., Tub.

typhoid: Ars., Bapt., Bell., Bry.,
Kali-c., Mur-ac., Op., Phos.,
Ph-ac., Rhus-t., Sulph.,
Tarax.

aborting: Bapt., Pyrog.

watery: Nit-ac., Rhus-t., Sabin.

mixed with clots: Arn., Bell.,
Caust., Puls., Sabin.

BLOOD-VESSELS: Acon., Aml-
ns., Apis, ARN., Bell., CARB-
V., Ferr., Fl-ac., Gels., Glon.,
Ham., Hyos., Lach., Lyc.,
Nat-m., Phos., PULS., Sang.,
Sec., Sep., Sul-ac., Sulph.,
Thuj., Vip-t., Zinc.

distended, full, visible, varicose,
etc.: Arn., Ars., Bell., Calc.,
Calc-f., Carb-v., Fl-ac.,
Glon., Ham., Lach., Phos.,
Plat., Puls., Sang., Sec., Sep.,
Sulph., Zinc.

insanity, with: Arn., Ars., Fl-
ac., Lach., Lyc., Sulph.,
Zinc.

followed by: Anac., Ant-c.,
Arn., Ars., Bell., Caust.,
Cupr., Hyos., Ign.,
Lach., Lyc., Nux-v.,
Phos., Sep., Sulph.,
Verat.

menses, Agg.: Ambr.

painful: Ham., Puls.,
Thuj., Zinc.

swelled: Paeon., Puls.

heat in: Ars., Bry., Calc., Med.,
Rhus-t., Syph.

painful: Ham., Zinc.

vascular: Lach., Lyc., Thuj., Tril-
p., Zinc.

writing in: Bell., Hydr-ac.

ACHING, etc.: Lith-c., Spong., Stroph-h., Tab., **Verat-v.**

ALTERNATING with: Benz-ac., Glon., Kalm., Nat-m., Nat-p., Stroph-h., Visc.

ANGER, **Agg.**: Cupr.

ANGINA: Ars., Cupr., **Latr.**, Ox-ac., Spig., **Tab.**

ANGUISH: Stroph-h., Ther.

ANXIETY, with: ACON., Arn., Ars., Aur., Calc., Carb-v., Dig., Merc-c., Murx., **Phos.**, Plat., Psor., 'Puls., Spig., Sulph., Verat.

waking, on: Spong.

APEX (region): Apis, Coc-c., Sulph.

ARMS, to: Alum., Bar-c., **Cact.**, **Carb-v.**, Dios., Glon., Kali-n., Kalm., Lat-m., Lyc., Phos., Spig., Stict.

left, to: Ars., **Acon.**, Cact., Cimic., **Dig.**, **Kalm.**, Lach., Lat-m., Lil-t., Phos., Puls., RHUS-T., SPIG., Stroph-h., Tab., TARENT., Thyr.,

to right: Borx., Kreos., Ox-ac., Phos., Phyt., Plb.

ASCENDING, **Agg.**: Ars., Calc.

AUDIBLE: Ars-i.

AXILLAE to: Kali-n., Lat-m., Thyr.

BACKWARD (l. **scapula**): **Agar.**, Aloe, Cimic., **Kali-c.**, **Kalm.**, Laur., **Lil-t.**, Mez., **Naja**, Rhus-t., Rumx., SPIG., Sulph., Tab., Ther., Thuj.

BALL, **as of a**: Lil-t.

BASE **to apex:** Syph.

BURNING: Acon., **Ars.**, Aur., Bry., Calc., Cupr., Hyos., Op., **Phos.**, Puls., Rhus-t., Sulph., Syph., Verat-v.

BURSTING, distended, etc.: Glon., Phos., Zinc.

CLUTCHING: Thyr.

COLD: Bov., **Helod.**, Kali-m., Sul-i.

COLDNESS in: ACON., Ars., Rhus-t., **Verat.**

COMPRESSION: Am-c., Ars., Colch., Spig., Zinc. (cap).

CONGESTION: Phos.

see **Generalities**

CONSTRICTION, grasped, squeezed, clutched and released alternately etc.: **Cact.**, Iod., Lach., Lil-t.

COUGHING, **Agg.**: Aur., Phos.

CRACKLING: Spig., Spong.

CUTTING: Colch., Verat., Zinc-chr. (apex).

DRINKING, **Agg.**: Con., Cupr.

DROPS: Hyper.

EARS to: Thyr.

EMPTY, hollow, as if: Croc., Graph., Kali-c., Med., Sulph., Tab.

ENDOCARDITIS: Aur., Lach., Spig., Zinc-i.

EXERTION, Agg.: Cact., Dig., Nit-ac., Staph.

EYES with: Lith-c., Spig.

FLOATS: Bov., Bufo, Crot-c., Kali-i., Pip-m., Sumb.

FLUTTERING, trembling, etc.: Calc., Chin., Cimic., Dig., Lil-t., Nat-m., Nux-v., Rhus-t., Spig.

FULL: Verat-v.

GOITRE heart: Ars., Bufo, Crot-h., Lach., Lat-m., Lycps-v., Phos., Spong., Thyr.

HANDS over: Bufo, Hydr-ac., Laur., Naja, Tarent.

HANGING by a thread, as if: Aur., Kali-c., Lach., Lil-t., Med., Merc., Nux-m., Sep.

HEAD, alternating with: Aml-ns., Glon., Nux-m., Stront-c., Stroph-h., Tab.

congested: Scopar.

extending to: Glon., Med., Nux-m., Phos., Sep., Spig., Spong., Stroph-h.

HEART-BEAT AND PULSE, audible: Ang., Apis, Arn., Bism., Puls., Sabad., Spig., Sulph.

body, over whole: Bell., Ferr., Glon., Kali-c., Lach., Nat-m.

ceasing, as if: Aur., Cic., Cimic., Conv., DIG., Gels., Lob., Rumx., Vib.

full: Ant-t., Bell., Bry., Calc., Canth., Coloc., Ferr., FERR-P., Gels., Glon., Graph., Hep., Hyos., Merc., Mez., Nux-v., Phos., Ran-s., Spong., Stram., Sulph., VERAT-V.

strong, and: Acon., Bell., Bry.

weak, and: Ferr-p., Gels., Verat.

changeable, variable: Cina, Dig., Laur., Naja.

dicrotic: Gels., Kali-c.

flowing : Ferr-p., Gels., Syph., Verat-v.

hard: Acon., Am-c., Bell., Bry., Canth., Chin., Colch., Coloc., Ferr., Graph., Hep., Hyos., Ign, Iod., Mez., Nit-ac., Nux-v., Phos., Plb., Sil., Spong., Stram., Sulph., Zinc.

single beats: Aur., Cact., Lach., Lil-t., Zinc.

heavy: Lycps-v.

intermittent, intermits, drops beats: Ars., Carb-v., Dig.,

Kali-c., Mur-ac. (3rd), **Nat-m.** (3rd), Nit-ac. (4th), Ph-ac., Tab., Verat.

every 3rd, beat: Nat-m., Nit-ac.

irregular: Ant-c., Ars., **Cact.,** Cann-s., **Dig.,** Ferr., Glon., Kali-c., Lach., **Nat-m.,** Op., Sep., **Spig.,** Stram., Stroph-h., **Verat.**

large: Acon., **Ferr-p.,** Lycps-v., Manc., Phos., Syph., Verat-v.

one hard: Sep., Zinc.

palpitation: Acon., Ars., Aur., Cact., **Calc.,** Cham., Chin., **Crat.,** Dig., Glon., **Iod.,** Kali-bi., Kali-c., **Lyc., Merc., Nat-m.,** Nit-ac., **Nux-v., Phos., Puls.,** Rhus-t., Sep., **Spig.,** Spong., **Stroph-h., Sulph.,** Thuj., Thyr., **Verat.,** Zinc.

anxious, nervous, etc.: Acon., Ars., Aur., **Coff., Crat.,** Dig., Lach., Nat-m., Ph-ac., **Puls., Spig.,** Valer., Verat.

attacks of: Cann-s., Olnd., Phos.

chill, during: Nat-m.

continuous: Calc., Carb-v., Crat., Sulph.

cough, Agg.: Ol-j.

exertion, from slight: Ars., Calc., Con., Rhus-t.

faintness, with: Crot-h., Hydr-ac., Lach., Laur., Lil-t., **Nux-m.,** Puls., Stroph-h., Thyr., Verat.

flowing: Ferr-p., Gels., Syph., Verat-v.

fright, Agg.: Dig.

hammering: Thyr.

lying, Agg.: Merc., **Puls.,** Sulph., Thyr., Zin-i. (1).

metastasis to: Abrot., Aur., Cact., Colch., Dig., Iod., Kalm., Lach., Naja, **Phos.,** Spig., Spong., Sulph.

motion, Amel.: Ferr., Lob.

nervous, anxious: Ol-an., **Phos.,** Stroph-h., Sumb.

occiput, to: Cimic., Sep.

painful: Spong.

sitting, when: Mag-m., Spig.

stiff, as if: Aur-m.

stooping, Agg.: Thyr.

sweat, with: Spong., Tab., Verat.

violent, shakes body: Crat., Gels., Lycps-v., Mur-ac., Puls., Verat-v.

quick: Acon., Ant-t., Ars., Bell., Glon., Lach., Nux-v., Phos., Rhus-t., Spong., **Sulph.**, **Verat.**

rapid: Ther.

more than heart: Spig.

shakingthe body: Nat-m., Rhus-t. Comp. **Visible.**

sharp: Rhus-t.

slow: Cic., DIG., Gels., **Kalm.**, **Myrt.**, Ol-an., Op., Sep., Stram., **Verat-v.**

and quick, alternately: Stroph-h.

small: Acon., **Ars.**, Camph., Carb-v., **Cupr.**, Hell., Rhus-t., Stroph-h., **Verat.**

soft: Ferr-p., Gels., Syph., Verat-v.

temperature, discordant: Pyrog.

thready: Tab., Verat.

tremulous: Ant-t., Calc., **Spig.**

thumping: Aur., Iod., Rhod.

unequal: Agar., Ign., Kali-chl., Op.

violent: Gels., Verat-v.

visible: Ars., Glon., Iber., **Kalm.**, Lach., Naja, Sep., **Spig.**, Sulph., Verat.

Comp. **Shaking.**

weak: Acon., **Ant-t.**, Ars., Carb-v., Colch., Kali-c., Lach.,

Merc., **Mur-ac.**, Naja, Op., **Ph-ac.**, Phos., **Rhus-t.**, Stroph-h., **Verat.**

HEAVINESS: Aur-m., Lil-t., Lycps-v., Puls., Spig., Tub.

HOLLOW: Med.

HYPERTROPHY: Thyr.

IMPEDED: Rumx.

INFLAMED, phlebitis, etc.: Acon., **Ars.**, Chin., Kali-c., Ham., **Lach.**, PULS., **Spig.**, **Sulph.**, Vip-t.

JUMPING: Aur., Merc-i-f.

LIVELY: Stroph-h.

LIVER SYMPTOMS, **with**: Agar., Aur., Cact., Calc., Dig., Lept., Mag-m., Myrt., Sang.

LOOSE, as if: Aur., Crot-h.

LYING **on r., side, Agg.**: Alum., Bad., Cimic., Kali-n., Lach.

METASTASIS **to**: Aur., Kalm., Lach.

MOTION, **Agg.**: Con., Mag-m., Spig.

Amel.: Gels., Mag-m., Rhus-t.

MUSCLE **exhaustion**: Zinc-i.

NECK **and throat to**: Ars., Bell., Glon., Naja, Phos., Phys., Scopar., Spig., Spong.

NEEDLES **at**: Cimic.

OPPRESSION: Nat-n., Scopar.

PURRING: Glon., Iod., Spig.

RADIATING: Acon., Glon., **Kalm.**, **Spig.**

REFLEX from: **Naja.**

RHEUMATISM: Aur., Benz-ac., Gels., **Kalm.**, **Lach.**, Spig.

RIGHT SIDE, as if on: Borx., Ox-ac., **Phyt.**

RISING, **as if:** Podo., Valer.

SCAPULA **to, left:** Kali-c., Kalm., Lach., Spig.

SHOCKS at: Calc., Lith-c., Nux-v.

SHORT **breath:** Stront., Thyr.

SHOULDER **to:** Scopar.

SIDE, **on right:** Borx.

SITTING, **Agg.:** Mag-m.

SORE, bruised: APIS, ARN., Bapt., BAR-C., Cact., **Cimic.**, Fl-ac., Lach., **Lith-c.**, **Lycps-v.**, Nat-m., Spig.

SPINE, **touch, Agg.:** Tarent.

SQUEEZING: Arn., Cact., Iod.

STAGNATED sensation; **circulation, stands still:** Acon., **Lyc.**, Sabad., Sep., Zinc.

STOOLING, **Agg.:** Con.

STOP, as if to: **Dig.**, Lob.

SURGING **upward:** Spong.

SWELLED, full, etc., as if: Asaf., Glon., **Lach.**, Pyrog., Sep., Sulph.

SYMPTOMS, **vary** with: Lycps-v.

TENSION: Rad-met.

THROB, **one:** Zinc.

TIRED FEELING: Nux-v., Pyrog., Rhus-t.

TOBACCO, **Agg.:** Cact.

TREMOR, **quiver:** Cic., Naja, Stroph-h.

TUMULTUOUS: Acon., Aml-ns., Lycps-v.

TURNS OVER, twists, etc.: Apis, **Arn.**, Cact., Caust., **Lach.**, Rhus-t., **Sep.**, Tab., Tarent.

TWITCHING: Aesc., Arg-met., Camph.

UNSTEADY: Tab.

VALVES: **Bar-c.**, Calc., **Kali-c.**, Lach., Laur., Phos., **Puls.**, Spong., **Stroph-h.**, **Tarent.**, Zinc-i.

WATER, as if in: Bov., **Bufo.**

BACK, SPINE AND CORD

AGAR., Ars., Aur., **Bell.**, CALC., Chinin-s., **Cimic.**, Cocc., Gels., Hyper., Kali-c., **Lach.**, Nat-m., Nat-s., **Nux-v.**, Par. (s), PHOS., Ph-ac., **Pic-ac.**, **Rhus-t.**, Sec., SIL., **Sulph.**, Ther. (s), Valer. (s), Vario. (s), **Zinc.**

RIGHT: Calc., Cic., Fl-ac., **Sulph.**, Zinc.

to left: Calc-p., Cocc., Kali-p., Sulph., Tell.

LEFT: Dros., Glon., Sil.

to right: Bell., Cund., Nat-c., Ox-ac.

ALTERNATING SIDES: Agar., Bell., **Berb.**, Calc., Calc-p., Kali-bi., Kalm.

with headache: Acon., Alum., Brom., Ign., Meli-a., Sep.

CATCHING IN: Dios.

CHANGING here and there: Berb., Cimic., Kali-bi.

CHEST, into: Acon. (r), Arn., Barc. (l), Berb., **Bry.** (l), Calc-p. (r), Camph., Kali-c. (r), Kali-n., Laur., Lyc. (r), Merc. (r), Mez. (l), Petr., Plat. (l), Samb., Sars., Sep. (r), Zinc. (l).

UPWARD: Gels., Lach., Lil-t., Nit-ac., Phos., Sulph.

SPINE, congested: Gels.

cracking: Sec.

cutting, up: Nat-s., Polyg-s.

descending: Pic-ac., Tab., Tell.

eructations, **Amel.**: Zinc.

hot iron: **Alum.**, Bufo, Camph.

icy needles, in: Agar., Cocc.

injuries: Con., Hyper., Sil., Zinc.

sensitive: **Chinin-s.**, **Lach.**, Nat-m., Phos., Ther., Zinc.

sexual excesses, Agg.: Calc., Croc.

standing, Agg.: Zinc.

tickling: Sumb.

up and down: Gels., Phyt.

COCCYX: Arn., Bel-p., **Hyper.**, Ruta, Sil.

thighs, to: Rhus-t.

ACHE: Eup-per., Phyt., Sanic., Staph., Vario., Zinc.
            Comp. **Spine.**

ACNE: Rumx.

ASCENDING: Ars., Rad-met., Zinc-val.

BED, early in: Staph.

BENDING backward: Ign.

Amel.: Plat., Med.

BLOW or sudden shock: Bell., Cic., **Sep.**, Stann.

BROKEN, as if: Arn., Bell., Ham., **Kali-c.**, Lyc., Nat-m., Phos., Senec.

BURNING, heat: Agar., Alum., **Ars.**, Bapt., Carb-an., Cocc. (s), Kali-bi. (s), **Lyc.** (s), **Phos.** (s), Phys. (s), Sec., Sil., Sulph., Tab. (s).

upward in: Bapt., Phos.

CHILLS: Caps., **Eup-per.**, Gels.

down: Am-c., Lac-c., Valer.

up: Ol-j., Ox-ac., **Sulph.**

and down: Eup-per., Gels., Ip., Puls., Sulph.

COITION, emissions, etc., **Agg.:** Cob., Ferr., Nat-m., Nit-ac.

COLD water trickles down: Caps.

COLDNESS: Merc., Nux-v., Puls., Sil., Sulph., Verat.

down: Canth., Eup-per., Lac-c., Stram.

spine (interscapular): Agar., Amm., Arg-n., Caps., Helon., Hyos., Lachn., Med., Petr., Polyp., Rhus-t., Sec.

burning sudden: Croc.

COLIC, with: Sars.

CONTRACTION: Hydr-ac., **Rhus-t.**

COUGHING, **Agg.:** **Bell.**, Bry., Nat-m.

CRAMP: Caust., **Chin.**

CRAWLING: Lac-c.

CYST, on: **Phos.**

EVERYTHING, **Agg.:** Kali-c., Lach., Sep.

FORWARD, **scapular region:** Bry., Sulph. (l), Zinc. (l).

lumbar region: Berb., Cham., Kali-c., Kreos., SABIN.

around pelvis: Sabin., Sep., Vib.

heavy: Aloe, Pall., Tarent.

thighs, to: Thyr.

GENITALS, to: Kreos.

KIDNEYS, **Agg.:** Cadm-s., Senec., Solid.

MENSES, **Amel.:** Senec.

MENTAL **exertion, Agg.:** Pic-ac.

MOTION, **Agg.:** Kali-c.

MUSCLES, **atrophy:** Thuj.

NUMBNESS: Acon., Agar., **Berb.**, Bry., Kali-bi., **Ox-ac.**, Plat., Sep.

PLUG, lump, nail, etc.: Anac., **Arn.**, Berb., **Carb-v.**, Chin., Cinnb., Cob., Kali-m., Lil-t., Lyc., Merc-d., Merc-i-r., Mosch., Phos., Plan., Senec., Teucr., Ust.

PRESSURE, **Agg.:** Agar., **Bell.**, **Chinin-s.**, Cimic., Phos.

Amel.: Bry., **Dulc.**, KALI-C., **Nat-m.**, Rhus-t., Ruta, **Sep.**

RAISING, **arms. Agg.:** Nat-m., Rhus-t., Sanic.

SHARP, darting, shooting: Kali-c., Nat-m., Ox-ac.

SHORT, as if: Agar., Aur., Hyos., Lyc., Sulph.

SITTING, **Agg.:** Agar., Rhus-t., Sep., Valer., Zinc.

SPASM: Sec.

SPOTS, **Agg.,** in: Agar., **Alum.,** Caust., Chel., Chin., Kali-bi., Lach., Nit-ac., Ox-ac., **Phos.,**

Ph-ac., Plb., Rhus-t., Thuj., Zinc.

STIFF: **Berb.**, **Caust.**, Dulc., Kali-c., Led., Nux-v., Puls., Rhus-t., **Sep.**, Sil., **Sulph.**

ascends: Ars.

STOMACH, to: Berb.

SWALLOWING, **Agg.**: Caust., Kali-c., **Rhus-t.**

THIGHS, **down**: Berb., Hep., Kali-c., Vib.

THROBBING: Bar-c., Bell., Lyc., Nat-m., Phos., Sep., Sil., Thuj.

URINATING, **Agg.**: Syph.

Amel.: Lyc.

UTERUS, to: Sep., Vib.

VERTERA, absent: Mag-p.

dorsal, upper: Kalm.

heat, agg.: Agar.

WALKING, **Amel.**: Tab.

WEAK: Ars., Bar-c., Calc., **Cocc.**, Graph., Kali-c., Nat-m., Nux-v., Phos., Ph-ac., Sel., Sep., Sil., Zinc.

SCAPULAR REGION

Bry. (r), **Chel.** (r), Chin., Dulc., Kali-c., Kreos., Jug-r. (r), Merc., Ol-an. (r), Rhus-t., Rumx. (r), **Sep.**, Zin-chr. (l).

BETWEEN: Am-m., Ars., Calc., Calc-p., Caps., Helon., Nit-ac., Phos., Sep.

UNDERNEATH: Calc., **Gels.**, Merc.

ACHE: Carb-ac., Helon., **Sep.**, Sulph.

BORING, **left**: Aur., Dig., Hyper., Meny., Mez., Nat-c., **Ph-ac.**, Ruta, Spig.

BROKEN, **as if**: Crot-c., Lil-t., **Mag-c.**, Nat-m., Plat., Verat.

BRUISED: Calen. (r), Crot-c. (r), Kali-c. (r).

BURNING: **Ars.**, Echi., Lyc., Lycps., Med., **Phos.**, Rob., Sulph.

CHILLY, **below**: Camph.

COLDNESS: Ars., **Caps.**, Caust., Pyrog., **Sep.**

CRAMP: Grat., Phos., Verat.

CRAWLING: Med. (l).

CUTTING: Canth., Lac-c., Med., Nat-s., Spig., Zinc.

edge of: Ran-b.

ERUCTATIONS, **Amel.**: Zinc.

FORWARD **from**: Bar-c., Merc. (r), Mez. (l), Phos., Ran-b. (l), Sulph.

HEART to: Bry., Sulph.

HEAVINESS: Calc., Chin., Gran., Lach., **Nux-v.**, Rhus-t.

ITCHING: Caust. (l).

LUMP: Chin., Lyc., Mag-c., Nux-v., Prun. (l), Rhus-t.

SORENESS: **Chin.**, Cimic., Hyper., **Phos.**, Quas., Sep.

SWALLOWING, **Agg.**: Kali-c., Rhus-t.

THROBBING: Mag-m. (l).

UNDER: Gels.

WEAK: Alum., **Apis, Cocc.**, Kali-i., **Nat-m.**, Rad-met., Raph., Sul-ac., Thlasp.

DORSAL REGION

Arn., Ars., **Bell.**, Calc., Caust., Chin., **Cocc.**, Gels., Ign., Lyc., **Nat-m., Nux-v.**, Phos., Pic-ac., **Puls., Rhus-t.**, Ruta, Sep., Sil., **Sulph.**

CURVATURE: Aur., Calc., Lyc., Merc., **Puls., Sulph.**

EMACIATED: Nux-v.

SENSITIVE, **spine: Agar.**, Bell., Chinin-s., Cimic., Hyper., Ign., Nux-v., Phos., Zinc.

STIFF: Caust., Rhus-t.

WEAK: Pic-ac.

　interscapular: Agar., Alum., Rad-met., Sars., **Thlasp.**

LUMBAR REGION

Aesc., Alum., **Ant-t.**, Ars., Berb., **Calc.**, Caust., Cimic., Kali-c., Nux-m., NUX-V., Puls., RHUS-T., Sanic., **Sep.**, Solid., Sulph., Vario., Zinc-ar.

AFFECTED **by everything:** Kali-c., Sep.

BREAKING, **as if: Bell.**, Eup-per., Kali-i., Lyc., **Nat-m.**, Ruta, Senec.

BURNING: Aeth., Podo.

CHEST, to: Berb., Sulph.

CHILL, **starts in:** Gels., Hyos., Lach., **Nat-m.**, Stront-c., Sulph.

COLD: Bry., Canth., **Eup-per.**, Gels., **Lach.**, Merc-c., Rhus-t., Sanic., **Sulph.**

COMPRESSION: Aeth.

COUGH, **Agg.:** Acon., Nit-ac.

CRACKING: Sec., Sulph.

CRAMP: Aur-t.

DISLOCATIVE **pain:** Eup-per., Lach.

EXERTION, **Agg.:** Zinc-ar.

FORWARD in: **Berb., Cham., Kali-c.**, Kreos., SABIN.

　around pelvis: Sabin., Sep., Vib.

HEAVY: Cimic.

HOT **iron:** Act-sp., Alum., Cann-s., Graph.

JARRING, **Agg.**: Zinc-ar.

LAME: Berb., Gels., Kali-i., Lach., Ox-ac., Ph-ac., Rhus-t., Sulph.

LUMBAGO: Ant-t., Bell., Kali-bi., Nux-v., Ox-ac., **Rhus-t.**, Sec.

NUMB: Acon., Apis, Berb., Graph., Lappa, **Plat.**, Sil.

PAIN: Aesc., Ant-t., Bry., Caust., Dulc., Graph., Led., Mur-ac., **Nux-v.**, **Rhus-t.**, Sel., Sep., Sulph.

PARALYSIS: Cocc., Kali-c., Sep.

PRESSURE, **Amel.**: Kali-c.

PUBES to: Phos., Sabin., Vib.

RADIATING **from**: Bapt., Berb., Laur., Sep.

RAW, **as if**: Nat-c.

RENAL **disease, in**: Calc-ar., Senec., Solid., Visc.

SHORT, **tense, as if**: Am-m.

SICKENS **all over**: Solid.

SITTING, **Agg.**: Zinc-ar.

STANDING, **Agg.**: Psor., Zinc., Zinc-ar.

STIFF: Bar-c., Caust., Lach., **Rhus-t.**

STITCHES: Berb., **Bry.**, Coloc., **Kali-c.**, Lyc., Puls.

STOMACH to: Sulph.

SWEAT: Naja.

TOUCH, **Agg.**: Cimic., Lil-t.

VERTEBRAE **of**: Kreos., Stann., Zinc.

WALKING, **Agg.**: Psor.

WIND, **as of a**: Sulph.

SACRUM

Graph., Hep., Hyper., Rhus-t.

BRUISED: Aesc.

THIGH, INTO: Colch. (r), Kali-c. (l).

UPPER LIMBS

Am-m., Ars., Bell., **Calc.**, **Caust.**, Cocc., Ferr., Kali-c., Lyc., Merc., Nux-v., Phos., Puls., RHUS-T., Sep., **Sil.**, SULPH.

RIGHT: Bell., Bism., Bry., Calc., Caust., Coloc., Graph., Nat-c., Ran-s., Sars., Sec., Sil., Stront-c.

LEFT: Anac., Arn., Asaf., Cact., Cimic., Kali-c., Nit-ac., Rhus-t., Sabin., Squil., Stann., Stram., Sulph.

ALTERNATING BETWEEN: Acon., Alum., **Calc.**, Caust., Cham., Chin., COCC., Colch., **Lac-c.**, Lyc., Mag-m., Mang., Plat., Sep., **Zinc.**

upper and lower limbs: Cocc., Fago., Kali-bi., Kali-m.,

Kalm., Nat-c., **Sil.**, **Valer.**, Visc.

clammy: Camph., Carb-v., Pic-ac.

cramp: Cimic., Vip-t.

diarrhea, with: Cupr., Jatr., Sec.

deep breathing, Agg.: Cann-s.

BEHIND HIM **Agg.:** Ign., Sanic.

BURNING: Ther., (up)., Verat.

CHEST, **on, Agg.:** Psor.

CRAMP: Olnd.

DEAD: Scopar. (r).

HANGING **down, Amel.:** Arn., Con., Lyc., Mag-m., Phos., Rhus-t.

HEAVY: Stroph-h.

JERKED **up:** Sabad.

LYING, **Agg.:** Kali-c.

NUMB: Aloe (l), Echi., Graph., Phyt. (r), Puls. (l), Rhus-t. (l), Zin-ar. (r to l).

PARALYSIS, **right:** Am-c., Cupr., **Lyc.**, Sulph., Zinc.

RESTLESS: Kali-br., Samb., Tarent.

RIGHT **in heart affections:** Ars., Kalm., Merc-i-f., Merc-i-r.

SWINGING: Cina.

VEINS: **Puls.**, Thyr.

WRITING, **Amel.:** Zinc-ar.

SHOULDER: Acon., Bry., Ferr., Ferr-p., Kali-c., Kalm., Mag-c., Puls., Rhus-t., Rumx. (l), Sang., Stict. (r).

right: Ferr., Kalm., **Sang.**, Stront-c.

left: Ferr., Ferr-p., Led., Mag-c., Nux-m., Sulph.

to right: Lyc.

alternating: Lyc.

cold: Viol-o.

cough, Agg.: Rumx. (l).

heavy: Anac., Chin., Lach., Phos., Puls., **Rhus-t.**, Staph., Sulph.

higher, as if: Hell. (l), Merc. (l).

night, Agg.: Fl-ac., Sang., Ust.

uneasy: Asclp.

UPPER ARM: Cocc., Ferr., Nat-m.

FOREARM: Calc., Caust., Merc., Rhus-t., Staph.

HANDS: **Calc.**, Caul., Lyc., Nux-v., Phos., **Sulph.**

backs of, dorsum: Kreos., Mur-ac. (eruption), Nat-c. (eruption), Pix (eruption), Puls. (eruption), Rhus-t., Sep.

palms: Anac., Graph., Petr., Ran-b., Sele., Spig.

abscess: Tarent.

contractions in: Graph.,
Guaj.

crack: Kreos.

cramp: Sabin.

desquamate: Elaps, Graph.,
Rhus-t.

dry: Ars., Bism., Cham.,
Nux-m., Sulph.

eczema: Sulph., Vario.

hot, burn: Crot-t., Diph., Ol-
j., Sulph.

and soles: Bism., Lil-t.,
Lyc., Petr., Phos., Sang.,
Stann., Sulph.

itch: Anac., Kreos., Sulph.

moist, sweat: Naja, Viol-o.

nodes: Caust., Ruta.

sore: Rhus-t.

vesicles: Kreos., Verat-v.

warts on: Sulph.

washing., Agg.: Rhus-t.

withered: Diph., Sang.

and feet, burning: Fl-ac.

cold sweat, on: Cimic., Ip.,
Kali-bi.

cramps: Lyss.

restless: Stict.

sweaty: Naja.

behind him: Ign., Sanic.

clammy: Sanic., Tarent., Thyr.

cold: Kali-m.

coldness of one: Chin., Dig., Ip.,
Lyc., Puls., Rhus-t., Sulph.,
Thyr. (l).

sweat, during: Thuj.

water in, Amel.: Fl-ac., Gels.

cracks, also fingers: Calc.,
Graph., Petr., Sars.

cramp: Anthraci., Mag-c., (dorsum)., Pyrog., Verat. (dorsum).

dry: Bism. (palms), Lyc., Sulph.

eczema: Cor-r., Nat-c., Pix, Sep.,
Zinc.

heat, burning, etc.: Agar., Asar.,
Carb-v., Lach., Mur-ac.,
Petr., PHOS., Sang., Sep.,
Spig., Stann., Sulph.

hot: Cocc., (then cold)., Kali-c.,
(chill with)., Mez., (one),
with cold feet: Sep.

icy: Thuj. (heat), Thyr.

lame: Caust.

numb: Echi. (alternating), Form.

offensive: Phys.

purple: Sep.

restless, busy: Kali-br., Sulph.,
Tarent., Thyr.

sweat, on: Calc., Nux-j., Sulph.,
Thuj., Tub.

cold on dorsae: Both.,
Chion., Zinc-s.

during heat: Am-c., Ferr-p., Nit-ac.

swelled, as if: Coll., Kali-n., Stront-c., Ter.

tremble: Lol-t., Tarent.

veins swelled: Am-c., Arn., Ham., Laur., Nux-v., Op., Phos., PULS.

vesicles: Kreos., Verat-v.

washes, the: Coca, Lac-c., Syph.

water, in, Agg.: Ign., Nat-m., Phos.

weak: Zinc.

wrings: Ars., Kali-br., Sulph., Ther.

FINGERS: Am-m., Lyc., Rhus-t., Sil., Sulph., Thuj.

   alternate with gastric symptoms: Kali-bi.

   around: Calc-p., Kali-bi., Lith-c.

      ulceration: Graph., Puls., Sil.

   backward: Sec.

   between: Graph., Sel.

   bites: Med., Plb.

   blue: Agar., Carb-v., Sec.

   burning: Mag-c.

   clenched thumbs: Cupr., Hyos., Merc,

   cold: Abrot., Agar.

   convulsions, spasms of: Agar., Chel., Cupr., Sec.

crossed: Carb-v., Graph.

desquamation: Am-m.

drawn together: Phos.

felon, runround, etc.: Apis, Anthraci., Ars., Fl-ac., Hep., Lach., Merc., Nat-s., Psor., Sil., Sulph., Syph., Tarent-c., Thuj.

   deep: Calc., Merc-c., Sil., Sulph.

formication: Sec.

heavy: Stroph-h.

itching: Psor.

jerking: Caust., Cycl., Rheum, Stann., Sulph.

joints, knuckles: Nat-m.

mashed: Hyper.

motions of: Kali-br., Mosch.

nodes: Abrot., Benz-ac., Berb., Calc., Caul., Kali-m., Led.

numb: Aran., Calc., Lyc., Phos., Rhus-t., Thyr.

pale: Kreos.

picks, plays with, etc.: Arum-t., Calc., Con., Crot-c., Kali-br., Lach., Ther.

               Comp. Carphology.

sensitive: Berb., Lac-c.

sides: Sars.

spread apart: Glon., Lac-c., Lyc., Med., Sec.

stiff: Kali-c.

sweat: Lyc.

tense: Mag-p.

writing, Agg.: Caust., Cycl., Kali-c., Mag-p., Stann., Sul-ac.

FINGERTIPS: Am-m., **Calc-p.,** Kali-c., Lach., Phos., Sec., Teucr., Thuj.

brown: Tub.

burn: Canth., Med., Nat-m.

bursting: Caust.

cracked: Aur-m., Bar-c., Bell., Caust., Cist., Cund., Fl-ac., **Graph.,** Med., Merc., Merc-c., Mez., Mur-ac., Nat-m., Petr., Ran-b., **Sars.,** Sil.

heavy: Plb., Stroph-h.

numb: Nat-m., Sulph.

painful: Calc., Cist., Lac-c., Sil., Sulph.

red: Acon.

sensitive: Berb., Calc-p., Cist., Lac-c., Nat-c., Sars., **Sulph.,** Tarent.

sweat on: Carb-an., Carb-v., Phos., Sep., Sulph.

ulcers: Psor.

NAILS: Ant-c., Graph., Merc., **Sil., Sulph.,** Thuj., Ust.

bites: Acon., **Ars.,** Arum-t., Cina, Lyc., Med., Senec., Stram.

blue: Nux-v., Verat.

brittle, crumbling, etc.: Clem., Cupr., Fl-ac., Graph., Lept., Merc., Par., Senec., Sil., Sulph.

corner of: Lach.

crumble: Fl-ac., Graph.

cutting: Petr., Sars.

deformed, thickened: Graph., Sep., Sil., Sulph.

discolored: Graph., Nit-ac., Thuj.

distorted., crippled: Ant-c., Graph., Sil., Syph., Thuj.

edge of: Calc-p., Rad-met.

falling off: Grap., Sil., Squil.

gnawing: Alum., Berb., Lach., Lappa.

hangnails: Calc., Nat-m., Nat-s., Rhus-t., Sulph.

ingrown: Fl-ac., **Graph,** Hep., M-aust., **Sil.,** Sul-i., Sulph., Teucr.

loose, as if: Apis, Pyrog.

ribbed: Fl-ac., Thuj.

painful: Caust., Graph., Merc., Nit-ac., Sil., Sulph.

run arounds: Nat-s., Syph., Thuj.

scaling: Alum.

soft: Thuj.

splitting: Ant-c., Fl-ac., Lept., Ruta, Sil., Thuj.

spotted: Nit-ac.

thin: Lept.

ulcers: Sil.

under: Alum., Berb.

yellow: Con., Sep., Sil.

JOINTS: Calc., Caust., Kali-c., Led., Lyc., Merc., Rhus-t., Sep., Sulph.

shoulder: Calc., Ferr., Ferr-p., Ign., Kali-c., Nat-m., Puls., Rhus-t., **Sang.**, Sep., Staph., Sulph.

elbow: Caust., Kali-c., Rhus-t., Sep., Sulph.

bend of: Kali-c.

tip of: Hep.

eruption: Syph.

herpes: Manc., Petr., Phos., Ran-b., Sep., Staph., Thuj.

numb: Nat-s., Puls.

paralysis: Rhus-t.

wrist: Bov., Calc., Caust., Kali-c., Rhus-t., Ruta, Sabin., Sep., Sulph., Viol-o. (r).

bruised: Rhod.

cold: Calc-fl.

finger: Ant-c., Calc., Calc-f., Caul., Caust., Lyc., Sep., Spig., Sulph.

ulcers on: Borx., Mez., Sep.

BONES: Asaf., Chin., Cocc., Rhus-t., Sil., Staph.

CLAVICLE, air: Chlor., Rumx.

stitch: Puls.

under: Calc-p., Rumx

HUMERUS, aches: Bry. (r), Gels. (r).

broken, seems: Bov., Cocc., Puls.

cramp: Valer. (l).

crushing: Stann.

DELTOID: Ferr., Ferr-p., Mag-c. (r), Phyt. (r), Sang. (r), Staph. (r), Syph.

RAISING ARM, **Agg.**, letting it hang, **Amel.**: Acon., Arn., Bar-c., CON., Ferr., Kali-c., Led., Lil-t., Med., Merc., Rhus-t., **Sang.**, Sanic., Sep., Sil., Sulph., Tell.

RESTLESS: Agar., Caust., Mur-ac., Tarent.

WEAKNESS: Anac., Bell., Calc., Cic., **Kali-c.**, Sulph.

LOWER LIMBS

Alum., **Ars.**, Bell., **Calc.**, CAUST., Graph., Kali-c., Lach., **Led.**, LYC., Merc., Nit-ac., Nux-v., PULS., RHUS-T., Sep., SIL., SULPH., Valer., Zinc.

RIGHT: Ars., Bell., Bry., Coloc., Graph., Lach., Nux-v., Phos., Puls., Rhod., Sars., Sec., Sep.

LEFT., Ambr., Asaf., Calc., Cina, Con, Ferr., Hep., Lyc., Nit-ac., Rhus-t., Sil., Stram., Sulph.

ALTERNATING BETWEEN: Acon., Aloe, Ars., BRY., Calc-p., Cham., Cic., Coloc., Cupr., Dios., Graph., **Kali-bi.**, Kali-c., Kali-n., Lach., Lil-t., Mag-p., **Nat-m.**, Nat-s., **Puls.**, **Rhus-t.**, Sep., Sil., **Sulph.**

HIPS AND LOINS: Arn., Caust., Euph., Lyc., Phyt., Plb., Rhus-t., Ruta, Sep., Sulph.

above: Caust.

alternating between: Euon.

bruised: Ruta.

burning, joins: Bar-c.

change of weather: Phyt.

contracted: Polyg-s.

cramp, in: Led.

forced apart, disjointed, etc.: Agar., Calc-p., Con., Sep., Sulph., Tril-p.

hip, to: Arn., Cimic., Coloc., Lac-c., Lil-t., Onos., Thuj, Ust.

hollow (loins): Pall.

iliacs, down thighs: Berb.

morbus coxarius: Acon., Ambr.,

Apis, Arg-met., Arn., Ars., Asaf., Aur., Bell., Bry., Calc., Canth., Caust., Cham., Coloc., Dig., Dros., Graph., Hep., Kreos., Led., Lyc., Merc., Mez., Nux-v., Olnd., Petr., Phos., Puls., Rhus-t., Ruta, Sabin., Sep., Sil., Staph., Sulph., Thuj., Zinc.

motion, Agg.: Ant-t.

Amel.: Am-m., Calc-p., Iris.

pregnancy, in: Calc-p.

rising., Agg.: Nat-s.

sticking in loins: Berb., Plb.

weak: Calc-p., Rat., Tril-p.

wrenched: Iris.

BUTTOCKS: Graph., Ph-ac., Staph., Sulph.

red: Carb-v., Cham., Sulph.

THIGHS: Ars., Chin., Clem Guaj., **Merc.**, **Nat-m.**, Phyt., Sep.

anterior: Anac., Spong., Xan.

posterior and sciatic nerve: Coloc., Graph., **Rhus-t.**, Sel., Sep., Sulph., Zinc.

outer side: Caust., Helon., **Ph-ac.**, Phyt.

inner side: Petr., Rhod., Stann., Sulph.

bone pains: Euph., Guaj., Ruta.

broken: Ruta.

cold: Berb.

cramp: Ant-t., Chel., **Cupr.**, Meny.

pains into: Cham., **Staph.**, Xan.

short, as if: Kreos.

sweat, cold: Caps., Spong.

twitching: Kali-m.

weak: Eup-per., **Gels.**, Lappa, Mur-ac., Urt-u.

LEGS: Am-c., Calc., Lyc., Puls., Sep., Sil., Staph.

left to right: Mag-c.

ache: Ars-i., **Eup-per.**, Guaj., Helon., Nit-ac., Pic-ac., **Phyt.**, Polyg-s., Rhus-t., Still., Sul-i., Vario.

blood rushes to: Arg-met., Aur., Meph., Phel., Thyr.

blue: Vip-t.

bruised, as if: Caust., Eup-per., Gels.

burning: Crot-h., Nat-s.

calf: Apis, Eup-per., Jatr.

bruised: Eup-per., Staph.

cramp: Cupr., Plat., Verat., Vib., Vip-t., Zinc-i.

clammy: Lil-t.

coition, Agg.: Calc., Nat-m.

cold: Carb-v., Lil-t. (night in bed).

cramp: Stront-c., Sulph.

crosses the: Gels., Lil-t., Murx., Rhod., **Sep.**, Thuj.

elongated: Coloc., Kreos., Rhus-t., Sulph.

eructations, Amel.: Puls.

floating: Acon., Spig., Zinc-i.

fulness, bursting: Ham., Vip-t.

heavy: Alum., Calc., Gels., Nat-c., Pic-ac., Rhus-t., Sulph.

numb: Graph., Plan., Thyr.

numb, r.: Cedr., Eup-per., **Kali-c.**, Nux-m., Zinc.

petechiae: Apis, Led., Solid.

presses foot to floor: Ign., Med., Zinc-i.

restless: Agar., Ars., Carb-v., Kali-c., Nit-ac., Rhus-t., Sulph., Tarent., ZINC.

rotation Agg.: Bry., Cocc., Coloc., Kali-c.

shooting up: Nux-v.

shortened: Ambr., Coloc., Mez., Olnd., Phos., Sep.

stool, Agg.: Apis, Sec., Verat.

stretching, Amel.: Med.

sweat, cold, on: Puls., Ter.

tremulus: Plan.

twitching: Phys., Tarent.

ulcer: Fl-ac., **Lach.**, Sul-i.

weak: Cocc., Cur., **Gels.**, Mang., Rhus-t., Zinc.

weather changes, **Agg.**: Phyt.

TIBIA, shin: Agar., **Asaf.**, Calc., Carb-v., Cinnb., Lach., Merc., Mez., **Phos.**, Phyt., Puls., Still.

nodes: Calc-f., Sul-i.

pains, in: Lach., Phyt., Still., Sul-i.

sticking, in: Puls.

syphilis: Merc., Phyt., still., Sul-i.

CALF: Alum., Arg-n., Ars., Calc., Graph., Ign., Nit-ac., **Nux-v.**, Puls., Sep., Stann., Staph., Sulph., Valer.

cramp in: Calc., **Cham.**, Coloc., **Cupr.**, Dulc., Ign., Lyc., Mag-p., NUX-V., Rheum, Scopar., Sec., **Sep.**, Stann., Staph., SULPH.

TENDO ACHILLES: Anac., Kalibi., **Mur-ac.**, Sep., Valer., **Zinc.**

FOOT: Arn., Ars., Bell., Bry., Caust., Kali-c., Lyc., **Puls.**, Sep., Sil., Zinc. (edge).

arches: Ruta, Sil.

bed, out out: Ars., Cham., Sang., Sec., **Sulph.**

bones: Chin., Cupr., Hyper., Led., Mez., Phyt., Pyrog., **Ruta**, Staph., Syph.

border of: Graph., Led., Lith-c.

braces: Ign., Med.

broken, as if: Hep., Zinc.

bunions: Graph., Lyc., Paeon., Sil.

clubby: Nux-v.

cold, **Agg.**: Bar-c., Con., Lach., **Nux-v.**, **Puls.**, Sil.

  bed, in: Ars. (l), Calc., Graph., Lyc. (r), Psor., Raph. (r), Senec., Sep., Sil., Tub. (l).

  icy: Bell.

wet **Agg.**: Puls.

cold water, as if in: Gels.

coldness of one: Bar-c. (r), Carb-v. (l), Chel., Con., **Lyc.** (r), Psor. (l), Puls. (r), Rhus-t. (l), Sabin. (r), **Sulph.** (l), Tub. (1).

cramp: Frax., Rumx., Verat-v.

  pregnancy, in: Calc.

damp: CALC.

desquamation: Manc.

dorsae: Led.

  cramp: anac., Lach., Verat-v.

  swelled: Bry., Puls., Thuj.

dry: **Sulph.**

edema: Kali-c. (l)

edge of: Kali-bi.

floating, as if: Spig.

hard floor, **Agg.**: Ruta.

heavy: Alum., Ars., Cycl., **Nat-m.**, Puls., Rhod., Ruta, Sulph.

higher than head, as if: **Spig.**

itching: Pic-ac., Stroph-h.

motion, Amel.: Zinc.

moves, for relief: Ars., Rhus-t., Zinc.

numb: Ars., Cocc., Form., **Nux-v.**, Plat., Sep.

right: Alum., Ant-c., Ars., Camph., Kali-bi., Mang., Rhus-t.

left: Graph., Kali-c., Med., Nat-m., Phos., Psor., Thuj.

paralysis: Caust.

restless: Ars., Rhus-t., **Zinc.**

spasm of: Bism., Verat.

sweat, acrid: Manc., **Sil.**, Thuj.

backs of: Iod.

cold: Bar-c., Calc., Kali-m., Tarent.

destroys shoes: Graph., Hep., Naja, Sanic., Sec., Sil.

foul: Lach., Ol-an.

sticky, hose stiff: Am-c., Calc., Kali-c., Lyc., Manc., Sanic.

suppressed: Bar-c., Sil., Zinc.

sweating: Bar-c., Calc., Carb-v., Iod., Lyc., Puls., **Sep.**, Sil., Sulph., Thuj.

foul odor: Bar-c., Kali-c., Nit-ac., Puls., **Sil.**, Thuj.

swelling, right: Bov., Lac-c., Lach., Lyc., Sars., Sec., Spong., Spig., Stront-c., Sulph.

left: Apis, Coloc., Como., Kreos., Lyc., Sang., Sil., Tell.

vesicles: Nat-c.

HEELS: Am-m., Calc., Caust., Con., Ferr., Graph., Ign., Led., Mang., Nat-c., Puls., Sabin., Sep.

cold: Merc., Sang., Sep.

elevating, Amel.: Phyt.

pain: Mang., Puls., Rhod., Valer.

sore: All-c., Lac-c., Led., Polyg-s.

stone, under: Aur., Berb., Brom., **Cann-s.**, Hep., **Lyc.**, Rhus-t.

throbbing: Nat-s.

DORSUM: Calc., **Caust.**, Hep., Puls., Spig., Tarax.

SOLES: Cupr., Ph-ac., Puls., Tarax.

ache: Zinc-ar.

burn: Calc., **Lach.**, Lyc., Psor., Sang., Sanic., SULPH.

callosities: Ant-c., Ars., **Bar-c.**, Graph., Rad-met., Sep., SIL., Sulph., Symph.

Comp. **Hardness.**

cramp: Calc., Cupr., Sulph., Verat-v.

itch: Cimic., Tarent.

painful: Kali-c., Kali-p., **Lyc.**, Med., Puls.

pressure, Amel.: Zinc-ar.

soft, furry: ALUM., Ars., Cann-s., Cocc., Helon., **Xan.**, Zinc.

swelled: Ferr., Lyc., Puls.

tender: Ant-c., Calc., Led., **Med.**, Nat-c., Thuj.

vesicles: Nat-c., Nat-s.

TOES: **Arn., Caust., Graph.**, Plat., Puls., Ran-s., Sabin., **Sulph.**, Thuj.

ache: Zinc. (tips).

broken: Lach.

corns: **Ant-c.**, Bry., Calc., Ign., Lyc., Rhus-t., **Sep.**, **Sil.** (soft), Sulph.

 inflamed: Sil.

cracked: Sabad.

cramp: Zinc-chr.

drawn down: Ars., Colch., Cupr., Hyos.

 up: Lach.

glistening: Sabin.

gout: Rhod., Sabin.

great: Arn., Asaf., Caust., Kali-c., Nat-s., Plat., Sabin. (podagra), Sil., Zinc.

inflamed: Sabin. (big).

numb, first: Ars., Calc., Cham., Nat-s.

red: Sabin.

swelled: Led. (big).

thighs to: Nux-v., Thal-met.

tips: Kali-c.

 balls of: Led., Petr., Puls., Spig.

 blisters: Nat-c.

 nails: Graph., Sabad.

touch, Agg.: Ars., Calc., Chin., Kali-c., Sep., Sulph.

tremor: Arn., Mag-c.

uncover, must: Fl-ac., Sulph.

vesicles: Sec.

JOINTS: Bry., Calc., Caust., Kali-c., Led., Lyc., Nat-m., Rhus-t., Sep., Sil., Stront-c., Sulph.

hip: Bry., **Caust.**, Led., Merc., Ph-ac., Rhus-t., Stram., Thuj.

knee: Apis, Aur., Benz-ac., Caust., Chin., **Gels.**, Led., Nat-m., Nux-v., Petr., Puls., Rhus-t., **Sep.**, Sulph.

 ascending and descending Agg.: Verat.

 cramp: Ter.

effusion: Apis, Iod., Sulph.

eruption: Led.

numb: Merc-i-f., Nat-p.

shocks through: Puls., Valer.

spread apart: Lyc., Plat.

tremble: Chin., Zinc.

tubercular: Calc., Iod., Lyc., Sulph.

weak: Cocc., **Gels.**, Sep.

popliteal space: Bell., Con., Mez., Nat-c., Nat-m., Onos., Phos.

sweat: Bry., **Carb-an.**, Con., Dros., Sep.

patella: Bell., Con.

plug, under: Cham.

ankles: Caust., Led., Lyc., Nat-m., Rhus-t., Rumx., Sep., Sulph.

break: Phos.

cold: Calc-f., Ign., Mag-m., Med.

cramp: Meny., Rumx., Zinc-i.

heavy: Ant-c., Crot-t., Led., Nit-ac., Sec., **Sulph.**

inflamed: Mang.

nervous: Mag-m.

sprain: Led.

sweat, on: Crot-h., Naja.

swelled: Stront-c.

weak: Carb-an., **Nat-c.**, **Nat-s.**, **Nit-ac.**, Ph-ac., Sec., Sil., Stront-c.

toe-joints: Aur., Caust., Kali-c., Led., Sabin., Sep., Sulph., Teucr., **Zinc.**

BONES: Merc., Phos., Phyt., Puls., Pyrog., Ruta, Sil., Staph., Syph.

BATHING, COOL, **Amel.**: Aur., **Led.**, Phys., Rat., Thuj.

CROSSING LIMBS, **Agg.**: Rhus-t.

   Amel.: Ant-t., Lil-t., Murx., Rhod., Sep., Thuj.

DOWN TO FEET, **pain**: Alum., Caps., Lyc., Rhus-t.

ELEVATING LIMBS, **Amel.**: Bar-c., Calc., CArB-V., Graph., Ham., Puls., Ran-s., **Sep.**, **Vip-t.**

HAMSTRINGS, **short, tense**: Bry., Dios., Nat-m.

INVERSION: Cic., Merc., Nux-v., Petr., PSOR., Sec.

JERKING UP: Lach., **Lyc.**, Myg.

PHLEGMASIA DOLENS: Apis, Ars., Bell., **Calc.**, Lach., Lyc., Merc., Puls., Sulph., Vip-t.

SCIATICA: Ars., **Coloc.**, Dios., Ign., Kali-bi., Nux-v., **Rhus-t.**, Ruta, Sel., Sep., Tell.

   ascending pain: Led., Nux-v.

   boring: Lach.

deep pain: Kali-bi., Ruta.

emaciated parts: **Calc.**, Caust., Plb.

heat, **Agg:** Ferr., Merc., Visc.

Amel: Ars., Mag-p.

move, must: Bry., Caust., Lyc., Mag-c., **Rhus-t.**, Zinc-val.

numbness, with: **Acon.**, Cham., Gnaph.

shootings: Acon., **Coloc.**, Iris, Mag-c.

sitting, **Agg.: Am-m.**, Bell., Hyper., Indm., Lept.

sprained., **Agg.:** Tell.

touch, **Agg.:** Chin., Coff., Plb., Visc.

wetting, after: Dulc., **Rhus-t.**

WEAKNESS, paralysis, etc.: Ars., Gels., Nat-m., Nux-v., Sep., Sulph.

SKIN

Apis, Ambr., **ARS.**, Bell., Bry., Calc., Caust., Graph., Hep., **Lach., Lyc., MERC.**, Nit-ac., Petr., Phos., Puls., Ran-b., Ran-s., **RHUS-T.**, Sabad., Sars., Sep., Sil., **SULPH.**, Thuj., Thyr., Ust., Viol-o., Viol-t.

under: Acon., Aesc., Agar., Alum., Bell., **Brom.**, Cic.,

Coca, Lach., Phos., **Sec.**, Thuj., **Zinc.**

ALTERNATING with: Ant-c., Ars., Calad., Graph., Hep., Staph., Sulph.

BITING: Syph.

BLEEDS on scratching: Arum-t., Lyc., Psor.

BOILS, arms, on: Petr.

axillae: Lyc., Phos.

blind: Lyc.

calf, on: Sil.

crops, of: Echi., Sil., Sulph., Syph.

eye, over left: Nat-m.

nates, on: Sulph.

nose, on tip: Acon., Anan.

on septum: Anthraci.

small and sore: Arn., Lappa, Pic-ac., Sec., Tub.

soles: Rat.

thighs: Hyos., Ign.

BUBO: Merc-i-f., Merc-i-r.

BULLAE: Ran-s., Syph.

BUNION: Agar., Sil.

BURNING, **heats, etc.:** Acon., Ars., **Bell.**, Fl-ac., Lach., Rad-met., Sulph., Ter., Ust.

CALLOSITIES: **Ant-c.**, Graph., Phos., Rad-met., Symph.

Comp. **Hardness.**

CLAMMY: Aeth.

COLD: Camph., Carb-v., Kali-n., Med., **Verat.**

Agg.: Agar., **Hep.**, Lac-d., Petr., Psor., **Rhus-t.**

bathing, Agg.: Ant-c., Thuj.

and dry: Camph., Nux-m.

CRACKS, see **Generalities.**

CRAWLING like a bug or worm under: Calc., Cocain., Oena., Stram., Vario.

CRUSTS: Ars., CALC., **Dulc.**, Graph., Lyc., Mag-m., Manc., Merc., **Mez.**, Nat-m Nit-ac., Petr., Psor., **Rhus-t.**, Sil., SULPH.

beneath (pus): Bov., Lyc., Mez., Thuj.

brown: Olnd.

conical: Sil., Syph.

cracked: Vio-t.

dirty: Psor.

falling: Nit-ac.

humid: Nit-ac., **Staph.**, Vinc., Vio-t.

shiny: Olnd.

tenacious fluid: Viol-t.

thick: Bov., **Calc.**, Kali-bi., Petr.

white: Ars.

yellow: Graph.

CYSTS and WENS: see **Generalities.**

DESQUAMATION: see **Generalities.**

DIRTY color: **Ars.**, Ferr., Ferr-pic., Merc., Petr., Phos., **Psor.**, Sec., Sulph.

DRY, sweat and moisture scanty: see **Generalities.**

DUSKY: Ars-i., Calc-p., Merc.

EDGES: Graph., Hep., Nat-p., Nit-ac., Petr., Psor., **Sulph.**

itching: Ambr., Caust., Petr.

ECCHYMOSES, petechiae, purpura, etc.: **Arn.**, **Ars.**, Bry., Colch., Crot-h., Ham., Kreos., **Lach.**, Led., Mur-ac., Phos., Pyrog., Rhus-t., Sec., Solid., Sul-ac., Tarent., Ter.

Comp. **Hemorrhages.**

EPITHELIOMA: **Ars.**, Ran-s., Sep., **Thuj.**

ERUPTIONS (tendency to): Acon., ARS., Bell., **Calc.**, Caust., Clem., **Dulc.**, **Graph.**, Lach., **Lyc.**, MERC., Mez., Nat-m., Nit-ac., Phos., Psor., Puls., RHUS-T., **Sep.**, **Sil.**, SULPH.

acne: Bell., Carb-v., Eug., Graph., **Hep.**, Kali-br., Merc., Nux-v., Sep., Sulph.

acuminate, conical: Ant-c., Ant-t., **Ars.**, Hydr., Puls., **Sil.**

black, tipped: Carb-v.

circular (ringworm): Calc., Clem., Nat-c., Nat-m., Ol-j., Sep., Sulph., Tell., Tub.

clustered: Calc., Crot-t., Nat-m., Rhus-t.

confluent: Bell., Cic., Rhus-t.

coppery: Ars., Carb-an., Kreos., Rhus-t.

delayed: Ant-t., Ars., Bry., Stram.

dry: Bar-c., Calc., Carb-v., Hep., Merc., Sep., Sulph., Verat.

dysentery, and: Rhus-t.

eczema: Alum., Ars., Bell., Bov., Carb-v., Clem., Dulc., Graph., Hep., Kreos., Lyc., Merc., Mez., Petr., Phos., Rad-met., Rhus-t., Solid., Sulph.

foul: Lappa, Vinc.

moist: Sul-i.

erythematous: Ars., Merc., Sulph.

exanthema; with fever, etc.: Acon., Bell., Bry., Coff., Merc., Phos., Puls., Rhus-t., Sulph.

favus: Ars., Sulph.

fine: Agar., Carb-v., Nat-m., Rhus-t., Sabad., Verat.

fish, after: Ars., Sep.

flat: Lach., Ph-ac., Sep.

granular: Ars., Carb-v., Hep.

hair, in apex of: Kali-bi.

herpetic: Acon., Ars., Bell., Dulc., Hep., Manc., Merc., NAT-M., Petr., Ran-b., Rhus-t., Sep., Sulph., Vario.

horny, horns: Ant-c., Ars., Borx., Graph., Ran-b., Sil., Sulph.

impetigo contagiosa: Ars., Ant-t., Arum-t., Calc., Graph., Rhus-t., Sulph., Tarent.

indented: Bov., Thuj., Vario.

intertrigo: Cham., Lyc., Merc., Sulph.

itch-like: Carb-v., Caust., Hep., Lyc., Merc., Sel., Sep., Sulph.

lichen: Acon., Agar., Bry., Cic., Cocc., Dulc., Lyc., Mur-ac., Nat-m., Sulph.

fiery: Cic., Lyc., Rhus-t.

measly, see Generalities, mentagra: Calc., Graph., Sep.

miliary: Acon., Ars., Bry., Coff., Dulc., Ip., Merc., Phyt., Sulph.

moist: Calc., Cic., Clem., Graph., Lyc., Merc., Rhus-t., Sep., Sulph.

nodular: Kali-i., Nat-s., Sil.

painful: Arn., Bell., Hep., Lach., Lyc., Merc., Phos., Ph-ac.

painless: Lyc.

papules: Acon., Bry., Dulc., Merc., Sulph.

pedunculated: Thuj.

pemphigus: Ars., Arum-t., Canth., Dulc., Hep., Ranb., Rhus-t.

petechiae, with: Ail., Mur-ac.

pimples: Ant-c., Caust., Nit-ac., Sep., Zinc.

prurigo: Sep.

psoriasis: Ars-i., Berb-a., Borx., Clem., Dulc., Graph., Merc., Phos., Psor., Radmet., Ran-b., SEP., Sulph., Thyr.

pustulating: Ant-c., Ant-t., Ars., Cic., Dulc., Lyc., Merc., Merc-d., Nat-c., Puls., Rhus-t., Sulph., Thuj., Thyr., Vario.

apices, black: Anthraci., Kalibi., Lach.

brown: Verat.

receding: Bry., Camph., Caust., Cupr., Lyc., Sulph., Zinc.

roseola: Kali-i., Bars.

rubella: Acon., Bell., Bry., Puls.

rupia: Ars., Cham., Graph., Merc., Petr., Sep., Sulph.

scabby, crusty: Calc., Con., Graph., Hep., Lyc., Mag-

m., Manc., Merc., Petr., Psor., Rhus-t., Sars., Sil., Sulph.

Comp. Generalities

bloody: Merc., Sulph.

sparse: Ail., Mur-ac.

touch, Agg.: Apis, Chin., Cocc., Coff., Hep., Lach., Mang., Plb., Thuj.

scaly: Calc., Clem., Phos., Sulph.

scarlatinous: Ail., Am-c., Apis, Bell., Cham., Merc., Murac., Phos., Phyt., Stram., Sulph.

maligna: Ail., Lach.

serpiginous: Ars., Sulph.

suppressed, undeveloped, etc.: Ail., Ars., Bry., Cupr., Mez., Stram., Sulph., Thuj., Verat., Zinc.

tettery: Alum., Ars., Bov., Calc., Cham., Con., Dulc., Graph., Lyc., Merc., Mez., Nat-m., Petr., Phos., Rhust., Sep., Sil., Sulph., Vib.

Comp. Eczema.

urticarious, hives, wheals, etc.: Ant-c., Apis, Calc., Caust., Dulc., Graph, Hep., Phos., Polyg-s., Rhus-t., Sep., Sil., Urt-u.

urticaria, with: Canc-f., Myr., Polyg., Urt-u.

ascarides, with: Urt-u.

liver symptoms, with: Calc-f., Myrt., Ptel.

receding: Stroph.

shell fish, from: Ter., Urt-u.

varicella: Acon., Ant-c., Ant-t., Bell., Led., Puls., **Rhus-t.**

variola: Ant-t., Ars., **Merc.**, Puls., **Rhus-t.**, Sulph., **Thuj.**, Vario.

vesicular, blisters, etc.: **Ars.**, **Arum-t.**, **Canth.**, Caust., **Crot-t.**, Dulc., Graph., Lach., Manc., Merc., **Nat-m.**, Phos., **Ran-b.**, **Rhus-t.**, Sec., Sep., Sulph., Urt-u.

dark: Anthraci.

zoster: Ars., Graph., Lach., Merc., Mez., **Ran-b.**, **Rhus-t.**, Vario.

EXCORIATED, denuded, raw: Arn., **Arum-t.**, Aur., Carb-v., **Cham.**, Chin., Cist., Fl-ac., **Graph.**, Hep., **Ign.**, Iod., Kreos., **Lyc.**, Meli-a., Merc., Nit-ac., Ol-an., Petr., Psor., **Puls.**, Sang., Sep., **Sulph.**

Comp. **Soreness.**

EXHALATIONS: Stroph-h.

FLABBY, relaxed: Calc., Merc-d., Spong., Verat.

FOLDS, flexures, etc.: Ars., Calc., Carb-v., GRAPH., Hep., Lyc.,

Merc., Mez., **Nat-m.**, Nit-ac., Ol-an., Petr., PSOR., Puls., Sep., Sel., Sil., Sulph., Zinc.

cracks: Graph., Merc., Petr.

FRECKLES: **Lyc.**, Phos., **Sep.**, **Sulph.**

FUNGUS GROWTH, excrescences, **warts,** figwarts, condylomata, polypi, proud flesh, hematodes, etc.: Alum., Ant-c., Ars., Bar-c., **Calc.**, **Carban.**, **Caust.**, Clem., Cocc-c., **Dulc.**, Lach., **Lyc.**, **Med.**, **Merc.**, Merc-c., Nat-c., **Nat-s.**, NIT-AC., Petr., **Phos.**, **Ph-ac.**, Psor., Rhus-t., **Sabin.**, Sang., Sil., **Staph.**, Sulph., THUJ.

bleeding: Nit-ac., Phos.

flat: Merc-i-f.

fleshy: Alum., Calc., Staph., Thuj.

granular: Calc., Nit-ac., Staph., Thuj.

horny: Ant-c., Sil.

pedunculated: Lyc., **Nit-ac.**, **Sabin.**, **Thuj.**

ragged: Nat-c., Ph-ac., Rhus-t., Thuj.

spongy: Calc., Lyc., Nit-ac., Staph., Thuj.

suppressed: Meny., Nit-ac., Staph., Thuj.

ulcerating: Hell.

GANGLION: Am-c., Benz-ac., Ruta.

Comp. **Cysts.**

GANGRENE: **Ars.**, Bell., **Carb-v.**, Chin., Kreos., **Lach.**, Plb., Sec., Sil., Solid., Tarent.

cold: Ars., Lach., Sec., Sil.

diabetic: Con., Lach., Solid.

hot: Acon., Ars., Bell.

moist: Chin., Hell., Phos.

threatened, with blue parts: Ars., Asaf., Aur., Con., Hep., Lach., Merc., Sil., Verat.

traumatic: Arn., **Lach.**

GOOSESKIN: Hell., **Nux-v.**, Par Verat.

HAIRY: Med., Thuj.

HARD: **Ant-c.**, Clem., Dulc., Graph., Petr., Phos., **Rhus-t.**, Sars., **Sep.**, Sil.

HEAL, won't, difficult, vulnerable: **Arn.**, **Ars.**, Calc., **Cham.**, Con., Graph., **Hep.**, Kali-bi., **Lach.**, **Lyc.**, Merc., Petr., Sil., **Sulph.**

Comp. **Suppuration.**

suppurates, unhealthy: Ant-c., Hep., Mez., **Sil.**, Sulph., thuj.

HIVES: Urt-u.

receding: Stroph-h.

shell fish, after: Urt-u.

INACTIVE: Anac., **Con.**, Kali-c., Lyc., **Ph-ac.**

INDENTED: Apis, Ars., **Bov.**, Caps., Phos., Verat.

INFLAMED: Cham., Hep., Petr., Sil., Sulph.

INTERNAL symptoms, alternating with: Ars., Crot-t., Rhus-t.

IRRITABLE: Rad-met.

ICHTHYOSIS: **Ars-i.**

ITCH, BAKER'S, barber's: Graph., Lith-c., Rhus-t., Sul-i.

ITCHING: Acon., Agar., Ambr., Ant-c., Apis, **Calc.**, **CAUST.**, Fago., **Lyc.**, **Merc.**, Phos., Psor., **Puls.**, **Rhus-t.**, Sep., **Sil.**, Staph., **Sul-i.**, Sulph.

affected part, over: Agar.

air, Agg.: Hep., **Rumx.**

Amel.: Stront-c.

bathing, after: Bov., Calc., Clem., Mag-c.

bed, in: Kali-ar., Led., Pic-ac., Sil., **Sulph.**

biting: Olnd., Staph.

burning: **Agar.**, Apis, Caust., Lach., Petr., Rhus-t., Sil., **Sulph.**

crawling: Tell.

discharges: Tell.

heated, when: Lyc.

here and there: Am-c.

internal: Apis, Calc., Phos., Rhus-t., Sang., Sumb.

painful: Bar-c.

pleasurable: Sulph.

scratching, Agg.: Crot-t.

bumps, form: Dulc., Mez., Rhus-t., Verat.

eruption follows: Am-c., Olnd.

moisture follows: Graph., Olnd., Rhus-t.

must: Agar., Arg-met., Coff., Psor., Staph.

uncovering, on: Nit-ac., Rum.

LEPROUS DISEASES: Ars., Sep., Sil., Sulph.

LOOSE: Carb-an.

LOUSINESS: Merc., Olnd., Sulph.

LUPUS: Ars., Calc., Graph., Lyc., Merc., Nat-m., Rhus-t., Sep., Sil., Staph., Sulph.

hypertrophicus: Ars., Graph.

vorax: Ars., Sep., Sil., Staph., Sulph.

MENSES, Agg., before: Borx., Carb-v., Dulc., Graph., Kali-c., Mag-m., Nat-m., Sang., Sars., Sep., Stram., Verat.

MOIST: Carb-v., Graph., Lach., Lyc., Rhus-t.

MOTTLED: Ail., Lach., Puls., Sulph.

NAEVI, birth-mark, etc.: Arn., Ars., Calc., Calc-f., Carb-an., Carb-v., Fl-ac., Lach., Lyc., Phos., Plat., Sep., Sulph., Thuj., Ust.

smooth, mottled: Con., Phos., Sep., Sulph.

spidery: Carb-v., Lach., Plat., Sep., Thuj.

NETTLE RASH: Dulc., Urt-u.

NODES, under: Alum., Mag-c.

NUMB, insensible: Anac., Arg-n., Nux-v., Olnd., Sec.

OILY, greasy: see Generalities.

OOZING: Calc., Graph., Lyc., Merc., Petr., Sulph.

PAINFUL: Ars., Calc., Carb-v., Cupr., Hep., Ip., Lach., Merc., Nit-ac., Nux-v., Ph-ac., Sil., Sulph., Verat.

cold to: Agar., Aur., Plb., Rhus-t.

Comp. Sensitive.

PARCHMENT-LIKE: Ars., Calc-f., Lyc., Petr., Sil.

PRURIGO: Acon., Bry., Calc., Carb-v., Con., Graph., Merc., Nat-m., Nit-ac., Nux-v., Op.,

Puls., Rhus-t., Sabin., **Sep.**, Thuj., Urt-u.

senilis: Ars., Merc., Mez., Olnd., Sulph.

PRURITIS senilis: Alum., Ars., Dulc., Fago., Mez., Urt-u.

of diabetes: Mang.

PUFFED, bloated: Ant-c., **Apis**, Calc., Caps., Cupr., Ferr., Kreos., Led., Phyt., Ust.

QUIVERING, twitching: Mang., Phos., Sec., Tab.

ROUGH, **ragged**: Ars., Bell., **Calc.**, Calen., Fl-ac., Iod., Nit-ac., **Petr.**, Phyt., Psor., Sabad., Sep., Sulph., Tub.

SCARS: see **Injuries.**

SCLERODERMA: Rad-met.

SCLEROSIS: Plb.

SCURFY, scaly, mealy: **Ars., Calc.**, Dulc., Kali-m., Kreos., Lyc., Manc., Med., Nat-c., Nit-ac., Phos., Rhus-t., Sep., **Sil.**, **Sulph.**, Thyr.

Comp. **Desquamation.**

SENSITIVE: Ars., Asaf., Bell., Calc., Carb-v., Chin., **Lach.**, Mang., Nat-m., Plan., Sil., Tub., Verat.

Comp. **Painful.**

SOFT, **boggy**: Ars., Caps., Kali-c., Lach., Sil., Thuj.

SOGGY, wilted: Rumx., Sil.

SPOTS, itching: Con., **Led., Sep.**, **Sil., Sul-ac.**, Zinc.

pigmented: Iod., Lyc., Sep.

red: Merc., Pic-ac., Rhus-t.

blood: Cor-r.

wine: Sep.

sore: Ferr., Hep.

white: Alum., Ars., Merc., Nat-c., Sep., **Sil.**, **Sulph.**

STICKY: Phos.

STIFF: **Rhus-t.**, Verat.

STINGING: Ther.

STRIPES, **streaks, etc., on**: Bell., Bufo, **Carb-v.**, Caust., Hep., Merc., Ox-ac., Phos., Pyrog., Sabin., **Sil.**

STROPHULUS: Merc., Sulph.

SWELLED: Syph.

SWELLINGS, on: Ant-c., Arg-met., Ars., Bar-c., Graph., Thuj.

TANNED: Tub.

TENSE: Cact., Caust., Nit-ac., **Phos.**, Stront-c.

THICK: Ant-c., Dulc., **Graph.**, Petr., Rad-met., **Rhus-t., Sep.**, Sil., Sulph.

TIC: Ars., Ran-b.

TINGLING, prickling: Acon., Kali-c., Kalm., Sec.

Comp. **Itching.**

ULCER: see **Generalities.**

UNHEALTHY: See **Heals.**

WARTS: see **Fungus Growth.**

WASHING, bathing, **Agg.:** Ars., Sulph.

WENS: see **Cysts.**

WINE colored: Sep.

WITHERED, shrivelled: Ars., Borx., **Calc., Chin., Cocc.,** Cupr., **Iod.,** Lyc., **Sec., Verat.**

WORMS: Ars., Coca, Merc., Nat-c., Nit-ac., Sel., Sil., Sulph.

WRINKLED: Abrot., **Calc.,** Camph., Ph-ac., Sars., **Sec.,** Sep., Verat.

SLEEP

YAWNING: Ant-t., **Caust.,** Cina, Croc., Hep., **Ign.,** Kreos., Lyc., Mang., **Nux-v.,** Op., Phos., Plat., Puls., **Rhus-t.,** Zinc-val.

accompaniment, as a: Castm., Cina, Kreos., Sars.

chill, with: Thuj.

eating, Agg.: Nat-s., Squil., Sulph.

evening: Arn.

headache, and: Form., Staph.

incomplete: Lach., Lyc.

violent: Hep., Ign., Plat., Rhus-t., Staph.

sleepy, and: Kali-n., Kreos.

stretching, and: Cham., Nux-v., Rhus-t.

tears, with: Staph.

SLEEPINESS (by day): Aeth., Ant-c., **ANT-T., Bapt., Calc., Chel.,** Clem., Croc., **Ferr-p., Gels.,** NUX-M., NUX-V., OP., **Ph-ac.,** Phos., Puls., Sulph.

yet sleepless at night: Puls., **Sulph.**

morning: Calc., Con., Graph., Nux-v., Sep.

forenoon: Ant-c., Sabad.

afternoon: Chin., Nux-v., Rhus-t., Sulph.

evening: Ars., Calc., Kali-c., **Nux-v.**

SLEEP **accompanied by:** Ant-t., Nux-m., Puls.

caused by other complaints: Ant-t., Nux-m., Op., Rhus-t., Verat.

eating, on: Chin., Nux-v., Rhus-t., **Sulph.**

exertion, Agg.: Sel.

lying on side: Thuj. (l).

menses, with: Mag-c.

absent: Senec.

migraine then: Sulph.

pneumonia, in: Ant-t., Chel., Op., Phos.

stool, after: Aeth.

sudden: Rumx.

SLEEP, answers, then sleeps at once: Bapt., Hep.

anxious: Acon., Ars.

broken: Zinc.

can't fall to: Laur., Phos.

care, worry, Agg.: Calc.

coma vigil: Acon., Op.

comatose, soporous: Croc., Nux-v., Op., Puls., Stram., Verat.

cries out in: Borx., Hyos., Lyc., Rheum.

day, by night wakeful: Ferr., Mosch., Op., Ph-ac., Rhus-t.

jerks on falling to: Ars., Bell., Ign., Nit-ac., Op., Sep.

   during: Carb-v., Dig., Kali-c., Op., Rheum.

laughter, during: Lyc.

light, hears every sound: Acon., Alum., Am-c., Ars., Coff., Ign., Lach., Merc., Op., Phos., Sel., Sulph.

pains, during: Ars., Aur., Bell., Carb-an., Cham., Graph., Lyc., Merc., Nit-ac., Sulph., Sul-ac., Til.

restless, tossing about, etc.: Acon., Ars., Bar-c., Bell., Chin., Puls., Rhus-t., Sil., Sulph.

sings, in: Sulph.

stupid, deep, etc.: Aeth., Ant-t., Bapt., Bell., Con., Led., Nux-m., Op.

unrefreshing, awakes tired, etc.: Bry., Chin., Con., Hep., Lach., Mag-c., Op., Rhus-t., Sulph., Zinc.

___

lying on back: Bry., Puls., Rhus-t., Stram.

with hands overhead: Lac-c., Nux-v., Puls.

strange positions in: Cina, Plb.

___

during, nightmare: Acon., Nux-v., Op., Paeon., Sep., Stram., Sulph.

chews and swallows: Cina, Ign.

saliva, flow of: Lach., Merc., Phos., Rhus-t.

shrieks, screams, etc.: Apis, Cina, Ign., Zinc.

snoring: Op.

somnambulism: Dict., Phos.

starting up, jerks, etc.: Acon., Ars., Bell., Calc., Cham., Cina, Ign., Lyc., Puls., Sep., Sil., Stram., Zinc.

talking: Lach., Puls.

WAKING, frequently, cat-naps: Calc., Hep., Op., Phos., Puls., Sep., Sulph.

can't sleep again: Nux-v.

confused: Bov., Chin., Petr., Phos.

dreams, awake: Bell., Lach., Sil., Sulph.

too early: Kali-c., Nat-c., Nux-v., Ran-b.

late: Calc., Graph., Nux-v., Sep.

anger, in: Cham., **Lyc.**

confusion, in: Chin.

fright, nightmare, etc., in: Bell., Borx., **Cina**, Hyos., **Ign.**, Lach., Nat-m., Sil., Stram., SULPH., Thuj., Zinc.

Comp., **Mind, Waking.**

jerk, with a: Bell.

SLEEPLESSNESS: Acon., **Ars.**, Bell., Calc., Cham., Cocc., COFF., **Hyos.**, Kali-c., Lach., Merc., **Nux-v.**, Op., Ox-ac., Phos., PULS., Rhus-t., Sep., Sil., **Sulph.**, Zinc-val.

after 3 a.m.: Nux-v., Sep.

early (late falling asleep): Ars., Bry., Calc., Carb-v., Chin., Graph., Merc., Nux-v., Phos., **Puls.**, Rhus-t., Sep.

late (after midnight): Caps., Coff., Kali-c., **Nux-v.**, Sil.

although sleepy: Apis, **Bell.**, Cham., Hep., Op., Phos., Puls., Sep.

caused by: Ars., Bry., Calc., **Cham.**, Chin., Coff., Merc., Phos., Puls., Rhus-t., Sep.

idea, fixed: Calc., Graph., Puls.

once awaking, on: Nat-m.

nervousness: Acon., Chin., COFF., Gels., Hyos., Lach., Lyc., Mosch., **Nux-v., Plat.**

restlessness: Acon., Ars., Cham., Iod.

rush of ideas: Calc., Coff., Gels., Hyos., Ign., Nux-v., Op., Puls.

twitchings: Ars., Bell., Ign., Sulph.

drunkards, in: Lach., Op.

excitement, nervous, Agg.: Calc., Coff., Hyos., **Nux-v.**, Teucr.

exhaustion, Agg.: Aven., Coca, Cocc., **Coff.**

heart symptoms: Crat.

lying on side: Card-m. (l), Thuj. (l).

DREAMS: Am-m., Arn., Ars., Bry., Calc., **Chin., Graph.**,

Lach., Lyc., **Mag-c., Nat-m.,**
NUX-V., PHOS., PULS.,
Rhus-t., Sil., Sulph., Thuj.

agreeable: Calc., Nat-c., Nux-
v., **Op.,** Puls., Sep.,
Staph., Viol-o.

anxious: Kali-m.

blood, fire, etc., **of:** Phos.,
Rad-met., Rhus-t.

of day's work, difficulties,
etc.: Bry., Nux-v., Puls.,
RHUS-T.

dead, of the: Ars., Mag-c.,
Phos., Thuj.

falling: Brom., Caust., Coll.,
Con., Kreos., Laur., Nat-
c., Ph-ac., Rat., Thuj.

fantastic: Calc-i.

flying, of: Latr.

frightful: Crot-h., Tub.

gloomy: Plan.

laborious, exhausting: Arn.,
Echi., Rhus-t.

loathsome: Lach.

lying on left side: Sep.

many: Ars., Senec.

nightmares: Paeon., Sep.,
Stram.

shame: Tub.

sleep, first: Sil.

true: Rad-met.

vivid, fire, etc.: Cann-s.,
Hyos., Phos., Puls., Rad-
met., Rhus-t., Sil.,
Sulph., Tub.

weeping: Plan., Stram.

CHILL, CHILLINESS, COLDNESS, ETC.

IN GENERAL: Ant-c., Aran.,
Arn., Ars., Aur., **Camph.,**
Caust., Chin., Chinin-s., Eup-
per., Graph., Ip., Kali-chl.,
Lac-d., LYC., Meny., **Mosch.,**
Nat-m., Nux-m., Phys. (wa-
ter), **Puls.,** Sabad., Sil., Staph.,
Symp., Thyr., **Verat.**

affected part: Ars., Bry., Cocc.,
Colch., Lach., **Led.,** Meny.,
Mez., Rhus-t., Sec., Sil.

partial or single parts: Ars.,
Calc., Carb-v., Chel., Chin.,
Ign., Kali-c., Meny., PULS.,
Sec., **Sep.,** Sil., **Spig.,** Sulph.,
VERAT.

one-sided: Bar-c. (r), **Bry.,** Carb-
v. (1), **Caust.,** Con., **Dros.,**
Lyc., **Mosch.,** Nux-v., Par.,
Puls., Rhus-t. (1), Sabin. (r),
Sulph. (l), Thuj.

external: Ign., Nux-v., **Verat.,**
Zinc.

internal: Ars., Calc., Laur.,
Sulph.

abdomen: Ambr., Ars., Phos., Sep., **Verat.**

back (starts in): Bell., **Caps.**, Caust., Cocc., Dulc., Eupper., **Gels.**, Hyos., **Lach.**, Lyc., **Nat-m.**, Puls., **Rhus-t.**, Sec., Sep., Staph., Stront-c., Sulph.

extremities: Ambr., **Bell.**, Carbv., Caust., Puls., Sec., Sil.

heat, alternating with: Am-m., Ars., Bell., Calc., Cham., Chin., Eup-per., **Gels.**, Hep., Lach., Merc., Nux-m., **Nux-v.**, Ol-an., Rhus-t., Samb.

BEARING-DOWN, WITH: Castm., Sec., Sil.

COLDS, **ascending:** Arum-t., **Brom.**, Lac-c., Merc., Sep.

CHILL **of snow and ice, from:** Ant-c., Dros., Iod., Laur., Puls., Seneg., Verat., Verb.

COVERS, **Agg.:** Apis, Calc-s., Camph., **Ip.**, Puls., Sec., Sep.

DESCENDING: Bry., Carb-v., Kali-c., Phos., Lyc., Sulph., Tub.

MENSTRUAL: Bar-c., Graph., Mag-c., Senec.

SOPOR, **with:** Ant-t., Chel., Gels., Nux-m., OP., Stram., Verat.

URINATING, **on:** Nit-ac., Plat., Thuj.

HEAT

HEAT, **fever, burning, etc.:** ACON., Apis, ARS., BELL., BRY., **Canth.**, Caps., **Carb-v.**, **Caust.**, Cham., Chin., Ferr-p., Gels., Ign., Kali-s., Lach., **Lyc.**, Med., **Merc.**, Merc-c., Merci-v., Nat-m., **Nux-v.**, Op., PHOS., Pic-ac., PULS., RHUS-T., Sang., **Sulph.**

external: Acon., Bell., Canth., Ign.

internal: Acon., Ars., Bell., Nuxv., Sul-i., Tab., Verat.

with cold external parts: **Acon.**, Ant-t., Apis, Arn., **Ars.**, Bell., Calc., **Camph.**, Carb-v., Cham., Coff., Cina, Dig., Dros., Hyos., Ign., Iod., Ip., Kali-c., **Mez.**, **Mosch.**, Nit-ac., Nux-v., Ph-ac., Plat., Rhus-t., Sulph., **Verat.**

partial: Acon., Apis, ARS., Bell., Bry., Calc., **Canth.**, Caps., Carb-v., Caust., Cham., Lyc., **Merc.**, **Nux-v.**, PHOS., **Puls.**, **Rhus-t.**, Sep., SULPH., Verat-v.

external: Ars., Bell., Merc., Phos., Ph-ac., Sulph.

internal: Acon., Bell., Bry., Canth., Laur., Phos., Sulph.

---

chest, into: Thuj.

chill, alternates with: Hydr.

> then: Thyr.

dry, burning: Acon., **Apis**, **Ars.**, Bell., Bry., Carb-an., Carb-v., Mez., Mur-ac., Nux-v., Op., Puls., Rad-met., Sec., Spig., **Tub.**, Vesp.

exhaustion: Acon., Helon., Verat-v., Zinc-i.

> Comp. **Sunstroke.**

feet, cold, with: Tarent.

fiery: Apis, **Ars.**, **Bell.**, Carb-an., Guaj., Kreos., Phos., Spig., Vesp.

> **Agg.**: Zinc-val.

> **Amel.**: Alum., **Ars.**, Caps., Carb-v., Lyc.

flushes, in: Calc., Coll., Fl-ac., Lach., Mang., Phos., Sang., Sep., Sulph., Sul-ac., Thyr., Tub.

> Comp. **Wave-like Sensations.**

hands, cold, with: Thuj.

intolerable: Sabin.

mental exertion, **Agg.**: Spong.

only: Valer.

painful: Canth.

partial: Apis, Borx., Par. (one side), Ph-ac.

pungent, glowing: Ruta, Tarent.

shivers with: Ars., Sec.

sleep, during: Calad., Samb.

spots: Tub.

sweat, then chill: Calad., Kali-bi.

> with: Med., Ph-ac., Psor., Spong. (thighs), Verat-v.

thirstless: Cham., Cina, Ign., Puls.

uncover, can't: Kali-i., Nat-s.

weakness, with: Spong.

FEVER, black-water: **Ars.**, Lyc.

cerebro-spinal: Bell., Gels., Verat-v.

gastric: Bapt., Ferr-p., Yuc.

hyperpyrexia: Bapt., Iod., Pyrog., **Sulph.**, Verat-v.

> intermittent: Aran., ARS., Caps., Cedr., EUP-PER., Ign., **Ip.**, Nat-m., Nux-v., Ph-ac., Puls., Sulph., **Verat.**

menses, with: Pyrog., Sep.

nightly: Ars., Bell., Calc., Cham., Hep., Iod., Petr., Phos., PULS., **Sil.**, Sulph., Urt-u.

painful: Bry., Rhus-t.

painless: Phos., Ph-ac.

suppression, **Agg.**: Cham.

sweat, **Amel.**: Ars., Lyc., Rhus-t.

> continues, after: Calc., Chin., Merc., Ph-ac., Sep., Sulph.

vertigo, with: Urt-u.

SWEAT

IN GENERAL, easy tendency to, etc.: **Agar.**, Ant-t., **Calc.**, **Chin.**, **Ferr.**, **Graph.**, **Hep.**, Kali-c., Lach., **Lyc.**, Med., Merc., Merc-cy., **Nat-c.**, Natm., **Nux-v.**, Op., **Phos.**, Phac., Samb., **Sep.**, **Stann.**, Staph., **Sulph.**, **Tub.**, Verat.

Comp. Moistness.

ACRID: Tarent., Fl-ac.

CHILL, alternating with: Ars., Chin., Mez., Nux-v., Spig.

followed by: Carb-v., Hep., Nux-v.

CHILL with: Tab.

CLAMMY: Lyc., Merc., Phos., Verat-v.

COLD: Ant-t., Ars., Camph., **Carb-v.**, Castm., Chin., Dros., Merc., Sec., **Verat.**

cough, Agg.: Ant-t., Verat.

on forehead: Ant-t., Carb-v., Cina, Merc-c., Op., VERAT.

COLDS from: Nit-ac.

COMPANY, Agg.: Thuj.

COUGHING, Agg.: Carb-v., **Hep.**, Tub.

COVERS, heat, etc., **Amel.**: **Clem.**, Hep., **Nux-v.**, Rhus-t., **Stront-c.**

F- 34

DEBILITATING: Calc-p.

Comp. Discharges.

GUSHES, in: Aml-ns., Apis, **Bell.**, **Colch.**, Jab., Ip., Lach., Merccy., Nat-c., Phos., Samb., Tab., Thuj., **Valer.**

HEART symptoms, with: Spong.

HOT, **burning: Bell.**, **Cham.**, Ign., Ip., **Op.**, Sabad., Sang., Sep., Stann., Stram., Viol-t.

ITCHING, causing: Cham., Op., Rhus-t.

LYING on right side, **Agg.**: Lach.

MENSES, **Agg.**: **Graph.**, Nux-v., Verat-v.

MOTION, **Agg.**: Merc-c.

MUSTY: Thuj., Thyr.

NERVOUS: Jab., Rhus-t.

NIGHT, at: Calc., Hep., Kali-c., Merc., Petr., Prun., Samb., Sil.

ONIONS, garlic, etc., like: Art-v., Bov., Kali-p., Lyc.

PAIN, **Agg.**: Cham., Merc., Rhust.

PARTIAL: Apis, Bar-c., CALC., Carb-v., Merc-c., Nux-v., Phos., **Puls.**, Sel., SEP., **Sil.**, Sulph., **Thuj.**, Verat.

PARTS, bare, on: Thuj.

upper: Calc., Thuj.

PHTHISIS, of: Ars., Bry., Calc., Carb-v., Chin., Ferr., Hep.,

Kali-c., Merc., Petr., Phos., Ph-
ac., Prun., Samb., Sep., Sil.,
Stann., Sulph.

first sleep, in: Ars.

after: Lach.

all night: Phos.

awaking, on: Samb.

PROFUSE, **drenching:** Calc-hyp.,
Chin., Coca, Jab., Ph-ac., Sil.,
Sul-ac., Tarent., Thyr., Til.

PROLONGED: Merc.

RELIEF, without: **Bell.,** Benz-ac.,
Chel., Dig., Form., Hep.,
MERC., Op., Phos., **Pyrog.,**
Tarent-c., Sal-ac., Tub.

SALTY **deposit:** Nat-m., Sel.

SCANTY: Alum., Graph.

see **Dryness.**

SPOTS, **in:** Merc., Petr., Tell.

STEAMING: Psor.

STICKY: Kali-bi., Lyc.

STIFFNESS, **hose, linen:** Nat-m.,
Sel.

STOOL, **Agg.:** Nat-c., Plb., Verat.

SUPPRESSED: Acon., Bell., Bry.,
Cham., Chin., Coloc., Dulc.,
Lach., Rhus-t., Sil., **Sulph.**

UNCOVERING, **intolerance of:**
Clem., Graph., Hep., Nat-c.,
Nux-v., Rhus-t., **Samb.,**
Stront-c.

Comp. **Discharges.**

UNILATERAL: **Bar-c.** (1), Chin.
(1), **Nux-v.,** Phos. (r), Puls. (r),
Sulph.

UPPER **parts:** Calc., Sil.

URINOUS: Canth., Nit-ac.

WAKING, **on:** Dros., Par., **Samb.,**
Sep., **Sulph.**

WASHING, **Amel.:** Thuj.

YELLOW, **staining:** Bell., Carb-
an., Graph., **Lach., Merc.,** Sel.

PART THREE

Comprising of:

(a) Table of the Approximate Duration of Action of Remedies.

(b) Complementary Remedies.

(c) Antagonistic Remedies.

(d) List of Remedies and their Abbreviations.

Table of the Approximate Minimum Duration of Action of Remedies by Weeks

Acon. Agar.^{3} Ag-c.^{1} Alum.^{4} Ambr.^{4} Am-c.^{4} Am-m.^{2} Anac.^{3} Ang.^{2} Ant-c.^{5} Ant-t.^{2} Arg-met.^{2} Arn.^{2} Ars.^{4} Asaf.^{4} Asar.^{1} Aur.^{4} Bar-c.^{5} Bell.^{3} Bism.^{3} Borx.^{2} Bov.^{4} Brom.^{2} Bry.^{2} Calad.^{4} Calc.^{5} Camph.^{1} Cann-s.^{1} Canth.^{2} Caps.^{2} Carb-an.^{4} Carb-v.^{4} Caust.^{5} Cham.^{1} Chel.^{1} Chin.^{3} Chinin-s.^{2} Cic.^{4} Cina.^{2} Clem.^{4} Cocc.^{3} Coff. Colch.^{3} Coloc.^{4} Con.^{3} Croc.^{1} Crot-h.^{3} Cupr.^{3} Cycl.^{2} Dig.^{3} Dros.^{2} Dulc.^{4} Euphr.^{2} Euph.^{4} Ferr.^{5} Fl-ac.^{3} Graph.^{5} Guai.^{3} Hell.^{3} Hep.^{6} Hyos.^{1} Ign.^{1} Iod.^{4} Ip. Kali-c.^{5} Kali-n.^{4} Kreos.^{1} Lach.^{3} Laur. Led.^{4} Lyc.^{5} Mag-c.^{5} Mag-m.^{4} Mang.^{4} Meny.^{2} Merc.^{2} Mez.^{4} Mosch. Mur-ac.^{3} Nat-c.^{4} Nat-m.^{4} Nit-ac.^{4} Nux-m.^{1} Nux-v.^{2} Olnd.^{3} Op. Par. Petr.^{5} Phos.^{5} Ph-ac.^{4} Plat.^{4} Plb.^{3} Prun.^{3} Puls.^{1} Ran-b.^{3} Ran-s.^{4} Rheum. Rhod.^{4} Rhus-t.^{4} Ruta.^{1} Sabad.^{3} Sabin.^{4} Samb. Sars.^{3} Sec.^{2} Sel.^{4} Seneg.^{3} Sabad.^{6} Sep.^{6} Sil.^{6} Spig.^{2} Spong.^{3} Squil.^{2} Stann.^{4} Staph.^{3} Stram. Stront-c.^{4} Sulph.^{5} Sul-ac.^{3} Tarax. Teucr.$_2$ Thuj.^{3} Valer.^{1} Verat.^{2} Verb.^{1} Viol-o.^{1} Viol-t.^{1} Zinc.^{4}

As long as old ailments reappear or are worse, without the appearance of essentially new symptoms which lie outside of its sphere of action, we should guard against a repetition of the remedy, or changing to a new one. — **Boenninghausen.**

Symptoms appearing last in a proving have the highest value.—**Hering.**

Complementary Remedies

ABROTANUM—Bry., Kali-bi., Lyc.

ACETICUM ACIDUM—Chin.

ACONITUM—**Arn.**, Bell., **Bry.,** Coff., Mill., **Phos., Spong., Sulph.**

AETHUSA—**Calc.**

AGARICUS—**Calc.**

ALLIUM CEPA—**Phos.,** Puls., Sars., Thuj.

ALLIUM SATIVUM—Ars.

ALOE—Sulph.

ALUMINA—**Bry.,** Ferr.

ANTIMONIUM CRUDUM— Squil.

ANTIMONIUM TART.—**Bar-c.**

APIS—Arn., Ars., Bar-c., Hell., Merc-cy., **Nat-m., Puls.**

ARGENTUM NITRICUM— Calc., Nat-m., Puls., Sep.

ARNICA—Acon., Calc., Nat-s., Psor., **Rhus-t., Sul-ac.**

ARSENICUM—All-s., Carb-v., Lach., **Nat-s.,** Phos., **Puls., Sulph., Thuj.**

ARUM TRIPHILLUM—Nit-ac.

ASA FOETIDA—Caust., **Puls.**

ASARUM—Caust., Puls., Sil.

BARYTA CARB.—Ant-t.

BELLADONNA—Borx., **Calc., Hep., Merc.,** Nat-m.

BRYONIA—Abrot., **Alum., Kali-c.,** Lyc., **Rhus-t.,** Sep., **Sulph.**

BUFO—Calc.

CACTUS—Ars.

CALADIUM—Nit-ac.

CALCAREA CARB.—Bar-c., **Lyc., Sil.**

CALCAREA FLUOR.—Rhus-t.

CALCAREA PHOS.—Ruta, Sulph., Zinc.

CALENDULA—Hep.

CANTHARIS—Apis.

CAPSICUM—Nat-m.

CARBO ANIMALIS—Calc-p.

CARBO VEG.—**Ars., Chin., Kali-c.,** Lach., Phos.

CAUSTICUM—Graph., Lach., Petr., Sep., **Stann.,** Staph.

CHAMOMILLA—**Bell.,** Calc., Mag-c., Sanic.

CHELIDONIUM—**Lyc.,** Merc-d.

CHINA—**Ars., Calc-p., Carb-v.,** Ferr., Kali-c.

CINA—**Calc.,** Dros., Sulph.

CINNABARIS—Thuj.

CLEMATIS—Merc.

COCCULUS IND.—Petr.

COFFEA—Acon.

COLCHICUM—Ars., Spig.

COLOCYNTHIS—Caust., Merc., Staph.

CONIUM—**Phos.**, Sil.

CORALLIUM RUB.—Sulph.

CROTALUS HOR.—Carb-v., Lycps-v.

CUPRUM—Ars., **Calc.**, Iod.

DROSERA—Carb-v., Nux-v., Sulph.

DULCAMARA—Alum., **Bar-c.**, Nat-s.

FERRUM—Alum., Ars., **Chin.**, Ham.

FERRUM PHOS.—Nat-m.

FLUORICUM ACIDUM—**Sil.**

GELSEMIUM—Arg-n., Sep.

GLONOINUM—Bell.

GRAPHITES—Ars., Caust., Ferr., Hep., Lyc., **Sulph.**

HAMAMELIS—Ferr., Fl-ac.

HELLEBORUS—Zinc.

HEPAR—Iod., **Sil.**

IGNATIA—**Nat-m.**, Ph-ac., Puls., Sep.

IODIUM—**Bad.**, Lyc., Sil.

IPECACUANHA—**Ars.**, **Cupr.**

KALIUM BI.—Ars., Phos., **Psor.**

KALIUM CARB.—Ars-i., **Carb-v.**, Nit-ac., **Phos.**

KALIUM MUR.—Calc-s.

KALMIA—Benz-ac., Spig.

KREOSOTUM—**Sulph.**

LACHESIS— Ars., Calc., **Carb-v.**, Hep., **Lyc.**, Nit-ac., **Phos.**, Zinc-i.

LACTICUM ACIDUM—Psor.

LEDUM—Chin., Sep.

LEPTANDRA—Phos.

LYCOPODIUM—**Calc.**, Graph., **Iod.**, Kali-c., **Lach.**, Phos., **Puls.**, **Sulph.**

MAGNESIUM CARB.—Cham.

MERCURIUS—Aur., Bad., **Bell.**, Hep., Sep., Sulph.

MEZEREUM—**Merc.**

NATRIUM CARB.—**Sep.**

NATRIUM MUR.—**Apis**, Arg-n., Ign., **Sep.**

NATRIUM SULPH—Ars., Thuj.

NITRICUM ACIDUM—Ars., Arum-t., Calad., **Calc.**, Lyc., Thuj.

NUX MOSCH.—Calc., **Lyc.**

NUX VOMICA—Bry., Cham., Con., Kali-c., **Phos.**, Puls., Sep., Sulph.

OPIUM—**Alum.**, Bar-c., **Bry.**, **Phos.**, **Plb.**

PALLADIUM—Plat.

PETROLEUM—Sep.

PHOSPHORICUM ACIDUM—**Chin.**

PHOSPHORUS—All-c., **Ars.**, **Calc.**, **Kali-c.**, Lyc., Sang., Sep., Sil., Sulph.

PLUMBUM—Rhus-t.

PODOPHYLLUM—Calc., **Nat-m.**, Sulph.

PSORINUM—Sep., **Sulph.**, Tub.

PULSATILLA—**Ars.**, **Bry.**, Kali-bi., Kali-s., Lyc., **Sep.**, Sil., Stann., Sulph., Sul-ac., **Zinc.**

RHEUM—**Mag-c.**

RHUS TOX.—**Bry., Calc.,** Caust., Lyc., Med., **Phos., Phyt.,** Puls., **Sulph.**

RUTA—**Calc-p.**

SABADILLA—Sep.

SABINA—Thuj.

SANGUINARIA—Ant-t., Phos.

SARSAPARILLA—Merc., **Sep.**

SECALE—**Ars.**, Thuj.

SEPIA—**Nat-m.**, **Phos.**, Psor.,

Puls., Sulph.

SILICEA—**Fl-ac.**, **Hep.**, **Lyc.**, Phos., **Thuj.**

SPIGELIA—Spong.

SQUILLA—**Ant-c.**

SPONGIA—**Hep.**

STANNUM—Puls.

STAPHYSAGRIA—Caust., **Coloc.**

SULPHURICUM ACIDUM—**Puls.**

SULPHUR—Acon., **Aloe,** Ars., Bad., **Bell., Calc., Merc., Puls.,** Psor., Pyrog., **Rhus-t.**, **Sep.**, **Sul-i.**

SUMBUL—Lactuca.

TABACUM—Op.

TARENTULA—Ars.

TEUCRIUM—Calc.

THUJA—**Merc.**, Nat-m., **Nit-ac.**, **Puls.**, Sabin., **Sil., Sulph.**

TUBERCULINUM—Calc., Kali-s., Sep.

VERATRUM ALB.—**Ars.**, Carb-v.

ZINCUM—**Puls.**, Sep., Sulph.

Antagonistic Remedies

ACETICUM ACIDUM—Borx.,
Caust., Nux-v., Ran-b., Sars.

AMMONIUM CARB.—Lach.

APIS—Rhus-t.

BELLADONNA—Dulc.

BENZOICUM ACIDUM—Cop.

CAMPHORA—Kali-n.

CANTHARIS—Coff.

CARBO VEG.—Kreos.

CAUSTICUM—Acet-ac., Coff.,
Coloc., Kali-n., Nux-v., Phos.

CHAMOMILLA—Zinc.

CHINA—Dig., Sel.

COCCULUS—Coff.

COFFEA—Canth., Caust., Cocc.,
Ign.

COLOCYNTHIS—Caust.

DIGITALIS—Stroph-h.

DULCAMARA—Bell., Lach.

IGNATIA—Coff., Nux-v.

IPECACUANHA—Chin., Op.

KALIUM NIT.—Camph., Caust.,

Ran-b.

LACHESIS—Am-c., Dulc., Nit-
ac., Sep.

LYCOPODIUM—Nux-m.

MERCURY—Lach., Sil.

NITRICUM ACIDUM—Lach.,
Nat-m.

NUX MOSCHATA—Lyc., Nux-
v., Puls., Rhus-t., Sil., Squil.

NUX VOMICA—Acet-ac.,
Caust., Ign., Nux-m., Zinc.

PHOSPHORUS—Caust.

PULSATILLA—Nux-m.

RANUNCULUS BULB.—Acet-
ac., Kali-n.

SARSAPARILLA—Acet-ac.

SELENIUM—Chin.

SEPIA—Lach.

SILICEA—Merc., Nux-m.

STAPHYSAGRIA—Ran-b.

SULPHUR—Nux-m., Ran-b.

ZINCUM—Cham., Nux-v.

List of Remedies and Their Abbreviations

1. Abies canadensis	Abies.
2. Abies nigra	Abies-n.
3. Abrotanum	Abrot.
4. Absinthium	Absin.
5. Acalypha indica	Acal.
6. Aceticum acidum	Acet-ac.
7. Aconitum napellus	Acon.
8. Actaea racemosa	Cimic.
9. Actaea spicata	Act-sp.
10. Adonis vernalis	Adon.
11. Aesculus hippocastanum	Aesc.
12. Aethusa cynapium	Aeth.
13. Agaricus muscarius	Agar.
14. Agnus castus	Agn.
15. Ailanthus glandulosa	Ail.
16. Aletris farinosa	Alet.
17. Allium cepa	All-c.
18. Allium sativum	All-s.
19 Aloe socotrina	Aloe
20. Alumina	Alum.
21. Ambra grisea	Ambr.
22. Ambrosia artemisiaefolia	Ambr.
23. Ammonium carbonicum	Am-c.
24. Ammonium muriaticum	Am-m.
25. Ammonium phosphoricum	Am-p.
26. Amylenum nitrrosum	Aml-ns.
27. Anacardium orientale	Anac.
28. Angustura vera	Ang.

29. Anantherum muriaticum	Anan.
30. Anthracinum	Anthraci.
31. Antimonium crudum	Ant-c.
32. Antimonium sulphuratum auratum	Ant-s-aur.
33. Antimonium tartaricum	Ant-t.
34. Apis mellifica	Apis
35. Apocynum cannabinum	Apoc.
36. Aralia racemosa	Aral.
37. Aranea diadema	Aran.
38. Argentum metallicum	Arg-met.
39. Argentum nitricum	Arg-n.
40. Arnica montana	Arn.
41. Arsenicum album	Ars.
42. Arsenicum iodatum	Ars-i.
43. Artemisia vulgaris	Art-v.
44. Arum triphyllum.	Aru-t.
45. Asafoetida	Asaf.
46. Asarum europaeum	Asar.
47. Asclepias tuberosa	Asclep.
48. Asterias rubens	Aster.
49. Atropinum sulphuricum	Atro-s.
50. Aurum metallicum	Aur.
51. Aurum muriaticum	Aur-m.
52. Avena sativa	Aven.
53. Badiaga	Bad.
54. Baptisia tinctoria	Bapt.
55. Baryta carbonica	Bar-c.
56. Baryta muriatica	Bar-m.
57. Belladonna	Bell.

58.	Bellis perennis	Bell-p.	90.	Carbo animalis	Carb-an.
59.	Benzoicum acidum	Benz-ac.	91.	Carbo vegetabilis	Carb-v.
60.	Berberis vulgaris	Berb.	92.	Carbolicum acidum	Carb-ac.
61.	Bismuthum metallicum	Bism.	93.	Carboneum	
62.	Blatta orientalis	Blatta-o.		sulphuratum	Carbn-s.
63.	Borax	Borx.	94.	Carduus marianus	Card-m.
64.	Bothrops lanceolatus	Both.	95.	Castoreum	Castm.
65.	Bovista	Bov.	96.	Caulophyllum	
66.	Brachyglottis repens	Brach.		thalictroides	Caul.
67.	Bromium	Brom.	97.	Causticum	Caust.
68.	Bryonia alba	Bry.	98.	Ceanothus americanus	Cean.
69.	Bufo rana	Bufo	99.	Cedron	Cedr.
70.	Bursa pastoris	Thlasp.	100.	Cenchris	Cench.
71.	Cactus grandiflora	Cact.	101.	Cepa	All-c.
72.	Cadmium		102.	Cereus bonplandii	Cere-b.
	sulphuricum	Cadm-s.	103.	Chamomilla	Cham,
73.	Caladium seguinum	Calad.	104.	Chelidonium majus	Chel.
74.	Calcarea acetica	Calc-acet.	105.	Chenopodium album	Chen-al.
75.	Calcarea arsenicosa	Calc-ar.	106.	Chimaphila	
76.	Calcarea carbonica	Calc.		umbellata	Chim.
77.	Calcarea fluorica	Calc-f.	107.	China officinalis	Chin.
78.	Calcarea		108.	Chininum	
	hypophosphorica	Calc-hyp.		arsenicosum	Chinin-ar.
79.	Calcarea iodata	Calc-i.	109.	Chininum	
80.	Calcarea phosphorica	Calc-p.		sulphuricum	Chinin-s.
81.	Calcarea picrata	Calc-pic.	110.	Chionanthus	
82.	Calcarea sulphurica	Calc-s.		virginica	Chion.
83.	Calendula officinalis	Calen.	111.	Chloralum	
84.	Camphora	Camph.		hydratum	Chlol.
85.	Cancer fluviatilis	Astac.	112.	Chloroformium	Chlf.
86.	Cannabis indica	Cann-i.	113.	Chlorum	Chlor.
87.	Cannabis sativa	Cann-s.	114.	Cicuta virosa	Cic.
88.	Cantharis	Canth.	115.	Cimex lectularius	Cimx.
89.	Capsicum annuum	Caps.	116.	Cimicifuga racemosa	Cimic.
			117.	Cina	Cina

118.	Cinchona officinalis	Chin.	152.	Daphne indica	Daph.
119.	Cinnabaris	Cinnb.	153.	Dictamnus albus	Dict.
120.	Cinnamonum	Cinnm.	154.	Digitalis purpurea	Dig.
121.	Cistus canadensis	Cist.	155.	Dioscorea villosa	Dios.
122.	Clematis erecta	Clem.	156.	Diphtherinum	Diph.
123.	Cobaltum metallicum	Cob.	157.	Drosera rotundifolia	Dros.
124.	Coca	Coca	158.	Dulcamara	Dulc.
125.	Cocculus indicus	Cocc.	159.	Echinacea angustifolia	Echi.
126.	Coccus cacti	Coc-c.	160.	Elaps corallinus	Elaps
127.	Codeinum	Cod.	161.	Elaterium	Elat.
128.	Coffea cruda	Coff.	162.	Epiphegus virginiana	Epip.
129.	Colchicum autumnale	Colch.	163.	Equisetum hyemale	Equis.
130.	Collinsonia canadensis	Coll.	164.	Erigeron canadense	Erig.
131.	Colocynthis	Coloc.	165.	Eryngium aquaticum	Eryng.
132.	Comocladia dentata	Com.	166.	Eucalyptus globulus	Eucal.
133.	Conium maculatum	Con.	167.	Eugenia jambos	Eug.
134.	Convallaria majalis	Conv.	168.	Euonymus europaea	Euon.
135.	Copaiva officinalis	Cop.	169.	Eupatorium perfoliatum	Eup-per.
136.	Corallium rubrum	Cor-r.	170.	Eupatorium purpureum	Eup-pur.
137.	Cornus florida	Corn.	171.	Euphorbium	Euph.
138.	Crataegus oxyacantha	Crat.	172.	Euphrasia	Euphr.
139.	Crocus sativus	Croc.	173.	Eupionum	Eupi.
140.	Crotalus cascavella	Crot-c.	174.	Fagopyrum esculentum	Fago.
141.	Crotalus horridus	Crot-h.	175.	Ferrum iodatum	Ferr-i.
142.	Croton tiglium	Crot-t.	176.	Ferrum metallicum	Ferr.
143.	Cubeba officinalis	Cub.	177.	Ferrum phosphoricum	Ferr-p.
144.	Culex musca	Culx.	178.	Ferrum picricum	Fer-pic.
145.	Cundurango	Cund.	179.	Fluoricum acidum	Fl-ac.
146.	Cuprum aceticum	Cupr-act.	180.	Formica rufa	Form.
147.	Cuprum arsenicosum	Cupr-ar.	181.	Fraxinus americana	Frax.
148.	Cuprum metallicum	Cupr.	182.	Gambogia	Gamb.
149.	Cuprum oxydatum	Cupr-ox.	183.	Gelsemium sempervirens	Gels.
150.	Curare	Cur.	184.	Ginseng	Gins.
151.	Cyclamen europaeun	Cycl.			

185. Glechoma hederacea	Glech.
186. Glonoinum	Glon.
187. Gnaphalium	
polycephalum	Gnaph.
188. Gossypium herbaceum	Goss.
189. Granatum	Gran.
190. Graphites	Graph.
191. Gratiola	Grat.
192. Grindelia robusta	Grind.
193. Guajacum	Guaj.
194. Gymnocladus	
canadensis	Gymno.
195. Hamamelis virginica	Ham.
196. Hecla lava	Hecla
197. Hedeoma	Hed.
198. Helianthus annuus	Helia.
199. Helleborus niger	Hell.
200. Heloderma horridus	Helo.
201. Helonias dioica	Helon.
202. Hepar sulphuris	Hep.
203. Hippomane mancinella	Hipp.
204. Homarus	Hom.
205. Hura brasiliensis	Hura
206. Hydrastis canadensis	Hydr.
207. Hydrocotyle asiatica	Hydrc.
208. Hydrocyanicum	
acidum	Hydr-ac.
209. Hyoscyamus niger	Hyos.
210. Hypericum perforatum	
	Hyper.
211. Ichthyolum	Ichth.
212. Ignatia amara	Ign.
213. Indigo	Indg.
214. Indium metallicum	Ind.
215. Inula helenium	Inul.

216. Iodium	Iod.
217. Iodoformium	Iodof.
218. Ipecacuanha	Ip.
219. Iris versicolor	Iris
220. Jaborandi	Jab.
221. Jacaranda caroba	Jac.
222. Jalapa	Jal.
223. Jatropha curcas	Jatr.
224. Juglans regia	Jug-r
225. Justicia adhatoda	Just.
226. Kalium arsenicosum	Kali-ar.
227. Kalium bichromicum	Kali-bi.
228. Kalium bromatum	Kali-br.
229. Kalium carbonicum	Kali-c.
230. Kalium causticum	Kali-caust.
231. Kalium chloricum	Kali-chl.
232. Kalium cyanicum	Kali-cy.
233. Kalium hydroiodicum	Kali-i.
234. Kalium muriaticum	Kali-m.
235. Kalium nitricum	Kali-n.
236. Kalium	
permanganatum	Kali-perm.
237. Kalium phosphoricum	Kali-p.
238. Kalium sulphuricum	Kali-s.
239. Kalmia latifolia	Kalm.
240. Kaolinum	Alumin-sil.
241. Kobaltum	Cob.
242. Kreosotum	Kreos.
243. Lac caninum	Lac-c.
244. Lac defloratum	Lac-d.
245. Lachesis trigono-	
cephalus	Lach.
246. Lachnanthes	
tinctoria	Lachn.

247.	Lactuca virosa	Lact.	276.	Mancinella	Manc.
248.	Lamium album	Lam.	277.	Manganum metallicum	
249.	Lapis albus	Lap-a.			Mang-met.
250.	Lappa major	Lappa	278.	Marum verum	Teucr.
251.	Lathyrus sativus	Lath.	279.	Medorrhinum	Med.
252.	Latrodectus mactans	Lat-m.	280.	Melilotus alba	Meli-a.
253.	Laurocerasus	Laur.	281.	Menispermum	
254.	Lecithinum	Lec.		canadense	Menis.
255.	Ledum palustre	Led.	282.	Mentha piperita	Menth.
256.	Lemna minor	Lem-n.	283.	Menyanthes trifoliata	Meny.
257.	Leptandra virginica	Lept.	284.	Mephitis	Meph.
258.	Lilium tigrinum	Lil-t.	285.	Mercurius auratus	Merc-aur.
259.	Linaria vulgaris	Lina.	286.	Mercurius corrosivus	Merc-c.
260.	Lithium carbonicum	Lith-c.	287.	Mercurius cyanatus	Merc-cy.
261.	Lobelia inflata	Lob.	288.	Mercurius dulcis	Merc-d.
262.	Lolium temulentum	Lol-t.	289.	Mercurius iodatus	
263.	Lycopodium clavatum	Lyc.		flavus	Merc-i-f.
264.	Lycopus virginicus	Lycps-v.	290.	Mercurius iodatus	
265.	Lyssinum	Lyss.		ruber	Merc-i-r.
266.	Macrotinum	Macro.	291.	Mercurius praecipitatus	
267.	Magnesium			ruber	Merc-p-r.
	carbonicum	Mag-c.	292.	Mercurius solubilis	Merc.
268.	Magnesium		293.	Mercurius sulpho-	
	muriaticum	Mag-m.		cyanatus	Merc-s-cy.
269.	Magnesium		294.	Mercurius	
	phosphoricum	Mag-p.		sulphuricus	Merc-sul.
270.	Magnesium		295.	Mercurius vivus	Merc.
	sulphuricum	Mag-s.	296.	Mezereum	Mez.
271.	Magnetis		297.	Millefolium	Mill.
	polus arcticus	M-arct.	298.	Mitchella repens	Mit.
272.	Magnetis polus		299.	Morphinum	Morph.
	australis	M-aust.	300.	Moschus tunquinensis	Mosch.
273.	Magnolia grandiflora	Magn-gr.	301.	Murex rurpurea	Murx.
274.	Malandrinum	Maland.	302.	Muriaticum acidum	Mur-ac.
275.	Malaria officinalis	Malar.	303.	Mygale lasiodora	Mygal.

304.	Myfica cerifera	Myric.
305.	Myrtus communis	Myrt-c.
306.	Naja tripudians	Naja
307.	Naphthalinum	Naphtin.
308.	Narcotinum	Narcot.
309.	Natrium arsenicosum	Nat-ar.
310.	Natrium carbonicum	Nat-c.
311.	Natrium muriaticum	Nat-m.
312.	Natrium nitricum	Nat-n.
313.	Natrium phosphoricum	Nat-p.
314.	Natrium sulphuricum	Nat-s.
315.	Niccolum metallicum	Nicc.
316.	Niccolum sulphuricum	Nicc-s.
317.	Nicotinum	Nicot.
318.	Nitricum acidum	Nit-ac.
319.	Nitro-muriaticum acidum	Nit-m-ac.
320.	Nuphar luteum	Nuph.
321.	Nux juglans	Nux-j.
322.	Nux moschata	Nux-m.
323.	Nux vomica	Nux-v.
324.	Ocimum canum	Oci.
325.	Oenanthe crocata	Oena.
326.	Oleander	Olnd.
327.	Oleum animalis	Ol-an.
328.	Oleum jecoris aselli	Ol-j.
329.	Onosmodium virginianum	Onos.
330.	Opium	Op.
331.	Opuntia vulgaris	Opun-v.
332.	Origanum	Orig.
333.	Osmium	Osm.
334.	Oxalicum acidum	Ox-ac.
335.	Paeonia officinalis	Paeon.
336.	Palladium	Pall.
337.	Pareira brava	Pareir.
338.	Paris quadrifolia	Par.
339.	Passiflora incarnata	Passi.
340.	Paullinia pinnata	Paull.
341.	Petroleum	Petr.
342.	Petroselinum	Petros.
343.	Phellandrium aquaticum	Phel.
344.	Phosphoricum acidum	Ph-ac.
345.	Phosphorus	Phos.
346.	Physostigrna venenosa	Phys.
347.	Phytolacca decandra	Phyt.
348.	Picricum acidum	Pic-ac.
349.	Picrotoxinum	Picro.
350.	Pilocarpinum	Pilo.
351.	Pinus palustris	Pin-p.
352.	Pinus sylvestris	Pin-s.
353.	Piper methysticum	Pip-m.
354.	Pix liquida	Pix
355.	Plantago major	Plan.
356.	Platinum metallicum	Plat.
357.	Plumbum metallicum	Plb.
358.	Podophyllum peltatum	Podo.
359.	Polygonum sagittatum	Polyg-s.
360.	Polymnia uvedalia	Polym.
361.	Polyporus officinalis	Bol-la.
362.	Populus tremuloides	Pop-t.
363.	Pothos foetidus	Ictod.
364.	Prunus spinosa	Prun.
365.	Psorinum	Psor.
366.	Ptelea trifoliata	Ptel.

367.	Pulex	Pulx.	400.	Scutellaria lateriflora	Scut.
368.	Pulmo vulpis	Pulm-v.	401.	Secale cornutum	Sec.
369.	Pulsatilla nigricans	Puls.	402.	Selenium	Sel.
370.	Pyrogenium	Pyrog.	403.	Senecio aureus	Senec.
371.	Quassia	Quas.	404.	Senega	Seneg.
372.	Radium bromatum	Rad-br.	405.	Senna	Senn.
373.	Radium chloratum	Radm-chl.	406.	Sepia	Sep.
374.	Ranunculus bulbosus	Ran-b.	407.	Serpentaria	Serp.
375.	Ranunculus scleratus	Ran-s.	408.	Silicea	Sil.
376.	Raphanus sativus niger	Raph.	409.	Sinapis nigra	Sin-n.
377.	Ratanhia	Rat.	410.	Solanum nigrurn	Sol-n.
378.	Rheum	Rheum	411.	Solidago	Solid.
379.	Rhododendron chrysanthemum	Rhod.	412.	Spigelia anthelmintica	Spig.
			413.	Spongia tosta	Spong.
380.	Rhus aromatica	Rhus-a.	414.	Squilla maritima	Squil.
381.	Rhus radicans	Rhus-r.	415.	Stannum metallicum	Stann.
382.	Rhus toxicodendron	Rhus-t.	416.	Staphysagria	Staph.
383.	Ricinus communis	Ric.	417.	Sticta pulmonaria	Stict.
384.	Robinia pseudacacia	Rob.	418.	Stillingia sylvatica	Still.
385.	Rumex crispus	Rumx.	419.	Stramonium	Stram.
386.	Ruta graveolens	Ruta	420.	Strontiana carbonica	Stront-c.
387.	Sabadilla	Sabad.	421.	Strophanthus hispidus	Stroph-h.
388.	Sabal serrulata	Sabal.			
389.	Sabina	Sabin.	422.	Strychninum	Stry.
390.	Salicylicum acidum	Sal-ac.	423.	Strychninum arsenicosum	Stry-ar.
391.	Sambucus nigra	Samb.			
392.	Sanguinaria canadensis	Sang.	424.	Strychninum phosphoricum	Stry-p.
393.	Sanicula aqua	Sanic.			
394.	Santoninum	Sant.	425.	Sulphur	Sulph.
395.	Saponaria officinalis	Sapo.	426.	Sulphur iodatum	Sul-i.
396.	Sarracenia purpurea	Sarr.	427.	Sulphuricum acidum	Sul-ac.
397.	Sarsaparilla	Sars.	428.	Sumbul	Sumb.
398.	Scilla maritima	Squil.	429.	Symphoricarpus racemosus	Symph.
399.	Scoparius genista	Scopar.			

430. Symphytum officinale Sym-r.
431. Syphilinum Syph.
432. Syzygium
       jambolanum Syzyg.
433. Tabacum Tab.
434. Tanacetum vulgare Tanac.
435. Tarentula cubensis Tarent-c.
436. Tarentula hispana Tarent-h.
437. Taraxacum Tarax.
438. Tellurium Tell.
439. Teplitz Tep.
440. Terebinthiniae Terb.
441. Teucrium marum
       verum Teucr.
442. Thallium metallicum Thal-met.
443. Thaspium aureum Ziz.
444. Thea chinensis Thea
445. Theinum Theine.
446. Theridion
       curassavicum Ther.
447. Thlaspi bursa
       pastoris Thlasp.
448. Thuja occidentals Thuj.
449. Thymolum Thymol
450. Thymus vulgaris Thymu-vg.
451. Thyreoidinum Thyr.
452. Tilia europaea Til.
453. Titanium Titan.
454. Trillium pendulum Tril-p.
455. Trombidium Trom.
456. Tuberculinum Tub.
457. Tussilago farfara Tuss-fr.
458. Uranium nitricum Uran-n.

459. Urtica urens Urt-u.
460. Ustilago maydis Ust.
461. Uva ursi Uva.
462. Vaccininum Vac.
463. Valeriana officinalis Valer.
464. Variolinum Vario.
465. Veratrum album Verat.
466. Veratrum viride Verat-v.
467. Verbascum thapsus Verb.
468. Vespa crabro Vesp.
469. Viburnum opulus Vib.
470. Vinca minor Vinc.
471. Viola odorata Viol-o.
472. Viola tricolor Viol-t.
473. Vipera torva Vip-t.
474. Viscum album Visc.
475. Wyethia helenoides Wye.
476. Xanthoxylum
       fraxineum Xan.
477. X-ray X-ray
478. Yerba santa Erio.
479. Yucca Yuc.
480. Zincum arsenicosum Zinc-ar.
481. Zincum chromatum Zinc-chr.
482. Zincum cyanatum Zinc-cy.
483. Zincum iodatum Zinc-i.
484. Zincum metallicum Zin.
485. Zincum phosphatum Zinc-p.
486. Zincum sulphuricum Zinc-s.
487. Zincum valerianicum Zinc-val.
488. Zingiber Zing.
489. Zizia aurea Ziz.

❖ ◯ ❖